ADULT-GERONTOLOGY AND FAMILY NURSE PRACTITIONER CERTIFICATION
Examination Review Questions and Strategies

FOURTH EDITION

Jill E. Winland-Brown EdD, APRN, FNP-BC
Professor and Family Nurse Practitioner
Christine E. Lynn College of Nursing
Harbor Branch Oceanographic Institute Campus
Florida Atlantic University
Boca Raton, Florida

Lynne M. Dunphy PhD, APRN, FNP-BC, FAAN
Professor and Routhier Chair of Practice
College of Nursing
University of Rhode Island
Kingston, Rhode Island

F. A. DAVIS COMPANY • Philadelphia

F. A. Davis Company
1915 Arch Street
Philadelphia, PA 19103
www.fadavis.com

Printed in the United States of America

Last digit indicates print number: 10 9 8 7 6 5 4 3 2

Publisher, Nursing: Joanne Patzek DaCunha, RN, MSN
Director of Content Development: Darlene D. Pedersen, MSN, APRN, PMHCNS
Project Editor: Echo Gerhart
Electronic Project Editor: Tyler Baber
Cover Design: Carolyn O'Brien

ISBN 10: 0-8036-2704-1
ISBN 13: 978-0-8036-2704-8

As new scientific information becomes available through basic and clinical research,
recommended treatments and drug therapies undergo changes. The author(s) and publisher
have done everything possible to make this book accurate, up to date, and in accord with
accepted standards at the time of publication. The author(s), editors, and publisher are not
responsible for errors or omissions or for consequences from application of the book, and
make no warranty, expressed or implied, in regard to the contents of the book. Any practice
described in this book should be applied by the reader in accordance with professional
standards of care used in regard to the unique circumstances that may apply in each
situation. The reader is advised always to check product information (package inserts) for
changes and new information regarding dose and contraindications before administering
any drug. Caution is especially urged when using new or infrequently ordered drugs.

Library of Congress Cataloging-in-Publication Data
Winland-Brown, Jill E., 1948-
  Adult-gerontology and family nurse practitioner certification examination : review
questions and strategies / Jill E. Winland-Brown, Lynne M. Dunphy. — 4th ed.
      p. ; cm.
  Rev. ed. of: Adult and family nurse practitioner certification examination / Jill E.
Winland-Brown, Lynne M. Dunphy. 3rd ed. c2009.
  Includes bibliographical references.
  ISBN 978-0-8036-2704-8 — ISBN 0-8036-2704-1
  I. Dunphy, Lynne M. Hektor. II. Winland-Brown, Jill E., 1948- Adult and family nurse
practitioner certification examination. III. Title.
  [DNLM: 1. Nursing Care—Examination Questions. 2. Advanced Practice Nursing—
Examination Questions. 3. Nurse Practitioners—Examination Questions. 4. Test Taking
Skills. WY 18.2]
  610.73076--dc23
                              2012046203

Dedication

I would like to dedicate this book to all my students who reinforce that learning is lifelong, we'll never know everything, but we know where to look or who to ask.

Jill E. Winland-Brown

To my dear husband, Jim, with thanks for his steadfastness, good humor, loyalty, and affection, and to Bradley James Arthur Hektor, the best teenager in the world!

Lynne M. Dunphy

Preface

When we originally began this process, review books were only available for physician assistants and physicians. As nurse educators who had been preparing undergraduates for the NCLEX exam for many years, we knew the importance of taking sample exams in the discipline that reflect the test content. Thus, the idea for this book was born.

Research shows that answering numerous sample test questions is the best way to prepare for taking a multiple-choice exam such as the current certification exam. We saw a tremendous need for a book that contained a large number of sample test questions with rationales, as well as reinforcement in test-taking skills. In the second edition, we updated information using new standards and guidelines. We also increased the number of questions. In the third edition, relying heavily on evidence-based practice, we updated content, added new medications, and utilized new practice guidelines. We increased the number of questions for each chapter, each practice examination in the back of the book, and the CD examination. This fourth expanded edition prepares both MS and DNP graduates for the exam. Additional gerontology content and questions were added to support the integration of adult and gerontology content. Success on multiple-choice exams is a skill that can be learned like any other skill—for example, playing tennis—and the outcomes improve with practice.

We suggest reading Chapters 1 and 2 first to get a feel for both taking the exam and setting up an individualized study plan. Next, you might want to take one of the practice tests in the back of the book to assess your baseline score. These practice tests simulate the certification examination in both content and the number of questions. Taking the practice test will help you identify your weaknesses and design your individual study plan. We then suggest you go to the chapter containing test questions for the content area in which you feel you are weakest.

Because nursing is rapidly changing and is an art, as well as a science, there are many conflicting viewpoints and practices regarding treatment options. Every effort has been made to ensure that the content is current and relevant, and several sources were used for the rationales of each question. For further information regarding content, the references used for the questions appear at the end of each chapter. We suggest that this book be used as a companion to our textbook, *Primary Care: The Art and Science of Advanced Practice Nursing*, which elaborate further on each rationale.

After you pass the certification exam, this book can be used as a study guide to continually refresh your knowledge base. We suggest writing comments next to each question that will assist you in remembering and noting ideas to be researched further. We sincerely wish you success on certification and hope that this book contributes in a small way to that success. Best of luck.

—*Jill E. Winland-Brown*
—*Lynne M. Dunphy*

Contributors

Sandra Allen, MSN, APRN-BC
American Mobile Dermatology
Boynton Beach, Florida

Lisa J. Bedard, MSN, APRN-BC, CNRN
Stroke and Neurodiagnostics Manager
Lawrence & Memorial Hospital
New London, Connecticut

Sharon K. Byrne, DrNP, CRNP, NP-C, AOCNP, CNE
Asst. Clinical Professor of Nursing &
Program Director Family Nurse Practitioner Track
College of Nursing & Health Professions
Drexel University
Philadelphia, Pennsylvania

Marcia R. Gardner, PhD, RN, CPNP, CPN
Associate Professor, Department of Family Nursing
College of Nursing, Seton Hall University
South Orange, New Jersey

Diane Gerzevitz, MSN, APRN, BC
Family Nurse Practitioner
Assistant Professor Emeritus
College of Nursing
University of Rhode Island
Kingston, Rhode Island

Donna Maheady, EdD, APRN-BC
Associate Graduate Faculty
Christine E. Lynn College of Nursing
Florida Atlantic University
Boca Raton, Florida

Kymberlee A. Montgomery, DrNP, WHNP-BC, CNE
Drexel University College of Nursing and Health
Professions
Philadelphia, Pennsylvania

Lynne Palma, DNP, FNP-BC, CDE
Nurse Practitioner Program Coordinator
Christine E. Lynn College of Nursing
Florida Atlantic University
Boca Raton, Florida

Karen A. Rugg, RN, BS, CDOE
Certified Diabetes Outpatient Educator
Graduate Assistant, FNP Candidate
College of Nursing
University of Rhode Island
Kingston, Rhode Island

Denese Sabatino, MSN, ARNP-C, CCRN
Nurse Practitioner/Clinical Educator
Department of Critical Care
Cleveland Clinic
Weston, Florida
Baptist Hospital
Miami, Florida

We would also like to thank the following
individuals for contributions to previous editions:
Denise Coppa
Allison M. Jedson
Janice S. Hayes
Deborah A. Raines
Lorraine M. Schwartz
Susan Elaine Sloan
Douglas H. Sutton
Sharon A. Thrush
Marcella R. Thompson

Reviewers

Sue Anne Bell, MSN, FNP, BC
Nurse Practitioner
Washtenaw County Public Health Department
Doctoral Student
University of Michigan School of Nursing
Ann Arbor, Michigan

Tami Jakubowski, DNP, MSN, APRN-Pediatric
Assistant Professor
The College of New Jersey
Ewing, New Jersey

Laurel Halloran, PhD, APRN
Professor
Western Connecticut State University
Danbury, Connecticut

Acknowledgments

I would like to thank Bruce Wishnov, DO, for his mentorship and having never been too busy or too irritable for any questions!!! You are a caring physician and an all-around great guy.

LMD

We would both like to thank the entire F. A. Davis team, especially Joanne DaCunha, publisher, for her enthusiasm, support, and friendship, Julie Scardiglia developmental editor, for her firm hand and expertise, and Jodi Kohl, project manager.

JW-B & LMD

Contents

INTRODUCTION

Chapter 1: *Achieving Success on a Certification Examination*

Lynne M. Dunphy

Congratulations! With the purchase of this book, you have taken your first step along the road to becoming a certified advanced-practice nurse (APRN). The earlier in your educational process you begin preparing for the certification examination, the greater your chance of success. If you are a nurse practitioner who has been "out there" for a number of years and never sat for certification, or need to recertify, this book will help you understand the certification process and the steps you need to take to succeed on the certification examination of your choice. Regardless of your situation, the important point is that you have begun! Remember, the longest journey begins with a single step.

Certification and Why It Is Important

There are basic differences between becoming licensed (something you achieved at the completion of your basic nursing program by sitting for the state boards or the National Council Licensure Examination for Registered Nurses [NCLEX-RN]) and becoming certified. An understanding of these differences is important to your ultimate success on the certification examination. Becoming "test savvy" demands a thorough comprehension of the underlying premises and purposes of the examination for which you are sitting.

LICENSURE

Licensure is a legal requirement. You must be licensed by a state to practice nursing in that state. The purpose of licensure is to protect the public from unsafe practitioners. Legal regulation of nursing practice is the joint responsibility of the state legislature and the state board of nursing. Minimum competency is assessed on a licensure examination, in the case of the new graduate nurse, the NCLEX. This examination asks: Have you met the basic criteria for safe and effective nursing practice? The test questions on the licensure examination are from frequently updated job analyses of entry-level nursing practice. They reflect the concepts and functions that a registered nurse (RN) needs to know and perform for safe entry-level practice.

Currently, the licensure examination is prepared and administered by the National Council of State Boards of Nursing (NCSBN). Composed of representatives from every nursing board in the United States and five of its territories, this body is responsible for setting a national standard for safe and effective entry-level nursing practice and assessing it through administration of a national licensing examination, the NCLEX-RN. Every state now mandates passage of this examination as a prerequisite for state licensure as a registered nurse.

CERTIFICATION

Certification is the process by which a nongovernmental agency or association grants recognition to an individual who has met certain predetermined standards for practice. It can be mandatory or voluntary. APRN certification is not mandated, although currently most states require passage of the appropriate certification examination as a prerequisite for licensure to perform advanced-practice nursing functions. As of this writing, only New York and California do not require certification prior to obtaining licensure to practice as an APRN. The nurse practitioner certification examinations measure role and population level competencies for entry-level practice, similar in function to the NCLEX.

Certification validates entry-level knowledge of an advanced nursing specialty in a defined population area; the process of recertification recognizes continued proficiency in that specialty. In 1974 the American Nurses Association (ANA) initiated a national voluntary certification process to recognize excellence in nursing practice. By 1978 the purpose had broadened to include the assurance of quality in advanced nursing practice. This was done partly to recognize professional achievement but also to identify nurses who were potentially eligible

for third-party reimbursement. By the 1990s, the regulation of advanced-practice nursing had become a topic of increasing concern within the nursing profession. Whether a secondary level of licensure, rather than certification, was the more appropriate regulatory mechanism was widely debated for some time. At the same time, licensure and certification requirements proliferated and varied widely from state to state, often causing issues for APRNs who chose to geographically relocate.

In 2006 the NCSBN released a draft of a vision paper titled "The Future Regulation of Advanced Practice Nursing." This began a formal dialogue among many stakeholders in nursing, which included regulation, education, certification, and practice. This dialogue, the work of the APRN Consensus Work Group and the NCSBN APRN Advisory Committee, culminated in the publication in 2008 of "The Consensus Model for APRN Regulation: Licensure, Accreditation, Certification, and Education," often referred to as "LACE." This document supported the continuation of certification administered through testing divisions of professional associations, specifically the ANA subsidiary, the American Nurses Credentialing Center (ANCC), and the American Academy of Nurse Practitioners Certification Organization (AANP), as the appropriate means of regulation of advanced-practice nursing. Future national certification examinations by both these bodies will designate an APRN role in a specific population. [See **Figure 1-1**] National certification

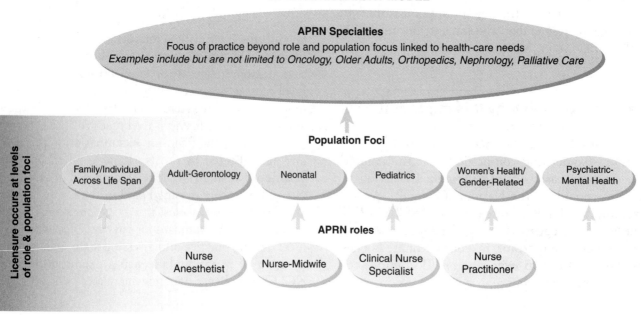

APRN REGULATORY MODEL

Figure 1-1

Figure 1-1

by one of these designated bodies serves as eligibility for licensure to practice in most states and is required for most third-party reimbursement, as well as institutional credentialing. Since 1998, certification has been a prerequisite to Medicare reimbursement. The Veterans Affairs Medical Systems now mandate national certification for advanced-practice nurses, as does the U.S. Military. National certification is also required to obtain a National Provider Identifier (NPI). An agency can limit scope of practice per their policies, but the scope of practice is defined in the nurse practice act of the respective state. Qualifications for licensure and nursing titles that are permitted, as well as scope of practice options, are spelled out by the state or territo's laws and regulations. [See Table 1-1]

The purpose of licensure is to assure the public that an individual has mastered a body of knowledge and has acquired the skills necessary to function as an entry-level advanced practice in a particular role caring for a specific population, building upon the foundation of basic nursing knowledge conferred with RN licensure. [See Figure 1-2] Consensus has increasingly emerged regarding what these competencies and skills are. In summary, the candidate for certification as an APRN should recognize that certification is a formal process, conducted by nongovernmental organizations, to validate *entry-level* advanced practice nursing knowledge, skills, and competencies, based on predetermined standards, and is a part of the requirement in most states to obtain licensure and status as an APRN. See **Table 1-2** for recognized certifying organizations for APRN practice.

TABLE 1-1. PURPOSES OF NATIONAL CERTIFICATION

- Required for advanced nursing practice licensure in most states.
- Indicates specific advanced role and population-based competencies at an entry-level building on foundational nursing knowledge.
- Provides greater career opportunities and mobility
- Required for third-party reimbursement in Medicare populations as well as most other insurers
- Often required for institutional credentialing
- Required by the Veterans Administration and the U.S. Military
- Required to obtain a National Provider Identifier (NPI).

BUILDING A CURRICULUM

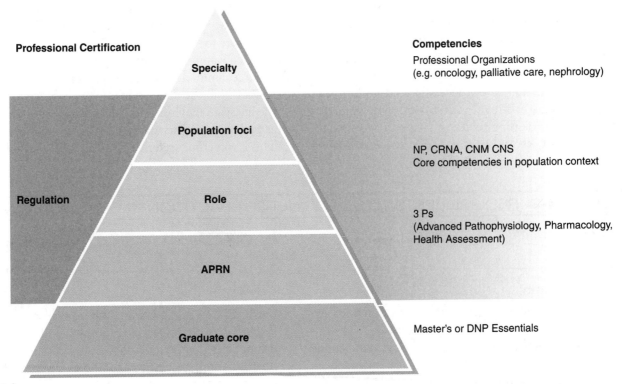

Professional Certification

Specialty

Population foci

Regulation

Role

APRN

Graduate core

Competencies
Professional Organizations
(e.g. oncology, palliative care, nephrology)

NP, CRNA, CNM CNS
Core competencies in population context

3 Ps
(Advanced Pathophysiology, Pharmacology, Health Assessment)

Master's or DNP Essentials

Figure 1-2

TABLE 1-2. RECOGNIZED NURSING ASSOCIATIONS AND ORGANIZATIONS OFFERING ADVANCED-PRACTICE NURSING CERTIFICATION FOR THE NURSE PRACTITIONER ROLE AS OF 2012

ASSOCIATION OR ORGANIZATION

American Academy of Nurse Practitioners (AANP)
AANP: http://www.aanp.org/certification
certification@aanp.org
American Nurses Credentialing Center (ANCC)
ANCC: http://www.nursecredentialing.org

YOUR ROLE

You are making an important, timely, and professionally astute decision by choosing to become certified. In 1998 Margretta Madden Styles, president of the ANCC, noted in *Credentialing News*, "As the global tide turns from governmental regulation and public protectionism toward competitive quality improvement of services and informed consumer choice, voluntary credentialing is a movement whose time has come." We concur.

Table 1-3 lists the requirements for nurse practitioner certification by the ANCC and AANP as of 2012. You must keep abreast of both of these credentialing Web sites for continued and changing information regarding the implementation of the 2008 APRN Consensus Model, or, as it is commonly referred to, LACE—*Licensure, Accreditation, Credentialing, and Education*. To qualify to take an examination and become certified at the APRN level, a nurse must (1) meet requirements for clinical or functional practice in a specialized field and (2) provide evidence of successful completion of an approved master's-level curriculum. After meeting these criteria as they relate to a given specialty, the nurse must take and pass the relevant certification examination. Only then will the nurse be certified in that specialty.

Certification Examinations

This book is geared toward the nurse who is seeking national certification as an adult-gerontological primary care nurse practitioner (AGNP) and/or a Family Care Nurse Practitioner (FNP). The AGNP certification examination is designed to assess your abilities as an APRN in the delivery of primary care services to an adult population, defined as adolescence through old age. The gerontological nurse practitioner (GNP) will no longer be offered by either ANCC or AANP. This change is in recognition of the need for more nurse practitioner with knowledge of the care of older adults, as well as adults. Part of the 2008 Consensus documents recommendations were to combine Adult-Gero competencies.

The Family Primary Care Nurse Practitioner certification examination is designed to assess your abilities as an APRN in the delivery of primary care services across the life span, including pre- and postpartum care, as well as pediatric primary care and the care of older adults. This is sometimes referred to as "cradle to grave."

TABLE 1-3. REQUIREMENTS TO SIT FOR NURSE PRACTITIONER CERTIFICATION

AMERICAN NURSES CREDENTIALING CENTER (ANCC)	*AMERICAN ACADEMY OF NURSE PRACTITIONERS (AANP)*
Requirements	
• Master's-level nurse practitioner program from an accredited institution of higher learning • Meet practice requirements specific to certification type, usually a minimum of 500 clinical hours in specific population	• Master's-level nurse practitioner from an accredited institution of higher learning (nurse practitioners without this degree may petition the certification board for permission to sit for the examination by endorsement *only* through 2012)

AMERICAN NURSES CREDENTIALING CENTER

The ANCC Web site contains a test content outline (TCO) that describes the major categories and domains of practice as well as related topics and subtopics that are covered on the examination. The examination currently consists of 175 questions, 150 of which are scored and 25 pretest questions that are not scored. The nonscored questions cannot be distinguished from the scored items.

The TCO includes information about how the content is weighted—that is, how many or what percentage of the test questions are in each of the major domains. **Table 1-4** lists the major categories or domains of practice for the FNP examination and includes an approximate number of questions and the overall percentage for each category. To facilitate understanding of each of the major domains, the ANCC also includes subcategories in a topical outline format. **Table 1-5** provides similar information for the ANP examination. **Table 1-6** lists the five major domains of practice, as defined by ANCC, as well as the related subcategories that are currently being tested on both the ANP and FNP examinations.

The importance of reviewing the current TCO before sitting for the examination cannot be overstated. It should be noted that there is some overlap in these categories. Additionally, all questions are classified according to life span and problem-focused content areas. The life span dimension for the ANP examination includes non–age-specific content as well as specific content pertaining to the adolescent, the adult, and the aging adult, specifically age 13 to elder. The FNP life span dimension includes the same content as the ANP examination plus content relating to children, infants, and childbearing women. The gerontologic population is defined as persons older than age 55.

The last dimension is related to problem areas and organizes question content by body system—for example, cardiovascular, endocrine, and respiratory.

What this means is that each test question is characterized across three dimensions. For example, a test question that asks about the treatment of a 70-year-old woman with a diagnosis of osteoporosis would be characterized as follows:

- Dimension One—Clinical Management
- Dimension Two—Life Span: Older Adult
- Dimension Three—Problem Area: Musculoskeletal

Be aware that the TCO may change from examination to examination, so you need to review your handbook carefully for the most current content breakdown.

TABLE 1-4. ANCC FAMILY NURSE PRACTITIONER CERTIFICATION EXAMINATION CONTENT OUTLINE DOMAINS OF PRACTICE (2012)

DOMAINS OF PRACTICE	NUMBER OF QUESTIONS	PERCENT QUESTIONS
Theoretical Foundations of Advanced Practice Nursing	37	25
Professional Role	23	15
Health Care Policy and Delivery	15	10
Clinical Assessment	30	27
Clinical Management	45	30
Total	**150**	**100**

TABLE 1-5. ANCC ADULT GERONTOLOGICAL PRIMARY CARE NURSE PRACTITIONER CERTIFICATION EXAMINATION CONTENT OUTLINE (2012)

DOMAINS OF PRACTICE	NUMBER OF QUESTIONS	PERCENT
Foundations of Advanced Nursing Practice	34	22.67
Professional Role	21	14
Health Care Policy and Delivery	16	10.67
Health Assessment	34	22.67
Clinical Management	45	30

TABLE 1-6. FNP/ANP EXAMINATION: Domain Related Subcategories

MAJOR CATEGORY OR DOMAIN OF PRACTICE	SUBCATEGORIES
Foundations of Advanced Nursing Practice	Therapeutic Communication
	Growth and Developmental Influences/Assessment
	Health Promotion
	Psychosocial Influences
	Socioeconomic, Cultural, and Spiritual Influences
	Teaching/Guidance
Professional Role and Policy	Scope and Standards of Practice
	Health Care Ethics, Including Advocacy and Negotiating
	Safe Practice—Minimizing Errors
	Interpreting and Critiquing Research, Including Levels of Evidence
Health Care Policy and Delivery	Regulatory Guidelines and Legal Issues
	Reimbursement
	Documentation
	Informatics
	HIPAA; OSHA
Clinical/Health Assessment	Epidemiology/Disease Control
	Anatomy and Physiology
	Pathophysiology
	Comprehensive and Focused History Taking
	Risk Assessment
	Diagnostic Reasoning
Clinical Management	Evidence-Based Practice (EBP)
	Advanced Clinical Decision Making
	Formulating and Evaluating a Treatment Plan and Outcomes
	Coordination of Care
	Health Promotion/Disease Prevention

To assess each examinee's level of specialty knowledge independent of the group taking the examination, a *criterion-referenced standard* is used. In this approach, each examinee's score is compared with an absolute number determined by the content experts who develop the examination. You want to answer every question. Even if you have no idea of the answer, by sheer chance alone you stand a 25% chance of guessing the correct answer. You are not penalized for incorrect answers.

The test development committee determines the passing score after careful consideration of the content of the test questions. The passing score is always expressed in terms of the number of questions you must correctly answer on the total test as well as statistical examinations of the reliability and validity of the "piloted" test questions. Additional statistical examination of the piloted questions is assessed for inclusion in the final graded pool of test questions on the next examination.

Your performance on the total test determines your success or failure. The examination is administered year round in a computerized testing center. You are permitted 3.5 hours to answer 175 questions. Plan an additional 30 minutes for check-in and practice time at the computer, including a tutorial. Because it is a computerized examination, you will receive your score approximately 3 to 5 minutes after completing the examination! A passing score is 350 or higher of a possible 500 points; 2011 statistics reveal 82% of ANP and 82.2% of FNP candidates pass, which translates to a minimum passing score of approximately 350. If not successful, a candidate can apply to retest after 90 days.

You will need to be recertified every 5 years. This may be accomplished by accumulating continuing education credits. Please check the ANCC Web site for the most current information because guidelines for recertification are subject to change.

AMERICAN ACADEMY OF NURSE PRACTITIONERS

The AANP currently offers competency-based national certification examinations for the ANP (soon to be AGNP), FNP, and GNP. AANP will also be "retiring" its GNP-specific examination; it has embraced the conceptualization of the role of the Adult APRN as including Adult-Gero competencies. Reflecting APRN knowledge and expertise, the content areas of these examinations include health promotion, disease prevention, and diagnosis and management of acute and chronic diseases. The examinations given by the AANP were developed in conjunction with the Professional Examination Service, a not-for-profit organization with more than 50 years of experience in developing and administering national licensing and certification examinations in health-related fields.

Both certifying examinations require a master's degree from an accredited program. This certification program is fully accredited by the National Commission for Certifying Agencies (NCCA).

The Academy Certification Program, in conjunction with the Professional Examination Service, conducted a role delineation study to determine areas of clinical knowledge to be tested. As a result of this study, the examination was structured around assessment (approximately 45 questions, or 33%), diagnosis (approximately 35 questions, or 26%), formulation and implementation of treatment plans (approximately 31 questions, or 23%), and evaluation and follow up (approximately 24 questions, or 18%). The Web site also provides a list of 20 knowledge areas. **Table 1-7** outlines this content. Examinees must be able to integrate knowledge of pathophysiology, psychology, and sociology with the assessment, diagnosis, and treatment of patients in primary care. Knowledge of health promotion and disease prevention, as well as management of acute/episodic and chronic illness in the primary care setting, are tested.

The ANP examination tests knowledge of late adolescence, adult, and geriatric primary care, and the FNP examination tests clinical knowledge of prenatal, pediatric, adolescent, adult, and geriatric primary care. The AANP examination defines *gero* as above age 65, in contrast to age 55 for ANCC. Additionally, content for the AANP examination includes young gerontologicals (age 65–84 years) and frail elderly (above age 85).

TABLE 1-7. ADULT, GERONTOLOGY, AND FAMILY NP EXAMINATIONS: Knowledge Areas Included on AANP Examination

1. Health promotion and disease prevention
2. Anatomy, physiology, and pathophysiology
3. Interviewing concepts and techniques
4. Health history
5. Signs and symptoms
6. Physical examination
7. Laboratory/diagnostic tests
8. Clinical decision making
9. Differential diagnosis
10. Pharmacological therapies
11. Nonpharmacological/complementary/ alternative therapies
12. Diagnostic and therapeutic procedures
13. Biopsychosocial theories
14. Patient and family education and counseling
15. Community resources
16. Health-care economics and practice management
17. Evidence-based practice
18. Legal and ethical issues
19. Cultural competence
20. Principles of epidemiology

This examination has an overall pass rate of approximately 87% according to 2010 data. It is also a computer-based examination offered year round. You know whether you have passed or failed at the end of the examination.

Achieving Success

Practitioner programs often focus on assessment, management, and evaluation of *disease*. Indeed, this is the role most of you perform in your respective work settings. The ability to diagnose and treat disease is paramount to your safe and effective functioning as an APRN, and certification examinations increasingly reflect this reality. However, it is important never to lose sight of the fact that these examinations are certifying your abilities as an APRN and as such have an underlying commitment rooted in nursing-based knowledge, health, health promotion, and human responses to health and illness. This is especially apparent on the TOC of the ANCC examination. Fully 25% of content is labeled "Theoretical Foundations of Advanced Nursing Practice."

As a nurse, your reaction to the various manifestations of health and illness phenomena is instinctively different from that of other primary care providers. This is manifested in different ways on each examination, but it is an important distinction to keep in mind as you ponder various distractors and wonder what answer is the best. Similarly, the test blueprints and type of questions asked reflect a continued commitment to concepts of health promotion and disease prevention as well as the underlying principles of therapeutic communication skills that are so essential to forging meaningful nurse-client relationships. Nursing-based elements of growth and development, nutrition, and therapeutic communication, as well as questions about cultural differences and cross-cultural communication, will be integrated with content concerning specific aspects of diagnosis, pharmacology, and disease management.

Questions testing physical assessment and history-taking skills, as well as content from advanced physical assessment, remain prominent. Although a certain amount of basic pharmacological content is included, the latest drugs and pharmacological interventions may not always appear because the examination questions are prepared and tested well in advance. (Note: Questions about your knowledge of safe prescribing for pregnant women almost always appear on the FNP examinations.)

If you have been in active practice for some time, you must exercise care as you take the examination. Distractors (see chapter 2) will not necessarily correlate with what you currently see and do. Remember, the examination reflects the *ideal* answer according to the certifying body; this ideal answer may not always mirror the realities of your practice. Test answers draw on national guidelines and standards of practice promulgated by a variety of bodies. Your practice is likely to be focused on a specialty and to reflect the practice patterns and priorities of your particular geographic region and site. The questions on the examination are looking for much more generalized responses and might well reflect phenomena that you very seldom experience. Allowing yourself to become frustrated with the distractors will not help you but rather will hinder your ability to succeed. This is why it is essential that you study large numbers of sample test items (see chapter 2).

Being test savvy and succeeding on a multiple-choice examination is a far different skill from the expert skills you bring to your practice. But these skills are not mutually exclusive. It is a matter of having the correct mind-set. This mind-set is predicated on an awareness of the *nursing base* of the certification examination coupled with an understanding of the *test blueprint*. Develop a determination not to select an anecdotal answer based on experience from your own practice but rather to select an answer based on nationally recognized, clinically based guidelines and rooted in clinical literature.

You have taken the first step toward certification by purchasing this book! Mentally review the important reasons to become nationally certified. Fix the end goal vividly in your mind. Imagine how you will feel when you receive that message on the screen saying PASSED, that you are a nationally certified APRN. It is a satisfying and worthwhile goal to achieve.

Take the next step on the road to success by turning to chapter 2. It will assist you in the development of important test-taking skills and provide guidelines for your individualized study plan.

You can succeed!

Bibliography

Advanced Practice Registered Nurse Consensus Model. Retrieved from http://nonpf.com/associations/10789/files/APRNConsensusModelFinal09.pdf.

American Academy of Nurse Practitioners: http://www.aanp.org/certification.htm, Certification examination program description, 2012, accessed February 20, 2012. http://www.aanpcertification.org/ptistore/resource/documents/Annual_Report_2011.PDF.

American Nurses Certification Corporation certification Web page: http://www.nursecredentialing.org, accessed February 3, 2012. http://www.nursecredentialing.org/Certification/FacultyEducators/FacultyCategory/Statistics/2011CertificationStats.aspx.

Dunphy, LM, Winland-Brown, JE, Porter, BO, and Thomas, D: *Primary Care: The Art and Science of Advanced Practice Nursing*, ed 4. FA Davis, Philadelphia, 2011.

National Council of State Boards of Nursing: https://www.ncsbn.org/Draft_APRN_Vision_Paper.pdf, Draft vision paper: The future regulation of advanced practice nursing, 2006, accessed July 23, 2007. https://www.ncsbn.org/.

National Organization of Nurse Practitioner Faculties: http://www.nonpf.com/NONPF2005/CoreComps-FINAL06.pdf, Domains and core competencies of nurse practitioner practice, 2006, accessed July 28, 2007.

National Organization of Nurse Practitioner Faculties. http://www.nonpf.com/NONPFJune2009/Clarification, Clarification of Nurse Practitioner *Speciality* and *Subspecialty* Clinical Track Titles, Hours, and Credentialing, accessed October 10, 2011.

Chapter 2: Test-Taking Skills and Designing Your Study Plan for APRN Certification

Lynne M. Dunphy

This chapter has several parts. The first part actively assists you in assessing your study and testing style. It prepares you to develop an individualized study plan that will enable you to achieve your goal: becoming a nationally certified advanced-practice nurse (APRN). Another part reviews the nature of the adult nurse practitioner and family nurse practitioner certification examinations (we use the term "exam" from this point on) and how that translates to actual test questions. The remaining parts deal with the specifics of answering multiple-choice test questions and the skills necessary to succeed on a multiple-choice exam. Evaluating test-taking skills, developing a formal study plan, and readiness on exam day are also covered.

Study Habits: Know Yourself

There are several approaches to developing good study habits and effective test-taking skills. Among them are recognizing what your preferred learning style is, realizing the importance of active versus passive studying, and following basic tips for getting started and developing test-taking skills.

WHAT TEST-TAKING TYPE ARE YOU?

This fun exercise allows you to diagnose your own studying and test-taking style. Are you a tortoise or a hare? Are you a peacock? Or are you more like a deer? Knowing your style can assist you in designing your study plan for the exam and answering test questions on exam day. For example, are you a tortoise, moving slowly and laboriously through each question, taking far too long, and then having to rush at the end, thereby increasing your chance of error? Or are you a hare, racing through the exam questions as fast as you can, often misreading information, and likely to make quick guesses rather than carefully thought-out responses?

Are you preoccupied with grades and personal achievement, viewing the certification exam as a threat? Do you procrastinate about studying rather than developing and sticking to a well-designed study plan, thus increasing your anxiety? Do you argue with some test questions, convinced that none of the options is right according to your practice? Then you may be a peacock. Remember, exam questions are *not* perfect but still require that you choose the *best* available option. Do *not* waste time and energy arguing mentally with a test question. Select what you feel is the best option and *move on!*

Or are you a deer? Do you easily lose self-confidence and tend to run away, doubting your initial response? Are you often academically successful but experience anxiety when information is presented in an unfamiliar format?

Table 2-1 assists you in identifying your test-taking personality.

TABLE 2-1. IDENTIFYING YOUR TEST-TAKING TYPE

HARE	*TORTOISE*	*PEACOCK*	*DEER*
Study Style			
• Crams • Feels anxious during study sessions	• Obsessive • Focuses on details; misses the bigger picture	• Procrastinates • Puts off studying; does not think there is a need to study	• Diligent • Smart; has good study habits but lacks self-confidence
Test-Taking Style			
• Often first to finish • Rushes; does not thoroughly read questions and answers • Makes quick guesses • Feels anxious when answer is not readily apparent	• Often last to finish • Spends too much time examining details and rereading questions and answers • May have to rush at end to complete exam in allotted time	• Reads own ideas into questions • Changes initial responses often because expected answer is not present • Selects answer based on anecdotal experience	• Questions own knowledge • Changes initial responses • Feels anxious when faced with information that is presented differently from expected way • Voices self-doubt during testing
Test-Taking Strategies			
• Develop and stick to a study plan; avoid last-minute cramming. • Focus on decreasing test-taking speed. • Read questions as though speaking them aloud in your head to avoid scanning. • Read all options. • Time yourself in practice tests; allow no less than 1 minute per question. • Keep a watch in front of you while taking the test; determine the halfway point and mark it on the exam.	• Focus on concepts and not details during study periods. • Use concept maps. • Focus on increasing testing speed. • Do not linger too long over one question. • Time yourself in practice tests; allow 45 to 60 seconds for each question.	• Develop and stick to a study plan. • Practice with sample tests. • Maintain objectivity; avoid adding own interpretation. • Avoid changing answers.	• Continue usual study activities. • Work on self-confidence. • Develop a self-confidence mantra to recite if you find yourself doubting your knowledge. • Use practice tests to increase confidence. • Avoid changing answers.

(continued)

HARE	TORTOISE	PEACOCK	DEER
Relaxation Techniques • Breathe deeply. • Practice positive visualization. • Avoid caffeine. • Develop a test-taking mantra to recite if you find yourself losing focus.	• Breathe deeply. • Practice positive visualization. • Avoid caffeine.	• Breathe deeply. • Practice positive visualization. • Avoid caffeine.	• Breathe deeply. • Practice positive visualization. • Avoid caffeine.

Source: Adapted from Sides, MB, and Korchek, N: *Successful Test-Taking Strategies,* ed. 3, Lippincott Williams & Wilkins, Philadelphia, 1998, p. 77; and Dickenson-Hazard, N: Test-taking strategies and techniques. In Kopac, CA, and Millonig, VL (eds): *Gerontological Nursing Certification Review Guide,* revised ed. Health Leadership Associates, Potomac, MD, 1996, pp. 3–5.

WHAT IS YOUR PREFERRED LEARNING STYLE?

Awareness of your learning style will also guide you in selecting study strategies. Learning styles are related to the pathways or channels through which you prefer to absorb information. The three types of learners are commonly identified as *visual, auditory,* and *tactile* (sometimes called *kinesthetic*).

Visual Learners

Visual learners learn better from reading and writing than from hearing and talking about information. They usually find background noise, such as music and television, distracting rather than helpful. Following are strategies for visual learners:

• Read texts in a quiet place.
• Watch appropriate videos.
• Use visual study aids such as concept maps, flash cards, and charts.
• Use highlighting markers or colored paper to take notes.

Auditory Learners

Auditory learners grasp information most effectively by listening and talking. Combining information with music often works well for auditory learners. Following are strategies for auditory learners:

• Read texts aloud.
• Listen to audiotapes of course material.
• Make up a song about the content and sing it aloud (especially helpful for assimilating difficult content).
• Listen to background music or other noise.
• Talk about the content with a study partner.

Tactile or Kinesthetic Learners

Tactile or kinesthetic learners prefer to learn "hands on." They have difficulty sitting still for long periods. During study sessions, they should stand and move around or take frequent stretch breaks. Integrating physical activity with study works well for these learners. Following are strategies for tactile learners:

• Move around while studying.
• Read while exercising on a stationary bicycle.
• Listen to tapes of learning material while walking or biking.
• Rewrite or type notes.

Although almost everyone is capable of learning through all of their sensory pathways, most have a preferred channel. Think about which of the three learning styles discussed works best for you. Time is often at a premium for nurses studying for certification, and capitalizing on your preferred learning style will help you study in the most efficient way. Keep strategies for your preferred learning style in mind as you develop your study plan.

ACTIVE VERSUS PASSIVE STUDYING

Regardless of your personal learning style, the more actively you are engaged in the material, the better your ability to retain and comprehend content. For example, many of us have had the experience of reading an entire chapter, or listening to a review CD, only to find that our mind drifted away sometime earlier and we have difficulty recalling even the most basic information. Time is a precious commodity, so it is far more efficient to learn actively the first time than to reread or relisten to an entire chapter a second time. Tips used to improve active learning include taking notes while reading, pausing after each heading or subheading, and summarizing the content. Can you identify the main idea that the author was attempting to impart? Did you pass over new terms without taking the time to become familiar with them? As you read a summary, do you realize that you really need to go back to a more detailed reference because your knowledge is insufficient? Although active engagement may slow you down initially, it will save you time in the long run because now you are involved in active learning and not simply hoping that something will stick as you speed by.

GETTING STARTED

Studying, like regular exercise, is good for the brain. As a health-care professional, you will find that it will always be your job to keep abreast of the professional literature and spend some time studying. To recertify, you are mandated to keep your practice current through a combination of a number of clinical hours and continuing education options. The earlier you begin to plan for certification or recertification, the better.

The principles of effective study are simple but often ignored. There is one central law about study—the law of mass effect. Any worthwhile studying takes time. And in todays world, time is a precious commodity. Therefore, if you want to study, you need to set aside adequate time and plan accordingly. Be prepared to delay the start of new projects until this one is complete and you have successfully taken the exam. There is no way around the hours involved. There are no shortcuts. But you need to make it easy to begin.

TIPS FOR STUDYING

Just as a cold engine will run a little rough, settling down to study when one is out of the habit can be difficult. The following suggestions should make it easier to begin studying and to return to it on a regular and consistent basis.

- **Create a pleasurable personal environment.** This is a very basic but frequently overlooked requirement for successful study. Organize all your study materials in one area. Try to create a pleasant and regular work space for yourself. Perhaps it will be just part of a room, but make it an inviting part. Decorate it with flowers, pictures, or whatever makes the area appealing to you. For the kinesthetic learner, an open area that allows free movement may be better than a small office. Some literature suggests that playing classical music, especially from the baroque era, in the background increases concentration and retention. Decide whether background music is helpful for you or distracting. Background music may be helpful for an auditory learner, whereas a visual learner may find it a distraction.

- **Plan your activities in advance and be realistic.** Plan in advance what you are going to work on and do not be overly ambitious. Blocks of 1 hours at most are recommended, with a 10-minute break every 45 minutes. List the tasks beforehand; otherwise, you might spend valuable time trying to decide what material to review. Set specific targets for the time available.

- **Keep focused on the goal: becoming certified!** Keep the benefits of studying clearly in mind—in this case, the joy of receiving your passing score, followed by your embossed certificate in the mail. Visualize and imagine what the envelope will look and feel like when it comes in the mail. Feel your relief and joy when you find out your passing score! Picture the certificate framed, hanging in your office. Write down a list of all the things you stand to gain from passing the exam and reread it when you are ready to begin to study. Maybe the list includes a raise, an advanced level of licensure, a new job, or prescriptive privileges. Focus on these results and how they make you feel. Close your eyes and allow the feelings to flood through you!

- **Use your knowledge of yourself and of basic tips.** There are a number of ways you can make studying more fun. Make use of your best time of day. For some, this might mean rising early while the rest of the household sleeps and stealing time alone, undisturbed, with a hot cup of tea or coffee. For others, evening is preferable. Study for short periods with frequent breaks.

Remember to integrate whatever learning modalities work best for you. For example, if you are an auditory learner, use audiotapes. Listening to tapes while you are walking is especially good for tactile learners.

- **Think in terms of "bite-size" pieces and structure your study plan accordingly.** Use the "salami" principle: Cut large tasks into smaller ones and digest them one at a time. This will keep you from becoming overwhelmed and defeated before you begin.

- **Variety is also essential.** For example, divide your time between test question review and content review, or break up the study period into a variety of different tasks. Take notes for part of the time and read for part of the time. Do not keep at any one activity—even your practice exams—for longer than 45 minutes. Try studying with a study group part of the time. Discussing the materials with others is an especially good strategy for auditory learners.

- **Study with your purpose in mind**—in this case, passing the certification exam. As stated earlier, research has shown that two-thirds of your study time will be most effectively spent taking sample test questions. Do not lose sight of this! Studying does not necessarily mean sitting and reading textbooks. Reading books in a linear fashion is often not the most effective way to master information. Always keep the end result in mind.

- **Leave the environment in readiness for your next session.** Leave your work environment inviting for the next time. Put your materials away so that they are easily accessible. Do not leave the area cluttered; instead, make it more pleasing. Spend the last few minutes of your study time tidying up so that your environment is all set for your next session. This is also an excellent time to plan what you will do the next time you sit down to study. Believe it or not, these small, concrete habits can make a big dent in your natural tendency to procrastinate.

- **Reward yourself.** Last but not least, reward yourself! Reward yourself for each study period. You might decide that if you spend 3 hours studying on Saturday, you will see a movie on Saturday evening, or go to the mall, or treat yourself to a long, leisurely bubble bath! Be good to yourself.

Now that you understand yourself better and know how to approach studying for the exam, we move on to providing some specific information about the certification exams.

Nature of the Exams

The ANCC consists of 150 scored questions and 25 items being piloted that do not count in your score. The AANP certification exams consist of 135 multiple-choice questions and may include up to 15 additional pilot questions. The exam is administered on a computer at a testing center, and you will know in a few minutes after you complete the exam if you have passed. The questions are at a variety of difficulty levels, administered in an integrated format. The exams are not computer adaptive at this time. Computer-adaptive testing is the technique used for the NCLEX licensure exam. With computer-adaptive tests, each answer, correct or incorrect, determines the difficulty level of the next question a participant receives, and each participant may answer a different number of questions to meet a minimum passing level.

The exams as of this writing are composed of multiple-choice questions *only*. This format means that you must be able to identify key words or phrases on a computer screen, not on the traditional paper format. Many test takers feel constrained when they are unable to underline or highlight key words and phrases. A helpful tip: Use the scratch paper and pencil provided to you when taking a computer-based examination to write down the key phrases if that helps you focus on the topic and/or issue being presented in the question. A reminder: Remember that the scratch paper is collected by the testing center staff before you may leave the testing area; this is done to maintain test question security. Additionally, plan time to familiarize yourself with the technology before the exam begins. There are tutorials that are simple in nature and will "warm you up," helping you feel more comfortable with the computerized format before beginning the actual exam questions. Another benefit of giving the exams via computer testing centers is flexibility as to the locations where the test is offered (more than 300) and the number of days when testing is available.

Test-Taking Skills: An Acquired Art

The ability to select the best response to each question is what determines your success on the exam. Knowledge of the content is, unfortunately, not enough to guarantee success. If you are not able to communicate your knowledge through the medium of a multiple-choice exam, you will not succeed in becoming certified. Succeeding on a certification exam is a "head set" and not always indicative of your actual practice ability or intellectual capability.

Achieving success on a multiple-choice test is a skill, and like any other skill, it can be improved. Remember how you improve your other skills, such as playing an instrument or a sport: **practice.** The same holds true for test-taking skills. The best way to succeed on the exam is through practice, practice, and more practice.

The more you practice answering sample test questions, the better you will become at it. That is why we have written this book for you. This book provides over 2,000 sample test questions. Research has shown that two-thirds of study time should be spent taking sample tests, and one-third of the time should be spent reviewing content. A number of exam-preparation books are available to you; however, very few contain nearly the number of test questions you need to develop and flex your test-taking muscles. This book provides enough questions to enable you to do that. Additionally, reading through the answers in the rationales—the WHY of the reason the selected answer is correct or incorrect—is an excellent way to expand your knowledge base in general. It also provides insight into how answers are keyed—why one answer is rated as correct over another answer that seems to make sense to you. Remember: You will not be able to argue with the certifying exam companies as to your theory about why one answer is more correct in your view. Allow yourself to "tune into" these rationales so that you become more familiar with the answers that are noted to be correct.

To begin strengthening your test-taking skills, we discuss two basic tools to use when taking the exam and some specific strategies.

BASIC TOOLS

Two basic tools that are used in nursing—and that you should employ when taking the certification exam—are the nursing process and Maslow's hierarchy of needs.

The Nursing Process

The nursing process is a great tool when taking your certification exam because it can guide you through problem-solving. The AANP certification exam structures very specific pieces of information around these areas (see table of contents of AANP exam on the Web site). As you recall from your basic nursing education program, the steps of the nursing process include assessment, diagnosis, planning, implementation, and evaluation. When a question provides you with a choice between assessment and implementation, you should remember these basic tips. The purpose of assessment is to validate or confirm the problem. When considering an answer choice that is an assessment, you should ask yourself, "Is this an assessment that is appropriate to the topic of the question?" If it is, you should carefully consider this as a very likely answer choice. If, however, you believe the correct answer choice is an implementation, you should ask yourself, "Do I have enough information to implement what it is the answer choice is asking me to do?" Lastly, if the answer choice is asking you to evaluate a situation, you should ask yourself, "What would be the outcome if I chose this answer?" The criteria for reference are always your textbook and/or guidelines, and you should avoid answer choices that are too narrow or reflective of an individual practice preference.

Maslow's Hierarchy of Needs

Another important tool is Maslow's hierarchy of needs. It is particularly helpful in making priority decisions. According to Maslow, there are five levels of human needs: physiological needs, a need for safety and security, a need for love and a sense of belonging, a need for self-esteem, and a need for self-actualization. Because survival is grounded in basic physiological needs, these needs take priority over any other human needs. It comes down to practicality. If you do not have oxygen to breathe or food to eat, your focus is not really on the stability of your love life. When trying to determine the priority between a physiological need of a client versus a psychosocial need, remember the priority is to meet the physical needs of the client. This doesn't imply that the correct answer is never psychosocial; it simply means that survival of the species requires us to address physiological needs first, before we advance through the other stages of human needs. Always think **ABCs**—**A**irway, **B**reathing, **C**irculation.

SPECIFIC STRATEGIES

The following strategies should help in answering the multiple-choice questions on the certification exam.

Strategy #1: Understand and Analyze the Anatomy of a Test Question

A multiple-choice test question consists of three parts:

- An *introductory statement*, which sets up the clinical scenario
- A *stem*, which poses a question
- *Options*, from which you must select the correct answer

The first step in analyzing a multiple-choice test question is to separate what the question *tells* you from what it *asks* you. The **introductory statement,** which may vary considerably in length, provides information about a clinical scenario, a disease process, or a nursing response. The **stem** poses a specific question, which you must answer on the basis of your advanced-practice nursing knowledge. Stems are worded in different ways. Some stems are in the form of a question; others are in the form of an incomplete statement that you must complete. You must select the one **option** that best answers the question or completes the incomplete statement from a number, usually four, of potential options, sometimes called distractors.

Knowing these components will assist you in analyzing the information presented and in focusing on the question's intent or issue. Let's look at an example that includes an introductory statement in the form of a clinical scenario. The stem, which in this example is in the form of an incomplete statement, is in bold print.

EXAMPLE 1

A 32-year-old woman comes to your office for a routine examination. Her blood pressure is 120/80. **You should recommend that the client have her blood pressure checked again in**

A. 6 months.

B. 1 year.

C. 2 years.

D. 5 years.

The first and most important step is to identify what the question is asking. You cannot expect to answer the question correctly until you understand the **topic** of the question. The introductory statement of Example 1 gives you information about the clinical situation—a 32-year-old female client came to your office for a routine exam and has a normal blood pressure; these are the topics. The stem asks you for a clinical judgment—when should she have her blood pressure checked again? You must select the option that provides the most accurate response—in this case, option C, according to current guidelines. This question is an example of a **recall (memory-based) question,** sometimes called a **knowledge-based question.** You need to *know* and *recall* the guidelines concerning the frequency of blood pressure measurements under different circumstances and within different populations.

Other test questions assess **comprehension.** This is defined as drawing inferences from information without necessarily relating inferences to other material—in other words, using only present information that is in the question. Test takers often fall into the trap of "reading material into" these types of questions—information that is not requested in the question.

EXAMPLE 2

A 41-year-old male comes to your office complaining of having hit his head. While assessing his eyes, you note that the left pupil constricts simultaneously when the right pupil receives direct light. His left pupil exhibits which reaction?

A. Direct papillary reaction

B. Consensual papillary reaction

C. Convergence reaction

D. Corneal light reflex reaction

In this case, the correct answer is option B. You were able to *comprehend* the requested information based on the exact information given in the question.

Nursing, however, is a practice-based discipline. Nurses must apply knowledge to specific situations. This ability is assessed through the *application* questions designed to assess your ability to implement, solve a problem, or perform a task. Application of nursing knowledge is essential to safe, competency-based, entry-level advanced nursing practice. Application sometimes implies **analysis** of information, meaning the question requires you to dissect and analyze information and/or distinguish between critical and noncritical data. The certification exam is a test of "minimum competency," and simply recalling facts would not provide the certification bodies with sufficient information to determine your abilities. As such, you can expect the majority of questions to be application and analysis type questions. These require you to integrate knowledge with the facts that are presented in order to choose the single best answer for each question. Review the following example.

EXAMPLE 3

Julie, age 18 months, is up to date with her immunizations and is due to receive her diphtheria, tetanus, and pertussis (DTP) and oral polio (OPV) vaccinations today. Her father is bedridden at home with AIDS. Which immunizations should Julie receive today?

A. DTP and OPV as scheduled

B. DTP and inactivated polio vaccine (IVP)

C. DTP; IPV; and measles, mumps, and rubella (MMR)

D. DTP, OPV, and MMR

You must synthesize several concepts regarding immunizations to select the correct answer (option B) for this question. You must integrate your recall knowledge regarding standard and current immunization schedules (e.g., that Julie should receive DTP and polio immunizations on this visit) with the specific clinical scenario, which, in this case, includes a family member—her father who has AIDS. This calls for you to modify the regular regimen for immunizations and to administer a dose of inactivated polio vaccine (IPV) rather than the standard OPV because of Julie's close proximity to her father, who may be susceptible to the live poliovirus found in the standard OPV.

A common error test takers make in a multiple-choice testing format is to analyze the questions and answer choices with their eyes. Analysis is, however, done with the brain. Be careful of "looks good" choices. The reference for each and every correct answer is

grounded in textbook and/or guideline knowledge. A common trap that test question writers use is to include answer choices that appear on the surface to be correct but are not.

You should also determine if the stem is requesting a **positive response** or a **negative response.** Positive-response stems request an answer that is true, appropriate, or accurate, whereas negative-response stems request an option that is incorrect, false, inaccurate, or inappropriate. Negative-response stems frequently contain words such as *except, not, false,* or *least.* Consider this example.

EXAMPLE 4

Risk factors for osteoporosis include all of the following **except**

A. alcohol.

B. obesity.

C. age.

D. sedentary lifestyle.

Example 3 is a straight recall question testing your knowledge about osteoporosis and its risk factors. The key word in the stem—*except*—is a negative. In other words, to select the correct response for this question, you must select the answer that is wrong or is *not* a positively correlated risk factor for osteoporosis. In this question, the correct response is B.

Strategy #2: Identify the Questions, Critical Elements, and Key Words

The ability to identify the **critical elements** and **key words** in a test question is crucial to a correct interpretation of the question. Critical elements, such as the key concepts and conditions, tend to appear in the introductory statement, whereas key words usually appear in the stem of the question. Regardless of the placement of these words, remember that everything you need to be able to answer this question correctly is provided for you.

Key words are important words or phrases that help focus your attention on what the question is specifically asking. For example, key words determine whether the stem is asking for a positive or negative response. Examples of key words include *most, first response, earliest, priority, on the first visit, on a subsequent visit, common, best, least, except, not, immediately,* and *initial.* Often, but not always, these words appear in bold or italicized print. Take a look at this example.

EXAMPLE 5

*Which of the following is an example of a **primary** preventive intervention?*

    A. Tetanus prophylaxis

    B. Screening sigmoidoscopy

    C. Papanicolaou smear

    D. Blood pressure screening

Example 5 is a recall question with a positive-response stem. Although all of the interventions are preventive, the key word is *primary*, allowing you to choose the correct answer, A.

After identifying the topic of the question, you must also identify the **issue** the question is asking about. For example, the question, as in Example 6, may be requesting information about a disorder.

EXAMPLE 6

Mr. Williams, age 76, is seen in the ambulatory care clinic. He is complaining about incontinence, suprapubic pain, urgency, and dysuria. A urinalysis reveals the presence of white blood cells (WBCs), red blood cells (RBCs), and bacteria. What is your assessment?

    A. Prostatitis

    B. Nephrotic syndrome

    C. Benign prostatic hypertrophy (BPH)

    D. Cystitis

By selecting the correct answer, D, you have demonstrated knowledge related to a disease process, the **issue** about which this question requested information. Other examples of issues include drugs, such as antibiotics or immunizations; diagnostic tests, such as urinalysis or serum glucose; toxic effects of a drug, such as rash or vomiting; problems, such as knowledge deficit or substance abuse; procedures, such as bone marrow aspiration or cardiac catheterization; behaviors, such as agitation or overeating; and, occasionally, a combination of these. Consider this example.

EXAMPLE 7

Which drug is not used in the treatment of acute gout?

    A. An NSAID

    B. Colchicine

    C. An antibiotic

    D. An analgesic

This is a **recall/knowledge-based** question with a negative-response stem. The **key word** is negative—*not*—and the **issue** is knowledge of drugs. The correct answer is C.

Strategy #3: Use Therapeutic Communication

In communication-type questions, you are always looking for a **therapeutic response,** the cornerstone of the nurse-client relationship. To communicate therapeutically, you need to use communication tools and avoid communication blocks. Remember your basic therapeutic nursing role. The nurse, whether at a generalist or advanced-practice level, is *always* therapeutic. Your role is *not* that of an authority figure. This may cause some confusion for practitioners from other cultures in which health-care providers are conceptualized as authority figures who give directions. Remember, this is a nursing-based exam. Your **initial response** is *always* the therapeutic response—the acknowledgment and validation of the client's feelings. This is really a safety issue. Are your responses to clients and families SAFE? In acknowledgment of the importance of this aspect of advanced nursing practice, the first domain on the ANCC Test Outline Content (TOC) actively includes therapeutic communication and the nurse-client relationship, critical aspects of **ALL** nursing practice.

EXAMPLE 8

Ms. Doe, age 55, is very fearful because of a breast lump you have just identified. She begins to cry and states, "I'm afraid of having a mammogram." Your initial response is

    A. "You must have the mammogram."

    B. "Don't worry; I'm sure it is nothing."

    C. "Wonderful advances have been made in breast cancer research."

    D. "You're feeling scared?"

The correct answer is D. Communication skills learned in Nursing 101 are important components of successful test-taking strategies. Table 2-2 reviews communication techniques that facilitate therapeutic communication and those that block therapeutic communication.

TABLE 2-2. COMMUNICATION TECHNIQUES

TECHNIQUES	EXAMPLES
Techniques That Facilitate Therapeutic Communication	
Offering self	"I'll stay with you..."
Showing empathy	"I see you are upset."
Silence	Remaining present but silent
Giving information	"You need to take this drug two times a day."
Restatement	"You feel hurt?"
Clarification	"You are saying that..."
Reflection	"You seem to be anxious."
Techniques That Block Therapeutic Communication	
False reassurance	"Everything will be OK."
Disapproval	"That was wrong."
Approval	"That was right."
Requesting an explanation	"Why did you do that?"
Giving advice	"I think you should..."
Deferring	"You need to talk with your doctor about that."
Defensiveness	"We are understaffed!"
Devaluing feelings	"That's silly; don't be upset!"

Another important component in selecting the correct answer to questions that address your ability to communicate therapeutically is prioritization of responses. More than one option may contain a therapeutic response. But which is the **first, best,** or **most therapeutic** response in that situation? Communication theory emphasizes that it is a priority to address the client's **feelings first.** Validate, validate, validate. "You seem to be very sad today, Mr. George." "I can see that you are upset." "You seem very anxious, Mrs. Smith." This should always be done *before* clarifying or presenting information. Is there a need to address the feelings? If so, this takes priority. Empathy, restatement, reflection, and being silent, as well as remaining with the client, are all excellent nursing strategies that can potentially validate client's feelings. The only exception to this rule would be the presence of a pressing or interfering physical problem.

Strategy # 4: Identify the Person Who Is the Focus of the Question

Another critical element is your ability to identify the person who is the focus of the question. This person might be the client or the person with the health-care problem, or a family member or neighbor of the person with the health-care problem, or another member of the health-care team. Take a look at this example.

EXAMPLE 9

Mr. Boyd, age 84, has dementia and is in a long-term care facility. His daughter and son-in-law are visiting. As they get ready to leave and begin to say good-bye, Mr. Boyd grabs his daughter's arm and begins to cry, saying "Don't leave me here. I will die in this place." As she leaves the room, his daughter is visibly upset and asks you if she should visit again soon because it has so upset her father. The best reply for you to make is

A. "You might try telephoning next time instead of visiting. Your father will know that you are thinking of him then."

B. "I will give you the number of the social worker. She will be able to arrange a team conference and family meeting."

C. "This is a very upsetting time for all of you. However, it is important that you continue to visit regularly. For now, I will go in and sit with your father for a little while."

D. "He needs time to adjust to this new setting. Perhaps it might be easier on you all if you just didn't visit for a few days."

In this question, the person who is the focus of the question is Mr. Boyd's daughter, not Mr. Boyd. The **key word** in the stem is **best** response. It is also helpful to identify the **issue** the question is asking about. The issue in this question is one of therapeutic communication, specifically, Mr. Boyd's daughter's feelings of concern about her father. C is the correct response because it validates the daughter's feelings first.

Strategy #5: Determine the Best Response

There may be more than one option in a test question that is correct. But which is the **best, first,** or **most therapeutically sound** response to the question posed? Application/analysis-based test questions often involve decision making, which is based on prioritization. Therapeutic communication skills teach the acknowledgment of feelings first. Teaching and learning theory reminds us that unless the client is motivated to learn, no client teaching will be successful. If the client is not motivated, this issue must be addressed first.

To assist you in the correct answer selection, follow a few tips:

- Assessment always comes before diagnosis and treatment.
- The key word *initial* usually implies the need to assess.
- Remember Maslow's hierarchy of needs.
- In communication-based questions, you must address the client's **feelings first.**
- In teaching and learning situations, learning is contingent upon **motivation.**

As stated earlier, according to Maslow, physiological needs always come first. In determining which physiological needs have priority, you might recall the ABCs for basic cardiopulmonary support—A for airway, B for breathing, and C for circulation. This is handy to remember for questions that present a sudden emergency situation or any situation that is potentially life threatening for the client. Once basic physiological needs are met, **safety** is the next priority, followed by **psychosocial** needs.

Strategy #6: Avoid Common Pitfalls

A very common cause of test-taking errors is misreading the test question. To avoid common pitfalls, follow these tips:

- Ask yourself, "What is this question *really* asking?"
- Look for the key words.

- Restate the question in your own words. Eliminate any options that require you to make assumptions about information that was not presented in the case scenario and any options that contain information not presented in the scenario. *Do not read anything new into or overanalyze the test question!* Go with your first, most straightforward response. It is usually your best bet for answering the test question correctly.
- Carefully review the question using the systematic format and strategies suggested in this book.
- Make a decision about each option as you read it; this is an efficient approach to test taking. Do not go back to that option once you have eliminated it, do not overcomplicate the case scenario presented, and do not rely on anecdotal data from your own practice. These are national exams with testing content based on national standards of practice.

Strategy #7: Select the Best Answer When You Do Not Know the Answer

We now discuss some more specific strategies for selecting the best answer. Certification exams do not penalize you for guessing. Imagine that you are beginning your exam. You have answered a few questions easily, but now you have come to a test question to which you do not know the answer. You have identified the introductory statement and the stem, have determined whether it is a positive-response stem or a negative-response one, and have read through the options. You have identified the issue and the person who is the focus of the question. But you are still uncertain of the answer. If this happens, follow these tips:

- **Eliminate incorrect options.** This is very important. Frequently, you will be able to eliminate two choices easily, and remember that if even a small part of the answer choice is incorrect, the whole answer choice is incorrect and you must eliminate it from further consideration. Eliminating incorrect answer choices improves your chances of choosing the correct response even when you are unsure of the exact answer choice. The key is to not panic. It is not realistic to expect to know everything that you will be tested on, but through careful preparation, use of test-taking tools and strategies, and analysis of the content presented in the question, you will improve your chances of successfully answering the question and passing the certification exam on the first attempt—a noteworthy goal!

- **Select the most global response option.** The option that offers the most comprehensive or general statement is often a better answer than an option that is more specific and thus more limited.

- **Eliminate similar options.** If two options say essentially the same thing, neither can be correct. If three of the four options sound similar, the "odd" one should win out. In other words, look for patterns or relationships within the answer choices to help you select the best answer.

- **Eliminate options that contain words like** *always* or *never.* Absolute options containing the words *always* or *never* are seldom correct.

- Look for words or phrases in the option that are similar to those in the introductory statement or stem. Try this strategy if you need to guess.

- Be alert to relevant information from earlier questions.

- Watch for grammatical inconsistencies between the stem and the options.

- **Look for the longest option.** It is often the correct response.

Key test-taking tips are given in Table 2-3.

TABLE 2-3. KEY TEST-TAKING TIPS

- Eliminate options you know are incorrect. If you can eliminate two options, even a guess has a 50% chance of being correct.
- Answer all questions as if the situations were ideal.
- Read the test question carefully.
- Separate what the question tells you from what it is asking.
- Identify all false-response stems.
- Select the most global response.
- Eliminate options that are incorrect or similar or that contain words such as *always* or *never.*
- Look for grammatical inconsistencies between the stem and the options, words in the options that have appeared in the stem, and the longest option.
- Be alert to information relevant to answering the question in the stem or in earlier questions.

Designing Your Study Plan

In creating your individual study plan, review and apply the phases of the nursing process: assess, plan, implement, and evaluate.

ASSESS AND DIAGNOSE

Begin by taking some sample exams. You might first try taking one of the practice exams that are in the back of the book. Only do 150 questions, and then assess your score. This will give you an idea of your baseline and how intensive your study plan needs to be. Then move onto the specific content areas in this book, beginning with your weakest areas first. For example, if your assessment of your practice test score indicates a specific weakness in Male Genitourinary content, begin with that chapter.

Reflect, as part of your assessment, on your test-taking type, preferred learning style, and personality. Remember, speed is not necessarily your best friend, and overanalysis can lead you to an incorrect answer choice, but careful analysis of each question is a prerequisite to success on the exam. The union of knowledge and strategy is what is needed to achieve a successful outcome on the certification exam. One complements the other, and both are imperative if you are to attain your goal of becoming a board-certified advanced-practice nurse.

Use the analysis of scoring in Table 2-4 to help you make an accurate assessment of why you missed the questions you did. Failure to analyze why you missed a specific question is a commonly missed

TABLE 2-4. ANALYSIS OF SCORING

Test-Taking Error
Review the sample test questions that you answered incorrectly and keep track of WHAT caused you to select the incorrect answer. Look for a pattern.
- Missed key word
- Did not read all of the distractors carefully
- Read into the question
- Misread or misunderstood the question
- Changed the answer
- Content weakness
- Forgot or did not recognize or understand the content
- Applied wrong concept or rationales

opportunity to improve your skills. Simply comparing your answer choice to the correct answer choice is a passive learning process. However, analyzing why you missed a question (assessment) and actively creating a strategy to correct the knowledge or skills deficit (implementation) will help you achieve the outcome you are seeking. For example, did you miss the correct answer because you did not know or remember the content? This is a knowledge deficit. Or did you miss a key word, read into the test question, or change the answer? If so, you need to continue to work on test-taking skills. You must become proficient at both—content knowledge and test-taking skills. Recognizing where you are vulnerable and then taking steps to improve in that area gives you a significant edge in preparing for your examination and building your confidence. These objectives are best achieved through ongoing self-testing with sample exam questions such as the ones provided for you in this book. Evaluate what percentage of questions you missed because of (1) content issues, (2) testing errors, or (3) confidence issues. Design your study plan accordingly. As you study, use the analysis of scoring to continue to track your progress.

Aim for an 85% grade on your practice exams to demonstrate a good level of mastery of each content area. Begin working on areas in which your knowledge may be lacking and progress to areas in which you are stronger. Opening a book and beginning on page 1 may not serve you well. However, recognizing that you may be weak in cardiovascular content and prioritizing your study time to concentrate on that content area to eliminate knowledge deficits will be very helpful.

Any test score below 80% indicates a need to initiate a more aggressive and intensive exam review. A score of 80% or higher, however, does not mean that you shouldn't prepare. You should still aim to review approximately 2,000 to 3,000 sample test questions before sitting for the exam, as well as do some basic content review. An initial score below 80% means you should aim to review a minimum of 5,000 sample test questions before the exam, as well as complete an intensive content review. Attending a certification review class is an additional way to shore up your knowledge base.

PLAN AND IMPLEMENT

The certification exam time line and study calendar (Table 2-5) provide a suggested 6-week time line, providing a countdown to exam time from the day you register for your exam. Use the salami technique. Study a little every day. Improve your self-image. Believe you are a good student and behave like one. Stick to your study plan. Set clear-cut goals and objectives.

Answer approximately 100 test questions in a specific content area. Assess your score. If it is between 85% and 95%, move on. Feel confident—but continue

TABLE 2-5. CERTIFICATION EXAM TIME LINE AND STUDY CALENDAR

SUNDAY	*MONDAY*	*TUESDAY*	*WEDNESDAY*	*THURSDAY*	*FRIDAY*	*SATURDAY*
Commitment • Register for the exam. • Evaluate your test-taking type and preferred learning style. • Take assessment exam. • Evaluate exam with analysis of scoring. • Develop study plan and gather study materials. • Fill out study calendar and begin. • Make arrangements for going to the exam.						
(Dates) **WEEK 1**	Content: Score:	Content: Score:	Content: Score:	Content: Score:	Content: Score:	Content: Score:
(Dates) **WEEK 2**	Content: Score:	Content: Score:	Content: Score:	Content: Score:	Content: Score:	Content: Score:

(continued)

SUNDAY	MONDAY	TUESDAY	WEDNESDAY	THURSDAY	FRIDAY	SATURDAY

Perseverance
- Continue studying.
- Take a week off from studying.

(Dates)

WEEK 3	Content:	Content:	Content:	Content:	Content:	Content:
	Score:	Score:	Score:	Score:	Score:	Score:

(Dates)

WEEK 4	Content:	Content:	Content:	Content:	Content:	Content:
	Score:	Score:	Score:	Score:	Score:	Score:

Focus and Reward
- Focus on content areas in which you scored less than 80% on sample questions.
- Make final arrangements for going to the exam.

(Dates)

WEEK 5	Content:	Content:	Content:	Content:	Content:	Content:
	Score:	Score:	Score:	Score:	Score:	Score:

(Dates)

WEEK 6	Content:	Content:	Content:	Content:	Content:	Content:
	Score:	Score:	Score:	Score:	Score:	Score:

* Source: Adapted from Hoefler, P: *Successful Problem-Solving and Test-Taking for Beginning Nursing Students*, ed 3. MEDS, Silver Spring, Md, 1997, p. 111.

to review sample test questions. If your score is lower than 85%, use the diagnostic grid.

As noted in chapter 1, both the ANCC and AANP exams cover pathophysiological content organized by body system. This is how you should organize your study time: by body system, by content areas associated with populations (usually age-driven), and by the specified domains on the exam. The body system content is specified by the chapter title. We suggest following the table of contents of this book, which is modeled on the practice domains spelled out by both certifying bodies. After assessing your baseline knowledge through use of the integrated practice exams provided in this book, move on to the content areas in which you scored the lowest. This will allow you to customize your study plan and make the best use of your time. Remember, for some people, this might be the neurological content; for others, it might be the endocrine or psychiatric content, and so on.

To review disorders and help you prioritize, use the following tips:

- Organize content by body system.
- Begin with the system you find the most difficult.
- Review the pathophysiology of that system, if necessary.
- List pertinent disorders of that system.

- Review incidence and contributing factors.
- Review early and late disease manifestations.
- Review the sequelae, prognoses, and life-threatening complications.
- Determine treatment; adjust for age.
- Review associated teaching and learning needs.
- Review coping techniques, prevention, and health promotion.
- Remember that the certification exam focuses on common diseases and disorders; use this information as a tool for success and avoid studying topics that are rarely seen in a primary care setting.

Using content maps is another approach to mastering content. Figure 2-1 is an example of a content map approach to reviewing disease processes. A content map is a picture or pattern of information. It also shows relationships between pieces of information. Developing content maps can help you to find content areas in which you are weak and avoid studying content you already know. People are drawn to study what they already know. They feel comfortable with that information, whereas new information can produce anxiety. In the long run, however, this is not a good strategy.

CONTENT MAP

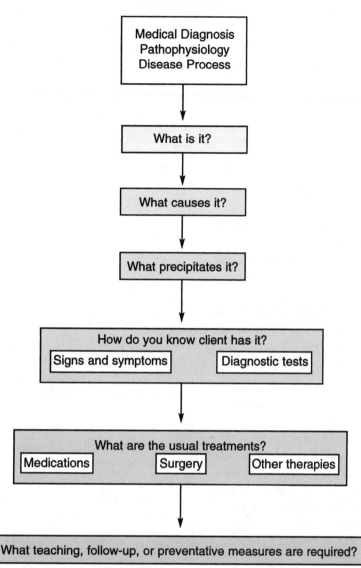

Figure 2-1

Few people can read a book and visualize the exact page, word for word, in their minds. A content map helps you find the information in your memory, where it is usually stored in patterns related to other memories. Using this structure, you can find out what areas you may not completely understand. Content maps start with general information and move to specifics. They can be helpful for people who spend so much time studying the details that they miss the bigger picture.

EVALUATE

To help you evaluate your progress, consider these tips:

- Take a sample test and use the test-taking analysis of scoring. Review one of your sample content area tests. Why did you answer the

questions that you got wrong incorrectly? Remember, active learning improves retention.

- If content is forgotten, use a content review. Did you not recognize or remember the content? This would indicate a need to review content using a book of condensed information or an outline-review text, or attending a certification review. It does not mean that you should return to your textbook or class notes.

- If a rationale is misunderstood, go back to textbooks. Did you not comprehend the content? For example, perhaps your basic understanding of the cardiac cycle was not thorough enough to include the severity and implications of various murmurs (i.e., which ones are relatively normal physiological events and which ones are indicative of more severe pathology). This would indicate a need to go back to one of your textbooks, or perhaps obtain audiotapes and/or videotapes with more detailed content, and review basic pathophysiological processes.

- If the error is in test taking or you need to build confidence, continue to take the sample exams. Did you answer a question incorrectly because you missed a key word? Did you not read all the options carefully enough? Did you read something into the question? Did you change an answer? Did you choose the correct answer but bubble in an incorrect response? All of these are indications of test-taking errors and indicate an ongoing need for you to continue practicing your skills using sample exams. If you are consistently scoring well on practice exams, it will make you feel more confident and comfortable with testing.

- Practice, practice, practice sample test questions. Using the analysis of scoring as you grade yourself on an integrated exam, followed by exams for specific body-system content, will enable you to design and update an individualized study plan that has specificity and relevance for you. For example, you may need to spend a week on neurological content but only a day on cardiac content. You *can* succeed in becoming certified!

Last-Minute Preparations: Relaxed and Ready

Well, you are finally there! The day of the exam has arrived. Several tried-and-true techniques can help you get through this day with success and confidence.

The night before the exam, get a good night's sleep. Last-minute all-night study sessions are *not* recommended. Since your examination will focus on comprehension and analysis, cramming the night before is not a test-taking strategy, and it often results in increased anxiety and lower test scores. However, taking time to review a few notes is acceptable. It might be better to do something relaxing and enjoyable like going to a movie.

Locate the exam site before the day of the actual exam and plan for possible traffic delays and bad weather on the day of the exam. Becoming lost or finding yourself stuck in traffic will only increase your anxiety. Know where to park and how long it will take you to get there.

The morning of the exam, do a few exercises to get your blood pumping to your brain. Eat lightly, but *do* have breakfast. Bring identification, your registration for the exam, at least two sharpened pencils if you are taking a paper-and-pencil exam, and a watch. Dress in layers. Avoid stimulants and depressants. Go light on the caffeine. Find the restroom, and use it before beginning the exam.

Pay careful attention to the instructions and tutorial for computer testing. Do deep-breathing and positive relaxation exercises to calm yourself. In a testing center, others will be taking different exams and will have started at different times, so do not panic if people come and go while you are testing. Stay focused!

Pace yourself—do not spend too long on any one test question—and it is usually best if you go with your first choice. You should understand that the certification exams are *not* computer adaptive, meaning that you will be able to mark a question and return to it later if time permits. (In computer-adaptive exams, like the NCLEX-RN, after submitting your answer choice, you are not permitted to return to a question and change your response.)

Use test-taking strategies when you do not know the answer. Identify distractions, such as backache or neck ache, noise, reading the same questions over and over, feeling tired, or thinking of your vacation. If these occur, *stop*, take a few deep breaths, refocus, then get back on track. Mental fatigue can certainly play a factor when you are taking a lengthy exam. We recommend that you pace yourself accordingly. For example, prepare ahead of time to rest between each set of 25 questions or so. Allow yourself to disengage even for 1 minute; then you will be better able to refocus and continue answering questions. Stretch as needed. Practice positive visualization if your mind begins to drift and you find it difficult to concentrate, thus reducing your ability to identify key words and topics and increasing the likelihood of your answering a question incorrectly. Do not overcomplicate or overanalyze the test questions—everything you need to know to answer the question correctly is included in the question stem or answer choices. Move on! Think positively about your success. Stay focused on your goal: becoming a nationally certified advanced-practice nurse.

Begin now by using this book as suggested. After all, the longest journey begins with a single step. Take that step now. Turn the page and begin.

Bibliography

American Academy of Nurse Practitioners: National competency-based certification examinations for adult and family nurse practitioners. American Academy of Nurse Practitioners, Austin, TX, 2007. http://www.aanpcertification.org/ptistore/control/index.

American Nurses Certification Corporation certification Web page: http://www.nursecredentialing.org, accessed April 2012.

American Nurses Certification Corporation Sample Questions. http://www.nursecredentialing.org/Certification/ExamResources/SampleQuestions/FamilyNP-Mar2010Test.htm, accessed April 2012.

Dunphy, LM, Winland-Brown, JE, Porter, BO, and Thomas, D: *Primary Care: The Art and Science of Advanced Practice Nursing*, ed 4. FA Davis, Philadelphia, 2011.

Miller, SK: *Adult Nurse Practitioner Review and Resource Manual*, ed 2. American Nurses Credentialing Center, Silver Springs, MD, 2005.

Sides, MB, and Korchek, N: *Successful Test-Taking*, ed 3. Lippincott Williams & Wilkins, Philadelphia, 1998.

EVALUATION AND PROMOTION OF CLIENT WELLNESS

Chapter 3: *Health Promotion*

Jill E. Winland-Brown

Questions

3-1 Herbert, a 69-year-old man, comes to your office complaining of nocturia. On questioning Herbert, you find that for the past 3 months he has been getting up at least five times a night to void. He came in to seek help today because of his wife's insistence that he be checked out. When you perform the digital rectal exam, you find that his prostate protrudes 3–4 cm into the rectum. What grade would you assign to Herbert's prostate enlargement?

A. Grade 1
B. Grade 2
C. Grade 3
D. Grade 4

3-2 Screening is considered a form of

A. health counseling.
B. primary prevention.
C. secondary prevention.
D. tertiary intervention.

3-3 Which industry is responsible for the most injuries?

A. Mining
B. Construction
C. Transportation and utilities
D. Manufacturing

3-4 Which immunization may prevent meningitis?

A. Hepatitis B
B. *Haemophilus influenzae* type B (Hib)
C. Measles, mumps, and rubella (MMR)
D. Varicella

3-5 When should a woman start getting Pap tests?

A. When she becomes sexually active
B. At age 21

C. During her first pregnancy
D. Before birth control is prescribed

3-6 Susie, age 5, comes to the clinic for a well-child visit. She has not been in since she was 2. Her immunizations are up to date. What immunizations would you give her today?

A. None; wait until she is 6 years old to give her booster shots
B. Diphtheria, tetanus, and pertussis (DTaP); *Haemophilus influenzae* type B (Hib); and measles, mumps, and rubella (MMR)
C. DTaP and IPV
D. DTaP, IPV, and MMR

3-7 Which tumor marker is specifically elevated in prostate cancer?

A. Prostate cancer tumor marker (PCTM)
B. Cancer antigen (CA) 125
C. Carcinoembryonic antigen (CEA)
D. Prostate-specific antigen (PSA)

3-8 Gerald, a 67-year-old male retired maintenance worker, comes to your office for a physical. On reviewing Gerald's history, you discover that he has had pneumonia twice in the past 5 years. When you question Gerald about his immunization history, he reveals that his last tetanus and diphtheria (Td) immunization was 6 years ago, and his last flu shot was 8 months ago during the last flu season. He denies ever having had a pneumonia vaccination. Which immunizations should you offer to Gerald today?

A. Td
B. Pneumococcal vaccine
C. Influenza
D. Td and pneumococcal vaccine

3-9 When should glaucoma screening be instituted?

A. When the client is age 65
B. When the client exhibits vision problems

C. At the client's annual exam

D. Starting at age 40

3-10   The U.S. government report, *Healthy People 2020, National Health Promotion and Disease Prevention Objectives*, lists which of the following as leading health indicators?

A. Obesity, substance abuse, and immunizations

B. Obesity, responsible sexual behavior, and driver education

C. Obesity, substance abuse, and driver education

D. Obesity, immunizations, and driver education

3-11   *Mimi, age 52, asks why she should perform a monthly breast self-examination (BSE) when she has an annual exam by the physician, as well as a yearly mammogram. You respond,*

A. "If you are faithful about your annual exams and mammograms, that is enough."

B. "More breast abnormalities are picked up by mammograms than by clinical exams or BSE."

C. "More than 90% of all breast abnormalities are first detected by self-examination."

D. "Self-examinations need to be performed only every other month."

3-12   *Alcohol, especially when used with tobacco, is a dietary factor in which type of cancer?*

A. Liver

B. Esophagus

C. Bladder

D. Breast

3-13   *When performing a sports physical exam on Kevin, a 16-year-old healthy boy, which question in the history is important to ask Kevin or his guardian?*

A. Did anyone in your family ever have sudden cardiac death?

B. Does anyone in your family have elevated cholesterol levels?

C. Did you ever have any injury requiring stitches?

D. Does anyone in your family have a history of asthma?

3-14   *Joseph, a 55-year-old man with diabetes, is at your office for his diabetes follow-up. On examining his feet with monofilament, you discover that he has developed decreased sensation in both feet. There are no open areas or signs of infection on his feet. What health teaching should Joseph receive today regarding the care of his feet?*

A. Wash your feet with cold water only.

B. See a podiatrist every 2 years, inspect your own feet monthly, and apply lotion to your feet daily.

C. Go to a spa and have a pedicure monthly.

D. See a podiatrist yearly; wash your feet daily with warm, soapy water and towel dry between the toes; inspect your feet daily for any lesions; and apply lotion to any dry areas.

3-15   *Harvey, age 55, comes to the office with a blood pressure of 144/96 mm Hg. He states that he did not know if it was ever elevated before. When you retake his blood pressure at the end of the examination, it remains at 144/96. What should your next action be?*

A. Start him on an ACE inhibitor.

B. Start him on a diuretic.

C. Have him monitor his blood pressure at home.

D. Try nonpharmacological methods and have him monitor his blood pressure at home.

3-16   *Sally, age 25, is of normal weight. She follows a diet of 70% carbohydrates, 10% fat, and 20% proteins. How do you respond when she asks you if this is a good diet?*

A. "Yes, this is a good diet."

B. "No, you should eat more proteins."

C. "You should be eating only about 55% carbohydrates."

D. "Make sure your fats are divided among saturated, polyunsaturated, and monounsaturated fats."

3-17   *What is the most common type of occupational (nonfatal) illness in the United States?*

A. Poisoning

B. Respiratory conditions caused by toxic agents

C. Repetitive stress injury

D. Skin disorders

3-18   *The primary objective of screening is to*

A. prevent a disease.

B. detect a disease.

C. determine the treatment options.

D. promote genetic testing to prevent passing on the disease.

3-19   *Tuberculin skin testing using the Mantoux test should be considered for*

A. high-risk adolescents, recent immigrants, and homeless individuals.

B. all clients every 2 years.

C. all clients at their annual physical.

D. all children before entrance into first grade.

3-20   *Josephine, a 60-year-old woman, presents to your office with a history of elevated total cholesterol, triglycerides, and low-density lipoprotein (LDL) cholesterol. She was started on a statin medication 4 weeks ago and is concerned about some muscle pains she has been experiencing. On questioning Josephine, you discover that she has had pain in both her thighs for the past 2 weeks. What possible complication of statin therapy are you concerned that Josephine might be experiencing?*

A. Liver failure

B. Renal failure

C. Rhabdomyolysis

D. Rheumatoid arthritis

3-21   *One of the major criteria for diagnosing chronic fatigue syndrome is*

A. generalized headaches.

B. unexplained, generalized muscle weakness.

C. sleep disturbance.

D. fatigue for more than 6 months.

3-22   *Margaret, age 29, is of medium build and 5 ft 4 in. tall. You estimate that she should weigh about*

A. 105 lb.

B. 110 lb.

C. 120 lb.

D. 130 lb.

3-23   *A heart-healthy diet should be recommended to clients*

A. with a low-density lipoprotein (LDL) cholesterol level greater than 160 mg/dL.

B. with a total cholesterol level greater than 200 mg/dL.

C. with a high-density lipoprotein (HDL) cholesterol level below 35 mg/dL.

D. regardless of age or risk.

3-24   *Dennis, age 62, has benign prostatic hyperplasia (BPH). He tells you that he voids at least four times per night and that he has read about a preventive drug called terazosin hydrochloride (Hytrin) that might help him. What do you tell him?*

A. "Its not a preventive drug, but it relaxes smooth muscle in the prostate and bladder neck."

B. "It changes the pH of the urine and prevents infections caused by urinary stasis."

C. "It relaxes the urethra."

D. "It shrinks the prostate tissue."

3-25   *Julia, age 18, asks you how many calories of fat she is eating when one serving has 3 g of fat. You tell her*

A. 12 calories.

B. 18 calories.

C. 27 calories.

D. 30 calories.

3-26   *When does the National Cholesterol Education Program recommend cholesterol screening for persons with no family history of coronary heart disease before age 55?*

A. Starting at age 20 and then at least every 5 years if the cholesterol level remains normal

B. Whenever any other blood test is ordered

C. At the annual routine physical

D. Starting at age 20 and then annually

3-27   *How do you respond when Jill, age 42, asks you what constitutes a good minimum cardiovascular workout?*

A. Exercising for at least 30 minutes every day

B. Exercising a total of 2 hours per week

C. Exercising for at least 20 minutes, 3 or more days per week

D. Exercising for at least 30 minutes, 5 days per week

3-28   *Ethnocentrism is*

A. being concerned about the health needs of all Americans.

B. putting the group being studied at the center of dialogue.

C. thinking that ethnic groups other than one's own are inferior.

D. keeping a central focus on commonalities, not differences.

3-29 *What is an example of an active strategy of health promotion?*

A. Maintaining clean water

B. Introducing fluoride into the water

C. Enacting a stress management program

D. Maintaining a sanitary sewage system

3-30 *Which of the following is a true contraindication to immunizations?*

A. Mild-to-moderate local reaction to a previous immunization

B. Mild acute illness with a low-grade fever

C. Moderate or severe illness with or without a fever

D. Recent exposure to an infectious disease

3-31 *What is the goal of a sports physical?*

A. To clear all athletes for full participation in their sport activity

B. To limit the number of athletes participating in a sport activity

C. To identify health risks that may be minimized or cured in order to allow participation

D. To identify students at risk for health problems and limit their sports participation

3-32 *When should children be screened for lead poisoning?*

A. Only if they are in high-risk groups

B. At age 12 months

C. At age 3 years

D. Only if they live in or regularly visit a house built before 1960

3-33 *Which is the leading cause of cancer deaths?*

A. Lung cancer

B. Prostate cancer

C. Colon cancer

D. Breast cancer

3-34 *Mark, a 56-year-old man, comes to your practice seeking help to quit smoking. You prescribe Chantix (varenicline), a prescription medication, to aid with his attempt. What instructions do you give Mark regarding how to stop smoking with Chantix?*

A. Start the Chantix today according to the dosing schedule and then quit smoking after the 12-week medication schedule.

B. Start the Chantix today according to the dosing schedule and then pick a date to stop smoking about 7 days after starting Chantix.

C. Pick a date to stop smoking and start Chantix that day according to the dosing schedule.

D. Start Chantix today, take it twice a day for 2 weeks, and then stop smoking.

3-35 *What is the ultimate goal of crisis intervention?*

A. To help persons function at a higher level than in their precrisis state

B. To help persons eliminate the crisis and get back to where they were

C. To prevent further crises

D. To eliminate stress altogether

3-36 *Who should get the annual flu vaccination?*

A. Patients who have asthma and COPD

B. Residents in a nursing home

C. All individuals, including infants

D. All persons aged 6 months and older

3-37 *Screening test recommendations for HIV infection include*

A. all clients.

B. persons getting married.

C. teenagers who have been sexually active for 1 year.

D. intravenous drug users and clients with high-risk behaviors.

3-38 *How can health-care providers help prevent the spread of antibiotic resistance?*

A. By ordering medications empirically

B. By ordering an antibiotic that is not commonly given

C. By ordering an antibiotic that the patient has not received before

D. By ordering an agent targeting the likely pathogens

3-39 *If a screening test used on 100 individuals known to be free of breast cancer identified 80 individuals who did not have breast cancer while missing 20 of the individuals, the specificity would be*

A. 80%.

B. 60%.

C. 40%.

D. 20%.

3-40 *You are sharing with your client the idea that he needs to get some counseling to deal with his severe stress because it is affecting his physiological condition. Which of the following hormonal changes occurs during severe stress?*

A. A decrease in catecholamines

B. An increase in cortisol

C. A decrease in antidiuretic hormone

D. A decrease in aldosterone

3-41 *How do you respond when Mattie, who is taking levothyroxine (Levothroid, Synthroid), says she has read that she should not eat brussels sprouts?*

A. "Brussels sprouts contain a high amount of iodine, and therefore you should not eat them."

B. "Brussels sprouts interfere with the absorption of the medication."

C. "There is no reason why you should not eat brussels sprouts."

D. "It is safe if you take the medication in the morning and don't eat brussels sprouts until the evening."

3-42 *Anorexia nervosa is a steady, intentional loss of weight with maintenance of that weight at an extremely unhealthy low level. Which statement is true regarding anorexia nervosa?*

A. The poor eating habits result in diarrhea.

B. It may cause tachycardia.

C. It may occur from prepubescence into the early 30s.

D. It may cause excessive bleeding during menses.

3-43 *Which of the following statements is true about the older adult?*

A. Older adults are at an increased risk for depression.

B. Depression is a normal part of aging.

C. Depression may just be the emotion felt when a spouse is grieving the loss of a loved one.

D. Most antidepressive drugs do not work without psychotherapy on older adults.

3-44 *Bone density studies to screen for osteoporosis should be performed on which of the following?*

A. Perimenopausal women who used to smoke but no longer do

B. Only on women after menopause

C. All women who have had hysterectomies

D. Women with drinking problems

3-45 *Which federal insurance program went into effect in 1966 to provide funds for medical costs for persons age 65 and older, as well as disabled persons of any age?*

A. Medicare

B. Title XIX of the Social Security Act

C. Medicaid

D. Omnibus Reconciliation Act

3-46 *Max states that he cannot give up drinking beer, but he will cut down. You suggest that his limit should be*

A. one can of beer a day.

B. two cans of beer a day.

C. three cans of beer a day.

D. four cans of beer a day.

3-47 *When is routine screening for hypothyroidism performed?*

A. When a client reaches age 65

B. Whenever a client exhibits symptoms

C. Never; it is not routinely recommended

D. When a client has a family history of thyroid problems

3-48   *When can Pap smears be safely discontinued?*

A. At age 80

B. At age 65 if the previous three Pap smears have been normal

C. Never; they should be continued throughout life

D. After menopause or hysterectomy

3-49   *Utilization review refers to a system*

A. of reviewing access to and utilization of health-care services.

B. that uses retrospective review of client records to reveal problems that may be addressed in the future.

C. to monitor diagnosis, treatment, and billing practices to assist in lowering costs.

D. that has clients use an identification card to be able to use health-care services.

3-50   *Which part of Medicare is basic hospital insurance?*

A. Medicare Part A

B. Medicare Part B

C. Medicare Part C

D. Medicare Part D

3-51   *Mary, a 70-year-old woman with diabetes, is at your office for her 3-month diabetic checkup. Mary's list of medications includes Glucophage XR 1,000 mg daily, an angiotensin-converting enzyme (ACE) inhibitor daily, and one baby aspirin (ASA) daily. Mary's blood work showed a fasting blood sugar of 112 and glycosylated hemoglobin (HgbA$_{1c}$) of 6.5. You tell Mary that her blood work shows*

A. that her diabetes is under good control and she should remain on the same medications.

B. that her diabetes is controlled and she needs to have her medications decreased.

C. that her diabetes is not controlled and her medications need to be increased.

D. that her diabetes has resolved and she no longer needs any medication.

3-52   *A conservative, preventive health approach for healthy adults is to recommend limiting salt intake to how many grams per day?*

A. 2 g

B. 4 g

C. 6 g

D. 8 g

3-53   *In women with HIV infection, there is a high prevalence of additional infection from*

A. *Chlamydia.*

B. syphilis.

C. human papillomavirus (HPV).

D. *Candida.*

3-54   *Twenty percent of colorectal cancers can be attributed to which dietary cause?*

A. High-fat diet

B. High-carbohydrate diet

C. Use of alcohol

D. Lack of fiber in the diet

3-55   *Which class of drugs causes the most adverse reactions?*

A. Chemotherapeutic agents

B. Anticonvulsants

C. Antibiotics

D. Antidepressants

3-56   *How much higher are health-care costs for smokers than for nonsmokers?*

A. 20%

B. 40%

C. 60%

D. 80%

3-57   *The National Cancer Institute recommends that adults eat how many grams of fiber a day?*

A. 10–20 g

B. 20–30 g

C. 30–40 g

D. 40–50 g

3-58 The broad-based initiative led by the U.S. Public Health Service (PHS) to improve the health of all Americans through emphasis on prevention, rather than just treatment, of health problems throughout the next decade is

A. the National Health Objectives Report.
B. Healthy People 2020.
C. the Surgeon General's Report.
D. the PHS Initiative.

3-59 The best defense against colds, flu, and respiratory syncytial virus is

A. the flu shot.
B. prevention.
C. increased dosage of vitamin C.
D. rimantadine HCl (Flumadine).

3-60 Marvin is a gay man who is ready to "come out." What is the last step in the process of coming out?

A. Testing and exploration
B. Identity acceptance
C. Identity integration and self-disclosure
D. Awareness of homosexual feelings

3-61 By 2030, the number of U.S. adults aged 65 or older will more than double to about 71 million. What percentage of older adults have one chronic condition?

A. 30%
B. 50%
C. 80%
D. almost 100%

3-62 Women tend to outlive men by an average of

A. 3–4 years.
B. 5–6 years.
C. 6–7 years.
D. 7 or more years.

3-63 Mildred, a 92-year-old independent woman, is moving into her daughter's home. Her daughter comes to see you seeking information to help keep her mother from falling. Which of the following interventions would you suggest she do to help prevent Mildred from falling?

A. Install an intercom system in Mildred's bedroom.
B. Limit the time Mildred is home alone.
C. Hire an aide to assist Mildred 24 hours a day.
D. Remove all loose rugs from floors and install hand grasps in bathtubs and near toilets.

3-64 A diagram that depicts each member of a family, shows connections between the generations, and includes genetically related diseases is called a

A. family assessment diagram.
B. family generation illustration.
C. generations diagram.
D. genogram.

3-65 The CAGE screening test for alcoholism is suggestive of the disease if two of the responses are positive. What does the E in CAGE stand for?

A. Every day
B. Eye opener
C. Energy
D. Ego

3-66 Jan's mother has Alzheimer's disease. She tells you that her mother's recent memory is poor and that she is easily disoriented, incorrectly identifies people, and is lethargic. Jan asks you, "Is this as bad as it gets?" You tell her that her mother is in which stage of the disease?

A. Stage 1
B. Stage 2
C. Stage 3
D. Stage 4

3-67 For which patient would you administer the HPV vaccination?

A. Susie, age 7
B. Janice, age 17, who had a baby 6 months ago and is breastfeeding
C. Alice, age 18, who is allergic to yeast
D. Jill, age 30, who is pregnant

3-68 When should children have their first visual acuity testing?

A. When they are able to read
B. When they enter kindergarten
C. At age 2
D. At age 3

3-69 Marie, a Russian Jew, married Endo, a Filipino, and is adapting to his culture. This is referred to as

A. acculturation.
B. biculturalism.
C. cultural relativity.
D. enculturation.

3-70 One of the most common causes of involuntary weight loss is

A. malignancy.
B. pulmonary disease.
C. endocrine disturbances.
D. substance abuse.

3-71 Who is the most important source of social support for an adult?

A. Spouse (if applicable)
B. Parents
C. Close friends
D. Children

3-72 The two main causes of death among U.S. adults aged 65 years or older are

A. heart disease and stroke.
B. stroke and suicide.
C. heart disease and Alzheimer's disease.
D. heart disease and cancer.

3-73 Most anal cancers are potentially preventable. Which of the following is a cause of anal cancer?

A. Sexually transmitted diseases (STDs)
B. A low-fiber diet
C. Hemorrhoids
D. Foreign bodies used as sexual stimulants

3-74 A child's head circumference should be measured until the child reaches what age?

A. 6 months
B. 12 months
C. 18 months
D. 24 months

3-75 Performing range-of-motion exercises on a client who has had a cerebrovascular accident (CVA) is an example of which level of prevention?

A. Primary prevention
B. Secondary prevention
C. Complications prevention
D. Rehabilitation prevention

3-76 The major public health and safety focus in the United States has shifted to

A. cardiovascular risk reduction.
B. domestic abuse and violence.
C. unintended pregnancies.
D. the threat of bioterrorism.

3-77 Sal is traveling out of the country and asks for a prescription to prevent traveler's diarrhea. What do you give him?

A. Trimethoprim with sulfamethoxazole (TMP-SMX) double strength daily
B. Bismuth subsalicylate, 2 tabs qid
C. Nothing, but tell him to "cook it, boil it, peel it, or forget it"
D. Nothing, but tell him to use bottled drinking water

3-78 Margo, age 50, is perimenopausal. She tells you she is taking dehydroepiandrosterone (DHEA) and wants to start on hormone replacement therapy (HRT). When she asks for your opinion, you tell her that

A. taking both DHEA and HRT is not recommended because it is like "double dosing."
B. DHEA is safe and will not affect prescribed medications.
C. she will be safe as long as she takes the minimum dose of both therapies.
D. DHEA has the same pharmacotherapeutic effects as HRT.

3-79   A 68-year-old woman presents to your office for screening for osteoporosis. Sandy states that her grandmother and mother both lost inches in their old age. Sandy has been postmenopausal for the past 15 years and never took any hormone replacement medications. She is Caucasian, weighs 108 lb, and is 5 ft 1 in. tall on today's measurement. When do women lose the greatest amount of bone density?

A. During adolescence

B. The first year of menopause

C. The first 10 years after menopause

D. Bone loss occurs continuously at the same rate from menopause to death.

3-80   Emily, a healthy 26-year-old woman, asks you how she can prevent bone loss as she ages. She is concerned because both her maternal grandmother and now her mother have severe osteoporosis. What guidance would you give to Emily?

A. Drink all the soda you like—it has no effect on your bone density.

B. It has not been proved that smoking affects bone loss.

C. Replace estrogen when you reach menopause.

D. Perform aerobic exercise at least three times a week.

3-81   Which individuals does the U.S. Preventive Services Task Force (USPSTF) recommend screening for depression?

A. Adults who are experiencing gender issues

B. Adults who have already tried unsuccessfully to commit suicide

C. All adults

D. If a provider suspects depression, the individual should be referred to a specialist rather than screening in the primary care office

3-82   The National Cancer Institute (NCI) recommends that mammography, as a method of screening for breast cancer, should be performed

A. every year after age 40.

B. only after a woman finds a lump when performing monthly breast self-examinations.

C. every 1–2 years after the age of 40.

D. After a clinical breast exam every 2 years

3-83   To quantify the margin of error in a screening instrument, the measure of validity is divided into two components: sensitivity and specificity. Sensitivity refers to a screening test's ability to

A. recognize negative reactions or nondiseased individuals.

B. identify persons who actually have the disease.

C. predict populations at risk.

D. give the same result regardless of who performs the test.

3-84   Which program aims to remove racial and ethnic disparities in health by addressing the screening and intervention needs of midlife uninsured women?

A. Public health screening programs

B. WISEWOMAN projects

C. American Heart Association screening protocols

D. Centers for Disease Control and Prevention

3-85   Molly, age 48, is healthy and has well-controlled asthma. She asks if she should get an annual flu vaccination. You tell her that she should

A. get it only after she reaches age 65.

B. get it only during the fall season when her asthma is bothering her.

C. get it on an annual basis.

D. not get it because she has a respiratory problem (asthma).

3-86   According to the Joint National Committee (JNC) on Prevention, Detection, Evaluation, and Treatment of High Blood Pressure guidelines, Jesse, who has stage 1 hypertension, should be placed on which treatment plan for control of his hypertension?

A. Thiazide diuretic

B. Diet and exercise

C. One drug from one of the following classes: ACE inhibitor, calcium channel blocker, or angiotensin receptor blocker (ARB)

D. Thiazide diuretic and either ACE inhibitor, calcium channel blocker, or an ARB

3-87   When should an African American man start to be screened for prostate enlargement by a digital rectal exam?

A. Age 60 and then yearly

B. Age 40 and then yearly

C. Age 40 and then every 2 years

D. Age 55 and then yearly

3-88   A lab value that is commonly decreased in older adults is

A. creatinine clearance.

B. serum cholesterol.

C. serum triglyceride.

D. blood urea nitrogen.

3-89   The U.S. Department of Health and Human Services recommends which of the following exercise guidelines for Americans to reduce the risk of chronic disease in adulthood?

A. Participate in 45 minutes of cardiovascular exercise at least three times per week.

B. Walk 1 hour every day.

C. Engage in vigorous intense activity 60 minutes most days of the week.

D. Engage in 30 minutes or more of moderately intense physical activity at least 5 days per week.

3-90   What are the two leading causes of death in the United States for all ages?

A. Cancer and stroke

B. Heart disease and cancer

C. AIDS and heart disease

D. Accidents and heart disease

3-91   Andrea, a 20-year-old nursing student, never had her second measles, mumps, rubella (MMR) immunization. What test must you do before giving Andrea her second MMR?

A. Complete blood count

B. Complete metabolic panel

C. Lipid profile

D. Urine pregnancy test

3-92   Which health-care system delivers comprehensive health maintenance and treatment services to members of an enrolled group who pay a prenegotiated and fixed payment?

A. Health maintenance organizations (HMOs)

B. Preferred provider organizations (PPOs)

C. Fee-for-service (FFS) independent practices

D. Exclusive provider organizations (EPOs)

3-93   For primary prevention of skin cancer, you would recommend a sunscreen with how much ultraviolet (UV) wave protection?

A. 15

B. 25

C. 30

D. 45

3-94   Marian's husband, Stu, age 72, has temporal arteritis. She tells you that his physician wants to perform a biopsy of the temporal artery. She asks if there is a less invasive diagnostic test. What test do you tell her is less invasive?

A. Computed tomography (CT) scan

B. Magnetic resonance imaging (MRI)

C. Electroencephalogram (EEG)

D. Color duplex ultrasonography

3-95   Susan is traveling to South America and wonders if she should get a tetanus and diphtheria (Td) vaccination. You tell her that

A. she needs one if she has not had a Td shot within the past 10 years.

B. she should have tetanus immune globulin administered before departure.

C. she should receive a tetanus shot now.

D. tetanus and diphtheria are no longer a serious problem in South America.

3-96   In discussing sexuality with the mother of a 4-year-old, you should be concerned with which of the following?

A. Has your child asked questions about anatomical differences between sexes?

B. Does your child touch his or her own genitals?

C. Does your child play "doctor" with children of the opposite sex?

D. A yes answer to any of these questions is of no concern.

3-97   Which of the following criteria is not diagnostic for a child with attention deficit-hyperactivity disorder (ADHD)?

A. The child frequently blurts out the answer to a question before the question is finished.

B. The child has difficulty following directions.

C. The child talks very little but is very restless.

D. The child often engages in physically dangerous activities.

3-98   An indicator of body fat measured by dividing weight in kilograms by height in meters is the

A. weight/height chart.

B. body mass index.

C. body fat measurement.

D. anthropometric measurement.

3-99   Martha, age 82, has an asymptomatic carotid bruit on the left side. What do you recommend?

A. ASA therapy

B. Coumadin therapy

C. Surgery

D. No treatment at this time

3-100   Harriet, a 76-year-old woman, comes to your office every 3 months for follow-up on her hypertension. Harriet's medications include one baby aspirin daily, lisinopril 5 mg daily, and calcium 1,500 mg daily. On today's visit, Harriet's blood pressure is 168/88. According to the Joint National Committee (JNC) VII guidelines, what should you do next to control Harriet's blood pressure?

A. Increase her dose of lisinopril to 20 mg daily.

B. Add a thiazide diuretic to the lisinopril 5 mg daily.

C. Discontinue the lisinopril and start a combination of ACE inhibitor and calcium channel blocker.

D. Discontinue the lisinopril and start a diuretic.

3-101   Which of the following definitions refers to the epidemiologic term of endemic?

A. Outbreaks of an illness/disease that occur occasionally and are unrelated in space and time

B. Presence of an event (illness or disease) at a much higher than expected rate based on past history

C. Presence of an illness/disease constantly present or present at a rate that is expected based on history

D. Presence of an event in epidemic proportions affecting many communities and countries in a short period of time.

3-102   Sandra, a 27-year-old nurse, states that she does not want to get the hepatitis B virus vaccine because of its adverse effects. You tell her that the most common adverse effect is

A. fatigue.

B. headache.

C. pain at the injection site.

D. elevated temperature.

3-103   Sam, age 30, has a total cholesterol level of 186 mg/dL. How often should he be screened for hypercholesterolemia?

A. Every 5 years

B. Every 2 years

C. Every year

D. Whenever blood work is done

3-104   A high sodium intake contributes to the risk of

A. cancer.

B. heart disease.

C. osteoporosis.

D. hypertension.

3-105   Many of the 78 million baby boomers have a hearing loss. In a survey, all of the following statements were reported by baby boomers. Which statement was shared by the greatest percentage?

A. Hearing loss is affecting the home life of baby boomers.

B. Baby boomers have problems hearing on cell phones.

C. Baby boomers are reluctant to admit the impact of their hearing loss.

D. Hearing loss is affecting the work/jobs of baby boomers.

3-106   Carol, a nursing student, is at your office for her nursing school admittance physical exam *and immunizations. On reviewing Carol's allergies, you find that she is allergic to baker's yeast. What would you tell Carol regarding the hepatitis B vaccine?*

A. You recommend that she receive the first hepatitis B vaccine today.

B. You advise her to wait until she is starting her clinical rotations to get the first hepatitis B injection.

C. You advise her that she cannot receive the hepatitis B vaccine because of her allergy to baker's yeast.

D. You instruct her to receive the first hepatitis B vaccine today, the second injection in 6 months, and the third injection in 1 year.

3-107 *Oral health problems are common and painful. Years ago, it was common to see almost all adults with complete dentures. Today, what percentage of U.S. adults aged 75 and older have lost all of their teeth?*

A. 10%

B. 25%

C. 50%

D. 75%

3-108 *Martin, an 83-year-old man, is at your office for his yearly physical exam. He has a history of hypertension, hyperlipidemia, cigarette smoking, and chronic obstructive pulmonary disease (COPD). Martin states that he has been feeling increased fatigue with minimal activity but denies any chest pain or shortness of breath. Martin's list of medications includes the following: one baby aspirin daily, one ACE inhibitor daily, diuretic daily, and statin medication daily. Martin's physical exam was normal. His blood pressure was 130/68, his heart rate was 88, and his respiratory rate was 22. Observing Martin during your examination, you detect that he utilizes pursed-lip breathing throughout the exam. What medication should he be started on for his COPD?*

A. Inhaled corticosteroid

B. Inhaled anticholinergic and inhaled beta-2 agonists

C. Oral steroids daily

D. Inhaled beta-2 agonists

3-109 *Which statement about gender disparities and suicide is true?*

A. Women take their own lives more often than men.

B. Men attempt suicide more often than women.

C. Suicide rates for males are highest among those aged 75 and older.

D. Poisoning is the most common method of suicide for both sexes.

3-110 *Which of the following is a major risk factor associated with osteoporosis and fragility fractures?*

A. Body weight less than 127 lb

B. Alcohol intake greater than 2 drinks/day

C. Estrogen deficiency occurring before 45 years of age

D. Low physical activity

3-111 *Which statement is true regarding testicular cancer?*

A. White men are at a higher risk.

B. All races are equally susceptible.

C. Although testicular self-examination (TSE) alerts the person to the presence of a tumor, it has not been shown to decrease mortality.

D. TSE should be taught to all middle-aged men.

3-112 *Postmenopausal women who are not on hormone replacement therapy need how much calcium per day to help prevent osteoporosis?*

A. 1,000 mg

B. 1,200 mg

C. 1,500 mg

D. 1,800 mg

3-113 *Harry is taking his entire family to Central America and is wondering about protection against mosquito bites causing malaria. What advice do you give him?*

A. Use an insect repellent with diethyltoluamide (DEET) for the entire family, applying it sparingly to small children.

B. Make sure the family is in well-screened or indoor areas from dusk to dawn.

C. Use an insect repellent with DEET for adults and permethrin for children, and stay inside from dusk to dawn.

D. Stay inside from dusk to dawn, and use an insect repellent with permethrin.

3-114 *Providers understand the effects of stress on the body. These effects go beyond the skin and can impair hair follicles. Which of the following conditions in a female can be described as hair "coming out in handfuls?"*

A. Telogen effluvium

B. Alopecia areata

C. Female pattern hair loss

D. Androgenic baldness

3-115 *Lewin's change theory involves fundamental shifts in person's behaviors to evoke and successfully implement change. The final phase is referred to as*

A. implementation.

B. refreezing.

C. finalizing.

D. change.

3-116 *Eileen, a 42-year-old woman, comes to your office with the chief complaint of fatigue, weight loss, and blurred vision. Eileen has a negative past medical history for any chronic medical problems. You obtain a fasting chemistry panel, lipid profile, complete blood count (CBC), and a HgbA_{1c}. The results of the blood work show Eileen's blood sugar to be elevated at 356 mg/ dL, total cholesterol elevated at 255, high-density lipoprotein (HDL) cholesterol low at 28, LDL elevated at 167, triglycerides 333, and HgbA_{1c} 12. On questioning Eileen further, you discover that both her grandmothers had adult-onset diabetes mellitus. You diagnose type 2 diabetes mellitus. Your treatment plan should include a cholesterol-lowering agent, an agent that lowers blood sugar, and which other class of medication?*

A. ACE inhibitor

B. Diuretic

C. Weight loss medication

D. Beta blocker

3-117 *The best strategy to promote personal health is to*

A. instill a sense of responsibility in persons for their own health.

B. provide complete health information in many languages.

C. encourage health-promoting habits.

D. teach clients about appropriate risk factors.

3-118 *Which of the following individuals should get the shingles (herpes zoster) vaccine?*

A. Jerry, who has a mild upper respiratory tract infection and is allergic to neomycin

B. Timmy, who has been on prolonged use of high-dose steroids for his COPD

C. Joan, whose husband recently had shingles, and who is trying to get pregnant

D. Joe, who has a stressful job

3-119 *The first step in alleviating the problem of homelessness is to*

A. increase available housing for low-income individuals.

B. make public assistance more readily available.

C. correct the public's perception of homeless persons.

D. provide community support for deinstitutionalized persons.

3-120 *What is the term used to describe a disorder characterized by excessive sleep?*

A. Insomnia

B. Narcolepsy

C. Nocturnal myoclonus

D. Cataplexy

Answers

3-1   Answer C

The degree of prostate enlargement is based on the amount of projection of the prostate into the rectum. The normal prostate protrudes less than 1 cm into the rectum. Grade 1 enlargement is a protrusion of 1–2 cm, grade 2 is 2–3 cm, grade 3 is 34 cm, and grade 4 is greater than 4 cm.

3-2   Answer C

Screening is considered a form of secondary prevention because it seeks to identify the presence of diseases, such as high blood pressure, glaucoma, and diabetes, at early stages when treatment would be most effective.

3-3   Answer B

The construction industry is responsible for the most injuries (15 injuries per 100 full-time workers per year). Next in line are the agriculture, fishing, and forestry industries, followed by the manufacturing, transportation and utilities, and mining industries.

3-4   Answer B

Meningitis is one of the most severe manifestations of *Haemophilus influenzae* infection, and the *H. influenzae* type B (HiB) immunization may help prevent its occurrence. The HiB vaccination is especially important for children age 5 years and younger. It should be given at ages 2 months, 4 months, and 6 months, with the fourth dose given between ages 12 and 18 months. Hepatitis B vaccination is important for all infants to help prevent liver disease as adults. A measles, mumps, and rubella (MMR) vaccination protects against measles, mumps, and rubella (German measles), and varicella vaccination protects against chickenpox.

3-5   Answer B

Women are advised to begin Pap testing either 3 years after the onset of vaginal intercourse or at the age of 21, whichever comes first. For a young teenager, birth control may be prescribed without first performing a pelvic exam.

3-6   Answer D

Because Susie has not been in for several years, one cannot assume that she will come in next year to get the immunizations that are due between the ages of 4 and 6; therefore, this opportunity to give her immunizations cannot be missed. Between the ages of 4 and 6, a child is due for diphtheria, tetanus, and pertussis (DTP); polio; and measles, mumps, and rubella (MMR) if all other immunizations are up to date.

3-7   Answer D

The tumor marker that is elevated in prostate cancer is prostate-specific antigen (PSA). Determined by a simple blood test, PSA is a tumor marker whose level in the bloodstream becomes elevated with prostate cancer, although it may also become elevated with benign prostatic hypertrophy (BPH). There is no prostate cancer tumor marker (PCTM). Levels of cancer antigen (CA) 125 are increased in the following cancers: epithelial ovarian, fallopian tube, endometrial, endocervical, hepatic, and pancreatic. It is also used to monitor for persistent or recurrent serous carcinoma of the ovary in the postoperative period or during chemotherapy. Measurement of the level of carcinoembryonic antigen (CEA) is used primarily for monitoring persistent, metastatic, or recurrent cancer of the colon after surgery and less frequently for breast or other cancers.

3-8   Answer B

Prevention of pneumococcal disease in older people is one of the health initiatives of the U.S. government report *Healthy People 2020, National Health Promotion and Disease Prevention Objectives*. The goal for health-care providers is to have 90% of all clients older than 65 years immunized against pneumococcal disease by the year 2020. The pneumococcal vaccine is a one-time injection that may need to be repeated in 8 years. Gerald does not need a Td booster because his last injection was only 6 years ago, and the Centers for Disease Control and Prevention recommends a Td booster every 10 years. The influenza injection would not be appropriate at this time. Influenza vaccine is adjusted yearly to address the type of influenza that is thought to be prevalent in that year. Also, the influenza vaccine is given just before flu season.

3-9   Answer D

While the USPSTF found insufficient evidence to recommend for or against screening adults for glaucoma, the American Academy of Ophthalmology recommends screening for glaucoma as part of the comprehensive adult medical eye evaluation, starting at the age of 20, with a frequency depending on an individual's age and other risk factors for glaucoma. The Department of Veterans Affairs recommends that every veteran over the age of 40 be screened for glaucoma in a primary care setting with a frequency depending on age, ethnicity, and family history. Glaucoma is an elevated intraocular pressure that is measured with the use of a tonometer.

Looking at all guidelines, answer D is the best choice. Waiting until the client exhibits vision problems may be too late.

3-10   Answer A

The U.S. government report *Healthy People 2020, National Health Promotion and Disease Prevention Objectives* cites obesity, substance abuse, and immunizations as leading health indicators. Driver education is not considered a leading health-care indicator. The fourth-generation plan, Healthy People 2020, builds on past achievements, reaffirms the two overarching goals from the past decade, and adds two more: promoting quality of life, healthy development, and healthy behaviors across life stages; and creating social and physical environments that promote good health.

3-11   Answer C

More than 90% of all breast abnormalities are first detected by self-examination. All women older than age 20 should examine their breasts monthly, a week after their period. After menopause, women should examine their breasts at the same time each month.

3-12   Answer B

Alcohol, especially when used with tobacco, is a dietary factor in cancer of the esophagus. Alcohol is also a factor in liver cancer. Dietary factors related to bladder cancer are unknown. A high-calorie diet (with high fat and low fiber) is a factor in breast cancer.

3-13   Answer A

The risk of sudden death during sports activities from hypertrophic cardiomyopathy may be greatly reduced with a thorough cardiac history and examination. If a child has a relative who died of sudden cardiac disease before age 55, that child could possibly have hypertrophic cardiomyopathy. Family history of asthma is not relevant to this exam question.

3-14   Answer D

The American Diabetes Association recommends careful inspection of a diabetic client's feet for corns, calluses, and open lesions to prevent further deterioration into diabetic foot ulcers. The client should wash his or her feet daily with warm soapy water and towel dry them, especially between the toes, to prevent fungal infections. Diabetic clients should see a podiatrist yearly. Encourage patients to use a mirror to inspect the bottom of their feet.

3-15   Answer D

Before drug therapy for hypertension is instituted, lifestyle modification and nonpharmacological methods such as salt restriction, weight reduction, biofeedback, and exercise should be considered. Aggressive treatment of all clients with a systolic pressure greater than 140 mm Hg and/or a diastolic pressure greater than 90 mm Hg is essential. The client should monitor his or her blood pressure at home and call the health-care provider if it exceeds the parameters discussed. In this case, Harvey should try nonpharmacological methods and monitor his blood pressure at home and then return in 1–2 weeks for follow-up. If his diastolic pressure is still 96 mm Hg after 2 weeks, a diuretic or an ACE inhibitor would be indicated.

3-16   Answer C

The National Cholesterol Education Program recommends that carbohydrates comprise about 55% of total calories, fat no more than 30% of total calories, and proteins about 15%–20% of total calories.

3-17   Answer C

Occupational repetitive stress injuries result from wear and tear on the body over a period of time. Repetitive stress injuries are one of the fastest growing workplace injuries and can happen any time there is a discrepancy between the physical requirements of a job and the physical capacity of the worker's body. Risk factors include repetitive motion, force, awkward posture, heavy lifting, or some combination of these factors. Teaching proper body mechanics is a good form of prevention. Skin disorders represent up to 20% of all occupational illnesses. Many incidences of workplace skin disease go unreported, and the true rate of occupational skin disease is probably much higher. The most common occupational skin disease is contact dermatitis, which may be classified as acute (weepy, edematous, vesicular, blistered) or chronic (dry, cracked, scaly, thickened). This is followed by respiratory conditions, then poisoning.

3-18   Answer B

The primary objective of screening is to detect a disease in its early stages to be able to treat it and change its progression. Treating a disease at the early asymptomatic period can significantly alter the course of the disease.

3-19   Answer A

Tuberculin skin testing using the Mantoux test should be considered in high-risk adolescents as well as recent immigrants and homeless individuals. For high-risk individuals, an induration of 10 mm or greater when read at 48–72 hours is considered positive.

3-20   Answer C

Rhabdomyolysis is a syndrome that results from destruction of skeletal muscle. It is usually diagnosed from laboratory findings that are characteristic of myonecrosis. Although there are no standard creatine kinase values that establish the diagnosis of rhabdomyolysis, elevations above 10,000 IU/L are usually indicative of clinically significant rhabdomyolysis. The syndrome usually affects muscles used in exercise, but it may present as generalized muscle weakness. It usually resolves on stopping the statin medication, but severe cases may lead to renal failure and death.

3-21   Answer D

Fatigue for more than 6 months and absence of other clinical conditions that may explain such fatigue are the two major criteria the client must demonstrate to be diagnosed with chronic fatigue syndrome. Other minor criteria include generalized headaches, unexplained generalized muscle weakness, sleep disturbances, sore throat, mild fever or chills, and migratory arthralgias without swelling or redness.

3-22   Answer C

To estimate a client's ideal weight, use the following formula: For women older than age 25, allow 100 lb for the first 5 ft, then add 5 lb for each inch thereafter. For men, allow 106 lb for the first 5 ft, then 6 lb for each inch thereafter. Multiply the number by 110% for a client with a large frame and 90% for a client with a small frame.

3-23   Answer D

A heart-healthy diet should be recommended for all clients regardless of age or risk. It is especially important that children learn healthy eating habits early in life. A heart-healthy diet follows the Dietary Guidelines for Americans developed by the U.S. Departments of Agriculture and Health and Human Services. It is designed for healthy people older than age 2 to maintain their health. The guidelines include eating a variety of foods; balancing the food you eat with physical activity; maintaining or improving your weight; choosing a diet with plenty of grain products, vegetables, and fruits; choosing a diet low in fat, saturated fat, and cholesterol; choosing a diet moderate in sugars; choosing a diet moderate in salt and sodium; and, if you drink alcoholic beverages, doing so in moderation.

3-24   Answer A

Terazosin (Hytrin) is an alpha-1 adrenergic blocker. It is not a preventive drug, but it does relax smooth muscle in the prostate and bladder neck and allows complete emptying of the bladder, relieving frequent nocturnal urination. Terazosin is begun at 1 mg at bedtime initially and then titrated upward to 10 mg once a day. Doxazosin (Cardura) is also effective as an alpha-1 adrenergic blocker. It is begun initially at 1 mg at bedtime, with the dosage doubled every 1–2 weeks to a maximum of 8 mg per day. Finasteride (Proscar), a 5-alpha reductase inhibitor, decreases the volume of the prostate within about 3 months. At 12 months, it seems to have reached its peak effectiveness. Finasteride is given 5 mg daily for at least 6 months; then the client is reevaluated.

3-25   Answer C

A gram of fat contains 9 calories, whereas a gram of either carbohydrates or proteins contains 4 calories. In this case, Julie was eating 3 g of fat, or 27 calories of fat (9 calories per gram of fat times 3 g of fat equals 27 calories).

3-26   Answer A

The National Cholesterol Education Program recommends cholesterol screening for persons with no family history of coronary heart disease before age 55. This should start at age 20 and then be done at least every 5 years. Earlier screening—at ages 10–15—should be considered for children with a family history of coronary heart disease that developed before age 55.

3-27   Answer C

A good cardiovascular workout consists of exercising large muscle groups for at least 20 minutes, 3 or more days per week, at an intensity of at least 60% of the maximum heart rate (220 beats per minute minus age). The American College of Sports Medicine recommends 3–5 days a week for most cardiovascular exercise programs. For cardiovascular benefits, aim for 20–60 minutes in your target heart rate zone, apart from the warm-up and cool-down period.

3-28   Answer C

Ethnocentrism is thinking that ethnic groups other than one's own are inferior. An ethnocentric perspective is a barrier to establishing and maintaining positive relationships with others.

3-29   Answer C

Enacting a stress management program is an active strategy of health promotion because it requires individuals to become personally involved. Maintaining clean water, introducing fluoride into the water, and maintaining a sanitary sewage system are all examples of passive strategies—those done for individuals and communities by others.

3-30   Answer C

The only true contraindications to immunizations, according to the American Academy of Pediatrics, are a moderate or severe illness with or without a fever and an anaphylactic reaction to a vaccine or a vaccine constituent. Illnesses themselves are not true contraindications to vaccinations. Early symptoms may be a prodrome of something else; however, risks of the diseases are usually greater than the complications of vaccination. Even a fever of 104.5°F (40°C) with a previous diphtheria, tetanus, and pertussis (DTP) immunization is not a contraindication to a subsequent DTP shot.

3-31   Answer C

The goal of the preparticipation sports exam is to protect the student from injury by identifying health risks and minimizing or curing them so that the student may participate in a sports activity. You might feel pressured by parents or coaches to pass the student regardless of your findings. Your responsibility is to further evaluate any abnormal findings on your exam before clearing the student to participate.

3-32   Answer B

The Centers for Disease Control and Prevention recommend that all children be screened for lead poisoning at age 12 months. If resources allow, children should then be screened again at age 24 months. Children ages 3–6 years should be tested for lead levels (using an assessment tool) every 6 months if they have a high risk of lead exposure. Those with normal lead levels should be retested once a year until age 6 years.

3-33   Answer A

Lung cancer is the leading cause of cancer death, and cigarette smoking causes almost all cases. Compared to nonsmokers, men who smoke are about 23 times more likely to develop lung cancer and women who smoke are about 13 times more likely. Smoking causes about 90% of lung cancer deaths in men and almost 80% in women. While breast, prostate, and colon cancer are widely prevalent, people don't die from them as frequently as from lung cancer.

3-34   Answer B

Chantix has shown to be more effective in helping smokers quit than Zyban, the only other nonnicotine prescription medicine for smoking cessation. While Chantix contains no nicotine, it works on the same receptors as nicotine. It's the addiction to nicotine inhaled from smoking that makes quitting so hard. The recommended dosing schedule for Chantix is as follows: day 1 to day 3: one tablet per day of 0.5 mg; day 4 to day 7: one 0.5 mg tablet twice a day (once in the morning and once in the evening); day 8 to the end of treatment: one tablet of 1 mg twice per day (once in the morning and once in the evening). Chantix should be taken with a full glass of water after eating. The client should choose a quit date when he/she will stop smoking. Chantix should be taken for 7 days before the quit date. This lets Chantix build up in the body. Smoking should cease on the quit day and Chantix should be continued for up to 12 weeks. If the client has not completely quit smoking by 12 weeks, another 12 weeks may help the client stay cigarette free. The most common side effect is nausea (30%), but not enough to make the client discontinue the medication.

3-35   Answer A

The ultimate goal of crisis intervention is to help people function at a higher level than their precrisis state. Eliminating the current crisis and returning people to the functional level where they were before the crisis will put them back in the same situation and make them susceptible to the crisis all over again.

3-36   Answer D

While A and B are correct, answer D is more inclusive. The Centers for Disease Control and

Prevention recommends a routine influenza vaccination for all persons aged 6 months and older. This represents an expansion of the previous recommendations for annual vaccination of all adults aged 19–49 years and is supported by evidence that annual influenza vaccination is a safe and effective preventive health action with potential benefit in all age groups.

3-37   Answer D

The Centers for Disease Control and Prevention recommend that all clients with high-risk behaviors be encouraged to be screened for HIV antibodies to identify those who are already infected so that interventions can be started to further halt the spread of the virus.

3-38   Answer D

Health-care providers can help prevent the spread of antibiotic resistance by only prescribing antibiotic therapy when it is likely to be beneficial to the patient, using an agent targeting the likely pathogens, and using the antibiotic for the appropriate dose and duration

3-39   Answer A

Specificity measures a screening test's ability to recognize individuals who are nondiseased or those with negative reactions (true negatives). It can be represented by a ratio of true negatives to the total number of known true negatives. In this case, the number of true negatives that the test recognized was 80, with the total number of known true negatives being 100. Therefore, 80 out of 100 (80/100) equals a specificity of 80%.

3-40   Answer B

During severe stress, the cortisol level increases, allowing mobilization of free fatty acids. This triggers a series of reactions. With the increased cortisol, glucose production from amino acids increases. During severe stress, as glucagon release increases, catecholamine levels increase. The insulin-to-glucagon ratio decreases, glycogen breakdown increases, and glucose production from amino acids increases. The release of antidiuretic hormone also increases during stressful periods, increasing the retention of water, and the level of aldosterone increases, leading to the increased retention of sodium.

3-41   Answer A

Clients taking levothyroxine (Levothroid, Synthroid) should avoid foods high in iodine such as brussels sprouts, cabbage, cauliflower, rutabagas, soy, and turnips because these foods, when added to the medication, raise client's iodine levels.

3-42   Answer C

Anorexia nervosa may occur from prepubescence into the early 30s and occurs most commonly from early to late adolescence. It occurs more frequently in women and may cause bradycardia, arrhythmias, and amenorrhea. Constipation is common in clients with anorexia because of their poor eating habits.

3-43   Answer A

Older adults are at an increased risk for depression because of the associated chronic health conditions that may also exist. Older adults are often misdiagnosed and undertreated. Depression is a true and treatable medical condition, not a normal part of aging. Depression is not just having "the blues" or the emotions one feels when grieving the loss of a loved one. It is a true medical condition that is treatable, like diabetes or hypertension. Most older adults see an improvement in their symptoms when treated with antidepression drugs alone, with psychotherapy, or with a combination of both.

3-44   Answer A

There is still debate as to the recommendations for screening for osteoporosis for women. Bone density studies to screen for osteoporosis are recommended for women at age 65. For women younger than 65, the literature supports screening only for perimenopausal women with risk factors that include Caucasian or Asian race, a history of bilateral oopherectomy before menopause, a slender build, smoking or having smoked tobacco, low calcium consumption patterns, a sedentary lifestyle, and a positive family history of the condition. Women who have had a hysterectomy but not an oopherectomy are not considered at particular risk. Alcohol negatively impacts bone health by interfering with the absorption and use of calcium and vitamin D and other bone nutrients. Because there are a number of negatives about drinking and bone density, it would be wise for persons with problems with bone loss to decrease or eliminate alcohol.

3-45   Answer A

Medicare was established in 1966 by the U.S. government as a federal insurance program to provide funds for medical costs for persons age 65 and older and disabled persons of any age. Medicaid, an amendment to Title XIX of the Social Security Act, went into effect in 1967 to provide basic health services to low-income persons. The Omnibus Budget Reconciliation Act was implemented in 1982, when 20 programs were combined into four block grants.

3-46   Answer B

The Committee on Diet and Health of the National Research Council recommends that alcohol consumption per day be limited to the equivalent of less than 1 oz of pure alcohol. This equates to two cans of beer, two small glasses of wine, or two average cocktails. This does not apply to pregnant women, who should avoid alcohol altogether.

3-47   Answer C

Screening for hypothyroidism is not routinely recommended. Because of the subtle presentation of hypothyroidism, health-care providers should order a thyroid-stimulating hormone level (TSH) test at their discretion. Most clinicians add a T4-level test to routine blood work and then, depending on the results, order a TSH test.

3-48   Answer B

Pap smears may be discontinued at age 65 if the previous three Pap smears have been normal. At or after the age of 30, women who have had three consecutive normal tests may have screening extended to once every 2–3 years. An exception to this is for women who are at higher risk of cervical cancer, such as women exposed to DES in utero or those who are HIV positive or immunocompromised for another reason. If a woman has had a hysterectomy, there is a need for a Pap smear only if the cervix has been left intact.

3-49   Answer C

Utilization review is a system to monitor diagnosis, treatment, and billing practices. It assists in lowering health-care costs by discouraging unnecessary procedures.

3-50   Answer A

Medicare Part A is basic hospital insurance. Medicare Part B is supplementary voluntary medical insurance supported by tax revenues and by additional monies paid by the insured to cover physician services, laboratory services, home health care, and outpatient hospital treatments.

3-51   Answer A

A person with diabetes mellitus type 2 should have a $HgbA_{1c}$ of 6.5 or less and a fasting blood sugar (fbs) less than 130 for optimal control. Because the clients lab results fall in those categories, she is under good control and her medications should stay the same.

3-52   Answer C

A conservative, preventive health approach for healthy adults is to recommend limiting salt intake to 6 g or less per day. This includes salt added to food during cooking or at the table, salt added as an ingredient to processed foods, and salt that occurs naturally in foods. Table salt is approximately 40% sodium by weight; therefore, a diet incorporating 6 g of salt contains about 2.4 g of sodium.

3-53   Answer C

Women with HIV infection have a high prevalence of human papillomavirus (HPV) infections. These infections are associated with an increased incidence of squamous intraepithelial lesions in HIV-seropositive women.

3-54   Answer D

Twenty percent of colorectal cancers can be attributed to a lack of fiber in the diet. A high-fat diet has also been secondarily implicated.

3-55   Answer C

Of all the drug classes, antibiotics cause the most adverse reactions. The other drug classes that cause a high number of adverse drug reactions are, in order, chemotherapeutic agents, cardiovascular agents, antihypertensive agents, anticonvulsants, and antidepressants.

3-56   Answer B

Health-care costs for smokers at any given age are as much as 40% higher than for nonsmokers. Although smokers have more diseases than nonsmokers, nonsmokers live longer and can incur more health costs at advanced ages.

3-57   Answer B

The National Cancer Institute recommends that adults eat 20–30 g of fiber a day to prevent colon cancer. The plant kingdom is the only source of fiber-containing foods.

3-58   Answer B

The broad-based initiative led by the U.S. Public Health Service to improve the health of all Americans through an emphasis on prevention and not just treatment of health problems throughout the next decade was initially called *Healthy People 2000, National Health Promotion and Disease Prevention Objectives*. It took its lead from the 1979 report *Healthy People: The Surgeon Generals Report on Health Promotion and Disease Prevention*. Although all the objectives in that report were not achieved, it had such a positive impact that *Healthy People 2000* was conceived. The major difference in the 2000 report was the primary emphasis on health promotion and individual responsibility. HP 2020 is now the fourth-generation plan.

3-59   Answer B

The best weapon against infections, such as colds, flu, and respiratory syncytial virus, is prevention, with basic measures of hand washing, good hygiene, and isolation of infected persons. The flu shot augments the basic preventive measures. Although many persons believe taking extra vitamin C and the herb echinacea will shorten the length of a cold, vitamin supplements have not been proved necessary in persons with balanced diets. Rimantadine HCl (Flumadine) is effective against influenza A only if given within 48 hours of symptom onset.

3-60   Answer C

The last step in the process of a gay man or lesbian "coming out" is that of identity integration and self-disclosure. The process of discovering and revealing one's sexual orientation can occur at any age and is known as "coming out." Stage theories for coming out have been summarized as a four-step process: (1) awareness of homosexual feelings, (2) testing and exploration, (3) identity acceptance, and (4) identity integration and self-disclosure. If the ultimate costs of self-disclosure are felt to be too high, an individual may become socially isolated or deny gay or lesbian identity.

3-61   Answer C

About 80% of older adults have one chronic condition. Fifty percent of older adults have at least two chronic conditions. Infectious diseases (such as influenza and pneumococcal disease) and injuries also take a disproportionate toll on older adults. Efforts to identify strategies to prevent or reduce these risks and to effectively intervene in these conditions must be pursued.

3-62   Answer C

In more developed countries, since the late 1970s, the difference in life expectancy for men and women has narrowed, but women still outlive men by 6–7 years.

3-63   Answer D

The correct answer is to allow Mildred her independence but provide a safe environment by removing loose rugs that she could easily trip over and installing handrails by the toilet and in the bathtub. The rails will provide support for her as she goes from a sitting to a standing position. Hiring an aide 24 hours a day would decrease Mildred's independence. Leaving Mildred home, alone or not, will not change her chance of falling.

3-64   Answer D

A genogram is a diagram that depicts each member of a family and shows connections among the generations, including all members of the extended family for several generations. It includes the health status of each member, including any genetic diseases.

3-65   Answer B

The *E* stands for eye opener, or the need for a drink early in the day. The C stands for cutting down, the A stands for annoyed by criticism of drinking, and the G stands for guilt feelings about drinking.

3-66   Answer C

Families of persons with Alzheimer's disease (AD) need to know that AD is a progressive disorder of the brain affecting memory, thought, and language. Although the progression of the stages is individual and changes may occur rapidly or slowly over the course of several years, knowing what stage a family member is in helps family members in planning and knowing what to expect. Stage 1 is the onset, which is insidious. Spontaneity, energy, and initiative are decreased; slowness is increased; word finding is difficult; the person angers more easily; and familiarity is sought and preferred. In stage 2, supervision with detailed activities such as banking is needed, speech and understanding are much slower, and the train of thought is lost. In stage 3, personality change is marked and depression may occur. Directions must be specific and repeated for safety, recent memory is poor, disorientation occurs easily, people are incorrectly identified, and the person may be lethargic. In stage 4, apathy is noticeable. Memory is poor or absent, urinary incontinence is present, individuals are not recognized, and the person should not be alone.

3-67 Answer B

HPV vaccination is not recommended for use in women who are pregnant. A contraindication to the HPV vaccines is a history of immediate hypersensitivity to yeast. Women who are lactating or immunocompromised are eligible to receive the vaccine. It is also recommended for females ages 9–25 years, whether or not they have had sex yet and even if the women already have a history of genital warts, a positive HPV test, or an abnormal Pap test.

3-68 Answer D

Children should have their first visual acuity testing at age 3. Visual acuity should be tested using a pictorial wall chart, and strabismus should be tested for using the cover-uncover test. Visual acuity testing should be repeated at age 5 or 6.

3-69 Answer A

Acculturation is the process of adapting to a culture belonging to someone else. Biculturalism is taking components of both cultures and making them fit one's lifestyle. Cultural relativity is the attempt to view the behavior of culturally different individuals within one's own framework. Enculturation is the process of acquiring one's cultural identity as it is transferred down from the older generation.

3-70 Answer A

Malignancies (lung, lymphoma, gastrointestinal tract), along with gastrointestinal diseases and psychiatric disorders, are the most common causes of involuntary weight loss. Other less common causes include pulmonary disease, endocrine disturbances, and substance abuse.

3-71 Answer A

The spouse has been shown to be the most important source of social support for an adult. If there is no spouse, family members are the next most important source. Research has shown that support from outside the family cannot compensate for what is missing within the family.

3-72 Answer D

The two main causes of death among U.S. adults aged 65 years or older are heart disease (28.2%) and cancer (22.2%). Stroke accounts for 6.6%, chronic lower respiratory disease 6.2%, Alzheimer's disease 4.2%, and diabetes 2.9%.

3-73 Answer A

Sexually transmitted diseases (STDs) are a cause of anal cancer. For women, other risk factors for anal cancer include an increased number (greater than 10) of sexual partners, having their first sexual experience before age 16, having four or more sexual partners before age 20, and anal intercourse. For men, other risk factors include having more than 10 sexual partners and being homosexual or bisexual.

3-74 Answer D

Head circumference should be measured until a child reaches age 2–4 months. It should be measured at birth; at 24 weeks; and at ages 2, 3, 6, 9, 12, 15, 18, and 24 months. Measuring growth and following its progression over the course of time can help identify significant childhood conditions. In addition to head circumference, height and weight should be measured at ages 3, 4, 5, and 6 months, then every 2 years thereafter.

3-75 Answer D

Performing range-of-motion exercises on a client who has had a cerebrovascular accident (CVA) is an example of rehabilitation prevention. Primary prevention would be eating a healthy diet as a young adult to prevent atherosclerosis, which might precipitate a CVA. Secondary prevention would include taking lipid-lowering drugs to prevent a CVA after having already developed hyperlipidemia. Although it is desirable to prevent any complications from the CVA, there is no level of prevention called complications prevention.

3-76   Answer D

Since 2001, the major public health and safety focus has shifted to safety from the threat of bioterrorism. Other health promotion concerns that are continuing include the threat of cardiovascular disease, cancer, childhood infectious diseases, sexually transmitted diseases, and unintended pregnancies. In addition, clients face problems related to domestic violence, abuse, poverty, and addictions. While nursing education programs have prepared providers to deal with these issues, it wasnt until recently that bioterrorism threats were integrated into curricula.

3-77   Answer C

Although antibiotics and bismuth subsalicylate are effective in the prevention of traveler's diarrhea, they are not generally recommended because of the potential side effects. Instead, advise clients to "cook it, boil it, peel it, or forget it."

3-78   Answer A

Dehydroepiandrosterone (DHEA) is a hormone that is abundant in the body and is naturally produced from cholesterol by the adrenal glands, with smaller amounts manufactured by ovaries. Taking both DHEA and hormonal replacement therapy (HRT) is not recommended because it is like "double dosing." It is not absolutely contraindicated, but because most clients do not adequately regulate the dosage of over-the-counter medications, the combination therapy may produce excessively high levels of estrogen. Additionally, because almost a third of clients today are taking some sort of herbal therapy, it is essential to ask in the history and physical what other therapies are being used.

3-79   Answer C

Bone loss begins at a rate of 0.5% a year in a woman's middle to late 40s. When menopause occurs, the rate increases up to 7% a year for the first decade after menopause. This increase in the rate of bone loss is directly related to a decrease in a woman's estrogen. After menopause, the bone loss decreases to 0.5%–1% a year until death. This patient should be encouraged to do weight-bearing exercises and have an adequate calcium intake of 1,000–1,500 mg/day with sufficient amounts of vitamin D.

3-80   Answer D

Emily is only 26 years old and has not reached her peak bone mass yet. It has been proven that aerobic exercise increases bone mass. Smoking and soda drinking both have been shown to decrease bone mass. Estrogen replacement therapy is no longer recommended for bone health; it is recommended only for short-term use to alleviate vasomotor symptoms of menopause.

3-81   Answer C

The USPSTF recommends screening all adults for depression in practices that have systems in place to assure accurate diagnosis, effective treatment, and adequate follow-up. Evidence shows that screening improves the accurate identification of depressed patients in primary care settings and that treating depressed adults identified in primary care settings reduces clinical morbidity. While the individuals in answers A and B should certainly be screened, answer C is more inclusive.

3-82   Answer C

The National Cancer Institute (NCI) recommends that mammograms, as a method of screening for breast cancer, begin at age 40 for women at average risk of breast cancer and continue every 1 to 2 years. The U.S Preventive Service Task Force (USPSTE) states that there is insufficient evidence that mammogram screening is effective for women age 75 and older.

3-83   Answer B

Sensitivity refers to a screening test's ability to identify persons who actually have a disease (true positives), whereas specificity measures a screening test's ability to recognize negative reactions or nondiseased individuals (true negatives). For example, if a screening tool were used on 100 individuals known to have prostate cancer and it detected 90 persons with prostate cancer, missing 10 of the individuals, the sensitivity would be 90%.

3-84   Answer B

Although the Public Health Department, American Heart Association, and Centers for Disease Control and Prevention all have excellent programs and screening protocols, only the WISEWOMAN program specifically addresses the needs of midlife uninsured women. The Well-Integrated Screening and Evaluation for Women Across the Nation (WISEWOMAN) program aims to remove racial and ethnic disparities in health by addressing the screening and intervention needs of midlife uninsured women. The program consists of 10 projects that have been successful at reaching financially disadvantaged and minority women who are at high risk for chronic diseases.

3-85   Answer C

Molly should get an annual flu vaccination because she has a long-term pulmonary problem. New guidelines from the Centers for Disease Control and Prevention state that everyone over the age of 6 months should receive an annual flu vaccination.

3-86   Answer A

The JNC guidelines for treatment of stage 1 hypertension recommend use of a thiazide diuretic as first choice for treatment of hypertension. Lifestyle modification with diet and exercise should already be in place.

3-87   Answer B

With respect to African American men, the American Cancer Society recommends that screening for prostate cancer with a digital rectal exam start at age 40 and be done yearly.

3-88   Answer A

The creatinine clearance value is commonly decreased in older adults because of impaired renal function. Serum cholesterol, serum triglyceride, and blood urea nitrogen values are usually increased in older adults.

3-89   Answer D

To reduce the risk of chronic disease in adulthood, engage in 30 or more minutes of moderately intense physical activity at work or at home at least 5 days per week. Greater health benefits may be obtained by participating in activity that is more vigorous in intensity or of longer duration. To help manage body weight and prevent a gradual increase in weight gain, 60 minutes of moderate to vigorous intensity activity may be done on most days of the week without increasing dietary caloric intake.

3-90   Answer B

The two leading causes of death in the United States for all ages are heart disease and cancer. Almost two-thirds of the deaths in the United States every year are from these causes.

3-91   Answer D

The MMR is a live attenuated vaccine, and therefore a female client must not be pregnant when she receives the vaccination. Female clients must also be informed that they need to refrain from becoming pregnant for the 3 months following MMR vaccination or risk birth defects to the fetus.

3-92   Answer A

Health maintenance organizations (HMOs) deliver comprehensive health maintenance and treatment services to members of an enrolled group who pay a prenegotiated and fixed price. Preferred provider organizations (PPOs) allow persons to go to any doctor in the network, whereas clients of HMOs must choose their doctor ahead of time. Fee-for-service (FFS) independent practices permit an individual to be treated in any facility, with the full fee paid by the client. Exclusive provider organizations (EPOs) limit clients to providers belonging to one organization. Some may be able to use outside providers at an additional out-of-pocket charge.

3-93   Answer A

For primary prevention of skin cancer, a sunscreen with an ultraviolet (UV) wave protection factor of 15 has been shown to be as effective as those with higher numbers. In addition, for primary prevention of skin cancer, all clients should be counseled to avoid UV waves from either the sun or tanning booths and to wear protective clothing.

3-94   Answer D

A biopsy of the temporal artery is usually required to confirm the diagnosis of temporal arteritis. Color duplex ultrasonography (a combination of ultrasonography and the flow-velocity determinations of a Doppler system) has been shown to examine even small vessels, such as the superficial temporal artery, and show a halo around the inflamed arteries when temporal arteritis is present. Therefore, it is a much less invasive procedure than biopsy. A computed tomography (CT) scan and magnetic resonance imaging (MRI) are done to detect neurological damage from hemorrhage, tumor, cyst, edema, or myocardial infarction. These tests may also identify displacement of the brain structures by expanding lesions. However, not all lesions can be detected by

CT scan or MRI. An electroencephalogram is used to evaluate the electrical activity of the brain. It can identify seizure activity as well as certain infectious and metabolic conditions.

3-95   Answer A

Because tetanus and diphtheria remain serious problems in South America, it is recommended that all travelers be current (within 10 years) on these vaccinations. Tetanus immune globulin should be administered to persons not previously immunized.

3-96   Answer D

A yes answer to any of these questions is of no concern. These are all normal behaviors for preschool children ages 3–6. These are the ways in which children express their concerns and explore their anatomy. Parents should honestly answer questions posed by their children regarding sexuality in terms the children can understand.

3-97   Answer C

Diagnostic criteria for the child with ADHD include frequently blurting out answers before a question is finished, difficulty following directions, engaging in physically dangerous activities (often without thinking of the consequences of actions), tending to talk excessively, and often interrupting others. Behavior in which the child talks very little but is very restless is not indicative of ADHD.

3-98   Answer B

The body mass index (BMI) is an indicator of body fat. It is derived by dividing weight in kilograms by height in meters. It shows a direct and continuous relationship to morbidity and mortality in studies of large populations. The weight/height chart gives a range of what the ideal weight is for each height, but it does not reflect body fat. Anthropometric measurement is the measurement of the size, weight, and proportions of the human body.

3-99   Answer D

Clients with asymptomatic carotid bruits have a 2% incidence of cerebrovascular accidents (CVAs) per year. Although ASA, anticoagulants, and surgery are frequently ordered, there are not sufficient data to prove that these treatments reduce the risk of CVA in clients with asymptomatic carotid bruits. Starting an asymptomatic older woman on ASA

therapy may produce more problems, such as skin bruising or gastrointestinal bleeding.

3-100   Answer B

The eighth report of the Joint National Committee on Prevention, Detection, and Treatment of Hypertension (JNC VIII) recommends that stage 2 hypertension be treated with a combination of a thiazide diuretic and an ACE inhibitor, ARB, calcium channel blocker, or beta blocker.

3-101   Answer C

The definition of Endemic is answer C. Answer A refers to Sporadic; B is an epidemic; and D is Pandemic.

3-102   Answer C

The most common adverse reaction to the hepatitis B virus vaccine is pain at the injection site (13%–20% in adults, 3%–9% in children). Other mild, transient systemic adverse effects are fatigue and headache (11%–17% in adults, 8%–18% in children) and temperature elevation (1%–6% of all injections).

3-103   Answer A

The National Cholesterol Education Program (NCEP), launched by the National Heart, Lung, and Blood Institute, recommends that persons with normal cholesterol levels be tested every 5 years. This is for individuals of average or low risk of developing CVD. Screening should occur more often for individuals whose levels are close to therapeutic thresholds.

3-104   Answer D

The Food and Drug Administration states that sodium may contribute to the risk of hypertension. Fat and fiber in grains, fruits, and vegetables decrease the risk of cancer, and insufficient calcium contributes to the risk of osteoporosis. Sodium intake should be reduced if there is a family health history of hypertension, diabetes, or any form of cardiovascular disease. Sodium intake should also be reduced if a personal health history indicates hypertension or glucose intolerance. Although hypertension is certainly a factor in heart disease, the best answer is hypertension because not all cardiovascular diseases are affected by the amount of sodium consumption.

3-105   Answer C

When the 78 million baby boomers were growing up, television, rock concerts, and other intense audio programs were coming of age. Earplugs were unheard of. This generation does not want to wear hearing aids or anything that marks them as being different or disabled. As a result, baby boomers frequently avoid seeking help from hearing aid professionals. The following statistics are from a national survey of baby boomers: 75% said they find themselves in situations in which people are not speaking loudly or clearly enough or they can't hear the TV, 53% said they have at least a mild hearing loss, 25% said their hearing loss affects their work, and 57% said they have trouble hearing on their cell phone.

3-106   Answer C

An allergy to baker's yeast is a definite contraindication to receiving the hepatitis B vaccine. Yeast is used in making the vaccine and is still present in the vaccine.

3-107   Answer B

Twenty-five percent of U.S. adults aged 75 and older have lost all of their teeth. Advanced gum disease affects 4%–12% of adults. Half of the cases of severe gum disease in the United States are the result of cigarette smoking. Three times as many smokers have gum disease as people who have never smoked. More than 7,600 people, mostly older Americans, die from oral and pharyngeal cancers each year.

3-108   Answer B

According to the Global Initiative for COPD guidelines, all symptomatic COPD clients should be started on an inhaled anticholinergic drug and a beta-2 agonist. Both are well tolerated by older adults and have few side effects.

3-109   Answer C

Suicide rates for males are highest among those aged 75 and older. Suicide rates for females are highest among those aged 45–54. Males take their own lives at nearly four times the rate of females and represent 78.8% of all U.S. suicides. During their lifetime, women attempt suicide about two to three times as often as men. Firearms are the most commonly used method of suicide among males (55.7%). Poisoning is the most common method of suicide for females (40.2%).

3-110   Answer A

Many major risk factors are associated with osteoporosis and fragility fractures. The major risk factors are body weight less than 127 lb, personal history of fracture as an adult, history of fracture in a first-degree relative, oral corticosteroid therapy of longer than 3 months, and current smoking. Minor risk factors include alcohol intake of more than two drinks per day, dementia, estrogen deficiency occurring before age 45 years, impaired vision, low lifelong calcium intake, low physical activity, poor health/frailty, and recent falls.

3-111   Answer A

White men are at a higher risk for testicular cancer than nonwhite men. Testicular self-examination (TSE), along with early detection and treatment, has decreased the mortality rates appreciably. TSE should be taught to all men ages 15–40. Testicular cancer is the most common solid tumor found in males ages 20–34.

3-112   Answer C

Postmenopausal women who are not taking hormone replacement therapy need 1,500 mg of calcium a day to help prevent osteoporosis. Because treatment for osteoporosis is limited, prevention is necessary to reduce the occurrence.

3-113   Answer C

Insect repellents with high concentrations (greater than 35%) of diethyltoluamide (DEET) are effective in preventing mosquito bites; however, DEET is not recommended to be applied to the hands or faces of young children. Permethrin is effective as a scabicide (at 5%) and as a pediculicide (at 1%). It is very effective at a low concentration against malaria-carrying mosquitoes and is safe for all ages. Other preventive measures include remaining in well-screened or indoor areas from dusk to dawn, using mosquito nets, and wearing clothing that covers most of the body.

3-114   Answer A

In telogen effluvium, clients usually describe this condition as hair "coming out in handfuls." Stress can cause some hair roots to be pushed prematurely into the resting state. Two months after an extremely stressful event, some clients report losing as much as 70% of scalp hair. The condition may resolve after the stress subsides. This is not the same as gradual genetic hair thinning. Alopecia areata is thought to be an organ-specific autoimmune disease that manifests as round or oval patches of nonscarring hair loss. Female pattern hair loss may be the result of alterations in androgen metabolism at the level of the hair follicle or in systemic hormonal changes. This balding pattern may develop during perimenopause or menopause.

3-115   Answer B

Lewin's change theory has three distinct and vital stages: "unfreezing"; "moving to a new level or changing" or "movement"; and "refreezing."

3-116   Answer A

Studies have shown the use of ACE inhibitors in clients with diabetes with or without hypertension has slowed the progression of nephropathy. You must monitor the client's creatinine and potassium levels routinely. If the client's renal function does decrease, elevated potassium levels may occur.

3-117   Answer A

The best strategy to promote personal health is to instill in people a sense of responsibility for their own health. Until people have made a commitment to assume personal responsibility for their own health, their health-promoting behaviors will not change. One of the nurse practitioner's functions is to effect changes in human behavior. Encouraging the adoption of personal responsibility is one way to do this.

3-118   Answer D

Joe, who has a stressful job, is a candidate for the shingles (herpes zoster) vaccine. All of the other conditions are contraindications for receiving the vaccine: allergy to neomycin, on prolonged use of high-dose steroids, and pregnant or might be pregnant. Women should not get pregnant until 4 weeks after receiving the vaccination.

3-119   Answer C

The first step in alleviating the problem of homelessness is to correct the public's perception of homeless persons. Current stereotypical opinions hinder effective delivery of health care as well as other resources that should be available. Lack of housing for low-income persons, restrictions on public assistance, and inadequate support for deinstitutionalized persons are all factors that have contributed to the problem of homelessness.

3-120   Answer B

Narcolepsy is a disorder characterized by excessive sleep. Narcolepsy with involuntary daytime sleep attacks may begin in adolescence. The person may have symptoms of this problem years before it is diagnosed. Insomnia is the inability to fall asleep or to stay asleep for a sufficient amount of time. Nocturnal myoclonus is a condition characterized by stereotypic kicking movements of the legs during sleep; it is more common in older adults. Cataplexy is often associated with narcolepsy. It is marked by abrupt attacks of muscular weakness and hypotonia triggered by an emotional stimulus such as anger or fear.

Bibliography

Centers for Disease Control and Prevention: http://www.cdc.gov/flu; http://www.CDCinfo@cdc.gov; http://www.cdc.gov/violenceprevention.

Dunphy, LM, et al: *Primary Care: The Art and Science of Advanced Practice Nursing*, ed 3. FA Davis, Philadelphia, 2011.

Hay, WM, Levin, MJ, Sondheimer, JM, and Deterding, RR: *Current Diagnosis & Treatment: Pediatrics*. McGraw Hill Lange, New York, 2011.

National Cancer Institute at the National Institutes of Health: *Mammograms*. http://www.cancer.gov/cancertopics/factsheet/detection/mammograms.

Population Reference Bureau: http://www.prb.org.

U.S. Department of Health and Human Services: *Healthy People 2020, National Health Promotion and Disease Prevention Objectives*. http://www.healthypeople.gov/2020.

How well did you do?

85% and above, congratulations! This score shows application of test-taking principles and adequate content knowledge.

75%–85%, keep working! Review test-taking principles and try again.

65%–75%, hang in there! Spend some time reviewing concepts and test-taking principles and then try the test again.

Chapter 4: *Care of the Emerging Family*

Donna C. Maheady
Jill E. Winland-Brown

Questions

4-1   Which of the following dietary changes would you recommend to Heather, who is experiencing nausea during her first trimester?

A. A bland diet taken frequently and in small amounts

B. An increase in fat intake

C. A decrease in carbohydrate intake

D. Restriction of fluid intake after 7 p.m.

4-2   Which of the following instructions should be included in the discharge teaching plan to assist the postpartal woman in recognizing early signs of complications?

A. The passage of clots as large as an orange is expected.

B. Call the office to report any decrease in the amount of brownish-red lochia.

C. Palpate the fundus daily to make sure it is soft.

D. Notify your health-care provider of a return to bright red vaginal bleeding.

4-3   Pregnant women should know that folic acid can help to prevent neural tube defects. For folic acid to be most effective, women should take it

A. before becoming pregnant.

B. during the second trimester.

C. during the third trimester.

D. soon after a positive pregnancy test.

4-4   Which of the following is the best description of the Lamaze method of childbirth education?

A. It focuses on the birth event and requires a dimly lighted room and a warm-water bath.

B. It uses no medical interventions such as fetal monitors, intravenous fluids, or medications.

C. It uses the child's father as a birthing coach and relies on deep abdominal breathing to handle the contractions.

D. It uses a focal point for concentration while the woman does controlled breathing techniques.

4-5   At birth, the anterior fontanelle has what shape?

A. Triangular

B. Oval

C. Round

D. Diamond

4-6   When is the brain configuration of a fetus roughly complete?

A. At 4 weeks' gestation

B. At 12 weeks' gestation

C. At 20 weeks' gestation

D. At 24 weeks' gestation

4-7   Mindy, age 42, is pregnant for the first time. She wants a chorionic villus sampling (CVS) performed for genetic testing. Which statement is true regarding CVS?

A. CVS may be offered at 11–14 weeks' gestation.

B. CVS detects only chromosomal anomalies and not anatomical aberrations such as open neural tube defects.

C. CVS is extremely safe.

D. CVS can be done in the physician's office.

4-8   Mr. Davis states, "I've had high cholesterol most of my life. I'm concerned about my daughter having it as well." The clinician knows that according to the National Cholesterol Education Program (NCEP) guidelines for children and adolescents, the acceptable range of total cholesterol (mg/dL) for children 2–18 years old is

A. less than 200.

B. less than 190.

C. less than 180.

D. less than 170.

4-9   *Sally, who is 18 weeks pregnant, had a maternal serum alpha-fetoprotein (MSAFP) level done. The results are elevated. What is the meaning of an elevated MSAFP level?*

A. The fetus has trisomy 21.

B. There is an increased risk that the fetus has an open neural tube defect.

C. The infant will be born with hydrocephalus.

D. The fetus has an increased risk of developing cerebral palsy.

4-10   *Eight-year-old Scott presents at the clinic with a rash. It is centripetal and began on his trunk. The very itchy lesions progressed from spots to "teardrop vesicles," according to his mother. The clinician considers which of the following infectious diseases?*

A. Measles

B. Roseola

C. Varicella

D. Fifth disease

4-11   *Sandra, who is 5 months pregnant and of average height and weight, asks you how many extra calories she should be adding to her diet per day. You tell her to add*

A. 200 calories.

B. 300 calories.

C. 500 calories.

D. 700 calories.

4-12   *Marisa was born with a red- to blue-purple nodule on her thigh that blanches dramatically with pressure. Over the past few months, it has increased in size. Her mother asks you what you think it is. You respond,*

A. "It may be a hemangioma."

B. "It may be a melanoma."

C. "It might be fibromatosis."

D. "It may be dermatofibrosarcoma protuberans."

4-13   *Jack and Jill present for a preconception health counseling session. Jack is 34, Jill is 33, and they have a 5-year-old son, Jake. Jake is the product of an uncomplicated pregnancy and labor.*

At birth, Jake had an open neural tube defect and now has spina bifida with a loss of function of his lower extremities. Jack and Jill want another child and ask if there is anything they can do to prevent the recurrence of a neural tube defect in future pregnancies. What is your best response to this couple?

A. "Take 60 mg a day of an iron supplement to enhance stores to support fetal development."

B. "It is a matter of genetics, and there is nothing you can do."

C. "Have a CVS performed at 12–14 weeks' gestation to determine the health of the fetus."

D. "Take 4 mg/day of folic acid, beginning before conception."

4-14   *What is the minimum number of café-au-lait spots that should be of concern?*

A. 1–3

B. 4–5

C. More than 5

D. Any number

4-15   *Marissa is a long-distance runner with 9% body fat. Which of the following findings is consistent with this situation?*

A. Regular menses and a basal body temperature that indicates ovulation

B. Irregular menses and a basal body temperature that indicates ovulation

C. Regular menses and a basal body temperature that indicates lack of ovulation

D. Irregular menses and a basal body temperature that indicates lack of ovulation

4-16   *Mildred is 6 months pregnant and presents with symptoms of urinary frequency, urgency, dysuria, and suprapubic discomfort. Her urine is cloudy and malodorous. She has no chills, fever, nausea, or vomiting. What is your diagnosis?*

A. Urinary calculi

B. Acute cystitis

C. Acute pyelonephritis

D. Interstitial cystitis

4-17   Growth hormone treatment for short stature remains controversial. The clinician should be aware of the following regarding the assessment of growth problems and idiopathic short stature.

A. Identification of a growth problem can be made based on one measurement.

B. Dysmorphic facial features will be present.

C. Identification of growth problems is usually made by an auxological evaluation, which compares the child's growth to standardized norms.

D. Measurements of children lying on the exam table paper are accurate.

4-18   Mrs. Nelms shares with you that her husband is on active duty with the National Guard. She states, "I'm left alone to care for three children." You know that children of active duty service members face many stressors (e.g., multiple deployments, relocations). These stressors can lead to

A. increased academic performance in children.

B. decreased behavior problems in children.

C. child maltreatment.

D. decreased incidence of depression in children.

4-19   Karen is taking oral contraceptive pills for fertility control. Karen calls the clinic and reports the presence of chest pain and shortness of breath. You instruct Karen to

A. eat smaller meals more frequently to prevent gastric distention.

B. stop taking the pills and use a nonhormonal contraceptive method.

C. wait for the physician to return a telephone call to the client.

D. go to the nearest emergency room immediately to be evaluated.

4-20   Aida, who is 29 weeks pregnant, received a blunt trauma to the abdomen during an argument with her boyfriend. She has no obvious injuries and denies pain. Aida needs to be monitored for the occurrence of

A. abruptio placentae.

B. liver hemorrhage.

C. ruptured spleen.

D. placenta previa.

4-21   Lynne comes to the clinic for her initial prenatal visit. Based on her menstrual history, the client is at 9 weeks' gestation and is scheduled to have an ultrasound for estimation of the gestational age of the fetus. Which fetal measurement is the best indicator of gestational age at this time?

A. Biparietal diameter

B. Femur length

C. Abdominal circumference

D. Crown-rump measurement

4-22   Which of the following should be avoided by the pregnant woman who is constipated?

A. Bulk-forming laxatives

B. Mineral oil

C. Stool softeners such as docusate sodium (Colace)

D. Drinking warm fluids on arising

4-23   Minnie is experiencing Braxton Hicks contractions. What should she do?

A. Take a cold shower.

B. Immediately call her health-care provider.

C. Go for a walk.

D. Lie down with her feet elevated.

4-24   What is the rationale for anemia seen throughout gestation?

A. Iron stores are depleted by the fetus.

B. It is difficult for the mother to consume as much iron as needed.

C. Mild dilutional anemia is seen as a result of an increased circulating blood volume.

D. Hepatic function is affected by the growing fetus.

4-25   An example of an X-linked recessive condition or trait is

A. muscular dystrophy.

B. hemophilia.

C. sickle cell anemia.

D. cystic fibrosis.

4-26 Jake is 8 years old. He is being seen for a routine physical. When reviewing his medications, you note that he is using the Daytrana transdermal patch for attention deficit/hyperactivity disorder (ADHD). What is the maximum length of time the Daytrana patch should be worn?

A. No longer than 9 hours a day

B. No longer than 6 hours a day

C. No longer than 12 hours a day

D. No longer than 16 hours

4-27 Marci has had several abortions in the past and has been unable to carry a pregnancy to full term because of an incompetent cervix. She states that the physician mentioned cerclage to her and asks you what that means. You tell her that cerclage is

A. a treatment of bedrest with frequent pelvic exams to make sure the cervix is not dilated.

B. a method in which an apparatus resembling a diaphragm is placed over the cervix to help it stay "tight."

C. a purse-string type of stitch placed around the cervix.

D. a treatment using intravaginal medicated sponges.

4-28 During Kim's first prenatal visit, she denies having had rubella or the rubella vaccine. Based on this information, which of the following is the most appropriate action?

A. Administer the rubella vaccine.

B. Take a blood sample to assess the rubella titer.

C. Tell the client to avoid infection with rubella during her pregnancy because it will result in a preterm birth.

D. Tell the client that, because rubella has little effect on the fetus, she should not worry about exposure to the disease.

4-29 What is a fetus's gestational age when its mother's uterus is palpable just above the pubic symphysis?

A. 4 weeks

B. 8 weeks

C. 12 weeks

D. 16 weeks

4-30 Which of the following tests is the diagnostic criteria for gestational diabetes according to the International Association of Diabetes and Pregnancy Study Group?

A. The presence of glycosuria on two urine samples within a 24-hour interval

B. A 50-g OGTT, with plasma glucose measurement fasting and at 1 and 2 h

C. A 75-g OGTT, with plasma glucose measurement fasting and at 1 and 2 h

D. A 100-g OGTT, with plasma glucose measurement fasting and at 1 and 2 h

4-31 Danger signs in the first trimester of pregnancy include

A. vaginal bleeding and absence of fetal movement.

B. edema extending to the upper extremities and vomiting.

C. presence of proteinuria and elevated blood pressure.

D. vaginal bleeding and persistent vomiting.

4-32 Nelda is breastfeeding her 6-week-old daughter. She comes today with pain, a lump in her right breast, and flu-like symptoms. You see that the breast is engorged, erythematous, and warm to the touch. Her temperature is 101.8°F (38.4°C). Your diagnosis is

A. breast abscess.

B. breast engorgement.

C. mastitis.

D. viral syndrome.

4-33 Heather, who is 5 weeks pregnant, is nauseous. She asks you how long this will last. You tell her the nausea usually disappears by the

A. 12th week.

B. 16th week.

C. 20th week.

D. 24th week.

4-34   A new mother asks, "Is it true that breast milk will prevent my baby from catching colds and other infections?" You should give which of the following replies based on current research findings?

A. "Your baby will have increased resistance to illness caused by bacteria and viruses, but he may still contract infections."

B. "You should not have to worry about your baby's exposure to contagious diseases until he stops breastfeeding."

C. "Breast milk offers no greater protection to your baby than formula feedings."

D. "Breast milk will give your baby protection from all illnesses to which you are immune."

4-35   Mrs. Garcia calls regarding her 18-month-old son's cough and cold. She asks the clinician, "Which medication should I give him?" Which of the following cough and cold products would you recommend?

A. Sudafed PE

B. Dextromethorphan

C. Guaifenesin

D. None

4-36   What is the simplest and safest method of suppressing lactation after it has started?

A. Administering oral and long-acting injections of hormonal preparations

B. Using breast binders

C. Gradually weaning the baby to a bottle or cup over a 3-week period

D. Stopping "cold turkey" (stopping breastfeeding immediately)

4-37   In evaluating a mother-and-infant breastfeeding situation, signs of an effective latch at the breast are

A. infant's cheeks sucked in and slow, shallow sucking.

B. infant's lips flanged out, cheeks full.

C. rapid, short, nonrhythmic sucking by infant.

D. maternal nipple discomfort throughout the feeding.

4-38   Ginny, who is planning on getting pregnant, is taking phenytoin (Dilantin). She states that she knows the drug is in category D and asks what that means. You know FDA category D indicates that

A. positive evidence of human fetal risk exists, but benefits may outweigh risks in certain situations.

B. animal studies have not demonstrated a fetal risk, but there are no human studies in pregnant women; or animal studies have shown an adverse effect that was not confirmed in human studies.

C. studies or experience have shown fetal risk that clearly outweighs any possible benefits.

D. controlled studies in women failed to demonstrate a risk to the fetus in the first trimester, and fetal harm appears remote.

4-39   Spontaneous abortion refers to the loss of a fetus of less than

A. 12 weeks' gestation.

B. 18 weeks' gestation.

C. 22 weeks' gestation.

D. 26 weeks' gestation.

4-40   When evaluating Marge during her first obstetric visit, you assess the shape of her pelvis. While drawing her a picture of her android-type pelvis, you explain that it has

A. a rounded, slightly ovoid, or elliptical inlet with a well-rounded forepelvis (anterior segment).

B. a wedge-shaped inlet, a narrow forepelvis, a flat posterior segment, and a narrow sacrosciatic notch with the sacrum inclining forward.

C. a long, narrow, oval inlet; an extended and narrow anterior and posterior segment; a wide sacrosciatic notch; and a long, narrow sacrum.

D. a distinct oval inlet with a very wide, rounded retropubic angle and a wider, flat posterior segment.

4-41   Early in pregnancy, all pregnant women need which of the following tests?

A. 3-hour glucose challenge test

B. Rh status

C. Direct Coombs' test

D. Pap smear

4-42   Margie, who has been breastfeeding for 4 weeks, has mastitis in her right breast and is taking Dicloxacillin. She asks you what she needs to do about feeding the baby. You respond,

A. "You need to stop breastfeeding and start with a bottle."
B. "You can still breastfeed on your left side and express the milk from your right side until the problem is resolved."
C. "There is no need to stop breastfeeding, but start with your left side."
D. "Stop breastfeeding for 2 weeks, then continue."

4-43   What is the recommended first-trimester weight gain for an underweight woman?

A. 2 lb
B. 3.5 lb
C. 5 lb
D. 7 lb

4-44   Marta asks you how pregnancy will affect her rheumatoid arthritis. You respond,

A. "There is a one-third rule: One-third get better, one-third remain the same, and one-third get worse."
B. "Pregnancy will have no effect on your rheumatoid arthritis."
C. "Seventy-five percent of women experience remission of the disease during pregnancy."
D. "It is advised that you don't get pregnant with this condition."

4-45   Risperdal has been approved by the FDA for treatment of the behaviors associated with autism in children over 5 years old. The clinician should be aware of the following common side effect.

A. Weight loss
B. Diarrhea
C. Nausea
D. Fatigue

4-46   When an infant is around 6 months of age, solid foods are usually added to the diet, generally in a recommended sequence. The first solid food recommended is cereal. What is the second type of solid food recommended?

A. Yellow vegetables
B. Strained meats
C. Green vegetables
D. Fruits

4-47   Nancy is concerned that her new breastfed baby is not getting enough fluid. What do you tell her so that she can assess for an adequate intake?

A. Weigh the infant every other day to see the weight gain in ounces.
B. If the infant is drinking and sleeping normally, an adequate intake is assumed.
C. If there are 6–10 wet diapers a day, intake is adequate.
D. If the infant is not irritable, an intake problem does not exist.

4-48   Molly has an appointment to see you for her annual well-child physical. The clinician knows that blood pressure screening is recommended at every preventive health care visit beginning at age

A. 4.
B. 5.
C. 3.
D. 2.

4-49   Children with Williams' syndrome typically have problems related to

A. brittle bones.
B. cardiovascular disease.
C. fear of strangers.
D. cleft lip and palate.

4-50   An asymmetric, softened enlargement of the uterine corner caused by placental development is a probable sign of pregnancy. What is it called?

A. Hegar's sign
B. Chadwick's sign
C. Goodrich's sign
D. Piskaçek's sign

4-51   Kim states that she has heard many old wives' tales of harmful things during pregnancy. Which of the following is harmful late in pregnancy?

A. Intercourse
B. Swimming

C. Douching

D. Dental visits

4-52   According to the International Association of Diabetes and Pregnancy Study Group, screening for gestational diabetes mellitus (GDM) should be done on which of the following clients?

A. All pregnant women at 24–28 weeks

B. Women age 40 or older

C. All women with threatened miscarriage

D. Women who report hypoglycemic symptoms

4-53   Lois is complaining of leg cramps during her pregnancy. What would you suggest to relieve them?

A. Take a calcium supplement daily.

B. Do several quick stretches to relieve the cramping.

C. Massage the cramping muscle.

D. Point your toes when exercising.

4-54   When should a child be moved from a car seat to a regular seat with a seat belt?

A. At age 4

B. At age 3

C. When the child weighs 40 lb

D. When the child weighs 30 lb

4-55   Sally and June report the news of their upcoming international adoption. The clinician should discuss the baby's need for follow-up examination within how long after arrival in the United States?

A. 2 weeks

B. 4 weeks

C. 6 weeks

D. 72 hours

4-56   At what age should children first be screened for lead toxicity?

A. 3 months

B. 6 months

C. 12 months

D. 3 years

4-57   The drug of choice for the pregnant woman with diabetes is

A. insulin.

B. glyburide (DiaBeta, Glynase, Micronase).

C. glipizide (Glucotrol).

D. metformin (Glucophage).

4-58   NSAID use during pregnancy has been linked to which condition in newborns?

A. Cardiac anomalies

B. Musculoskeletal weakness

C. Pulmonary hypertension

D. Central nervous system disorders

4-59   Tameka has an appointment for a well-baby checkup. The clinician knows that she will be due for her measles, mumps, and rubella immunization at age

A. 9 months

B. 6 months

C. 12 months

D. 4 months

4-60   Sarah, who just found out she is pregnant, is taking prenatal vitamins with extra daily supplements of iron. She may be a candidate for

A. a high-birth-weight baby.

B. vaginal spotting during the second trimester.

C. premature delivery.

D. excessive skin bruising.

4-61   Mrs. Peterson found pinworms on 8-year-old Randy. The clinician knows that treatment for pinworms with pyrantel pamoate includes treating

A. Randy and all of his siblings.

B. Randy and the siblings who share the same bathroom.

C. Randy and the siblings who share the same bedroom.

D. The entire household.

4-62   When is a pregnant woman at risk for developing congenital rubella syndrome?

A. During the first 4 weeks of pregnancy

B. During the first 16 weeks of pregnancy

C. During the last trimester

D. Any time during the pregnancy

4-63   Rh$_o$(D) immune globulin (RhoGAM) should be administered

A. when an infant is in distress at birth.

B. after a mother gives birth to a macrosomic infant.

C. when a D-negative mother has received a transfusion of D-positive blood.

D. when an infant with type A blood is born to a mother with type O blood.

4-64   What components make up the biophysical profile?

A. Nonstress test, amniotic fluid composition, fetal breathing, and fetal tone

B. Fetal tone, breathing, motion, and contraction stress test

C. Amniotic fluid composition, contraction challenge test, fetal breathing, and motion

D. Fetal tone, breathing, motion, amniotic fluid volume, and nonstress test

4-65   Hegar's sign, a physiological sign of pregnancy, is

A. cervical blueness.

B. softness of the uterus and ballottement at the isthmus.

C. cervical softness.

D. quickening.

4-66   Glenda gave birth to Jack 4 weeks ago. Her postpartum course was complicated by an intrauterine infection that was successfully treated with antibiotics. Today Glenda calls the office because Jack has white patches on his tongue and gums. She is concerned that her milk has become "sour" and is causing the white patches in Jack's mouth. Based on these data, what diagnosis do you suspect for Jack?

A. Oral chlamydia infection

B. Oral candidiasis

C. Mastitis

D. Epstein's pearls

4-67   Which of the following drugs should be used with extreme caution in breastfeeding mothers?

A. Azithromycin (Zithromax)

B. Phenobarbital (Luminal, Solfoton)

C. Propranolol (Inderal)

D. Cisplatin (Platinol)

4-68   Susie, who is 16 weeks pregnant, is having mild cramps with persistent and excessive bleeding. On examination, you find that some portion of the products of conception (placental) remain in the uterus, but the fetus has been expelled. What type of abortion is Susie having?

A. Incomplete

B. Threatened

C. Inevitable

D. Missed

4-69   Liza is 34 weeks pregnant and has mild hypertension. You are performing a nonstress test (NST). What is the criterion for a reactive NST?

A. A minimum of two fetal activity patterns in a 20-minute test period

B. The presence of two contractions with no fetal heart decelerations in a 20-minute test period

C. At least two fetal heart rate accelerations in response to fetal movement in a 20-minute test period

D. The absence of uterine contractions following fetal stimulation during a 20-minute test period

4-70   When asking a family member if the family generally gets the things they want out of life, if there are any "rules" in the family that everyone believes are important, and what role religion plays in the family, you are trying to assess which functional health pattern?

A. Role-relationship pattern

B. Cognitive-perceptual pattern

C. Value-belief pattern

D. Health-perception/health-management pattern

4-71   Mrs. Marcello calls you in a panic because her 8-year-old daughter has head lice. Which of the following medications is not recommended as a first line therapy?

A. Lindane shampoo

B. Nix

C. Rid

D. Ovide

4-72   What is the best description of Bishop's score?

A. It is a series of four maneuvers to determine fetal position.

B. It is a multiparameter evaluation of fetal condition following a nonreactive nonstress test.

C. It is an assessment of the cervix's readiness for elective induction.

D. It is an evaluation of fetal lung maturity and readiness for birth.

4-73   To obtain the daily calcium intake recommended during pregnancy, what should a woman consume per day?

A. One quart of cow's milk

B. Two cups of yogurt

C. Four slices of cheddar cheese

D. One cup of cottage cheese

4-74   Bea delivered vaginally 36 hours ago. You made rounds this morning and determined that she is ready to be discharged. You are at the nurses' station completing your documentation when Bea's husband comes up to you and states that his wife is very sick. Upon arrival at her room, you find Bea sitting up in bed. She states, "I cannot breathe! My chest hurts so much!" What do you suspect?

A. Myocardial infarction

B. Panic attack

C. Bacterial pneumonia

D. Pulmonary embolism

4-75   Susan is keeping a basal body temperature (BBT) graph as part of her infertility treatment. Today she shares the BBT graph with you. The BBT graph shows a nearly straight line. Which of the following is the best interpretation of Susan's BBT graph?

A. The client is not ovulating.

B. The client is not having intercourse.

C. The client is ovulating late in her menstrual cycle.

D. The client is not taking her temperature correctly.

4-76   A low-risk woman who is 16 weeks pregnant should be instructed to return to the prenatal clinic in

A. 1 week.

B. 2 weeks.

C. 3 weeks.

D. 4 weeks.

4-77   Gloria just delivered her baby and wants to start a vigorous exercise program to get back in shape. You advise her that she can start strenuous exercises

A. in 1 week.

B. in 3 weeks.

C. in 6 weeks.

D. whenever she wants.

4-78   Care of the infant experiencing neonatal abstinence syndrome due to maternal substance abuse should include which of the following?

A. Placing stuffed animals and mobiles in the crib to provide visual stimulation

B. Positioning the infant's crib in a quiet corner of the nursery

C. Avoiding the use of pacifiers

D. Spending extra time holding and rocking the baby

4-79   The G in APGAR stands for

A. gross appearance.

B. grunting.

C. grimace.

D. gas exchange.

4-80   Which one of the following behavior ratings is not included on the Denver Developmental Screening Test?

A. Compliance with examiner's requests

B. Alertness

C. Fearlessness

D. Attention span

4-81 *Pregnancy following the rapid weight loss and weight stabilization phase of bariatric surgery appears to be safe. Which nutritional deficiency is the most common problem related to pregnancy following bariatric surgery?*

A. Vitamin A

B. Anemia

C. Vitamin K

D. Vitamin C

4-82 *What is the presumptive symptom of pregnancy that involves tingling or frank pain of the breasts?*

A. Montgomery's tubercles

B. Colostrum secretion

C. Melasma

D. Mastodynia

4-83 *During the 6-week visit after a stillbirth, Mary states, "Sometimes I feel like I left my baby somewhere, and I can't remember where she is. Then I remember that she isn't alive." What is this is an example of?*

A. Anticipatory grieving

B. Disorientation

C. Reorganization

D. Searching and yearning

4-84 *What are the clinical characteristics consistent with a diagnosis of trisomy 21?*

A. Low birth weight, small jaw with recessed chin, muscle rigidity, and short sternum

B. Cleft lip and palate, polydactyly, malformed ears, and absence of the iris

C. Lymphedema of the hands and feet, webbed neck, coarctation of the aorta, and urinary tract abnormalities

D. Hypotonia, simian creases, epicanthal folds, and Brushfield spots

4-85 *Samantha, who has genital herpes, just found out that she is pregnant. Although she has not had a recurrence in years, she states that she has heard that genital herpes might cause a spontaneous abortion. You know that genital herpes*

A. might cause a spontaneous abortion at any time if the client has an active occurrence.

B. might cause a spontaneous abortion if the primary infection was early in the pregnancy.

C. might cause a spontaneous abortion if the recurrence is during the second trimester.

D. will not cause a spontaneous abortion.

4-86 *You see G5P4015 written on a client's history form. You surmise that*

A. the woman has been pregnant five times and has five living children.

B. the woman has five living children, including a set of twins, and she has had one abortion.

C. the woman has four living children and had one abortion, for a total of five pregnancies.

D. the woman is pregnant now and has five living children, including a set of twins.

4-87 *Allie, who has asthma, just found out she is pregnant. She is wondering whether she should continue taking her medications. Which of the following is true regarding asthma and pregnancy?*

A. Only inhaled (rather than oral) medications should be used.

B. In the event of an acute exacerbation, glucocorticoids should not be used.

C. Management differs little from management in nonpregnant women.

D. All medications may be used except for theophylline.

4-88 *A newborn delivered by a mother with no prenatal care exhibits the following: dysmorphic facial features including short palpebral fissures, a thin upper lip, an elongated and flattened philtrum, and a flattened midface region. You suspect that the mother engaged in what behavior during pregnancy?*

A. Excessive alcohol intake

B. Cocaine abuse

C. Chain smoking

D. Excessive high-impact aerobics

4-89 *Joyce, who experienced some transient emotional disturbances around her third postpartum day, is just now feeling like herself again after about 2 weeks. It is most likely that Joyce experienced*

A. maternity or "baby" blues.

B. postpartum depression.

C. postpartum psychosis.

D. postpartum anxiety disorder.

4-90   Which of the following statements about lesbian relationships is true?

A. Battering is a concern only in heterosexual relationships, but in lesbian relationships, there may be emotional or financial abuse instead of physical abuse.

B. Support from family, friends, and coworkers may be lost.

C. HIV infection is not a concern with two women who are in a committed relationship.

D. Childbearing issues do not affect lesbian couples.

4-91   Which of the following recommendations should you provide to parents about reducing the risk of sudden infant death syndrome (SIDS)?

A. Two small stuffed animals in the crib is the recommended limit.

B. A bare crib with a firm sleep surface; no soft objects, wedges, or ruffles.

C. Co-sleeping with parents is advised.

D. A plush, soft mattress with bumper pads is recommended.

4-92   Which screening test has the highest sensitivity and specificity for diagnosing iron deficiency in anemic clients?

A. Ferritin

B. Hemoglobin

C. Hematocrit

D. Reticulocyte count

4-93   Which of the following antibiotics is the best choice for acute pyelonephritis when it occurs during the seventh month of pregnancy?

A. Nitrofurantoin (Furadantin)

B. Trimethoprim and sulfamethoxazole (Bactrim, Septra)

C. Ampicillin (Principen, Polycillin)

D. Tetracycline (Panmycin, Achromycin V)

4-94   Which of the following statements is true regarding infant car seats?

A. An infant car seat should be placed facing backward until the infant's toes touch the seat.

B. An infant car seat should be placed facing backward until the infant weighs 20 lb.

C. An infant car seat should be placed facing forward until the infant outgrows it.

D. An infant car seat should be placed facing forward until the infant weighs 20 lb.

4-95   Mrs. Jones calls you about her 10-year-old daughter's dental pain. Parents should be informed that the maximum recommended number of daily doses and duration of use of acetaminophen for pain in pediatric patients is

A. four doses per day and 5 days.

B. five doses per day and 5 days.

C. four doses per day and 3 days.

D. five doses per day and 2 days.

4-96   According to Naegele's rule, if a woman's last normal menstrual period (LNMP) was September 23, what is her estimated date of delivery?

A. June 30

B. June 16

C. June 1

D. May 30

4-97   Heather is scheduled for a well-child visit. Her mother asks, "How much milk should she be drinking now?" The clinician states that the American Heart Association recommendation for milk intake after 12 months of age is

A. 8 ounces per day.

B. 12 ounces per day.

C. 16 ounces per day.

D. 24 ounces per day.

4-98   During nursery rounds, you examine a 12-hour-old newborn. The infant has a yellow tint to the skin and sclera. What lab test will you order to further evaluate this infant?

A. Blood glucose

B. Direct Coombs' test

C. Blood cultures

D. Arterial blood gas

4-99   *Nettie, who is pregnant, is suffering from an exacerbation of peptic ulcer disorder. Which is the best medication to order for her?*

A. Cimetidine (Tagamet)

B. Ranitidine (Zantac)

C. Sucralfate (Carafate)

D. Bellergal-S

4-100   *Allison is being seen today because of a follow-up request from the school nurse. During a routine scoliosis screening, Allison was found to have questionable findings. The clinician knows the following about idiopathic scoliosis.*

A. Idiopathic scoliosis does not run in families.

B. Idiopathic scoliosis is generally painless.

C. The scapula are equal with idiopathic scoliosis.

D. The curve associated with idiopathic scoliosis is left sided.

4-101   *Mrs. Sullivan shares concerns about her son's frequent bedwetting. She asks you about medication she has read about on the Internet. The clinician know that Desmopressin acetate (DDAVP) can be used for primary nocturnal enuresis in children older than*

A. 6 years.

B. 5 years.

C. 4 years.

D. 3 years.

4-102   *After 28 weeks' gestation, all women should perform fetal movement counts (FMCs). Which of the following statements is true regarding FMCs?*

A. Counts should be done as the woman is going about her work.

B. Ten movements should be obtained in 1 hour.

C. Ten movements should be obtained in 2 hours.

D. If decreased activity is perceived, a nonstress test (NST) should be performed at the next obstetric visit.

4-103   *What is the primary site of drowning for children younger than age 3?*

A. The ocean

B. A backyard pool

C. A lake

D. A bathtub

4-104   *Cydney, who is 30 weeks pregnant, is planning to travel outside of the United States. She asks you which immunizations she should or should not have. Which immunization do you recommend she NOT receive?*

A. Pooled gamma globulin

B. Chloroquine for malaria prophylaxis

C. Yellow fever

D. Inactivated polio vaccine (IPV)

4-105   *Carrie is due to deliver her second baby. During your work-up, you note that she hemorrhaged after delivering her first baby 2 years ago, has always had menorrhagia, and bruises easily. Her lab work reveals a normal blood work-up, including a normal prothrombin time and activated partial thromboplastin time. What do you suspect?*

A. Von Willebrand's disease

B. Hemophilia

C. Sickle cell anemia

D. Unfortunate coincidences

4-106   *Kawasaki's disease is the leading cause of acquired heart disease in children in the developed world. The clinician should be aware that the minimum length of treatment with low-dose aspirin is*

A. 4 weeks

B. 2–3 weeks

C. 6–8 weeks

D. 6 months

4-107   *In an infant, when you flex the hips and knees at a 90° angle and attempt to slip the femur heads onto the posterior tips of the acetabulums by lateral pressure of the thumbs and by rocking the knees medially with the knuckles of the index fingers, you are testing for normal hip movement. This test or maneuver is known as*

A. Ortolani's maneuver.

B. Barlow's test.

C. Spock's test.

D. Moro maneuver.

4-108   *Diane is the mother of a child diagnosed with autism. After the clinician recommends the seasonal flu vaccine for the family, Diane asks, "Does the flu vaccine contain thimerosal"? The clinician knows that*

A. the nasal spray does not contain thimerosal.

B. multidose vials do not contain thimerosal.

C. all flu vaccine vials do not contain thimerosal.

D. trace amounts of thimerosal are found in single-dose units.

4-109   *The clinician is seeing a toddler for a follow-up visit. The chart indicates that the previous examiner noted an innocent murmur. You should suspect a possible pathologic murmur if the examination reveals the following:*

A. Murmur is grade I-II/VI.

B. Murmur changes with toddler's position.

C. Murmur is musical in quality.

D. Murmur is diastolic.

4-110   *The reason most often cited to explain why women who have had a usual length of stay and normal delivery discontinue breastfeeding before 8 weeks postpartum is*

A. that the mother returned to work or school.

B. the perception that the infant is not receiving enough milk.

C. the ease of formula use.

D. maternal or infant illness.

4-111   *Jack is 4 weeks old and has oral candidiasis because his mother had an intrauterine infection that was successfully treated with antibiotics. What would you anticipate treating Jack with?*

A. Vinegar and water

B. Nystantin

C. Fluconazole

D. Antibiotics

4-112   *Talya is 2 years old and presents with signs and symptoms (s/s) of acute otitis media. Mom reports that she experienced a rash after the administration of penicillin in the past.*

If a "wait-and-see" approach is not indicated, which of the following antibiotics should be prescribed?

A. Augmentin

B. Amoxicillin

C. Omnicef

D. Trimox

4-113   *Mr. Johnson calls your office from the soccer field. His 10-year-old son, Joshua, was hit in the mouth during the game. One of Joshua's front teeth was knocked out. The clinician advises Mr. Johnson to*

A. rinse the tooth gently in cold milk, saline, or room temperature water and then replant it.

B. rinse the tooth gently in cold milk, saline, or room temperature water and put it in a clean cloth.

C. rub the root surface clean and rinse with saline or room temperature water.

D. rub the root surface clean and keep as dry as possible.

4-114   *Sheila is pregnant and fearful of getting cervical cancer as her sister recently did. She asks about receiving the HPV vaccine. How do you respond?*

A. "Yes, as long as you're in your first trimester, the HPV vaccine is safe and effective."

B. "Research has not shown this vaccine to be effective against preventing cervical cancer."

C. "After the age of 20, the HPV vaccine is not recommended."

D. "You should not receive the vaccination when you're pregnant."

4-115   *Development delay, lack of speech, seizures, walking and balance disorders, and a happy demeanor characterized by frequent smiling, laughter, and excitability describes which of the following syndromes?*

A. Cornelia de Lange syndrome

B. Prader-Willi syndrome

C. Angelman's syndrome

D. Flathead syndrome

4-116 *Shana shares concerns about her unborn child. She states, "My sister's child is diagnosed with autism." The clinician knows the following to be true about autism spectrum disorder (ASD):*

A. There is no genetic predisposition to autism.

B. Females are four times more likely to have an ASD than males.

C. About 20%–30% of children with an ASD develop epilepsy by the time they reach adulthood.

D. Mental retardation occurs in all cases.

4-117 *A poorly defined, flat, blue-black macule, present at birth and usually on the trunk and buttocks, is a*

A. blue nevus.

B. drug-induced blue macule.

C. Mongolian spot.

D. malignant melanoma.

4-118 *When can you hear fetal heart tones with a conventional fetoscope?*

A. At 7–8 weeks' gestation

B. At 10–12 weeks' gestation

C. At 18–20 weeks' gestation

D. At more than 20 weeks' gestation

4-119 *Patricia presents for her regularly scheduled prenatal visit at 34 weeks' gestation. During the interview, you determine that Patricia has not felt fetal movement for the past week. On examination, you are unable to auscultate the fetal heart tones. Which of the following would be useful in the diagnosis of an intrauterine fetal death?*

A. Chadwick's sign

B. Piskaçek's sign

C. Spalding's sign

D. Homan's sign

4-120 *Betsy is breastfeeding and complains of tenderness of the nipples all the time. You recommend that she*

A. apply ice to the nipples between feedings.

B. apply dry heat to the nipples between feedings.

C. use nipple shields.

D. stop breastfeeding.

4-121 *A woman with hyperemesis gravidarum would most likely benefit from a plan of care designed to address which of the following nursing diagnoses?*

A. Imbalanced nutrition, more than body requirements, related to pregnancy

B. Anxiety, related to effects of hyperemesis on fetal well-being

C. Anticipatory grieving, related to inevitable pregnancy loss

D. Ineffective coping, related to unwanted pregnancy

Answers

4-1 Answer A

Nausea during pregnancy may be helped somewhat by dietary changes, such as eating a bland diet taken frequently and in small amounts, increasing carbohydrate intake, decreasing fat intake, and trying to stay away from food odors. Good hydration is important in pregnancy; therefore, fluid restriction is never recommended.

4-2 Answer D

A return to bright red vaginal bleeding is a sign of a complication and potentially a late postpartum hemorrhage. The client should not be passing clots. It is expected that the amount of lochia will decrease over time. The fundus should be firm; a soft uterine fundus would result in increased vaginal bleeding.

4-3 Answer A

Folic acid should be taken before getting pregnant and during the first few weeks of pregnancy, often before a woman may even know she is pregnant. Folic acid is important throughout pregnancy, but to be most effective in preventing neural tube defects it needs to be taken prior to becoming pregnant.

4-4 Answer D

The Lamaze method of childbirth education uses patterned, controlled breathing with concentration on a visual focal point during labor. A focus on birth in a dimly lighted room and a warm water bath is the Leboyer method. Natural childbirth uses no medical interventions. The Bradley method is father-coached childbirth.

4-5   Answer D

At birth, the anterior fontanelle has a diamond shape, whereas the posterior fontanelle has a triangular shape. The fontanelles are soft and flat and may bulge when the infant cries.

4-6   Answer B

The brain configuration of a fetus is roughly complete at 12 weeks' gestation. Therefore, it is important to teach the pregnant client to avoid all drugs, alcohol, smoking, and other teratogenic agents that may cause neurological harm to the infant, unless the client checks first with her health-care provider.

4-7   Answer B

Chorionic villus sampling (CVS) detects only chromosomal anomalies and not anatomical aberrations such as open neural tube defects. CVS may be performed at 10–12 weeks' gestation, whereas amniocentesis may be performed at 15–18 weeks' gestation. Although safe, CVS has a slightly higher risk of loss of the pregnancy than does amniocentesis and is performed only in large facilities that offer experienced practitioners and real-time ultrasound imaging.

4-8   Answer D

According to the National Cholesterol Education Program (NCEP) guidelines for children and adolescents, the acceptable range of total cholesterol (mg/dL) for children 2–18 years old is less than 170. The borderline range for total cholesterol (mg/dL) is 170–199, and 200 or more is considered high.

4-9   Answer B

Maternal serum alpha-fetoprotein (MSAFP) testing is a screening procedure used to detect an increased risk for neural tube defects and ventral wall defects. MSAFP screening should be considered for all pregnant women at 16–18 weeks' gestation because 90% of neural tube defects occur in the absence of a positive history. MSAFP is elevated in 80%–90% of women whose fetuses have open neural tube defects or other fetal anomalies, such as omphalocele, congenital nephrosis, and fetal bowel obstruction, and in women with multiple fetuses. MSAFP levels are not elevated with closed neural tube defects such as hydrocephalus. Birth trauma is the most common cause of cerebral palsy, so there is no available screening test. It is diagnosed after birth.

An MSAFP is part of a triple screening test, and low values on triple screening testing are indicative of an increased risk for trisomy 21.

4-10   Answer C

The rash associated with measles first appears on the forehead and behind the ears. Papules enlarge and move downward to the face, neck and arms. The rash associated with roseola is nonpruritic, rose colored, and maculopapular. The rash associated with varicella is classic. It is centripetal and begins of the scalp, face, or trunk. Highly pruritic, the lesions progress from spots to "teardrop" vesicles. Fifth disease usually produces a distinctive red rash on the face that makes a child appear to have a "slapped cheek." The rash then spreads to the trunk, arms, and legs.

4-11   Answer B

A woman of average height and weight needs an additional 300 calories a day during pregnancy and an additional 500 calories a day when breastfeeding to ensure an adequate intake of essential nutrients for the child.

4-12   Answer A

Hemangiomas are single or multiple red to blue-purple nodules that blanch dramatically with pressure. Diffuse redness, increased hair growth, and scaling might occur over the lesions. They may occur anywhere and may be in a dermatomal distribution. Although usually present at birth, they may also increase in size during the first few months of life. Laser treatment can be done in selected cases. A melanoma may be multicolored but will not blanch. A fibromatosis is a firm, flesh-colored nodule with normal overlying epidermis that may occur anywhere. In infancy, these nodules are usually on the trunk and shoulder. Surgical excision is usually performed, but the lesions may recur. A dermatofibrosarcoma protuberans is an erythematous, firm nodule that occurs more frequently on the trunk and more commonly in boys than in girls. The treatment consists of a wide local excision.

4-13   Answer D

Adequate levels of folic acid supplements before conception and during the early stages of pregnancy have been shown to decrease the incidence of neural tube defects. Iron stores and supplementation do not affect neural tube development. A CVS procedure can identify chromosomal alterations but not structural abnormalities.

4-14   Answer C

The presence of more than five café-au-lait spots suggests neurofibromatosis. Café-au-lait spots are uniformly pigmented tan, nonscaly, and oval or irregularly shaped macules. The lesions are usually less than 0.5 cm in diameter and most commonly occur on the trunk but can occur anywhere, although they are not usually found on mucosal surfaces. Ten percent of normal individuals have one to three café-au-lait spots. No treatment is necessary for normal individuals, although the spots may be associated with pulmonary stenosis and mental retardation.

4-15   Answer D

Fourteen percent body fat is considered adequate if a woman is to have regular menses and regular ovulation. A woman with less than 10% body fat will ovulate and menstruate very irregularly or not at all.

4-16   Answer B

Symptoms of urinary frequency, urgency, dysuria, and suprapubic discomfort in the absence of chills, fever, nausea, and vomiting, along with cloudy, malodorous urine, are clinically diagnostic of acute cystitis. Acute cystitis and acute pyelonephritis are common renal disorders in pregnancy. Renal calculi may cause intermittent flank pain or pain that radiates around to the abdomen. Maternal symptoms of pyelonephritis include fever, shaking chills, malaise, flank pain, nausea and vomiting, headache, increased urinary frequency, and dysuria. Interstitial cystitis is a chronic, painful bladder disorder in which the course is unpredictable. The symptoms include urinary frequency, urgency, nocturia, and suprapubic pain in the absence of urinary pathogens. Although the etiology of interstitial cystitis is unknown, most attribute it to an initial insult to the bladder wall by a toxin, allergen, or immunologic agent that causes an inflammatory response.

4-17   Answer C

Identification of growth problems is usually made by an auxological evaluation which compares the child's growth to standardized norms. One of the most common reasons for abnormal growth concerns is inaccurate measurement. Measurements of children lying on the exam table paper are not accurate. Children with idiopathic short stature lack dysmorphic features. Identification of short stature is not an isolated measurement but an assessment of growth over time.

4-18   Answer C

The stressors of lengthy deployments can lead to child maltreatment. Risk factors include preexisting psychiatric problems of the child or stay-at-home parent, highly stressed nondeployed parents, and a lack of social connections or resources for those in military service. Academic performance is often decreased in children, and behavior problems often increase. Children of deployed parents have higher degrees of emotional difficulties.

4-19   Answer D

Shortness of breath and chest pains are potentially life-threatening complications associated with the use of oral contraceptives. This situation requires immediate attention. Waiting for the physician's return phone call will delay treatment. Changing contraceptive method and eating patterns does not address the immediate life-threatening problem.

4-20   Answer A

Trauma to the pregnant abdomen can result in abruptio placentae (premature separation of the placenta). Abruptio placentae is a life-threatening event. The enlarged uterus and its contents actually provide some protection to the other abdominal organs from trauma.

4-21   Answer D

Before 12 weeks' gestation, length as measured from crown to rump is the most accurate measure of gestational age. Biparietal diameter and femur length are used to monitor fetal growth in the second trimester of pregnancy. Abdominal circumference is useful in identifying some congenital anomalies.

4-22   Answer B

Mineral oil should be avoided by the pregnant woman who is constipated because it decreases the absorption of fat-soluble vitamins. Cathartics are also contraindicated because they may cause preterm labor. Bulk-forming laxatives and stool softeners can be used along with dietary interventions, such as drinking warm fluids on arising, eating foods high in bulk, and drinking 6–8 glasses of water per day to stimulate bowel motility.

4-23   Answer C

Braxton Hicks contractions (painless uterine contractions felt as tightening or pressure), which usually begin at about 28 weeks' gestation, usually disappear with walking or exercise. If they were true labor contractions, they would become more intense.

4-24   Answer C

Mild dilutional anemia is seen throughout gestation as the result of an increased circulating blood volume. Plasma volume expansion, which begins at 6–8 weeks' gestation, precedes and exceeds red cell volume. The circulating blood volume of a pregnant woman increases by 45%. Iron stores are not depleted by the fetus and hepatic function is not affected during gestation.

4-25   Answer B

Hemophilia is an example of an X-linked recessive condition, occurring more commonly in men than in women. Muscular dystrophy is an example of an autosomal-dominant condition in which the trait appears with equal frequency in both sexes. For inheritance to take place, at least one parent must have the trait unless a new mutation has just occurred. Sickle cell anemia and cystic fibrosis are both examples of autosomal-recessive conditions in which the trait appears with equal frequency in both sexes. For inheritance to take place, both parents must be carriers of the recessive trait.

4-26   Answer A

Daytrana should not be worn for more than 9 hours a day. It should be applied to a different hip each day. If the patch is worn longer than 9 hours in a day, or if more than one patch is worn at a time, too much medicine has been applied.

4-27   Answer C

Cerclage is a purse-string type of stitch placed around the cervix. A variety of suture materials can be used to create the stitch around an incompetent cervix. Cerclage is used in conjunction with restriction of activities and should be used cautiously when there is advanced cervical dilation or membranes are prolapsed into the vagina. Rupture of the membranes and infection are specific contraindications to cerclage.

4-28   Answer B

You need to determine immune status. Rubella during pregnancy can cause miscarriage or congenital anomalies. The woman should not be vaccinated during pregnancy because the fetus can be affected by the live virus. Immunity is best determined by assessing the rubella titer.

4-29   Answer C

The gestational age when the uterus is palpable just above the pubic symphysis is 12 weeks. At 12 weeks, the uterus becomes an abdominal organ, and at 15 weeks, it is usually at the midpoint between the pubic symphysis and umbilicus. The uterus is palpable at the umbilicus at 20 weeks, and after that, the fundal size correlates roughly with the gestational age up until about 36 weeks. At 36 weeks, the fundal height may decrease as the fetal head descends into the pelvis.

4-30   Answer C

After deliberations in 2008–2009, the International Association of Diabetes and Pregnancy Study Group developed revised diagnostic criteria recommendations. The diagnostic standard for the diagnosis of gestational diabetes is an abnormal 75-g OGTT with plasma glucose measurement fasting and at 1 and 2 h.

4-31   Answer D

Vaginal bleeding may be a sign of impending pregnancy loss; persistent vomiting may result in dehydration and ketosis, which, in turn, can affect organogenesis during the first trimester. During the first trimester, fetal movement is not perceptible. Quickening (the perception of fetal movement) occurs at 18–20 weeks' gestation. Edema of the hands and face is a sign of a constricted intravascular space and worsening pregnancy-induced hypertension (PIH), which occurs in the last trimester of pregnancy. Other signs of PIH are proteinuria and elevated blood pressure. In the first trimester, there is no change in the maternal blood pressure.

4-32   Answer C

With a history of 6 weeks of breastfeeding, pain, and a lump in the breast; flu-like symptoms; a temperature of 101.8°F (38.5°C); and physical examination revealing an engorged, erythematous, and warm-to-the-touch breast, your diagnosis is mastitis, an infection of the breast. Mastitis, which occurs in about 5% of lactating women, may be caused by tight clothing, missed infant feedings, poor drainage of the duct and alveolus, or infection with *Staphylococcus aureus, Escherichia coli,* or *Streptococcus.* A clogged duct, simple breast engorgement, breast abscess, and viral syndrome are differential diagnoses. A clogged duct and simple breast engorgement may be painful but not erythematous or warm to the touch. Also, flu-like symptoms would not be present. A breast abscess should be suspected if there is no resolution of symptoms after several days of antibiotic therapy. If an abscess is present, pitting edema over the affected area is possible. An abscess is usually treated with both antibiotics and drainage.

4-33   Answer C

Nausea and vomiting affect 50%–90% of all pregnant women. Nausea, ranging from mild to severe, typically begins at about the 4th week of pregnancy, peaks around weeks 8–12, and disappears by the 20th week of pregnancy. Severe nausea, known as hyperemesis gravidarum, affects about 1%–2% of all pregnant women.

4-34   Answer A

Breastfeeding increases resistance, but it does not protect the infant from all illnesses. Passive immunity is acquired through antibodies passed across the placenta.

4-35   Answer D

The use of cough and cold medications in infants and young children under 2 years is not recommended. The FDA strongly recommends that over-the-counter (OTC) cough and cold products should not be used for infants and children under 2 years of age because serious and potentially life-threatening side effects could occur.

4-36   Answer C

The simplest and safest method of suppressing lactation after it has started is to wean the baby to a bottle or cup gradually over a 3-week period. The milk supply will decrease with the decreased demand and with minimal discomfort. Oral and long-acting injections of hormonal preparations used to be the practice to suppress lactation. Because of their questionable efficacy and associated adverse effects such as thromboembolic episodes and hair growth,

this practice has been abandoned. In addition, bromocriptine (formerly used to suppress lactation) is not used because of the potential for severe hypertension, seizures, strokes, and myocardial infarctions associated with its use. The use of a snug bra, along with ice packs and analgesics, might help. If for some reason the mother must stop breastfeeding immediately, nipple stimulation should be avoided and the expression of milk should be discouraged.

4-37   Answer B

Signs of an effective latch-on are lips flanged out and cheeks full. Rapid, short, nonrhythmic sucking is consistent with nonnutritive sucking. With an effective latch-on, if maternal nipple discomfort is present, it subsides quickly because the pressure of the infant's sucking motion is on the areola, not the nipple.

4-38   Answer A

The Food and Drug Administration (FDA) has five categories into which it ranks drugs for their potential to harm a fetus if taken during pregnancy. Category D indicates that there is positive evidence that the drug has risk for the human fetus, but the benefits of the drug for the pregnant woman may outweigh risks in certain situations, such as when the pregnant woman is using phenytoin (Dilantin). The other four FDA pregnancy categories are as follows: Category A indicates that controlled studies in women failed to demonstrate that the drug poses a risk to the fetus in the first trimester and fetal harm appears remote. Category B indicates that animal studies have not demonstrated a fetal risk, but there are no human studies in pregnant women; or animal studies have shown an adverse effect that was not confirmed in human studies. Category C indicates that animal studies show that the drug causes adverse effects on the fetus, and there are no controlled studies in women. Category E indicates that studies or experience have shown that the drug causes fetal risk that clearly outweighs any possible benefits.

4-39   Answer C

Spontaneous abortion refers to the loss of a fetus of younger than 22 weeks' gestation and a weight less than 500 g. A delivered fetus of about 22–28 weeks' gestation and weighing 500–1,000 g is called immature. A delivered fetus of about 28–36 weeks' gestation and weighing 500–2,000 g is called premature. A full-term fetus is one that has attained 3–7 weeks' gestation and weighs at least 3,500 g.

4-40   Answer B

An android-type pelvis has a wedge-shaped inlet, a narrow forepelvis, a flat posterior segment, and a narrow sacrosciatic notch with the sacrum inclining forward. A woman's pelvis may be one of four types or a combination of them. A gynecoid-type pelvis has a rounded, slightly ovoid or elliptical inlet with a well-rounded forepelvis (anterior segment). An anthropoid-type pelvis has a long, narrow, oval inlet; an extended and narrow anterior and posterior segment; a wide sacrosciatic notch; and a long, narrow sacrum, often with six sacral segments. A platypelloid-type pelvis has a distinct oval inlet with a very wide, rounded, retropubic angle and a wider, flat posterior segment.

4-41   Answer B

Early in pregnancy, all pregnant women need their blood type and Rh status determined and need an atypical antibody titer (indirect Coombs' test) done. Although there are more than 400 antigens of the Rh factor, 90% of cases of Rh isoimmunization are caused by the D antigen. Women lacking antigenic determinant D require two exposures to the Rh antigen to produce significant sensitization, unless the first exposure was massive. A direct Coombs' test is performed on a blood specimen from the fetus/neonate, usually obtained from the umbilical cord. The 3-hour glucose challenge is diagnostic of gestational diabetes and is done in the second half of pregnancy. A Pap smear is performed only if the woman has not recently had one. As a result of normal pregnancy-related changes to the pregnant cervix, the reliability of the Pap smear is changed during pregnancy.

4-42   Answer C

When a woman who is breastfeeding develops mastitis, there is no need to stop breastfeeding unless the mastitis is very severe. The woman should begin breastfeeding on the unaffected side because the infant's first sucking is the strongest and would be more painful on the affected side. This also allows the affected breast to "let down." Sulfa drugs should not be prescribed if the nursing infant is younger than 1 month old. Dicloxacillin sodium (Dynapen, Dycill, Pathocil), cephalexin (Keflex),

and acetaminophen (Tylenol) may be safely prescribed.

4-43   Answer C

An underweight woman (less than 90% of ideal body weight) should gain 5 lb during the first trimester, for a total recommended weight gain of 28–40 lb. A woman of normal weight should gain 3.5 lb during the first trimester, for a total recommended weight gain of 25–35 lb. An overweight woman (greater than 120% of desirable pregravid weight for height) should gain 2 lb during the first trimester, with a total recommended weight gain of 15–25 lb. A severely overweight (greater than 135% of desirable pregravid weight) woman should gain 2 lb during the first trimester, for a total recommended weight gain of at least 15 lb during the pregnancy. These recommendations are from the U.S. Institute of Medicine, Subcommittee on Nutritional Status and Weight Gain During Pregnancy.

4-44   Answer C

For women with rheumatoid arthritis, 75% will experience remission of their disease during pregnancy. Activities of daily living are easier to perform because of decreased joint stiffness and swelling and an increase in grip strength. However, women with rheumatoid arthritis usually do experience major fatigue, and during labor and delivery, joint contracture may limit their positioning. Pain needs to be carefully assessed, and 95% of these women will experience a flare-up of their condition during labor and delivery.

4-45   Answer D

Weight gain, constipation, and fatigue/drowsiness are common side effects of Risperdal. Nausea is not a common side effect. The fatigue or drowsiness is sometimes a "good" side effect, as many children with autism do not sleep well, which adds to their behavior problems.

4-46   Answer D

The recommended sequence for adding solid foods to an infants diet at 6 months of age is as follows: (1) cereal, particularly rice because it is nonallergenic; (2) fruits, such as peaches, pears, and applesauce; (3) yellow vegetables, such as squash and carrots; (4) green vegetables, such as peas or beans; and (5) strained meats, such as nonallergenic lamb or veal.

4-47   Answer C

To help assess for an adequate intake in a breastfed baby, tell the mother that if there are 6–10 wet diapers a day in the first few months of life, the baby's intake is adequate. During the first few weeks, the infant's weight fluctuates greatly and is not an adequate indicator of fluid intake. If an infant is drinking and sleeping normally, it might be assumed that he or she is getting sufficient intake, although these assumptions may lead to problems. The infant may not be getting enough nourishment and actually may be sleeping because of decreased energy levels. An infant who is not irritable may be flaccid because of numerous other problems, such as neuromuscular conditions. Again, an adequate intake cannot be assumed.

4-48   Answer C

Blood pressure screening is recommended at every preventive health-care visit beginning at age 3 and should continue with each health-care visit. This is the recommendation from the American Academy of Pediatrics and the American Heart Association.

4-49   Answer B

The majority of individuals with Williams' syndrome have some type of heart or blood vessel problem. Typically, there is narrowing in the aorta (producing supravalvular aortic stenosis) or narrowing in the pulmonary arteries. Brittle bones are associated with osteogenesis imperfecta. Individuals with Williams' syndrome are typically unafraid of strangers. Cleft lip and palate is not associated with Williams' syndrome.

4-50   Answer D

A probable sign of pregnancy—Piskaçek's sign—is an asymmetric, softened enlargement of the uterine corner caused by placental development. Hegar's sign is softening of the uterine isthmus. Chadwick's sign is a bluish or cyanotic color to the cervix and upper vagina. There is no Goodrich's sign.

4-51   Answer C

Douching, which is seldom necessary, may be harmful during pregnancy. Intercourse late in the pregnancy may initiate labor, possibly because an orgasm might cause a uterine contraction reflex. Intercourse is usually cautioned against only in women who have had a previous premature delivery or are currently experiencing uterine bleeding. Water does not enter the vagina; therefore, swimming is not contraindicated. However, diving should be avoided because of the possibility of trauma. Good dental care is important during pregnancy; however, the dentist should be told that the woman is pregnant.

4-52   Answer A

After deliberations in 2008–2009, the International Association of Diabetes and Pregnancy Study Group recommend screening for GDM for all women not known to have diabetes at 24–28 weeks. Age 40 or older is considered a risk factor. Other risk factors include obesity, history of miscarriage or fetal death, history of premature infant, family history of diabetes, polyhydramnios, history of infant with macrosomia (greater than 4,000 g) or congenital malformation, pre-eclampsia, excessive weight gain, and glycosuria. A threatened miscarriage without a history of a previous miscarriage is not a risk factor. The term *hypoglycemic* could be interpreted in a variety of ways. This complaint would have to be evaluated before a decision about screening is made.

4-53   Answer A

For a pregnant woman complaining of leg cramps, use of a daily calcium supplement may help. Leg cramps are a normal discomfort experienced during pregnancy. They are caused by a lack of calcium, pressure of the enlarged uterus on the blood vessels, fatigue or chilling, sudden stretching or overextension of the foot, and/or excessive phosphorus in the diet. Some nursing suggestions that might relieve the leg cramps are using calcium supplements, practicing gentle steady stretching to relieve the cramp, avoiding massage of the cramping muscle, and avoiding toe pointing when exercising.

4-54   Answer C

A child should be moved from a car seat to a regular seat with a seat belt when he or she weighs 40 lb. Until the child weighs 70 lb, ideally, he or she should be in a booster seat. If the shoulder belt crosses the child's face or neck when buckled, it should not be worn but tucked behind the shoulders with just the lap belt in place. Children should not ride in the cargo area of a pickup truck, van, or station wagon. They should be in the rear seat of the vehicle, preferably in the middle of the seat.

4-55   Answer A

The Centers for Disease Control and Prevention recommend a physical examination within 2 weeks of arrival in the United States unless the child has a fever, vomiting, rash, or diarrhea. Four or six weeks would be too long a wait, and 72 hours would be too short a period of time.

4-56   Answer C

The Centers for Disease Control and Prevention recommends blood lead screening as part of routine health supervision for children at 12 months of age and again at 24 months of age. If a screening tool used results in all negative responses to all the questions, a child is considered at low risk for high doses of lead exposure but must receive a blood lead test at 12 months and 24 months of age.

4-57   Answer A

If medication is needed, the drug of choice for pregnant women with diabetes is insulin. Oral hypoglycemics such as glyburide, glipizide, and metformin should be avoided because they are all teratogenic. Diet remains the cornerstone of treatment for pregnant women with diabetes.

4-58   Answer C

NSAID use during pregnancy has been linked to pulmonary hypertension in newborns. Women commonly use these drugs during pregnancy. Other research studies have indicated a connection between NSAID use and an increased risk of miscarriage.

4-59   Answer C

The minimum age for administering the measles, mumps, and rubella immunization is 12 months. Children ages 2, 4, and 9 months are too young to receive the measles, mumps, and rubella immunization.

4-60   Answer C

Excessive iron intake during pregnancy may result in premature delivery and low-birth-weight babies. Healthy, nonanemic women who are planning to become pregnant should take 60 mg of iron once weekly and then double that dose to 120 mg weekly during pregnancy.

4-61   Answer D

Treatment for pinworms includes the entire household. Disinfecting the toilet and changing and washing underwear, bed linens, towels, clothes, and pajamas daily is recommended along with frequent hand washing and avoidance of scratching the infected area or placing fingers in the mouth.

4-62   Answer B

A pregnant woman is at risk for developing congenital rubella syndrome during the first 16 weeks of pregnancy. The risk of congenital rubella syndrome is related to the gestational age of the fetus at the time the pregnant woman is exposed to the infection. If the infection occurs 0–12 weeks after conception, there is a 51% chance the infant will be affected. If the infection occurs 13–26 weeks after conception, there is a 23% chance the infant will be affected. Infants are not generally affected if rubella is contracted during the third trimester, or 26–40 weeks after conception. Prenatal testing should be performed to determine if a woman is seronegative, in which case she should avoid anyone with a rash or viral illness.

4-63   Answer C

RhoGAM (Rh$_o$[D] immune globulin) should be administered when a D-negative mother has been given a transfusion of D-positive blood and whenever a potential for mixing Rh-positive fetal and Rh-negative maternal blood exists, such as with an abortion, ectopic pregnancy, amniocentesis, antepartum hemorrhage, fetal blood sampling, fetal death, or fetal surgery. If there is any doubt about whether or not to administer RhoGAM, it should be given.

4-64   Answer D

The biophysical profile (BPP) consists of the four parameters of fetal well-being—fetal tone, breathing, motion, and amniotic fluid volume—along with a nonstress test (NST). In high-risk pregnancies, the BPP is necessary for a comprehensive fetal assessment.

4-65   Answer B

Hegar's sign is softness of the uterus and ballottement at the isthmus. Other physiological signs of pregnancy are Chadwick's sign (cervical blueness), Goodell's sign (cervical softness), and quickening (feeling fetal movement, usually at 18–22 weeks gestation).

4-66 Answer B

Patchy, white areas in the mouth of a breastfed infant are consistent with a diagnosis of oral candidiasis, or thrush. The mother may also have a candidiasis infection of the breast nipple or areola, which, if left untreated, may progress to mastitis. Neonatal *chlamydia* infections manifest as conjunctivitis or pneumonitis. Epstein's pearls are small white or yellow cystic papules (1–3 mm in size) typically seen on the roof of the mouth and filled with fluid. They occur in 65%–85% of newborns, are completely harmless, and do not require treatment because they spontaneously resolve over the first few weeks of life.

4-67 Answer B

Phenobarbital should be used with extreme caution because of the slow rate of barbiturate metabolism by the nursing infant. It may cause sedation. The pharmacologic activity of medications depends on absorption, distribution, metabolism, and elimination by the infant. When choosing medication for nursing mothers, many factors should be considered. A medication with the shortest half-life and highest protein-binding ability should be used as well as medications well studied in infants. Advise mothers to administer single daily-dose medications just before the longest sleep interval for the infant. Advise breastfeeding immediately before medication dose when multiple daily doses are needed. Also, use a drug reference source with recent updates.

4-68 Answer A

An incomplete abortion occurs when some portion of the products of conception (usually placental) remains in the uterus. Usually, only mild cramps are reported, but bleeding is persistent and often excessive. A threatened abortion occurs when there is bleeding or cramping but the pregnancy continues. The cervix is not dilated. An inevitable abortion occurs when the cervix is dilated. The membranes may be ruptured, but passage of the products of conception has not occurred. Bleeding and cramping persist and passage of the products of conception is considered inevitable. A missed abortion occurs when the pregnancy has ceased to develop, but the conceptus has not been expelled. There is no bleeding, but a brownish vaginal discharge is present. Usually no pain is involved. Symptoms of pregnancy disappear and the uterus becomes smaller and irregularly softened, with the adnexa being normal.

4-69 Answer C

A nonstress test examines fetal heart reactivity in response to fetal movement. The criterion for a reactive test is the presence of at least two fetal heart-rate accelerations of at least 15 beats in amplitude and lasting at least 15 seconds in response to fetal movement during a 20-minute testing window. The relationship between uterine contraction and fetal heart response is the basis of a contraction stress test.

4-70 Answer C

The value-belief functional health pattern includes the following questions to be asked during the family assessment: Does the family generally get things it wants out of life? What are the important things for the future? Are there any "rules" in the family that everyone believes are important? What role does religion play in the family? There are 11 different functional health patterns that are applicable to the assessment of families, as well as individuals: health perception/health management, nutritional-metabolic, elimination, activity-exercise, sleep-rest, cognitive-perceptual, self-perception–self-concept, role-relationship, sexuality-reproductive, coping-stress tolerance, and value-belief. These guidelines provide information on family functioning that will assist the provider in setting goals with the family.

4-71 Answer A

Lindane is an organochloride. The American Academy of Pediatrics (AAP) no longer recommends it as a pediculocide. Although Lindane shampoo is approved by the FDA for the treatment of head lice, it is not recommended as a first-line therapy. Overuse, misuse, or accidentally swallowing Lindane can be toxic to the brain and other parts of the nervous system. Nix and Rid are common over-the-counter products. Ovide requires a prescription.

4-72 Answer C

Bishop's score is an assessment of the cervix's readiness for elective induction. Leopold's maneuvers are used to determine fetal position. The multiparameter evaluation following a nonreactive nonstress test is a biophysical profile. A lethicin/sphignomyelin (L/S) ratio is used to evaluate fetal lung maturity.

4-73   Answer A

To obtain the daily calcium intake recommended during pregnancy, a woman should consume at least 1 quart of cow's milk per day. Calcium must be supplemented during pregnancy to meet fetal needs and preserve maternal calcium stores. Milk is relatively inexpensive, and 1 quart of cow's milk contains 1 g of calcium, which is almost the 1.2 g recommended daily during pregnancy. The milk can be in forms other than liquid, such as in custards. However, caution your client that large quantities of milk, meat, cheese, and dicalcium phosphate (a supplement) may cause excessive phosphorus levels, which may result in leg cramps. If a woman is lactose intolerant, as in the case of many Native Americans, foreign-born African Americans, and certain Asians, protein, calcium, and vitamins must be supplied in other forms.

4-74   Answer D

Pregnancy is a hypercoagulable state, which increases the risk of clot development and formation of an embolism. The sudden onset of chest pain and shortness of breath is consistent with a pulmonary embolism. Because of the life-threatening nature of a pulmonary embolism, it is the first entity that needs to be ruled out. A myocardial infarction and bacterial pneumonia would have a more gradual onset.

4-75   Answer A

A flat BBT graph indicates lack of ovulation. If ovulation were occurring, the BBT would rise 0.5°F–1.0°F 24–48 hours after ovulation.

4-76   Answer D

The low-risk client is seen every 4 weeks until the 28th week of pregnancy. Between 28 and 34 weeks, the woman is seen every 2 weeks. After 34 weeks, she is seen weekly until delivery.

4-77   Answer B

After delivery, exercises to strengthen the muscles of the back, pelvic floor, and abdomen are advocated, but strenuous exercises should be postponed until about 3 weeks after delivery. This allows the abdominal muscles to partially regain their original length and tone and prevents undue client fatigue.

4-78   Answer B

Neonatal abstinence syndrome or drug withdrawal results in hyperstimulation of the infant's nervous system. Nursing care focuses on decreasing environmental and sensory stimulation during the period of withdrawal.

4-79   Answer C

The G in APGAR stands for grimace. The acronym APGAR helps in the assessment of the five components of a neonate's responses: appearance, pulse, grimace, activity, and respiration.

4-80   Answer C

The Denver Developmental Screening Test (DDST) does not include fearlessness as a behavior rating. The behavior ratings included on the DDST are fearfulness (on a rating of none, somewhat fearful, or very fearful), compliance with examiner's requests (on a rating of complies, usually complies, rarely complies), alertness (on a rating of interest in surroundings: alert, somewhat alert, or seriously disinterested), and attention span (on a rating of attentive, somewhat distractible, and very distractible).

4-81   Answer B

Anemia is the most common problem. Vitamin K, C, and A deficiencies are uncommon. All nutrient deficiencies should be identified before pregnancy if possible and corrected.

4-82   Answer D

The presumptive symptom of pregnancy that involves tingling or frank pain of the breasts is called mastodynia. Mastodynia (breast tenderness) may range from tingling to frank pain and is caused by hormonal responses of the mammary ducts and alveolar system. Similar symptoms may also occur just before menses. Other presumptive symptoms, or early manifestations of pregnancy, are as follows. Montgomery's tubercles (enlargement of the circumlacteal sebaceous glands of the areola) occur at 6–8 weeks' gestation and are caused by hormonal stimulation. Colostrum secretion is a symptom that may begin after 16 weeks' gestation. Melasma (the mask of pregnancy) is darkening of the skin over the forehead, bridge of the nose, or cheekbones and is most marked in women with dark complexions. It usually occurs after 16 weeks' gestation and is more prevalent in women who spend a lot of time in the sun.

4-83   Answer D

This is characteristic of the searching and yearning phase. The parent yearns for the deceased infant, is preoccupied with thoughts of the lost child, and may have physical manifestations such as aching arms, hearing the infant's cry, or looking for the infant.

4-84   Answer D

Characteristics of trisomy 21 (Down syndrome) include hypotonia, simian creases, epicanthial folds, and Brushfield spots. Findings of low birth weight, small jaw and recessed chin, muscle rigidity, and short sternum are consistent with a diagnosis of Edwards' syndrome (trisomy 18). Patau syndrome is indicated by the presence of a cleft lip and palate, polydactyly, malformed ears, and absence of the iris. Clinical findings of lymphedema of the hands and feet, webbed neck, coarctation of the aorta, and urinary tract abnormalities are indicative of Turner's syndrome.

4-85   Answer B

If a primary infection of genital herpes simplex occurs early in a pregnancy, a spontaneous abortion may result. Primary infection or a recurrence later in a pregnancy is not associated with an increase in pregnancy loss or fetal malformation. Before the initiation of labor, a woman who has a history of genital herpes simplex should have a thorough inspection of the vulva and lower genital tract. If active lesions are found, a cesarean section should be performed.

4-86   Answer B

G5P4015 written on the client's chart indicates that the woman has been pregnant five times (G for gravidity or total number of pregnancies), had four delivery experiences (P for parity or birth [alive or dead] of an infant or infants weighing more than 500 g; multiple gestation is counted as a single occurrence), and had one abortion. Because she has five living children, she must have had a set of twins because one of the pregnancies ended in an abortion. An abortion is a pregnancy that terminates before the 22nd gestational week or in which the fetus weighed less than 500 g. Another way to remember this is to think of FPAL (Florida Power and Light) as the four numbers following P. The first number (F) stands for full-term births (with multiple gestation counted as a single occurrence), P for premature births (preemies),

A for abortions, and L for the number of living children.

4-87   Answer C

The management of asthma in pregnant women differs little from management in nonpregnant women. Beta-2 agonists, theophylline, epinephrine, cromolyn, and glucocorticoids are all safe to use. Whenever possible, inhalation rather than oral medications should be used. During exacerbations, IV and oral glucocorticoids may be used in the usual manner. Typically, asthma during pregnancy follows the one-third rule: One-third of the women have improved symptoms; one-third have no change; and one-third have worse symptoms.

4-88   Answer A

An infant with dysmorphic facial features, including short palpebral fissures, a thin upper lip, an elongated and flattened philtrum, and a flattened midface region, has fetal alcohol syndrome (FAS). A diagnosis of FAS typically is warranted when a baby or child exhibits growth deficiency, the dysmorphic facial features, central nervous system effects, and a history of prenatal alcohol exposure. Maternal cocaine abuse may result in premature labor and delivery, lower birth weight, smaller head circumference, and decreased length at birth. Maternal smoking will result in a lower birth weight. High-intensity exercise programs result in decreased birth weight, whereas low- to moderate-intensity exercise programs may increase the birth weight.

4-89   Answer A

Maternity blues, sometimes called "baby blues," affect about 50%–70% of postpartum women. They are usually transient emotional disturbances that occur around the second to fourth postpartum day and may last from a few hours to several weeks. Postpartum depression, which affects about 10%–15% of postpartum women, is characterized by a depressed mood, irritability, fatigue, feelings of worthlessness, sleeping and eating changes, and changes in personality. It usually begins slowly and insidiously within 2–3 weeks after birth and may last up to a year. Postpartum psychosis, which affects about 1 or 2 of every 1,000 new mothers, is severely impaired ability to perform activities of daily living. Its onset is within a few weeks up to 3 months postpartum, with primiparas being at greater risk. Maternity blues, postpartum depression, and postpartum psychosis are three psychiatric disturbances that may occur during the puerperium. There is not a specific disorder named "postpartum anxiety disorder."

4-90   Answer B

Lesbian concerns include the loss of support from family, friends, and coworkers. Battering and physical, emotional, or financial abuses are possible in any relationship, and there are no boundaries regarding gender. However, a lesbian woman may not want others to be aware of her sexual preference because she may not be able to obtain needed help and counseling. HIV infection is possible in a casual lesbian relationship if one partner has used intravenous drugs or been in a relationship with an HIV-infected man or woman. In addition, women may exchange body fluids by using a dildo without a condom. If HIV infection is a concern, the health-care provider should counsel the women about safe sex practices. Other concerns of lesbian women relate to childbearing issues such as in vitro fertilization, donor sperm, who is the "real" mother, adoption issues, and custody issues.

4-91   Answer B

Recommendations from the American Academy of Pediatrics for sleep safety and SIDS risk reduction include putting the baby on his or her back for every sleep; sleeping on a firm surface with no soft objects, wedges, ruffles, blankets or bumper pads. Co-sleeping or bed sharing is not recommended.

4-92   Answer A

Ferritin has the highest sensitivity and specificity for diagnosing iron deficiency in anemic clients. Serum hemoglobin or hematocrit are the primary screening tests for identifying anemia. Venous hemoglobin is more accurate than capillary hemoglobin. A reticulocyte count is helpful to evaluate bone marrow function or to monitor marrow function and response to treatment.

4-93   Answer C

The antibiotic of choice for acute pyelonephritis occurring during the seventh month of pregnancy is ampicillin (Principen, Polycillin) because the most common offending pathogen is *Escherichia coli*. Ampicillin is safe for the mother and fetus and has minimal side effects. Earlier in the pregnancy, sulfonamides, nitrofurantoin, and cephalosporins

may be prescribed along with ampicillin. Nitrofurantoin should be avoided in the last trimester because it may induce hemolytic anemia in the newborn. Sulfa drugs must be avoided in mothers with glucose-6-phosphatase deficiency and are best avoided late in pregnancy because of the increased likelihood of neonatal hyperbilirubinemia. Trimethoprim is a folic acid antagonist; therefore, trimethoprim-sulfamethoxazole should be avoided in pregnancy.

4-94   Answer B

Infant car seats should be placed facing backward until the infant weighs 18–20 lb and is able to sit up well. Infant car seats should also be placed in the rear seat of the car, preferably in the middle of the seat.

4-95   Answer B

Potentially fatal hepatic necrosis is a dose-dependent adverse effect of acetaminophen overdose. The maximum recommended number of daily doses and duration of the use of acetaminophen for pain (other than sore throat) in this age group is five doses per day and 5 days. Sore throat should not be treated for more than 2 days without consulting a clinician because it may be the result of streptococcal infection. Acetaminophen should not be taken for fever for more than 3 days.

4-96   Answer A

According to Nagele's rule, the estimated date of delivery (EDD) can be figured by adding 7 days to the first day of the last normal menstrual period (LNMP) and then subtracting 3 months. If a woman's LNMP was September 23, her EDD would be June 30 (23 + 7 = 30; 9 − 3 = 6; = 6/30).

4-97   Answer C

The American Heart Association recommends two cups of milk (16 ounces) per day for a 1-year-old child. Intake of 8 or 12 ounces is not an adequate amount. Intake of 24 ounces exceeds the recommendation.

4-98   Answer B

The infant is showing signs of jaundice. Jaundice in an infant younger than 24 hours of age is often caused by Rh or ABO incompatibility. A direct Coombs' test will determine the presence of maternal antibodies in the baby's blood.

The other laboratory tests are not related to hyperbilirubinemia.

4-99   Answer A

H_2-receptor antagonists such as cimetidine can be prescribed for pregnant clients who have peptic ulcer disease. Ranitidine should not be used during the first trimester of pregnancy because of possible teratogenicity. Sucralfate should be avoided because it has not been adequately studied during pregnancy. Bellergal-S, an anticholinergic agent, contains phenobarbital and is contraindicated. Symptoms of peptic ulcer disease should be treated initially by avoidance of irritating foods and by antacids. Supportive advice may be given regarding cessation of smoking; eating small, bland meals; avoidance of stress; and so forth.

4-100   Answer B

Idiopathic scoliosis has a familial pattern. Pain associated with a curvature suggests an inflammatory or neoplastic etiology. With idiopathic scoliosis, the scapula are unequal. The majority of adolescents with idiopathic scoliosis have a right thoracic curve.

4-101   Answer A

Desmopressin acetate (DDAVP) is not recommended for primary nocturnal enuresis in children younger than 6 years. Desmopressin can cause a low level of sodium in the blood, which can be serious and possibly life threatening.

4-102   Answer C

After 28 weeks' gestation, when the woman is performing fetal movement counts (FMCs), 10 movements should be obtained in 2 hours. Usually, 10 movements are felt within 30 minutes, but 10 movements in 2 hours are considered acceptable. FMCs should be performed at the same time every day, preferably after a meal or when the fetus is most active. The woman should be lying in the left lateral position when doing the FMCs. If the woman senses decreased activity, a nonstress test (NST) or, at the very least, fetal surveillance should be initiated within 12 hours.

4-103   Answer D

Drowning is a major cause of death in toddlers. For children younger than age 3 years, bathtubs are the primary site of drowning. Toddlers should not be left unattended in the tub. They should also not be permitted to lean over the tub to play with water toys because they may fall in, hit their head, and not be able to get out. All swimming pools should be fenced in and have high latches on the gates. Children should be taught to swim as early as possible.

4-104   Answer C

Live-virus immunization products, such as yellow fever, measles, and rubella vaccines, are contraindicated in pregnant women. Pooled gamma globulin to prevent hepatitis A and chloroquine for malaria prophylaxis have been proved safe to administer to a pregnant woman. Inactivated polio vaccine (Salk) can be administered instead of the oral vaccine. If a woman has a normal, low-risk pregnancy, travel can be accomplished safely between the 18th and 32nd weeks. Commercial airlines have pressurized cabins that do not pose a threat to the fetus. It is not advisable to travel to endemic areas of yellow fever in Africa or Latin America or to areas of Africa or Asia where chloroquine-resistant falciparum malaria is a hazard because complications of malaria are more common in pregnancy.

4-105   Answer A

Von Willebrand's disease is the most common hereditary bleeding disorder, occurring in about 1% of the population. It is inherited as an autosomal dominant trait, so it is equally prevalent in men and women. Hemophilia is usually diagnosed during the first few years of life, and sickle cell anemia, if not diagnosed then, is usually diagnosed in childhood. Von Willebrand's disease is usually not diagnosed until after a severe hemorrhagic episode following surgery, trauma, dental procedures, or childbirth. Clients with von Willebrand's disease should be referred to a hematologist for coagulation studies. The treatment goal is to prevent bleeding or achieve hemostasis. Treatment depends on the severity of the disease and may range from intranasal desmopressin acetate spray (DDAVP nasal spray) to replacement of factor VIII or blood transfusions.

4-106   Answer C

Low-dose aspirin is continued until no evidence of coronary change is found by 6–8 weeks. Administration of aspirin is continued indefinitely in children who develop coronary abnormalities.

4-107 Answer B

Flexing the hips and knees at a 90° angle in an infant and attempting to slip the femur heads onto the posterior tip of the acetabulums by lateral pressure of the thumbs and by rocking the knees medially with the knuckles of the index fingers is known as Barlow's test. A palpable or audible hip click is not normally heard. With Barlow's test, the action is up and back like a piston. You are testing for normal hip movement. With Ortolani's maneuver, you are also testing for normal hip movement, but the action is to abduct: up and out. You flex the knees and hips, placing fingers bilaterally on the greater trochanters, thumbs gripping the medial aspect of femurs, then adduct and abduct. There is a positive jerking motion as the femur passes over the acetabulum. Very frequently, hip "clicks" are an indication for radiographic or orthopedic consultations. As in adults, clicks are caused by the movement of articular and periarticular parts, but the "clunks" attending subluxation and rearticulation are easily felt and often even grossly visible. There is no Spock's test. The Moro (startle) reflex is elicited by physical shocks and sudden changes in support of the infant.

4-108 Answer A

Seasonal influenza vaccine is produced in large quantities for annual immunization campaigns. Some of the vaccine is produced in multidose vials and contains thimerosal to safeguard against possible contamination of the vial once it is opened. The single-dose units are made without thimerosal as a preservative because they are intended to be used only once. The nasal spray vaccine is produced in single-dose units and does not contain thimerosal.

4-109 Answer D

Innocent murmurs are usually grade I-II/VI, change with position, and are musical or vibratory in quality. Pathologic murmurs are diastolic.

4-110 Answer B

The most often cited reason why women who have had a usual length of stay after normal delivery discontinue breastfeeding before 8 weeks postpartum is the perception that the infant is not receiving enough milk. The other reasons, in descending order, are the mother's return to work or school, ease of formula use, maternal or infant illness, infant liking the bottle better, and breast pain. This is important to know when teaching new mothers about the benefits of breastfeeding and what to expect.

4-111 Answer B

The treatment for oral candidiasis is Nystantin. A vinegar and water solution is used to rinse the breast nipples between feedings. Fluconazole is used for ductal candidiasis infection of the breast. Candidiasis is a fungal infection; therefore, antibiotics are not effective as a treatment.

4-112 Answer C

In the United States, acute otitis media (AOM) is the most common affliction necessitating medical therapy for children younger than 5 years. Omnicef is indicated for individuals who are penicillin-sensitive. Amoxicillin or Trimox is the drug of choice for AOM but is not appropriate for Tayla because of her penicillin sensitivity. Augmentin is not indicated because of her penicillin sensitivity.

4-113 Answer A

An avulsed tooth should be replanted as soon as possible. If the tooth is dirty, rinse it gently with cold milk, saline, or room temperature water, then replant it. Do not rub the root surface. If unable to replant, the tooth can be kept in cold milk, saline, or room temperature water and wrapped in plastic wrap to prevent dehydration. The prognosis for successful reimplantation decreases with time.

4-114 Answer D

HPV vaccination is not recommended for use in pregnant women. The vaccine is indicated for all teenagers (males and females) at age 11–12. Women who are lactating or immunocompromised may receive the vaccination.

4-115 Answer C

Angelman syndrome is characterized by development delay, lack of speech, seizures, walking and balance disorders, and a happy demeanor characterized by frequent smiling, laughter and excitability.

Cornelia deLange syndrome (CdLS) includes thin eyebrows; long eyelashes; a short, upturned nose; and thin, down-turned lips. Other characteristics include low birth weight, slow growth, small stature, and small head size. Medical issues include gastroesophageal reflux disease, heart defects, seizures, feeding difficulties, vision and hearing loss. Limb differences, behavioral issues, and developmental delays often exist. Prader-Willi syndrome typically causes low muscle tone, short stature, incomplete sexual development, and a chronic feeling of hunger that, coupled with a metabolism that utilizes drastically fewer calories than normal, can lead to excessive eating and life-threatening obesity. Flat-head syndrome refers to babies with misshapen heads from lying on their backs too long. They may be at heightened risk for developmental delays.

4-116   Answer C

About 20%–30% of children with an autism spectrum disorder (ASD) develop epilepsy by the time they reach adulthood. Males are four times more likely to have ASD than females. Twin and family studies strongly suggest that some people have a genetic predisposition to ASD. About 40% of people with ASD have average to above average intellectual abilities.

4-117   Answer C

Mongolian spots (congenital dermal melanocytosis) are poorly defined, flat, blue to blue-black lesions. They are usually found on the trunk and buttocks of the newborn but may occur anywhere. Mongolian spots are common in Asians and blacks. A biopsy reveals dermal melanocytes. They are usually asymptomatic, may fade with age, and do not require treatment. Some blue or blue-black macules that are acquired and not present at birth include blue nevus, a drug-induced blue macule, and malignant melanoma. A blue nevus usually occurs in an adolescent or adult and is asymptomatic. A biopsy reveals dermal melanocytes, and there is usually an excision of the macule for cosmesis or concern about melanoma. A drug-induced blue macule most commonly occurs on sun-exposed areas of the body when the person takes phenothiazines, chloroquine, hydroxychloroquine, gold, minocycline, or silver-containing medications, as well as some others. A biopsy reveals increased melanin and deposition of the drug. There is very slow fading with time, and usually the focal lesions are removed surgically. Malignant melanomas may be assessed using the ABCDs: A for asymmetry (melanomas tend to be asymmetrical), B for border irregularity (the border of a melanoma lesion tends to be irregular), C for color (a melanoma is usually multicolored, blue-black, or black-brown), and D for diameter (a melanoma is usually greater than 6 mm in diameter).

4-118   Answer C

Fetal heart tones can be heard with a conventional fetoscope at 18–20 weeks' gestation. At 7–8 weeks' gestation, a transabdominal ultrasound will show fetal heart movement. At 10–12 weeks' gestation, fetal heart tones can be heard with a Doppler stethoscope. At 20 or more weeks' gestation, fetal movements can be felt by the examiner.

4-119   Answer C

Spalding's sign is overriding (overlapping) of the fetal cranial bones, as seen on ultrasound. It is a result of the decreased tissue turgor that occurs after fetal death. Chadwick's sign is a deep blue-violet color of the cervix and vagina due to increased vascularity and is a presumptive sign of pregnancy around the fourth week of gestation. Piskacek's sign is a palpable lateral (asymmetrical) bulge or soft prominence where the uterine tube meets the uterus around the seventh to eighth week of gestation. A Homan's sign of eliciting pain when dorsiflexing the foot is indicative of a deep vein thrombosis (DVT).

4-120   Answer B

If a woman is breastfeeding and complains of constant tenderness of the nipples, suggest that she apply dry heat to the nipples between feedings. A common symptom during the first days of breastfeeding, tenderness of the nipples usually begins when the baby starts to suck and then subsides as soon as the milk begins to flow. If maternal tissues are unusually tender, dry heat usually helps. Ice tends to increase nipple tenderness. Nipple shields should be used only as a last resort because they interfere with normal sucking. If it is necessary to wear nipple shields, suggest glass or plastic shields with rubber nursing nipples rather than all-rubber shields. This is a temporary problem that can be resolved. Stopping breastfeeding for a temporary problem is an irreversible solution.

4-121   Answer B

The woman with hyperemesis gravidarum is anxious about the effect of her condition on the fetus. The etiology of hyperemesis is unknown, but the incidence is associated with conditions of elevated hCG levels, such as pregnancy. Although there may be an emotional component, there is no indication that the pregnancy is unwanted. With appropriate treatment and support, the fetal prognosis is favorable. Because of the excessive vomiting, a nursing diagnosis focused on nutrition would be Imbalanced Nutrition, Less Than Body Requirements.

Bibliography

American Diabetes Association: Standards of medical care in diabetes—2011. *Diabetes Care* 34:S15, 2011.

Dunphy, LM, et al: *Primary Care: The Art and Science of Advanced Practice Nursing*, ed 3. FA Davis, Philadelphia, 2011.

Gerding, R: Kawasaki disease: A review. *Journal of Pediatric Health Care* 25(6): 379–387, 2011.

Kennedy, MS: New evidence on vitamins, minerals, and pregnancy. *American Journal of Nursing* 107(2):19, February 2007.

March of Dimes. Folic acid. http://www.marchofdimes.com/pregnancy/folicacid_before.html, accessed 11/26/11.

Moon, RY, and Task Force on Sudden Infant Death Syndrome: SIDS and other sleep-related infant deaths: expansion of recommendations for a safe infant sleeping environment. *Pediatrics* 128(5):1341–1367, November 2011. http://pediatrics.aappublications.org/content/128/5/e1341.full, accessed 12/22/11.

National Center on Birth Defects and Developmental Disabilities (Centers for Disease Control and Prevention) et al.: *Fetal Alcohol Syndrome: Guidelines for Referral and Diagnosis*. Department of Health and Human Services, Atlanta, GA, 2005. http://www.cdc.gov/ncbddd/fasd/documents/fas_guidelines_accessible.pdf, accessed on 11/11/11.

National Institutes of Health, Office of Dietary Supplements: Folate. http://ods.od.nih.gov/factsheets/folate, accessed on 11/26/11.

Steinhorn, R., Berger, S: Persistent newborn pulmonary hypertension. http://emedicine.medscape.com/article/898437-overview#a1, accessed on 12/21/12.

U.S. Food and Drug Administration: Public health advisory: FDA recommends that over-the-counter (OTC) cough and cold products not be used for infants and children under 2 years of age. http://www.fda.gov/drugs/drugsafety/postmarketdrugsafetyinformationforpatientsandproviders/drugsafetyinformationforheathcareprofessionals/publichealthadvisories/ucm051137, accessed 12/22/12.

U.S. Preventive Services Task Force: Screening for iron deficiency anemiaincluding iron supplementation for children and pregnant women. http://www.uspreventiveservicestaskforce.org/uspstf06/ironsc/ironrs.htm, accessed 11/10/11.

Wilton, G, and Plane, M: The family empowerment network: a service model to address the needs of children and families affected by fetal alcohol spectrum disorders. *Pediatric Nursing* 32(4):299–306, 2006.

How well did you do?

85% and above, congratulations! This score shows application of test-taking principles and adequate content knowledge.

75%–85%, keep working! Review test-taking principles and try again.

65%–75%, hang in there! Spend some time reviewing concepts and test-taking principles and try the test again.

Chapter 5: *Growth and Development*

Marcia R. Gardner
Lynne M. Dunphy

Questions

5-1   At what age would a child be expected to remember a string of six numbers and repeat them backward?

A. 3 years

B. 6 years

C. 9 years

D. 12 years

5-2   The diet of a healthy nondiabetic older adult female is based on which guidelines?

A. Energy needs are 2,500–3,000 kcal/day.

B. 5–10% of calories should come from fats, especially monounsaturated fats.

C. 20–30% of calories should come from protein sources.

D. Calcium requirements decrease after age 70.

5-3   Nine-year-old Mark is a highly active child with limited self-control. He is easily distracted and has difficulty staying on task and working toward a goal. You determine that he should have a neurodevelopmental evaluation because he is showing signs of

A. ADHD.

B. dyslexia.

C. autism.

D. impaired hearing.

5-4   Developmental tasks of early adulthood (ages 20–45) include which of the following?

A. Psychological separation from parents and developing a capacity for intimacy with a partner

B. Starting a family

C. Achieving desired performance in a career

D. Graduating from college or a vocational school

5-5   Cyndy is 5 years old and cannot understand how the half-cup of vegetables on her plate is the same amount as the half-cup of vegetables in the saucepan. According to Piaget, she is at which stage of cognitive development?

A. Preoperational

B. Sensorimotor

C. Formal operations

D. Concrete operations

5-6   What is the first male secondary sexual characteristic to emerge?

A. Testicular enlargement

B. Growth of axillary and pubic hair

C. Growth of facial and chest hair

D. Deepening of the voice

5-7   Which theory of aging focuses on older adults' development of specific strategies to manage losses of function over time?

A. Disengagement theory

B. Activity/developmental task theory

C. Person-environment fit theory

D. Selective optimization with compensation theory

5-8   A 2-year-old is brought to the clinic for his annual exam. His mother tells you that he can speak approximately 5–10 single words but that she can understand what the child is saying only 25% of the time. To make his needs known, he typically resorts to gesturing rather than trying to use words. He appears to understand half of her commands. The child does not live in a bilingual household. Which steps are indicated?

A. Conduct an ear examination with pneumatic otoscopy and refer to audiology/speech clinic for evaluation.

B. After a normal ear examination with a pneumatic otoscopy, reevaluate the child in 6 months.

C. Treat with an antibiotic for presumptive chronic otitis media with effusion.

D. Give the child an articulation screening examination.

5-9   *Fine motor coordination improves during the middle childhood years. A person's ability to manipulate objects reaches adult capacity by which age?*

A. 6 years

B. 9 years

C. 12 years

D. 21 years

5-10   *As people age, they try to maintain previous lifestyles that have contributed to their personalities. This is an example of*

A. activity theory.

B. continuity theory.

C. disengagement theory.

D. age stratification theory.

5-11   *Sleep in older adults is characterized by which pattern?*

A. Increased time spent in REM sleep

B. Increased overall sleep time

C. Increased sleep latency

D. Increased proportion of deep sleep

5-12   *What is the term used when the last child leaves home, either for school or to move out on his or her own?*

A. Longed-for freedom

B. Silent guilt

C. Empty nest

D. Abandonment

5-13   *Adolescent thinking is egocentric, and adolescents sometimes perceive that they are the focus of everyone else's attention. This has been called the*

A. imaginary audience.

B. personal fable.

C. invulnerable self.

D. ego ideal.

5-14   *While assessing the skin of an infant, you note café-au-lait spots. Which disease should be ruled out?*

A. Tuberous sclerosis

B. Neurofibromatosis

C. Sturge-Weber syndrome

D. Fetal alcohol syndrome

5-15   *At what age does a child usually develop the ability to mentally reverse actions that have been completed?*

A. 2 years

B. 4 years

C. 6 years

D. 10 years

5-16   *Delayed development can be the result of malnutrition from a deficiency of protein, calories, or both. This is referred to as protein energy malnutrition, kwashiorkor, or*

A. protein-wasting disease.

B. hypermetabolic disease.

C. cachexia.

D. marasmus.

5-17   *Middle-aged persons who still have responsibilities for their children's care and are now caring for their own aging parents are sometimes said to*

A. have institutional guilt syndrome.

B. have the "full-nest" syndrome.

C. be in the "sandwich" generation.

D. be members of Generation X.

5-18   *The body and the senses typically reach their peak during which stage of life?*

A. Adolescence

B. Early adulthood

C. Middle adulthood

D. Late adulthood

5-19   *The tasks of middle adulthood include all of the following except*

A. affiliating with one's age group.

B. accepting and adjusting to the physical changes of middle age.

C. reviewing and redirecting career goals.

D. achieving desired performance in a career.

5-20   Jon, age 13, has some enlargement of the scrotum and testes, a reddened scrotal sac, and some hair texture alteration, but his penis is not enlarged. He is in Tanner stage

A. I.

B. II.

C. III.

D. IV.

5-21   Justin, age 18 months, crosses his legs when lifted from behind rather than pulling them up. His legs are also hard to separate, making diaper changing difficult. He persistently uses only one hand. What condition do you suspect?

A. Cerebral palsy

B. Mild hydrocephalus

C. Mild spinal cord defect (spina bifida occulta)

D. Fetal alcohol syndrome

5-22   You are examining a 58-year-old man who complains of recent onset of erectile dysfunction (ED). The approach to his concern should be guided by which principle?

A. There are multiple physical conditions associated with the development of ED.

B. Almost all men will develop ED by the time they reach their 60s.

C. Most ED is caused by hormonal imbalance

D. ED is correlated with the development of benign prostatic enlargement

5-23   Common medications for treating ADHD include

A. aminophylline and antihistamines.

B. methylphenidate, amphetamine, and their derivatives.

C. amphetamines and Accutane.

D. codeine and Valium.

5-24   Victoria's mother brings her for her 1-year checkup. As you are weighing her, you remember that at 1 year, her weight should be

A. twice her birth weight.

B. triple her birth weight.

C. four times her birth weight.

D. at least 25 pounds.

5-25   Which tooth is the first to erupt in an infant?

A. A lower central incisor

B. A lower lateral incisor

C. Lower canine

D. Upper lateral incisor

5-26   Which one of the following is a normal physiological change of aging?

A. A decrease in strength and speed of muscle contraction in the extremities

B. Degenerative arthritis

C. Rheumatoid arthritis

D. Bulging intervertebral disks

5-27   Johnny, age 3, is at the clinic for his well-child visit. He has trouble removing his own shirt as requested. His mother yanks off his shirt after smacking his wrist and saying, "You must do as you're told—quickly." Which action is indicated?

A. Ignore the behavior because both Johnny and his mother are probably nervous about being there.

B. Tell the mother that Johnny's behavior is perfectly normal.

C. Observe Johnny for signs of child abuse.

D. Report the mother to child protective services.

5-28   To best help parents foster social-emotional development in their preschooler, age 4, you advise them to

A. give instructions rather than choices to the child.

B. set strict limits for behavior and quickly discipline for misbehavior.

C. provide frequent opportunities to interact with other children.

D. ask questions that direct the child to think about how others are feeling.

5-29   A 6-year-old would most likely view a friend as

A. someone to share enjoyable activities with.

B. someone who has the traits that satisfy the child's needs and wants.

C. someone to share loyalty with.

D. someone to be intimate with.

5-30   *According to Piaget, the ability to develop abstract thinking occurs during which stage of life?*

A. Early childhood

B. Middle school age

C. Adolescence

D. Early adulthood

5-31   *Older adults face greater risks for fluid imbalance than young and middle adults due to which age-related factor?*

A. Increased amounts of intracellular fluid and total body water

B. Higher proportion of fat to muscle cells

C. Faster speed of metabolism

D. Increased intestinal motility

5-32   *David, a new father, expresses his concern that his newborn son does not smile at him when he talks to him. What do you tell him?*

A. "True social smiles usually do not emerge until 4–9 weeks of age."

B. "Continue to watch his response so we can be certain that he is seeing."

C. "Babies usually have a preference for the mother's face. That's probably why he doesn't smile at you."

D. "This may just be his personality."

5-33   *Developmental tasks of adolescence include which of the following?*

A. Searching for one's identity and growing independent from parents

B. Graduating from high school

C. Learning to establish meaningful relationships with siblings

D. Engaging in community service projects to assist acceptance into college

5-34   *Which of these language behaviors would be cause for concern at a primary care visit?*

A. A 1-year-old cannot say more than two words with meaning.

B. An 18-month-old uses unintelligible jargon and has only a few words that are intelligible to family members.

C. A 2-year-old uses only two- to three-word sentences.

D. A 3-year-old does not use three- to five-word sentences.

5-35   *Male reproductive system changes during middle and later adulthood result in which manifestation?*

A. Slight decrease in sperm production

B. Testicular enlargement

C. Decrease in estrogen-like hormone production

D. Stable levels of testosterone

5-36   *Why are younger children more predisposed to acute otitis media than older children?*

A. They are more susceptible to the new bacteria that they encounter.

B. Their eustachian tubes are more flaccid and more horizontal than those of older children.

C. They have more viral infections, which precipitate otitis infections.

D. They have more allergies, which are a frequent cause of serous otitis media.

5-37   *Debbie is developing self-assertion, spontaneity, self-sufficiency, direction, and purpose as her mother encourages, reassures, and cheers her on. Which of Erikson's stages of ego development best characterizes Debbie?*

A. Trust versus mistrust

B. Autonomy versus shame and doubt

C. Initiative versus guilt

D. Industry versus inferiority

5-38   *Susie is 18 months old and does not seem the least bit interested in being toilet trained. What do you tell her mother?*

A. Susie's behavior is typical, because most children are not ready for toilet training until age 2.

B. The majority of children Susie's age have started showing readiness behaviors related to toilet training by this age.

C. She can use reinforcement conditioning to discipline Susie whenever she soils her diapers and reward her when she stays dry.

D. She should have Susie spend time around other toddlers who are toilet trained so that she can learn from them.

5-39   Mrs. Groome calls the clinic to say she is distressed that her 3-month-old baby is still not sleeping through the night. Your best response to her would be

A. "At this age infants are typically sleeping at least 10 hours at night without waking."

B. "It may be helpful to give some rice cereal right before bedtime, because she probably is waking up at night due to hunger."

C. "The length of sleep for young babies is variable, but most sleep through the night by the end of the first year."

D. "Babies never sleep through the night until they are at least 6 months old."

5-40   Infants, born at term, are expected to sit well without support by what age?

A. 1–2 months

B. 3–4 months

C. 5–6 months

D. 7–8 months

5-41   A 14-year-old girl's BMI is plotted between the 85th and 95th percentiles. Based on developmental characteristics, which strategy is best to use when educating her about self-care changes that are needed?

A. Emphasize the benefits of diet and activity changes that she identifies as most important.

B. Describe the relationship between current health choices and later health risks.

C. Encourage her parents to share their recent experiences with weight management.

D. Tell her frankly that her weight is too high, and she must make changes to decrease risks for developing chronic illness like diabetes.

5-42   While assessing the eyes of baby Thomas, you observe inner canthal folds and Brushfield spots. What do you suspect?

A. Trisomies

B. Turner's syndrome

C. Down syndrome

D. Neurofibromatosis

5-43   Beginning at about age 55, most people can expect which of the following changes?

A. A 1- to 2-in. decline in height

B. Stable body weight

C. Sharper vision and hearing

D. Increased strength

5-44   Which cardiac finding can be normal in children and young adults?

A. Third heart sound (S_3)

B. Fourth heart sound (S_4)

C. Ejection click

D. Diastolic murmur

5-45   At what age should a normally developing child be able to use a pincer grasp and pick up small cereal pieces, raisins, and finger foods?

A. 2–3 months

B. 5–6 months

C. 9–10 months

D. 12–14 months

5-46   Self-actualization is the goal of personality development for which of the following theories?

A. Peck's expansion of Erikson's theory

B. Maslow's hierarchy of human needs

C. Jung's theory of individualism

D. Erikson's eight stages of life

5-47   Suzanne's 8-year-old daughter, Natasha, has attention deficit-hyperactivity disorder (ADHD). She asks if Natasha will "outgrow" her ADHD. You respond,

A. "Yes; when they become young adults, most children outgrow the problem."

B. "No; unfortunately, Natasha will have this for the rest of her life."

C. "No, but there are many treatments available that we need to start now."

D. "About 50% or more of affected children will continue to have some difficulty as adolescents and adults."

5-48   *Fragile X syndrome is usually diagnosed when a child*

A.   is a newborn.
B.   begins to walk.
C.   is past the toddler stage.
D.   begins puberty.

5-49   *At what age/stage of development would you expect a boy to reach his adult height?*

A.   One year after the enlargement of the testicles
B.   When his voice changes
C.   By the time he is 17
D.   He may continue to grow past his teenage years.

5-50   *Hattie, age 6, appears to be masturbating when she rubs herself back and forth against the rug. Her mother asks you for advice because she believes masturbation may cause emotional problems and blindness. What is your best response?*

A.   "Masturbation causes no physical, sexual, or mental problems."
B.   "Stop her now because she may progress to other sexual behaviors."
C.   "There is no research to show that masturbation causes blindness."
D.   "Don't worry; Hattie will be fine."

5-51   *Which of the following is a result of changes in the cell-mediated immune function that occur from aging?*

A.   Fewer neutrophils, so older adults do not respond to local infections quickly
B.   Increases in autoantibodies as a result of altered immune function
C.   Fewer thrombocytes
D.   The pancytopenia of aging

5-52   *Amanda states that her baby will not go to bed without her bottle. You tell her that if the baby must have a bottle at night, it should be a bottle containing*

A.   formula.
B.   breastmilk.
C.   diluted juice.
D.   plain water.

5-53   *Marta, age 16, is not happy with the size of her breasts. She asks if her breasts will continue to enlarge. How do you respond?*

A.   "Full breast growth occurs around age 15."
B.   "No, this is probably the size your breasts will remain."
C.   "Your breasts will continue to develop until about age 18."
D.   "Your breasts will continue to develop until about age 20."

5-54   *Evaluating an older adult client according to the successful aging paradigm involves assessment of*

A.   cognition, problem-solving, physical skills, and memory.
B.   health, social engagement, mental activity, and life satisfaction.
C.   vision, hearing, balance, and strength.
D.   coping, social support, financial resources, and living arrangement.

5-55   *Children begin to develop real friendships at the age of*

A.   18 months.
B.   3 years.
C.   6 years.
D.   10 years.

5-56   *Photosensitivity of the epidermis increases in older adults due to which of the following normal developmental changes of aging skin?*

A.   Reduction of Langerhans cells
B.   Decrease in vitamin D synthesis
C.   Decrease in enzymatically active melanocytes
D.   Significant decrease in vascular supply

5-57   *Erikson's stage of intimacy versus isolation occurs between what ages?*

A.   12 and 16
B.   16 and 20
C.   20 and 30
D.   50 and 60

5-58 *Shannon, age 4 months, is waiting in the exam room with her mother. When you walk into the room, you expect Shannon to*

A. begin crying.

B. turn her head toward the sound of the door or your voice.

C. not notice you.

D. smile at you.

5-59 *The diagnosis of ADHD is made using which of these?*

A. Comparison of child's characteristics with criteria in the *Diagnostic and Statistical Manual of Mental Disorders*, 4th edition (DSM-IV-TR)

B. Blood assays demonstrating elevated lead levels

C. Identification of EEG abnormalities

D. Scores on the Connors Parent and Teacher rating scales

5-60 *Which of these infant characteristics is associated with readiness for the introduction of solid foods into an infant's diet?*

A. At least one tooth has emerged.

B. Extrusion reflex has faded.

C. Infant is at least 3 months of age.

D. Infant wants to nurse every 3–4 hours.

5-61 *Assessment of an adolescent using the HEADSS framework involves asking the teen about*

A. habits.

B. exercise.

C. school.

D. disabilities.

5-62 *Erikson's final ego stage in older adults occurs when successful resolution results in these adults feeling comfortable with their life choices and the knowledge that they would have done everything the same way again. What is this ego stage called?*

A. Generativity versus stagnation

B. Workaholism versus retirement

C. Success versus failure

D. Integrity versus despair

5-63 *Four-year-old Jamie believes that there is more juice in a tall, thin glass than in a shorter, wider one. Jamie has not yet achieved which of the principles of Piaget?*

A. Conservation

B. Object permanence

C. Formal operations

D. Abstract reasoning

5-64 *Your 66-year-old patient is able to correctly interpret the meaning of the proverb "a penny saved is a penny earned." This helps to establish the patient's expected ability to*

A. access long-term memory.

B. engage in abstract reasoning.

C. execute concrete operations.

D. follow complex instructions.

5-65 *Sally Ann is concerned that she cannot afford special walking shoes for her baby, who is beginning to pull himself up to his feet. What do you tell her?*

A. "High-top shoes are necessary to prevent any ankle injuries when your baby falls."

B. "Don't worry; special shoes are not necessary. The more flexible the shoe, the better."

C. "Try to keep him off of uncarpeted floors until you can obtain shoes."

D. "The sock-type booties you have are fine."

5-66 *In a game of hide-and-seek, 3-year-old Michael hides his face and believes that no one else can see him. This behavior is an example of*

A. conservation.

B. object permanence.

C. egocentric thought.

D. concrete operations.

5-67 *Jason is in first grade. His mother expresses concern because he pronounces the th sound as f. For instance, he says "free" for "three." You respond to his mother,*

A. "This is normal at his age."

B. "He may have a hearing problem and does not know how it should sound."

C. "You should correct him when he does this, or he will not learn the proper way to say it."

D. "He should be referred to a speech therapist for evaluation."

5-68   You are watching a baby play with a toy in the examining room. You move the toy and cover it with a cloth. The baby removes the cloth and reclaims the toy. This is an indication that the baby has achieved which of the following?

A. Object permanence

B. Conservation

C. Basic trust

D. Initiative

5-69   While examining a 12-month-old boy whose family recently immigrated to the United States from Mexico, you notice that his weight is in the 95th percentile and his height is in the 50th percentile. You begin to discuss the implications of maintaining a healthy weight, and the mother tells you that she is very proud of her son's size. Your response to her is guided by your understanding that

A. some cultures believe that a fat baby is a healthy baby.

B. she is probably overfeeding the baby to stop his crying.

C. she does not understand the nutritional value of foods.

D. the relationship of obesity to childhood health risks has not been explained to her.

5-70   Germaine, age 12 years, comes to see you for her checkup. After weighing her, you note that her BMI is at the 96th percentile on the National Center for Health Statistics graph. Your response to this will be guided by the knowledge that

A. her size is acceptable for her age, and you will continue to follow up weight during subsequent checkups.

B. she has been in a phase of rapid growth, and it will slack off within a year.

C. she is healthy but may be at risk for an eating disorder.

D. she is obese and at risk for hypertension and diabetes.

5-71   Sue takes her young son Michael to day care every day. He has begun to cry loudly and try to cling to her when she leaves. Michael is likely what age?

A. 4–5 months

B. 8–9 months

C. 12–15 months

D. 15–18 months

5-72   When does the onset of menses usually occur?

A. Between ages 10 and 11

B. Between ages 12 and 13

C. Between ages 14 and 15

D. Between ages 16 and 17

5-73   Donna is breastfeeding her 3-month-old infant exclusively. She expresses concern to you that the baby's growth seems to be slowing down, and she wonders if she should supplement the diet with other foods. What would be your response?

A. "You are probably not producing enough milk. Try introducing several tablespoons of rice cereal, in addition to breastfeeding, once each day."

B. "As long as you are well nourished, the baby will get what she needs. Her growth pattern is normal for an exclusively breastfed baby."

C. "Other foods are not needed now, but supplement breastfeeding by offering about eight ounces of formula each day."

D. "This indicates it is time to begin weaning from breast to bottle and to begin to introduce solid foods."

5-74   You suspect autism in the young child of a client of yours, but the client says the child is just shy. For a diagnosis of autism, you know the Diagnostic and Statistical Manual of Mental Disorders requires that three criteria be present. Which of these behaviors would lead the nurse practitioner to suspect autism in a young child?

A. Receiving immunizations that use thimerosal as adjuvants

B. Abnormal verbal and nonverbal communication

C. Reliance on an imaginary friend for all interactions by a preschooler

D. Inability of a newborn to track mother's face from left to right

5-75   Which age-related changes in the respiratory system make drugs like albuterol (Proventil) and salmeterol (Serevent) less effective in older adults?

A. The vital capacity of the lungs decreases.

B. Residual lung volume increases.

C. There is a decrease in cellular oxygen uptake in lung tissue.

D. There is a decrease in the number of beta receptors.

5-76   What is the major determinant of sexual activity in older adults?

A. Physical and mental health

B. Social sanctions

C. Religious beliefs

D. Age

5-77   Davy, age 4, is here for a well-child visit. To assess for age-appropriate fine motor skills, what activity would you ask him to perform?

A. Copy a circle.

B. Cut on a line with scissors.

C. String beads.

D. Copy a square.

5-78   The feature(s) of fragile X syndrome that should be evaluated during well-child examinations include

A. being easily overwhelmed by stimuli and language delays.

B. shorter linear growth.

C. increased frequency of ear infections.

D. difficulty swallowing.

5-79   Which strategy for care of older adults is inconsistent with an approach supportive of aging in place?

A. Make changes to the home environment that can accommodate an individual's changing needs.

B. Refer for home care and adult day-care services.

C. Hire assistants to help with activities of daily living.

D. Emphasize the individual's limitations and likely need for long-term care placement.

5-80   Physiologic changes of aging can affect functional mobility. Screening for functional mobility of older adults involves which screening tool?

A. Katz Index

B. Get Up and Go Test

C. Functional Independence Measure

D. Mini Mental State Exam

5-81   The mother of your 3-year-old client is concerned because the child stutters. What should your approach be?

A. Refer to a speech clinic for a full evaluation.

B. Refer to a pediatric neurologist.

C. Explain that this can be normal until 4 years of age.

D. Perform an articulation test on the child.

5-82   Risks for automobile accidents are increased in older adult drivers due to which normal changes associated with aging?

A. Decreased ability to understand the driving-related dangers

B. Lack of recognition of their own physical challenges

C. Magnified physiological response to stressful situations

D. Increased reaction time

5-83   A 6-year-old has just been diagnosed with attention deficit hyperactivity disorder. His parents report that he is doing poorly in school and is often disruptive in the classroom. They ask what they can do. Your best response is:

A. "Children usually outgrow a high activity level."

B. "Use a consistent approach with behavioral 'cues' both at home and at school."

C. "Medications are the only interventions that can help with ADHD."

D. "You can have him tested for food and environmental allergies."

5-84   *At what stage of sexual development should a boy expect to begin to have nocturnal emissions?*

A. When he starts to get facial hair

B. When his scrotal sac begins to darken in color

C. Approximately 6–12 months after his penis begins to enlarge

D. At 15 years of age, regardless of his sexual development

5-85   *You are examining a previously healthy 6-month-old who was delivered by cesarean section at 32 weeks' gestation. Examination reveals the presence of Moro, Babinski, and Landau reflexes. Which interpretation of findings is accurate?*

A. Findings are normal.

B. Findings suggest developmental delay.

C. Findings indicate persistence of primitive reflexes often associated with neurological dysfunction.

D. Findings are imprecise due to the infant's age.

5-86   *To determine your client's emotional and cognitive level of functioning when you are performing a mental status examination, you assess several individual behaviors. What is the term used when one ponders a deeper meaning beyond the concrete and literal?*

A. Thought process

B. Abstract reasoning

C. Consciousness

D. Perception

5-87   *Josephine, age 6, is just learning to hop on one foot. You know that*

A. she should have been able to do this at age 3.

B. she should have been able to do this at age 4.

C. she should have been able to do this at age 5.

D. this is a normal age-related activity for her.

5-88   *Which of these musculoskeletal changes accompany older adulthood?*

A. Change in stature

B. Increased stride length

C. Improved fine motor skill

D. Stretching of muscle fibers

5-89   *Jane, age 45, is having her annual physical. She wants to know when she can expect to go through menopause. Your response to her would be*

A. "You should not have any more periods after the age of 50."

B. "Most women begin having irregular periods in their late 40s, but age can range from 40–60."

C. "It is typical to complete the process of menopause at your age. I'm surprised you haven't gone through it yet."

D. "You should think about hormone replacement therapy now."

5-90   *Miranda is playing with clay and realizes that she can roll a lump of clay into a long snakelike shape and then return that snakelike shape to a lump. She is exhibiting cognitive development typical of which of Piaget's stages?*

A. Sensorimotor

B. Preoperational

C. Concrete operations

D. Formal operations

5-91   *You are examining 14-year-old Bobby. He tells you he is embarrassed to undress in the school locker room because his "chest is swollen." You observe very slight breast enlargement and palpate small subareolar disks of soft, slightly tender tissue bilaterally. There are no other significant findings. His BMI is between the 75th and 85th percentile for his age. He takes no medications, supplements, or other substances. Which response to Bobby's concern is indicated?*

A. "This is called gynecomastia. It is normal, and many boys develop it during early adolescence. It usually resolves on its own within a year or so."

B. "You do have some excess tissue on your chest. It's because of your weight. Once you lose some weight, the swelling will go away."

C. "It's due to a condition called precocious puberty and means puberty is a bit too early. It will be important to do some blood tests to check your hormones."

D. "Swollen breasts in boys need further evaluation to make sure there's nothing wrong. You will need to have some x-rays, imaging, and blood tests."

5-92   When assessing growth and development from a cross-cultural perspective, health-care providers need to be aware that

A. there may be differences in normal growth curves.

B. children with immigrant parents have a difficult time developing social relationships in their age groups.

C. cognitive development may be delayed if children live in a bilingual household.

D. children from Asian households have higher IQs than American children.

5-93   When an adolescent girl's breasts and areolae are enlarged and there is no contour separation, which Tanner stage is she in?

A. I

B. II

C. III

D. IV

5-94   At what age can a baby usually say two to three words with meaning?

A. 8 months

B. 10 months

C. 12 months

D. 24 months

5-95   After conducting the Tumbling E Snellen eye test on a verbal 4-and-a-half-year-old boy, you determine that his vision is 20/30 in both eyes. Your next step is to

A. refer to a pediatric ophthalmology clinic to be evaluated for glasses.

B. recheck vision at the next well-child exam.

C. notify the preschool he will be attending in the fall that he needs to be seated in the front of the classroom.

D. reevaluate the child's vision in 3 months.

5-96   Your 49-year-old female client reports that she has not had a menstrual period in 3 months. She uses contraception. She is experiencing occasional poor sleep, sweating, and flushing. She believes she is entering menopause. Which step is appropriate to take next?

A. Initiate calcium supplementation

B. Obtain pregnancy test results

C. Send blood samples for follicle-stimulating hormone (FSH) and estradiol levels

D. Refer for bone density test

5-97   Some psychologists have suggested that at the end of adolescence, a kind of thinking emerges that goes beyond logic to encompass interpretive and subjective thinking. What is this called?

A. Postformal thought

B. Mature thinking

C. Adult cognition

D. Ephemeral perception

5-98   The mother of your 12-year-old female client is concerned because all of her daughter's friends have started their periods, but her daughter has not. Upon physical exam, you note that her pubic hair and breast development are both at stage III (Tanner). Your next step should be to

A. refer to an endocrinologist.

B. start the girl on birth control pills to encourage her menses to start.

C. order bone age x-rays.

D. explain to the mother and child that this appears to be normal for this child.

5-99   Why is Alzheimer's disease (AD) considered a specific disease, distinct from the normal developmental changes of aging?

A. There are types of AD that are inherited and present before age 60.

B. There are changes in biological processes that occur with normal aging.

C. There is a notable decline in cognitive functioning as people age.

D. There are multiple changes in organ functioning, especially in the brain.

5-100   When performing a mental status examination, you should keep in mind the ABCTs. What does the C stand for?

A. Cognition

B. Consciousness

C. Capabilities

D. Conscience

5-101 *The benefits of exercise during middle adulthood include which of the following?*

A. Less need for an increase in dietary calcium

B. Slower decline in central nervous system processing

C. A delay in the onset of menopause in women

D. A delay in development of vision problems

5-102 *The statement that mature adults look beyond themselves and are concerned about more global issues is an example of which stage of Erikson's theory?*

A. Ego integrity versus despair

B. Ego differentiation versus work role preoccupation

C. Ego transcendence versus ego preoccupation

D. Generativity versus self-absorption

5-103 *A 75-year-old man comes to your office for concerns about memory loss. He is worried that he has Alzheimer's disease. Which finding in the patient would be cause for concern?*

A. Often misplaces his car and house keys

B. Has difficulty remembering some of the names of people he has recently met

C. Sometimes forgets the names of his children

D. Recalls the names of only seven of the nine medications he is currently taking

5-104 *By the end of the first year of life, normal infants demonstrate interest in an object that a caregiver points out. Absence of this behavior is associated with which disorder?*

A. Cerebral palsy

B. Deafness

C. Autism

D. Down syndrome

5-105 *The mother of a 2-year-old toddler is concerned about her child's frequent temper tantrums and asks how to decrease their frequency. To address her concern, you advise her to*

A. firmly tell the child "no" when a tantrum is beginning

B. place the child in a time out during every tantrum

C. talk with the child about appropriate ways to communicate anger or disappointment

D. try to avoid situations that tend to provoke tantrums such as hunger, fatigue, and frustration

5-106 *Jake, 8 years old, is brought in by his mother for evaluation of school problems. When he was 4 years old, his preschool teacher had expressed concern regarding his high activity level interfering with play with other children. Now, in third grade, he is underachieving in both math and reading. His teacher says that he constantly fidgets and bothers the other children. The school counselor has recommended that he be evaluated for attention deficit hyperactivity disorder (ADHD). Which question would provide important additional information regarding the possible diagnosis of ADHD?*

A. "How do you think his behavior compares to the other 8-year-olds you know?"

B. "How does his teacher handle his behavior in school?"

C. "What is he like at home?"

D. "Has anyone in your extended family had a diagnosis of ADHD?"

5-107 *At what age can the health-care provider stop measuring head circumference in normal, full-term children whose growth has been normal to this point?*

A. When head circumference reaches 40 cm

B. When the anterior fontanel begins to close

C. At 3 years of age

D. After 12 months of age

5-108 *When completing the health history and review of systems for a healthy 88-year-old woman, you would expect which age-related change to be reported?*

A. Mildly blurry vision

B. Chronically dry and itchy eyes and eyelids

C. Increasing presbyopia

D. Tearing and photophobia

5-109   *Jonathan, 2-and-a-half years of age, has come to see you because his mother says he has been very fussy and irritable. When you examine his ears, you note that the tympanic membrane is red and bulging. He has a fever at 102.2°F. You look at his record and notice he has had three episodes of acute otitis media within the past 6 months. You are concerned about this because*

A. children younger than 3 years of age with recurrent otitis media are at increased risk for impaired speech and language development.

B. children with opaque tympanic membranes are probably deaf.

C. the infection is highly likely to spread to the meninges.

D. he will not be able to be immunized for at least 6 months.

5-110   *Byron is 36 months old. His mother asks you what toys she should have for him to play with at home. Your suggestions to her could include*

A. blocks and simple shape puzzles with few pieces.

B. a tricycle and a Wiffle (lightweight) ball and bat.

C. pop beads and Matchbox cars.

D. a mobile and a cloth book.

5-111   *Daisy, age 2, has a "blankie" that she carries with her at all times. Her mother is concerned that if she does not get rid of it, Daisy will remain attached to this blanket forever. What do you tell her?*

A. "Yes, it is important to eliminate dependence on the blanket. Her attachment to it is also probably related to her thumb sucking."

B. "Children should be weaned from their favorite toy or blanket gradually so that going without it is not so traumatic."

C. "Not to worry. This normal attachment may last throughout the preschool years."

D. "Try to reason with the child that this habit needs to be broken."

5-112   *What is the most common inherited cause of mental retardation in children?*

A. Down syndrome

B. Fragile X syndrome

C. Meningomyelocele

D. Hydrocephalus

5-113   *Cross-cultural studies of Piaget's theory of cognitive development provide which of the following conclusions?*

A. The stages and sequence of cognitive development are universal.

B. The rate of physical growth has a positive influence on cognitive development.

C. Some cultural groups achieve the task of conservation earlier than American and European children.

D. Piaget's theory was concerned with the prediction of psychological rather than cognitive development.

5-114   *The parent of a newborn asks you about the relationship between the infant's development and early experiences. Which theory guides your response?*

A. Neurons and the connections among them continue to develop throughout early childhood.

B. The immature nervous system and brain imprint on early, repeated experiences in early childhood.

C. Inborn temperamental patterns have the largest influence on infant and early childhood development.

D. All of the sensory and perceptual capabilities are well developed at birth, priming newborns for multiple types of early childhood experiences.

5-115   *Because children are curious about sexual feelings and developmental changes in their bodies from the preschool years onward, education about these feelings and changes should begin during*

A. the first year of life.

B. the preschool years.

C. the school-age years.

D. adolescence.

5-116   *At what age can children use scissors successfully and fasten and unfasten simple buttons?*

A. 2 years

B. 3 years

C. 4 years

D. 5 years

5-117   Which cognitive change is expected in healthy older adults age 65 and older?

A. Decrease in IQ

B. Slower information processing

C. Low capacity for learning

D. Decreased attentional focus

5-118   You are performing a physical examination of a 3-year-old who is new to your clinic. Which finding requires immediate further evaluation?

A. Heart rate increases during inspiration and decreases during expiration

B. Has an equal A-P and transverse chest diameter

C. Can stand briefly on one foot but cannot skip and hop

D. Weight plots in the 50th percentile, while height plots at the 75th percentile

5-119   What is the approximate annual weight gain of a school-age child?

A. 1–3 lb

B. 3–5 lb

C. 5–7 lb

D. 7–9 lb

5-120   Preferring peer group activity over adult activities, conforming to group rules, using secret codes, and desiring acceptance are common at ages

A. 2–4.

B. 4–6.

C. 6–10.

D. 12–15.

5-121   During the school-age years (6–11), children usually grow how many inches annually?

A. ½ in.

B. 3 in.

C. 5 in.

D. 6–8 in.

5-122   According to the American Academy of Pediatrics, what is the earliest age that visual acuity screening in primary care practice should be included in the overall well-child assessment?

A. 3 years

B. 4 years

C. 5 years

D. Visual acuity screening is only valid if performed by an optometrist.

5-123   At birth, a baby's head circumference should

A. range from 40–42 cm.

B. measure about 2 cm greater than the chest circumference.

C. be 25% larger than the height and weight percentiles.

D. measure 25% smaller than the height and weight percentiles.

5-124   Sally, age 12, asks you when you think her periods will start. What do you tell her?

A. "They should have started by now."

B. "They will probably start any day now."

C. "There is a range of normal for girls from 11–16."

D. "It might not happen until you're 15."

5-125   Most children display a clear tendency for right- or left-handedness by what age?

A. 2 years

B. 4 years

C. 6 years

D. 12 years

5-126   The parent of Jorge, a 27-month-old, is concerned because Jorge insists on going through the same sequence of washing his hands and face, sitting at the table, and using the same cup at every meal and snack, even at the mall's food court. He cries or has a tantrum when it's not possible. Your response to his parent should be based on which rationale?

A. These are normal and expected behaviors for the age.

B. Behavior modification techniques can help quickly extinguish these behaviors.

C. A child should be able to be more adaptable at this developmental stage.

D. These behaviors suggest the child is having difficulty coping with change.

Answers

5-1   Answer D

Short-term memory improves significantly during middle childhood. By the beginning of the preschool period, children can remember and reverse a sequence of two numbers. By the beginning of adolescence, they can perform the task with as many as six numbers.

5-2   Answer C

Older adults typically require between 1,600 and 2,200 calories per day to meet nutritional needs: 45–65% of calories should come from complex carbohydrates, 20–30% from lean proteins, and 25–30% from fats. Adults age 51 and older should have 1,200 mg of calcium daily.

5-3   Answer A

ADHD is marked by inattention, impulsiveness, a low tolerance for frustration, and a great deal of inappropriate behavior. This can be exhausting for parents and teachers. In some cases, ADHD can be managed by medications, but the use of medications is controversial. A specialist should evaluate a child suspected of having ADHD.

5-4   Answer A

Developmental tasks of early adulthood (ages 20–45) include becoming independent from the parents' home and care, learning to cooperate in a marriage relationship, and forming a meaningful philosophy of life. Achieving desired performance in a career comes later (in middle adulthood). Other developmental tasks of early adulthood include establishing a career or vocation, forming an intimate bond with another and choosing a mate, setting up and managing one's own household, making friends and establishing a social group, assuming civic responsibility and becoming a citizen in the community, and beginning a parenting role. Establishing a family and graduating from a postsecondary school are not necessary for completing developmental tasks in this age group.

5-5   Answer A

Cyndy is at the preoperational stage (ages 2–7) of cognitive development as formulated by Piaget. She cannot conserve (understand that things remain the same even if their material is rearranged). She is also egocentric (unable to take another person's viewpoint) and uses transductive reasoning (reasoning from one specific fact to another specific fact). The sensorimotor stage is from birth to age 24 months. At this stage, there is object permanence (things continue to exist even when out of sight) and the beginning of verbal language. The stage of concrete operations occurs from ages 7–11. It is typified by the belief in the here and now, the ability to recognize the importance of rules, and the idea of conservation (not being fooled by the rearrangement of matter). Formal operations (from ages 12–18) is the stage of having the capacity for abstract thought, the ability to use hypothetical and deductive reasoning, and the ability to generate many possible solutions to a given problem.

5-6   Answer A

Secondary sex characteristics occur in boys before puberty and may take 2–5 years to complete. Testicular enlargement is the first change, followed by penis and scrotal enlargement, deepening of the voice, growth of axillary and pubic hair, and finally growth of facial and chest hair.

5-7   Answer D

Selective optimization with compensation theory, a theory of psychological development and aging, states that to move through the older years in a satisfied and self-fulfilled way, people must develop strategies to manage the emotional effects of loss over time. They must increase selection and channel certain functions while reducing others and compensating for their loss. Disengagement theory holds that separation of older people from active roles in society is normal and appropriate and benefits both society and older individuals. Activity/developmental task theory theorizes that when individuals engage and interact with their environment, tools (exteriorized forms of mental processes) are produced that result in the people becoming more readily accessible and communicable to other people, bettering social interaction. The person-environment fit theory holds that outcomes are a function of the interaction between individuals and their environments, where good fit typically results in positive outcomes for the individual.

5-8   Answer A

Normal children at 24–30 months should have two- to three-word sentences, be able to ask simple questions, and be able to repeat simple phrases and sentences. They should be able to use more words than gestures to express themselves, and the words should be intelligible most of the time to the parents. The child should be referred to an audiology/speech clinic for evaluation.

5-9   Answer C

By the age of 8, a child can use each hand independently. The ability to manipulate objects continues to be refined and reaches adult capability by 11 or 12 years of age.

5-10   Answer B

Continuity theory describes the latter part of a person's life as a continuation of the earlier part of life. This is seen as one of the developmental theories of aging and proposes that as people age they try to continue as many of the aspects of their lifestyles as possible. Activity or developmental task theory assumes that older adults need to stay active to be successful emotionally and physically as they age. Disengagement theory states that as people age they withdraw from society and society expects it. Age stratification theory states that people in specific age group cohorts age at the same time.

5-11   Answer C

Older adults typically have prolonged sleep latency or longer period of time between going to bed and falling asleep. Other sleep characteristics associated with aging include more frequent nighttime awakening, less REM sleep, less deep sleep, earlier awakenings, and less overall sleep time.

5-12   Answer C

Empty nest is the term used when the last child leaves home, either for school or to move out on his or her own. It is a time when parents are alone as a couple once again.

5-13   Answer A

Adolescent egocentrism is a state of self-absorption in which the world is viewed from one's own point of view. This leads adolescents to believe that everyone else is watching them and is concerned about them. This is called imaginary audience.

5-14   Answer B

Café-au-lait spots and neurofibromas would indicate neurofibromatosis. Hypopigmented macules and adenoma sebaceum would indicate tuberous sclerosis, whereas facial port-wine hemangiomas would indicate Sturge-Weber syndrome, and nail hypoplasia or dysplasia would indicate fetal alcohol syndrome and trisomies.

5-15   Answer C

The concept of reversibility typically develops early in the transition to concrete operations as defined by Piaget. At this point children are able to mentally undo an action. For example, they can understand that adding two marbles to a set of three marbles results in five marbles, and that if you then take two marbles away, three marbles are left. In this stage, a child begins to apply logical processes to concrete problems.

5-16   Answer D

Delayed development can be the result of malnutrition from a deficiency of protein, calories, or both. Marasmus is related to kwashiorkor and is a form of protein calorie malnutrition, occurring chiefly in the first year of life. It may be partly caused by a hypermetabolic disease. Muscle wasting is one of the symptoms.

5-17   Answer C

Middle-aged persons who still have responsibility for their children and are now caring for their aging parents are considered (as a group) to be the "sandwich" generation because they are caught between the demands of their children and those of their parents. Although many individuals are hoping for the "empty nest" when children leave home, many, in reality, have a full house because their parents move in with them.

5-18   Answer B

In most respects, physical development and maturation are complete in early adulthood. Most people are at their peak in physical capabilities. The senses are as sharp as they ever will be. Even though there are changes in the elasticity of the eye, their effects at this point are usually minor.

5-19   Answer A

The tasks of middle adulthood include accepting and adjusting to the physical changes of middle age, reviewing and redirecting career goals, and achieving desired performance in one's career. Affiliating with one's age group occurs later—in late adulthood when individuals retire and have more time to socialize. Other tasks of middle adulthood include developing hobby and leisure activities, adjusting to aging parents, helping adolescent children in their search for identity, accepting and relating to the spouse as a person, and coping with an empty nest at home.

5-20   Answer B

Enlargement of the scrotum and testes, a reddened scrotal sac, some hair texture alteration, and a penis that is not enlarged are all characteristics of Tanner stage II. For boys, the sexual maturity rating scale developed by Tanner consists of five stages based on characteristics of pubic hair and genitalia. In stage I, the penis, testes, and scrotum are preadolescent in development. In stage III, there is further growth of the testes and scrotum, and the penis enlarges and becomes longer. In stage IV, there is an increase in the size of the penis with a growth in breadth and development of the glans, further enlargement of the testes and scrotum, and increased darkening of the scrotal skin. The pubic hair resembles that of an adult in type, but with the distribution considerably smaller than in the adult. In stage V, the genitalia are adult in size and shape, and the pubic hair is adult in quantity.

5-21   Answer A

You should suspect cerebral palsy whenever an infant crosses his or her legs when lifted from behind rather than pulling them up or bicycling like a normal infant does. Cerebral palsy should also be suspected if the child has legs that are hard to separate, making diaper changing difficult; persistently uses only one hand or, as he or she gets older, uses the hands well but not the legs; has difficulty sucking or keeping a nipple or food in his or her mouth; seldom moves voluntarily; or has arm or leg tremors with voluntary movement. Cerebral palsy needs to be detected early for effective treatment. Mild hydrocephalus should be noticed at an infant's well-baby checkup when measuring the head circumference. Spina bifida occulta is characterized by a depression or raised area and a tuft of hair over the defect in the spinal cord. A port-wine nevus may also be present. In many cases, neurological status is normal because spina bifida occulta does not always cause neurological dysfunction. Fetal alcohol syndrome would probably have been diagnosed earlier.

5-22   Answer A

Erectile dysfunction (ED) occurs in about one quarter of men aged 65 and older. There are many potential causes of ED, including hormone dysfunction, vascular insufficiency, antihypertensives and other medications, and psychological issues. Sexual dysfunction is a sensitive topic which may be embarrassing or difficult for the patient to disclose. Evaluation of ED should include a detailed history and review of systems, and a thorough physical examination.

5-23   Answer B

Amphetamine (Dexedrine, Adderall) and methylphenidate (Ritalin, Concerta, Methylin, Focalin, and so on) are preferred drugs for pediatric ADHD. Ritalin is a CNS stimulant that blocks the reuptake of norepinephrine and dopamine into the presynaptic neurons and increases the release of these monoamines into the extraneuronal space. Dexedrine probably causes the nerve endings to produce more norepinephrine at the synapse. Dysfunction in the actions of the neurotransmitters dopamine and norepinephrine may be key to the pathophysiological mechanisms of ADHD. These medications are likely effective in many cases of ADHD because they allow for these chemicals to be reabsorbed and recirculated.

5-24   Answer B

The average infant doubles his or her birth weight by 5 months and triples it by 1 year. Growth slows over the second year but is still continuous; the child should weigh about four times his or her birth weight at age 2 years.

5-25   Answer A

The lower central incisors are the first teeth to erupt in an infant, usually at around age 5–11 months. The lower lateral incisors erupt at age 6–15 months, the upper central incisors at age 6–12 months, and the upper lateral incisors at age 7–18 months. The lower canine incisors erupt from 16–20 months.

5-26   Answer A

A decrease in agility of older adults is due in part to a decrease in the speed and strength of muscle contractions in the extremities. Degenerative arthritis, rheumatoid arthritis, and bulging intervertebral disks are caused by specific disease processes in the skeletal system and are not the result of normal aging.

5-27   Answer C

Although both Johnny and his mother are probably nervous about being in the clinic, this behavior is not normal. If the mother spanks a child in front of an authority figure for an inconsequential act, it is possible that her behavior is indicative of child abuse. Although reporting the mother to a child protective services agency is a little drastic after only one encounter, you should document the incident and be alert to any other subtle or overt cues of child abuse.

5-28   Answer C

The preschool-age child (ages 3–6) develops initiative by interacting with others in socially acceptable ways. The child also develops initiative by learning to accomplish things, such as tasks given by a preschool teacher or age-appropriate household chores. Initiative also develops by feeling satisfaction with the successful completion of such activities. Preschoolers should be given choices when appropriate, such as choosing which cup they prefer to drink from or choosing between two acceptable pairs of socks to wear. Due to their egocentrism, they are unable to consider others points of view and will have difficulty understanding how others are feeling. Discipline for preschoolers should involve reinforcing desired behaviors.

5-29   Answer A

The development of friendship abilities involves three stages during middle childhood. In the beginning, children see friends as people who like them and whom they can have fun with. The next stage begins to take other people's traits and qualities into consideration, and the third stage begins to view friendship as entailing more closeness and mutual disclosure.

5-30   Answer C

According to Piaget, the ability to think abstractly develops during adolescence, as do the abilities to focus on formal operations, analyze situations, and use scientific reasoning. This is considered the formal operational period in Piaget's theory. In early childhood, children are in the preoperational period of cognitive development, when thinking is egocentric. The child of middle school age attains the concrete operational period when he or she can understand logical operations and principles and apply them to help interpret specific experiences or perceptions. The young adult should be capable of abstract thinking because the formal operational period begins with adolescence.

5-31   Answer B

Older adults' bodies have fewer muscle cells and more fat cells than those who are younger. Fat cells contain less fluid than muscle cells; thus the intracellular compartment has less fluid. Both total body water and intracellular fluid volumes are lower than in younger individuals, placing the older adult at higher risk for fluid imbalance.

5-32   Answer A

By age 4–9 weeks, babies smile at the sight of things that please them. The earliest smiles are fairly indiscriminate, becoming more selective over time. A true social smile is given in response to particular individuals.

5-33   Answer A

The developmental tasks of adolescence include searching for one's identity, appreciating one's achievements, and growing independent from one's parents. Other developmental tasks of adolescence include forming close relationships with peers, developing analytic thinking, evolving one's own value system, developing a sexual identity, and choosing a career. Not graduating from high school will not interfere with attainment of developmental tasks as long as the adolescent has a career plan not requiring a high school diploma. Although the other choices are important to some adolescents, they are not considered specific tasks for all adolescents to move successfully into young adulthood.

5-34   Answer D

By 36 months of age, normal children should be able to speak in short sentences, give their full names, use plurals, know two to three prepositions, and tell a story.

5-35   Answer A

Reproductive system changes seen in men as they age include slightly decreased sperm production, decreased semen volume, testicular softening, and decreasing testosterone levels.

5-36   Answer B

Younger children are more predisposed than older children to acute otitis media, primarily because their eustachian tubes are more flaccid and more horizontal than the tubes of older children. Although younger children are more susceptible to the new bacteria they encounter, have more viral infections, and have more allergies, the central role is played by the horizontal eustachian tube, which is anatomically predisposed to acute otitis media. The eustachian tube connects the nasopharynx with the middle ear, and organisms migrate through a shorter, more pliable tube more readily than they do in the more angled eustachian tubes of adults.

5-37   Answer C

Debbie, who is learning self-assertion, spontaneity, self-sufficiency, direction, and purpose, is in the stage of initiative versus guilt in Erikson's stages of ego development. Her mother is appropriately stimulating her, and she is developing a sense of initiative. This stage usually occurs around ages 3–5 years. Debbie has already progressed through the trust versus mistrust stage (birth through age 15 months) and the autonomy versus shame and doubt stage (ages 1–3 years). After her current stage—initiative versus guilt—Debbie will progress to industry versus inferiority (around age 6 through early adolescence).

5-38   Answer A

Although some babies are toilet trained earlier than age 2, most are not ready until then because bladder and bowel control requires a great deal of coordination and maturity of the nervous system. Starting toilet training too early is frustrating for both parents and children.

5-39   Answer C

New parents are often very tired and distressed when their infant does not sleep for an extended period of time. There are wide variations in the amount of sleep during infancy, but most infants sleep through the night by the age of 1 year. Early introduction of solids has not been shown to improve sleep duration in young infants.

5-40   Answer D

Most infants can sit with support at 4 months; all normal infants sit well without support by 8 months, and many are able to sit without support by 6 or 7 months.

5-41   Answer A

Adolescents are concerned with their developing independence and emerging sense of identity. They are most responsive to those health concerns that are immediate, not in the future, and that they themselves identify as important. Determining the issues and outcomes that this patient sees as important may facilitate adherence to the needed lifestyle changes. Teens identify most with struggles of their peers than with those of their parents.

5-42   Answer C

If you notice inner canthal folds and Brushfield spots, you should suspect Down syndrome. Slanted palpebral fissures are seen with other trisomies, blue sclera and osteogenesis imperfecta with Turner's syndrome, and Lisch nodules with neurofibromatosis.

5-43   Answer A

Maximum height is reached in the 20s and remains stable until about age 55. Bones becomes less dense at that point, and a slow loss of height begins, averaging 1 in. for men and 2 in. for women. "Middle-age spread" continues, visual and hearing acuity drop, and strength diminishes.

5-44   Answer A

The third heart sound is caused by forceful blood flow being pushed out of the atria and hitting the wall of the ventricle. It is normal in young children with healthy hearts and thin chest walls. The fourth heart sound means there is poor compliance in the ventricles. Ejection clicks can mean a faulty heart valve. Diastolic murmurs are always organic.

5-45   Answer C

Motor development in children proceeds sequentially as the muscles of gross and fine motor movements mature. Therefore, the health-care provider should note that the larger muscles of the hands develop before the smaller muscles. This enables the baby to grasp large items, like rattles, at 3–4 months. However, the fine motor coordination necessary to develop a pincer grasp does not develop until the child is 9–10 months old.

5-46   Answer C

Jung's theory of personality development describes the goal to be self-actualization. His theory purports that people strive for a balance between their inner experiences (introversion) and their outer expressions (extroversion). As people age, they sometimes question their beliefs, values, and possible goals, which can lead to a period of transition fraught with turmoil (midlife crisis).

5-47   Answer D

Long-term studies have shown that school-age children and adolescents with attention deficit-hyperactivity disorder (ADHD) experience school failure, aggression, antisocial behavior, poor social skills, emotional immaturity, low self-esteem, and interpersonal conflicts. The same studies revealed that more than 50% of adults who had ADHD as children continue to exhibit anxiety, low self-esteem, personality disorders, alcohol and substance abuse, and interpersonal difficulties.

5-48   Answer C

It is rare for a child to be diagnosed with fragile X syndrome during the first year of life. Although it is possible to detect the syndrome by amniocentesis, that screening is not routinely done unless there is a family history of the disorder. The child is often past the toddler stage when a diagnosis is made.

5-49   Answer D

Males can continue to grow into early adulthood. Testicular growth occurs approximately 6 months before the development of any pubic hair. The growth spurt in boys is usually 2 years after that of girls and doesn't reach its peak velocity until Tanner stage V in many cases. The deepening of the voice happens during the growth spurt.

5-50   Answer A

Masturbation is a common activity and should be ignored. It does not cause any physical, sexual, or mental problems. Drawing attention to the matter may make a child act out in other ways. Comforting the mother by telling her "not to worry" is not addressing the mother's concern.

5-51   Answer B

Due to the change in function of T and B lymphocytes in older adults, the formation of antibodies shifts to form antibodies against a person's own immune system. Normal aging does not in and of itself cause a decrease in thrombocytes or the other cell lines.

5-52   Answer D

To prevent milk-bottle syndrome and dental caries, infants and children should not go to bed with a bottle. If one is absolutely necessary on occasion, it should be a plain water bottle.

5-53   Answer B

The approximate average age for full breast growth in girls is age 16.

5-54   Answer B

The successful aging paradigm suggests that physical health, stimulation of cognitive capabilities, social involvement and engagement, productivity, and life satisfaction are major components of a healthy aging process. Assessment of these components can help the clinician understand an individual's aging process, typical patterns of daily living, and unmet needs.

5-55   Answer B

At about age 3 years, children begin to enjoy interaction with other children. Before this, they may have played alongside other children (parallel play) but have not engaged in real social interaction.

5-56   Answer C

Increased sensitivity to sunlight exposure increases in older adults as the number of melanocytes (pigment-carrying cells) decreases. This results in graying hair, reduced capillary blood supply, and fading skin color. Langerhans cells do decrease by 40%, but this is generally assumed to account for the increased hypersensitivity of skin in older adults, not increased photosensitivity.

5-57 Answer C

Erikson's stage of intimacy versus isolation occurs during early adulthood, and for some individuals it lasts into the 30s. The adult is seeking a mature relationship involving mutual trust, cooperation, sharing, and complete acceptance. Without this relationship, the person is withdrawn and lonely.

5-58 Answer B

By 4 months, the infant shows attention to sights and sounds by turning the head toward the source of the sound. Infants startle to sound. By 4 months, they begin to localize to the general direction of the sound. By 9 months, they can localize to the precise direction of the sound (up or down, not just in the general direction).

5-59 Answer A

A formal diagnosis of ADHD is made using the criteria in the DSM-IV. The DSM is being revised, and a new version is expected in May 2013.

5-60 Answer B

Signs of readiness for beikost (solids) include achieving the age of 4–6 months, fading of the extrusion reflex, control of head and neck muscles, ability to sit with support, and development of interest in what others are eating. The first tooth usually appears between ages 5 and 7 months, but teeth are not needed for introduction of solids.

5-61 Answer C

The HEADSS assessment framework guides the APRN to consistently ask teens about their Home life, Education, use of Alcohol and Drugs, Sexual activity, and thoughts about Suicide. These issues need to be considered at each health-care encounter with a teen in order to accurately assess physical and emotional health and health risks.

5-62 Answer D

Erikson's last ego stage in older adults is integrity versus despair. It is the stage when successful resolution results in adults feeling comfortable with their life choices and the knowledge that they would have done everything the same way again. Older adults who have successfully completed this phase in their life are in Erikson's integrity phase. When reviewing their life events, experiences, and relationships, they realize that these have been mostly good, and they have cherished memories. Failure to reach this point results in the despair phase, when older adults feel resentment, futility, hopelessness, and a fear of death.

5-63 Answer A

Conservation is the realization that quantity is unrelated to arrangement. Even when they view equal amounts poured into glasses of different shapes, young children cannot understand that the amount remains the same even when the level in the glasses is not the same.

5-64 Answer B

Interpretation of ambiguous or complex statements such as proverbs reflects abstract reasoning ability. Individuals with impaired cognitive functioning, such as those with dementia, are unable to correctly interpret these.

5-65 Answer B

When an infant begins to walk, special walking shoes are not necessary. Bare feet, sneakers, or other shoes are fine. A proper fit is much more important than hard soles or high-tops. Sock-type booties should not be used because they are slippery.

5-66 Answer C

Preschoolers are unable to take someone else's perspective and believe that others must see things as they see them. This is egocentric thought.

5-67 Answer A

By the time they reach first grade, most children pronounce words fairly accurately. However, phonemes such as *th, zw, j,* and *v* remain difficult for some time.

5-68 Answer A

In Piaget's theory of cognitive development, the child in the sensorimotor period achieves object permanence. Before this achievement, the child will not search for a toy that is hidden right before his eyes. Later, he or she will search for it even though it is out of sight, indicating that he or she knows it exists even when it is not in sight.

5-69 Answer A

In some poorer countries, stoutness is associated with good health and prosperity. Malnutrition is endemic in some areas, so fat stores are associated with health.

5-70   Answer D

Obesity is the condition of having excess body fat and is defined as having a BMI in the 95th percentile. Childhood obesity is an increasingly prevalent problem and places children at risk for many health problems, including hypertension and type 2 diabetes. It is a problem that needs to be addressed immediately because research strongly suggests that the earlier a child is obese, the more obese the child will become; furthermore, a child who is obese is likely to become an obese adult.

5-71   Answer B

Separation anxiety is the distress displayed when the usual caregiver leaves. It begins around 8 or 9 months and peaks at about 14 months.

5-72   Answer B

The onset of menses (menarche) usually occurs at age 12 or 13; however, it may begin before or after that age.

5-73   Answer B

Human milk is the ideal food for human infants because it has nutritional characteristics that are matched to the needs of human infants. A well-nourished mother can meet all her infant's nutritional requirements with breast milk alone for the first 4–6 months of life as long as the infant did not begin life with a deficit and has no other problems. The addition of solid foods or formula only displaces the amount of breast milk taken and thus does not supplement the diet. The typical pattern of weight gain in breastfed babies is rapid gain for the first couple of months, followed by a downward trend that leads some to question whether the intake is adequate. The World Health Organization (WHO) growth charts account for growth patterns of breastfed babies during the first year of life.

5-74   Answer B

The DSM-IV specifies the three core deficits of autism. These are impaired reciprocal social interactions, abnormal verbal and nonverbal communication, and a diminished repertoire of activities and interests, with the onset during infancy or childhood. Reliance on an imaginary friend for all interactions is not a diagnostic criterion of autism. There is no conclusive evidence supporting the increased incidence of autism in populations that receive immunizations containing mercury. The amount of thimerosal has been greatly reduced in vaccines. Neonates normally can follow an object or face to midline, not across midline.

5-75   Answer D

All of the answers include actual changes that occur in the respiratory systems of older adults. However, albuterol and salmeterol are beta-2 agonists, which require beta-2 receptor sites to act.

5-76   Answer A

Evidence suggests that people are sexually active well into their 80s and 90s. The two major factors determining sexual activity are good physical and mental health and previous regular sexual activity. The phrase "use it or lose it" seems to be relevant.

5-77   Answer B

To assess fine motor skills in a child, it is important to know that at age 3, a child can copy a circle; at age 4, a child can cut on a line with scissors; and at age 5, a child can string beads and copy a square, letters, and numbers.

5-78   Answer A

The behavioral features of fragile X syndrome include being easily overwhelmed by stimuli, excessive chewing on clothes, and frequent tantrums. Other features include hand biting, hand flapping, hyperactivity, mood instability, perseveration (repetition) and delays in speech, poor eye contact, short attention span, shyness, social anxiety, and tactile defensiveness. Linear growth, the incidence of ear infections, and difficulty swallowing are not affected by fragile X syndrome.

5-79   Answer D

Aging in place involves modification of the home environment and provision of support to keep aging adults in their homes. Research demonstrates that most older adults wish to remain in their homes and die at home.

5-80   Answer B

The Get Up and Go Test is a structured observation to evaluate functional mobility. To assess a patient, have the person rise from a chair, walk 10 feet forward, turn, and return to the chair and sit down again. Strength, balance, gait, pace, and coordination in turning are evaluated by the observer.

5-81   Answer C

Between the ages of 2 and 4, stuttering or dysrhythmia (which includes hesitations, repetitions, prolongations) is normal. It reflects the rapid acquisition of new vocabulary. The diagnosis of stuttering should be made only if it persists into the school years.

5-82   Answer D

Slowed reaction time can make it difficult for older drivers to respond to a recognized danger while driving. Other factors associated with aging, including decreased peripheral vision and difficulty sensing speed and distance of oncoming vehicles, also increase the risks for motor vehicle injury in this population. Most older drivers recognize their own driving challenges and adjust their driving patterns to accommodate for them. For example, they may avoid driving at night because of poor night vision or adaptation to glare.

5-83   Answer B

Studies have shown that a consistent approach with rewards and behavioral cues to remind the child when his behavior has exceeded acceptable limits is helpful to assist him in succeeding with schoolwork.

5-84   Answer C

Nocturnal emissions ("wet dreams") usually begin during sleep at about age 14. The first ejaculation of seminal fluid usually occurs about 1 year after the penis begins its adolescent growth.

5-85   Answer A

Preterm infants' development should be assessed using corrected rather than chronologic age. A 6-month-old born at 32 weeks' gestation is neurologically as mature as a 4-month-old infant. Moro, Babinski, and Landau reflexes would be present in a 4-month-old. Moro should fade by 6 months, Babinski is considered normal up to 18 months, and Landau emerges at about 3–4 months. Persistence of primitive reflexes past the age when they are expected to fade is cause for concern.

5-86   Answer B

Abstract reasoning is the term used to describe the activity of pondering a deeper meaning beyond the concrete and literal. Thought process is the way a person thinks—the logical train of thought.

Consciousness is being aware of one's own existence, feelings, thoughts, and environment. This is the most elementary of mental status functions. Perception is an awareness of objects through any of the five senses.

5-87   Answer B

Although a child should be able to learn to hop on one foot by age 4, the ability to perform one particular activity is not sufficient to determine if the child is developing normal motor skills. A more complete assessment is required. At age 5, a child should be able to skip on alternate feet and jump rope.

5-88   Answer A

Aging is accompanied by decreased muscle strength, decreased endurance, loss of flexibility and connective tissue elasticity, decreased bone mass, and decreases in stature due to changes in spine architecture.

5-89   Answer B

The age of menopause can vary widely. There is usually a 2-year period of irregular periods beginning in the late 40s, but it occurs earlier for some and may be as late as age 60 for others. After a year goes by without a menstrual period, menopause is considered complete.

5-90   Answer C

In the concrete operations stage, a child begins to apply logical processes to concrete problems and can apply the concept of reversibility. This is the idea that the process that changed an object can be applied to reverse the process.

5-91   Answer A

These are typical of gynecomastia, which is a normal finding in adolescent boys. Gynecomastia in adolescents is very occasionally associated with medical problems such as cancer and is seen in males who use anabolic steroids, marijuana, or other drugs.

5-92   Answer A

Cross-cultural studies of child development reflect differences in the achievement of growth and development milestones. Factors that may influence these differences include nutrition, preferred activities, and lifestyle differences. There should be no difference in the cognitive development of children in bilingual households. There is no evidence that any cultural/racial group is innately more intelligent than another.

5-93   Answer C

The sexual maturity rating scale developed by Tanner consists of five stages based on pubic hair and breast development for girls and pubic hair and genital development for boys. For girls, the middle stage, stage III, is characterized by the enlargement of breast and areola, with no contour separation and darker, coarser, and more curled pubic hair. Tanner stage I is preadolescent, with an elevation of papilla only and no pubic hair. In stage II, there is a breast bud; elevation of the breast and papilla as a small mound with enlargement of the areolar diameter; and a sparse growth of long, slightly pigmented downy hair, straight or only slightly curled, along the labia. In stage IV, there is projection of the areola and papilla to form a secondary mound above the level of the breast, and the pubic hair resembles an adult's in type, but with the distribution considerably smaller. In stage V, the breasts are at the mature stage and the pubic hair is adult in quantity, with distribution of the horizontal pattern.

5-94   Answer C

At age 12 months, a baby can usually say two or three words with meaning. At age 9–10 months, a baby can imitate the sounds of others but probably doesn't understand them. At age 24 months, a child can say two-word phrases.

5-95   Answer B

Although children of this age can be expected to have 20/20 to 20/25 vision, they do not have to be referred to ophthalmology until the results are 20/40 or worse, as long as they have no eye abnormalities on physical examination and they are having no visual difficulties during normal activity at home and school.

5-96   Answer B

Although amenorrhea and hot flashes are signs associated with the onset of menopause, a period of amenorrhea for the prior 12 months is necessary for the diagnosis. Women in the perimenopause phase may experience intermittent ovulation and irregular or widely spaced menstrual periods. It is still possible for this individual to become pregnant, and pregnancy should be ruled out. Beyond that,

laboratory tests are not needed for women whose menstrual periods have ended and who have associated signs such as hot flashes. Calcium supplements and bone density screening are recommended after menopause has occurred.

5-97   Answer A

Postformal thought goes beyond logic and encompasses interpretive and subjective thinking. Developmental psychologist Gisela Labouvie-Vief has suggested that thinking changes qualitatively during the early adult years. She asserts that the complexity of society and the increasing challenges of getting through that complexity require more than logical thought. Thinking becomes more flexible and interpretive.

5-98   Answer D

Typically, menarche occurs 2 years after the onset of thelarche, at the end of Tanner stage III. The average age for girls to reach menarche is 12.5 years.

5-99   Answer A

Some types of AD are inherited and present before age 60. There are also other forms of dementia, such as Pick's disease, that have the same outcome as AD but can be found as early as the fifth decade. These diseases have a genetic predisposition and may not be a result of the aging process. It should be remembered, however, that half of all people older than 85 are affected by AD.

5-100   Answer A

The ABCTs are the four main headings of a mental status assessment. The A stands for appearance, the B for behavior, the C for cognition, and the T for thought processes.

5-101   Answer B

Exercise can result in a slower decline in central nervous system processing, assist in the maintenance of muscle strength, lower low-density lipoprotein (LDL) and decrease cardiovascular risk factors, and decrease the risk of osteoporosis and fractures. It does not result in a reduced need for dietary calcium. The onset of menopause is not affected by the amount of exercise a woman engages in. Visual acuity declines are related to changes in the shape and elasticity of the lens, which are not related to exercise.

5-102   Answer D

Erikson's theory was enhanced in the early 1990s when he added the influence of social and cultural issues on the psychological development of middle-aged and older adults. According to Erikson, as people move through middle age, they have to resolve the conflict between continuing to grow in all ways (generativity) and slowing down physically, with fewer social contacts, as they retire from lifelong work, perhaps lose a spouse, and so on (stagnation).

5-103   Answer C

Some difficulty with recall is an expected age-related cognitive change. However, impaired recall of common words or loved one's names may indicate significant decline associated with dementia, including Alzheimer's disease. Further tests of cognitive function and referral to neurology or geriatric specialist are indicated.

5-104   Answer C

The absence of joint attention in older infants and toddlers is associated with autism.

5-105   Answer D

Tantrums are common occurrences in toddlers. They often occur in situations where the child is frustrated due to demands he or she cannot meet; when language skills are not adequate to communicate the child's needs or feelings; or when the child is hungry, fatigued, or similarly stressed. The most effective ways to minimize tantrums are to make sure the child is fed and well-rested, to have age-appropriate expectations for behavior, and to intercede early when the child's frustration is building. Using time out (placing the child in a low-stimulation, safe environment to calm down) can be effective in shortening the duration of a tantrum but is not a deterrent to the emergence of a tantrum. Toddlers lack the cognitive skills for reasoning and have limited language skills and impulse control, so discussing alternative communication methods is not appropriate for this age group.

5-106   Answer C

ADHD is among the most common neurodevelopmental disorders in children. Its hallmarks are hyperactivity, impulsiveness, and inattention beyond the norm for the child's age. Signs of ADHD are typically seen across settings rather than only in one setting or environment. Therefore, it is important to understand if the concerning behaviors are seen at home as well as at school. The diagnosis is reliable if made by a standardized approach.

5-107   Answer C

Head circumference by 1 year is almost one-third larger than at birth. The anterior fontanel is usually closed by 18 months of age. From ages 1–3, head circumference continues to increase by approximately 3 cm per month, whereas after age 3, head size increases only about 1 inch per year. Head circumference is typically assessed until age 3.

5-108   Answer C

Worsening near vision, or presbyopia, is an expected age-related change. Blurring may indicate the development of cataracts. Chronic itching and tearing, or photophobia, can be related to many disorders.

5-109   Answer A

Acute otitis media is characterized by middle ear effusion in the presence of symptoms such as fever, ear pain, and irritability. When there is effusion, the tympanic membrane is opaque and has limited mobility. Prolonged or recurrent middle ear effusion is associated with cognitive delay and hearing deficits, which lead to speech and language delays.

5-110   Answer B

By 2–2.5 years, the child has enough fine motor skill to assemble simple shape puzzles and build a tower with blocks or line up blocks to form a train. By 3 years of age, a child should be pedaling a tricycle and has the beginning dexterity to work with a bat and lightweight ball.

5-111   Answer C

Infants and toddlers often become attached to a particular toy or blanket and seem especially attached to it at night or when they are upset. This attachment may last through the preschool years and should not be interfered with because it does provide comfort during stressful situations.

5-112 Answer B

The most common inherited cause of mental retardation in children is fragile X syndrome. Mental retardation occurs in most boys with the syndrome and in more than 25% of girls with the syndrome. The syndrome was first described in 1969 and is responsible for about 30% of all cases of X-linked retardation. Involvement may range from mild learning and behavior difficulties to severe mental retardation. Other causes of mental deficiency include metabolic causes such as hypothyroidism (cretinism), hyperbilirubinemia, and hypoglycemia; chromosomal or genetic causes such as Down syndrome, Turner's syndrome, Klinefelter's syndrome, autosomal-dominant inheritance, and autosomal-recessive inheritance; and acquired causes such as maternal infection (rubella, toxoplasmosis, syphilis, and cytomegalovirus), maternal illness or drug use, birth injury, hypoxia, and trauma. Meningomyelocele and hydrocephalus are not chromosomal disorders.

5-113 Answer A

Cross-cultural studies strongly support that the sequence of stages in Piaget's theory is universal but that there can be differences in the rate at which these stages are mastered. There is no direct link between the rate of physical development and the rate of cognitive development in *normal* children.

5-114 Answer A

The first year of life is hallmarked by significant brain growth, including development of synaptic connections between and among neurons. Synaptic pathways that are stimulated continue to develop, while those that are unused do not continue to develop (neuronal pruning). Thus, early experiences have an important effect on development by stimulating and maintaining neuron connections. This is a "use it or lose it" situation.

5-115 Answer B

Because children are sexually curious at different ages, sex education should begin during the preschool years and continue thereafter. Children need truthful and factual information, and their questions should be answered with age-appropriate, honest answers. Studies have shown that children who have received sex education at home before schooling and during the school years are less likely to get pregnant or have casual sexual experiences in adolescence.

5-116 Answer C

At age 4, children can fasten and unfasten simple buttons, draw stick figures with three parts, successfully use scissors, and lace shoes.

5-117 Answer B

Slowing of processing and accessing information is a cognitive change associated with aging.

5-118 Answer B

Infants have a rounded appearance with relatively equal A-P and transverse diameter measurements. Past infancy, a barrel chest is abnormal. All other findings are considered normal in a child of this age.

5-119 Answer C

The approximate annual weight gain in the school-age child is 5–7 lb. During the school-age years, children become slimmer, with longer legs and a lower center of gravity. On average, boys are taller and heavier than girls until the adolescent growth spurt, which occurs earlier in girls.

5-120 Answer C

Preferring peer group activity over adult activities, conforming to group rules, using secret codes, and desiring acceptance are significant for the school-age child (ages 6–10). Children ages 2–4 have a difficult time sharing with each other and prefer parallel play. At ages 4–6, children are focused on themselves. They play with others but have a difficult time abiding by the rules, particularly if it means "losing" a game. At 12–15, early adolescents have one special friend and think that the rest of the world is thinking about them. They have "idols," usually sports or entertainment stars.

5-121 Answer B

During the school-age years, when physical growth is relatively slow and smooth, children usually grow about 3 in. in height annually.

5-122 Answer A

Early examination and vision screening should begin at the earliest age practical, which is usually at 3 years of age. Early detection of visual problems is important for the prevention of permanent visual impairment.

5-123   Answer B

At birth a baby's head is about one-third the size of an adult's head. For accurate measurement, the tape is placed over the most prominent part of the occiput and brought to just above the eyebrows. The circumference of a newborn's head ranges from 32–37 cm and is about 2 cm greater than the circumference of the chest. It will maintain that proportion for the next few months. The head circumference should also be at the same or nearly the same percentile as the child's length and weight percentiles.

5-124   Answer C

Most girls experience menarche at around the same age as their mothers did; however, the average age for American adolescents today is 12.5 years, with a standard deviation of 1.3 years. If a girl has not begun to have breast changes by age 13 or has not started her periods by age 16, she should be referred for evaluation.

5-125   Answer C

During infancy, some children show a preference for the use of one hand over the other. However, by the end of the preschool period, handedness is usually clear.

5-126   Answer A

This is a manifestation of ritualism, when the toddler wants things done in the same way each time. This is normal behavior in a toddler.

Bibliography

American Academy of Pediatrics: Use of photoscreening for children's vision screening. *Pediatrics* 109(3):524–525, 2002.

American Psychiatric Association: *Diagnostic and Statistical Manual of Mental Disorders: DSM-IV-TR*, ed. 4, text rev. American Psychiatric Association, Washington, DC, 2000.

Baltes, PB: *Lifespan Development and Behavior*, Vol. 7. Lawrence Erlbaum, Hillsdale, NJ, 1960.

Biro, FM: Pubertal assessment method and baseline characteristics in a mixed longitudinal study of girls. *Pediatrics* 126(10): e583–e590. http://pediatrics.aappublications.org/content/early/2010/08/09/peds.2009-3079.

Boyd, B, and Bee, H: *Lifespan Development*, ed. 6. Pearson, Saddle River, NJ, 2012.

Burke, MM, and Laramie, JA: *Primary Care of the Older Adult, A Multidisciplinary Approach.* Mosby-Elsevier, St. Louis, 2004.

Burns, CE, et al: *Pediatric Primary Care.* Saunders-Elsevier, Philadelphia, 2009.

Drachman, DA: Aging of the brain, entropy, and Alzheimer disease. *Neurology* 67:1340–1352, October 2006.

Dunphy, LM, et al: *Primary Care: The Art and Science of Advanced Practice Nursing*, ed 3. FA Davis, Philadelphia, 2011.

Elkind, D: *The Hurried Child, Growing Up Too Fast Too Soon*, ed 3. Da Capo Press, Cambridge, MA, 2001.

Hale, G, et al: Endocrine features of menstrual cycles in middle and late reproductive age and the menopausal transition classified according to the staging of reproductive aging (STRAW) staging system. *Journal of Clinical Endocrinology and Metabolism* 92(8), 2007.

Havighurst, RJ, Neugarten, BL, and Tobin, SS: Disengagement, personality and life satisfaction in the later years. In Hansen, P (ed.), *Age With a Future.* Munksgaard, Copenhagen, Denmark, 1963.

Hockenberry, MJ: *Wong's Clinical Manual of Pediatric Nursing*, ed 8. Mosby, St. Louis, 2012.

Hussain, J, et al: Environmental evaluation of a child with developmental disability. *Pediatric Clinics of North America* 54(1):15–29, 2007.

Jung, C: The stages of life. In *Collected Works: Vol. 8, The Structure and Dynamics of the Psyche.* Pantheon Books, New York, 1960.

Leibson, C, et al: Use and costs of medical care for children and adolescents with and without attention deficit hyperactivity disorder. *Journal of the American Medical Association* 285(1):60–66, 2001.

Linton, AD, and Lach, H: *Matteson & McConnell's Gerontological Nursing: Concepts and Practice*, ed 3. WB Saunders, St. Louis, 2007.

Marshall, WA, and Tanner, JM: Variations in the pattern of pubertal changes in boys. *Archives of Diseases in Children* 45(239):13–23, 1970.

Marshall, WA, and Tanner, JM: Variations in the pattern of pubertal changes in girls. *Archives of Diseases in Children* 44(235):201–303, 1969.

McDonald, RE, and Avery, DR: *Dentistry for the Child and Adolescent*, ed 6. Mosby, St. Louis, 1994.

Moss, SB, et al: ADHD in adults. *Primary Care Clinics of North America* 34(3), 2007.

Seidel, HM, et al: *Mosby's Guide to Physical Examination*, ed 7. Mosby, St. Louis, 2011.

Tanner, JM: *Growth at Adolescence*. CC Thomas, Springfield, IL, 1955.

Touhy, TA, and Jett, KF: *Gerontological Nursing and Healthy Aging*, ed 3. Mosby, St. Louis, 2010.

Tsudy, M, and Arcara KM: *The Harriet Lane Handbook*, ed 19. Mosby, St. Louis, 2012.

How well did you do?

85% and above, congratulations! This score shows application of test-taking principles and adequate content knowledge.

75%–85%, keep working! Review test-taking principles and try again.

65%–75%, hang in there! Spend some time reviewing concepts and test-taking principles and try the test again.

Chapter 6: *Health Counseling*

Lynne M. Dunphy
Karen Rugg

Questions

6-1 *Elyssa, age 69, lives alone. When talking about personal safety activities, you tell her,*

A. "Wear your slippers at all times, and don't walk barefoot."

B. "Wear your reading glasses when walking around so you'll have them when you need them."

C. "When smoking in bed, be sure to turn on the light to keep you awake."

D. "Wear wide-base, low-heel shoes with corrugated soles to help prevent slips and falls."

6-2 *Shelley, 65 years old, sees you for the first time. She has demonstrated osteopenia on a bone density test, and you have prescribed the appropriate medication for her. What additional lifestyle changes should you counsel for this client?*

A. She should begin a rigorous swimming program to actively build bone.

B. She should cut down on coffee, but tea is OK.

C. She needs to take a multivitamin every day.

D. She should begin weight training.

6-3 *Ralph, age 66, comes to your office with concerns regarding declining sexual function. He states that it takes him much longer to get an erection and sometimes he cannot get or maintain an erection. He has also noticed a diminished desire for sexual activity. He denies any change in his relationship with his wife of 35 years, with whom he has always enjoyed a satisfying sexual relationship. What do you do?*

A. Explain that you must investigate possible underlying causes of his problem, some of which are reversible and some of which are not.

B. Explain that diminished sexual desire and function are natural sequelae of aging.

C. Advise sexual counseling and prescribe Viagra.

D. Suggest that Ralph may be suffering from a low-grade depression and prescribe an antidepressant.

6-4 *Your 75-year-old client with osteoarthritis of the knee will be starting on a course of NSAIDs for pain management. The most important teaching point for your patient at this time is:*

A. You should start with a high dose first and taper down the dose as needed.

B. You should continue to take your Coumadin as you have been.

C. Report any excessive stomach upset or if you notice that your stools become dark or bloody.

D. At this point, it will not be helpful to lose weight.

6-5 *Jake, age 10, comes to your primary care office with his mother. You are in a rural area. What is a priority area for health counseling?*

A. Assessing the physical education program provided in Jake's school

B. Finding out whether the family has any pets

C. Determining whether Jake is able to swim

D. Asking about the occupation of the family, and if it is farming, providing adequate health counseling

6-6 *A new mother is refusing to vaccinate her infant because she is concerned about mercury in vaccines. What do you advise her?*

A. The risk of dying from childhood disease is greater than the health risks of thimerosal.

B. If thimerosal were dangerous, there would be an FDA warning on the label.

C. Thimerosal is not used as a preservative in routinely recommended childhood vaccines except for some forms of the influenza vaccine.

D. She should not be concerned about this.

6-7   Ilene brings in her 14-year-old daughter, Tracie, because she fears that Tracie may be sexually active. What do you do?

A. Start her on medroxyprogesterone acetate (Depo-Provera) immediately.

B. Perform a vaginal exam.

C. Ascertain in private from Tracie if she is contemplating becoming or is sexually active.

D. Call child protective services.

6-8   Nathan, a long-distance runner, says he heard that a high-protein diet would increase his endurance. When you counsel him, which type of diet do you tell him will increase an athlete's endurance?

A. A fat-and-protein diet

B. A normal mixed diet with fat, protein, and carbohydrates

C. A high-carbohydrate diet

D. A fruit-and-vegetable diet

6-9   Jane comes to your office shortly after the death of her husband of 40 years. You should be concerned if she expresses complaints of

A. waves or periods of depression.

B. loss of appetite.

C. crying when she talks with friends.

D. extreme guilt.

6-10   The most effective interventions available to health-care providers for reducing the incidence and severity of the leading causes of disease and disability in the United States are

A. screening tests.

B. immunizations.

C. counseling interventions that address the personal health practices of clients.

D. chemoprophylaxes such as the use of drugs and nutritional and mineral supplements.

6-11   Mike was given three stool cards at the lab and told how to do a fecal occult blood test at home, but he was not counseled as to what foods or drugs to eat or avoid. What do you tell him to do?

A. Do not take aspirin for 7 days before and during the collection period, and avoid red or processed meat for 3 days before and during the collection period.

B. Avoid eating clams and other shellfish.

C. Do not engage in vigorous physical exercise for 5 days prior to the test.

D. Avoid fruit juices.

6-12   You are teaching a client about his gout. Which of the following should you include in your teaching?

A. Once gout is treated, there is no danger of permanent damage.

B. Diet and alcohol may remain the same.

C. He should drink at least 1 quart of fluid per day.

D. Kidney stones and kidney damage may result if gout is not adequately managed.

6-13   Which of the following healthy lifestyle choices has been shown to improve the functioning power of a man's heart?

A. Improving diet

B. Taking vitamins

C. Doing aerobic exercise

D. Having a restful sleep at night

6-14   It is important to counsel your clients of all ages regarding prevention strategies for cancers of the colon and rectum. These strategies include

A. fecal occult blood testing on an annual basis after age 50.

B. emphasizing the importance of regular physical exercise and colonoscopy after age 50.

C. stressing the importance of regular physical exercise; a diet rich in vegetables, fruit, and fiber; and regular use of aspirin.

D. weight loss, smoking cessation, and a diet rich in fiber.

6-15   Sylvia has scleroderma and asks for counseling related to measures to help manage its effects. You tell Sylvia to

A. avoid becoming chilled.

B. cut down on smoking.

C. wear tightly layered clothing to keep the skin warm in winter.

D. begin physical therapy at the first signs of joint stiffness.

6-16   Melinda brings in her daughter Shirley, age 2, with an ear infection. She asks why Shirley gets such frequent infections. You respond that

A.   Shirley must be putting something in her ear.

B.   a high-fat diet results in higher cerumen production; the cerumen traps bacteria, causing the infection.

C.   her eustachian tubes are horizontal, which does not allow drainage.

D.   Melinda must dry Shirley's ears more thoroughly after bathing.

6-17   Joanne is a second-grade teacher and is frustrated that her students do not seem to be getting any physical exercise at home. She asks you for advice. What do you recommend?

A.   "Advise parents to play outside with their children after dinner."

B.   "Tell parents to let their children play outside after school."

C.   "Assign homework to students that must be done with their parents and involves physical activity."

D.   "Advise parents to turn the TV off for a week to get the children used to doing something else."

6-18   You must tell Joe, age 66, that the biopsy results from his lung tumor were positive for lung cancer and that his prognosis is poor. Which of the following is the best way to deliver this message?

A.   "Whatever I tell you in a moment, I want you to remember that the situation is serious, but there is plenty that we can do. It is important that we work closely together over the next several months. I am sorry, but your tests were positive for lung cancer."

B.   "I am sorry, but your test confirmed that you have lung cancer. Although the situation is very serious, there is still plenty that we can do. It is important that we work closely together."

C.   "Joe, can I ask that you have a family member or close friend with you when we talk?"

D.   "Joe, we need to work together. I am sure that we can provide help for you."

6-19   Mary is caring for her 83-year-old father at home. He has dementia and is unsteady on his feet. You recommend that Mary

A.   put her father in a nursing home so that she can have a life of her own.

B.   take in another elderly person so that her father can have company.

C.   get information on home safety and community resources.

D.   lock her father's bedroom door at night so that he will not wander into the street.

6-20   Asthma is increasing in all ages of the population. Primary prevention strategies include which of the following?

A.   Screening workers for hypersensitivity to lung irritants and counseling them to avoid jobs where they are exposed to irritants that affect them

B.   Providing masks for all industrial workers

C.   Providing pulmonary function tests for all industrial workers

D.   Providing yearly chest x-rays for all industrial workers

6-21   Your 68-year-old client presents with a herpes zoster rash (shingles) that radiates from the left axilla across to his spine. It is red, oozing, and painful. You tell your client

A.   to fill this prescription of acyclovir right away and begin using it as soon as possible.

B.   to fill the prescription when he can, but use calamine until he can get to the drugstore.

C.   that steroids are the only medication that will be helpful at this time.

D.   not to worry if he notices some eruptions on his face.

6-22   You counsel the mother of 2-year-old twins who live near a hazardous waste site that exposure to pesticides, polychlorinated biphenyls (PCBs), and dioxins has been linked to

A.   endocrine disruption.

B.   autism.

C.   asthma.

D.   leukemia.

6-23   *James, a 32-year-old medical student, received two of three hepatitis B vaccinations last year. He is wondering if he needs to start the schedule all over again. What do you tell him?*

A. "We'll give the third dose now because it's been at least 4 months since the first dose."

B. "Yes, all three vaccinations need to be repeated if it's been longer than 1 year."

C. "No, but we'll need to repeat the second injection."

D. "If the third injection wasn't given within 6 months after the first one, all three will have to be repeated."

6-24   *Susan is a new mother and hesitant about vaccinations for her baby. You tell her why they are essential and that by the time her child is 5 years of age, she should receive*

A. 10 vaccines.

B. 15 vaccines.

C. 20 vaccines.

D. more than 25 vaccines.

6-25   *A client who is an engineer flies frequently to Asia from the United States. Why should you educate this client about deep vein thrombosis (DVT)?*

A. Because Asian food is linked to DVT

B. Because the Asian time zone is 11 hours ahead

C. Because Asia is known to have endemic disease

D. Because an Asia–U.S. flight takes more than 8–10 hours

6-26   *Your 60-year-old client calls your office complaining of swollen joints, fatigue, and malaise. You confirm a diagnosis of rheumatoid arthritis. She will see a specialist but not for 1 month. Your best first course of action/recommendation would be:*

A. Continue to keep as active as possible and incorporate high-impact aerobics to keep your weight down, as your extra weight will wear on your joints.

B. Rest completely, as this disease can progress rapidly and you need to conserve your energy.

C. Alternate exercise such as walking or swimming with periods of rest.

D. Exercise is not very important, but you really should lose a few pounds to relieve your joint stress.

6-27   *Betty brings her 2-year-old in for a routine visit and mentions that her husband has a gun at home for protection. In counseling her, which is most appropriate?*

A. Tell her that you are obliged to report this to the police.

B. Recommend that the bullets and gun be kept separately, discuss other home protection devices, and suggest a combination lock on the trigger.

C. Ask her, "Why on earth would you keep a gun in the house with a 2-year-old?"

D. Tell Betty that you must speak to her and her husband together about this situation.

6-28   *Bob, age 46, has insulin-dependent diabetes mellitus. He asks your advice about foot care. You tell him to*

A. use alcohol daily to keep his feet dry.

B. soak his feet in warm water daily to keep them from cracking and drying.

C. inspect the bottoms of his feet frequently with a mirror.

D. use emollients to prevent drying and cracking.

6-29   *George, age 62, is taking a diuretic to control his blood pressure. What foods should he be eating in addition that might help?*

A. Bananas and milk

B. Ribs and coleslaw

C. Avocados and soda

D. Popcorn and peaches

6-30   *Darlene, age 55, is shocked when she is weighed during her visit to your office. "I can't believe that I have gained so much weight! What should I do?" What stage in health behavior change is Darlene in?*

A. Contemplation

B. Preparation

C. Action

D. Maintenance

6-31 Annie, age 26, has recently been diagnosed with multiple sclerosis. When advising her and her family, you say which of the following?

A. "You should avoid flying in airplanes because the altitude could trigger an exacerbation of your symptoms."

B. "You should initiate a vigorous exercise schedule to maintain function."

C. "You need to avoid all spicy foods, caffeine, and peppermints."

D. "You need to avoid hot showers."

6-32 Tim, age 66, has chronic obstructive pulmonary disease (COPD). He comes in for counseling regarding a flu shot. He states that he thinks he needs one but has heard some horror stories about the shot related to Guillain-Barré syndrome. What do you tell him?

A. "You have to weigh the advantages against the disadvantages."

B. "Your chances of getting the flu are 10 to 1, and your chances of getting Guillain-Barré are 1,000,000 to 1."

C. "If you are worried, you shouldn't receive the flu shot."

D. "There is no relationship between the flu shot and neurological complications."

6-33 When is it appropriate to discuss smoking cessation techniques with a client who smokes?

A. When the client presents with a smoking-related disease

B. At every visit

C. When the client indicates a readiness to stop smoking

D. Only when the client asks about them

6-34 Melanie wants to start working on a tan before her Caribbean cruise. You warn her about the hazards of sun exposure, but she is still insistent about getting a tan. What do you recommend?

A. Brief tanning periods using a sunscreen

B. Use of a tanning salon for several weeks before the cruise

C. Use of a self-tanning lotion or cream

D. Intervals of a half hour in the sun and a half hour out of the sun

6-35 Gene, who has insulin-dependent diabetes mellitus, is an avid tennis player. When counseling him about insulin and exercise, you tell him,

A. "When your blood sugar is consistently high, you need to exercise more to try to lower it."

B. "After injection with regular insulin, the peak time to exercise is 2–4 hours later."

C. "Inject the insulin into your arms so that it will be absorbed well while you are playing tennis."

D. "Eat within an hour after exercising."

6-36 What is the most common cause of injuries, the leading cause of hospital admissions for trauma, and the second leading cause of injury-related deaths for all age groups?

A. Motor vehicle accidents

B. Falls

C. Bicycle or motorcycle accidents

D. Rollerblading and roller skating accidents

6-37 Marvin has just been given a diagnosis of diabetes. To increase his adherence to a healthful lifestyle, you

A. initially have him come in every week for a urinalysis and fingerstick blood glucose test to see how he's doing.

B. tell him you will do a glycohemoglobin test every 3 months to assess his control of his blood sugar.

C. instruct him on self-monitoring of blood sugar.

D. tell him to call a nutritionist.

6-38 Your client, whom you recently treated for a sexually transmitted disease, has returned with a reinfection. At this point, you

A. reeducate.

B. stress the importance of "safe sex" in more emphatic terms.

C. instruct the client to avoid all sexual contacts.

D. expect that the client will need to come back for more than one visit.

6-39   Joy wants to stop smoking but is afraid that she will gain weight like all of her friends did when they stopped. What might you say to her that will encourage her to stop?

A. "Forget the weight gain; at least you'll live longer."

B. "The average weight gain is 5 pounds; it's worth it."

C. "Let's talk about several strategies you might use to prevent weight gain."

D. "Eat what you want and just exercise more."

6-40   Sam, age 26, likes to enter long-distance bicycle races. He asks you about carbohydrate loading to trick his muscles into storing energy before a competition. You advise him to

A. eat a high-carbohydrate diet for the first 4 days of the week before the competition, then a moderate-carbohydrate diet for the remaining 3 days.

B. increase his training time for 3 days before the competition to assist in releasing the stored energy.

C. avoid the practice of carbohydrate loading because it is very dangerous to his health.

D. cut back on activity and eat a very high-carbohydrate diet for the 3 days before the competition.

6-41   A client has questions about the chemicals at his or her workplace. Which initial action would you recommend?

A. Obtain a sample of the chemical(s) for laboratory analysis.

B. Request a material safety data sheet (MSDS) from the employer.

C. Terminate employment as soon as possible.

D. Call the local fire department.

6-42   Having routine mammograms after age 50 is an example of

A. health promotion.

B. disease prevention.

C. screening.

D. tertiary prevention.

6-43   Sam asks about saturated fats or "bad" fats, as he calls them. Which of the following is not a saturated fat?

A. Soybean oil

B. Coconut oil

C. Palm oil

D. Cocoa butter

6-44   Thomas, age 10, is sent home from school with pediculosis. You tell his mother that the cheapest and easiest remedy is to

A. use regular shampoo on his hair three times a day.

B. apply petroleum jelly (Vaseline) to the scalp and hair.

C. apply mayonnaise to the scalp and hair.

D. cut the hair very short or shave the head.

6-45   Which of the following seafoods do you not recommend for women who might become pregnant, are pregnant, or are nursing?

A. Swordfish, albacore tuna

B. Light white tuna, salmon

C. Haddock, halibut

D. Shrimp, pollock

6-46   Alicia, age 22, is in your office for her first prenatal visit. Recommended preventive services for all pregnant women include

A. blood typing and HIV and hypertensive screening.

B. assessment of height and weight and screening for HIV and asymptomatic bacteriuria.

C. Chlamydia screening, hypertension screening, and Rh(D) incompatibility screening with blood typing.

D. screening for syphilis, Chlamydia, hepatitis B, alcohol and tobacco abuse, asymptomatic bacteriuria, and Rh(D) incompatibility; blood typing; and discussing the importance of breastfeeding.

6-47   Marcie is very depressed because she has fibromyalgia. She states that her husband thinks she is just lazy. How can you help her deal with this problem?

A. Tell her husband that fibromyalgia is a real syndrome, and although it cannot be cured, it can be managed.

B. Have her husband come in with her during her next visit, and talk with them together.

C. Have him see a therapist because most husbands do not understand the condition.

D. Tell Marcie she just has to understand that her husband has made up his mind and will never change.

6-48   In counseling an obese client to lose weight, which of the following is the best recommendation you could make?

A. "Keep a diet history."

B. "Increase your activity."

C. "Cut down on the foods you eat."

D. "There is nothing to recommend because your obesity is hereditary and you will always be overweight."

6-49   You should advise any client who has received which of the following immunizations to use contraception for the next 3 months to avoid pregnancy?

A. MMR, yellow fever, or varicella vaccines

B. Rabies postexposure prophylaxis

C. Tetanus-diphtheria

D. Hepatitis B

6-50   Harold, who is 77, complains that he can't hear as well as he once used to and is reluctant to go to his weekly card game for fear of not hearing the conversation fully. You advise him to

A. go to your card games, but sit so that you can read the lips of other players.

B. see an audiologist and get fitted for a hearing aid.

C. not bother to do anything because this type of hearing loss seen with aging is normal and can't be corrected.

D. skip the card game and take up reading because it is more stimulating.

6-51   You are working in the emergency room when a firefighter arrives directly from the fire scene with increasing chest pain and shortness of breath. For which chemical exposure would you recommend biological monitoring?

A. Carbon monoxide (CO)

B. Carbon dioxide (CO_2)

C. Hydrogen cyanide (HCN)

D. Methane (CH_4)

6-52   Maury, age 77, asks for advice on interventions that he can try to alleviate the discomfort of his arthritis. What do you tell him to do?

A. Apply an ice pack to his stiff joints before exercising to reduce the discomfort.

B. Place a rolled towel under his knees when he lies on his back.

C. Rest at intervals throughout the day.

D. Eat more dairy products to increase the amount of calcium in his diet.

6-53   Joe has just started on a heart failure management program. With what finding should you alert him to call his nurse case manager?

A. Some swelling around his ankles

B. Shortness of breath when taking the stairs up to bed

C. A weight gain of 4 pounds since the previous week

D. Some loss of appetite

6-54   Which of the following is the primary reason given by health-care professionals as to why inadequate attention is paid to health counseling in the primary care setting?

A. Lack of motivation because working with clients to achieve behavioral change is difficult and often frustrating for the health professional

B. Skepticism about the effectiveness of health promotion and counseling

C. Uncertainty about which approaches may be most helpful with individual clients and problems

D. The fact that counseling is not "billable" and is therefore not cost effective

6-55   Your client has a hearing loss, probably a result of exposure to noise when working as a machine operator. What do you advise this client?

A. There is no need to wear hearing protection because there is already a hearing loss.

B. Stay out of work; noise-induced hearing loss is reversible with time.

C. Continue to wear hearing protection at work.

D. Wear hearing protection whenever exposed to loud noise.

6-56　*Nelda wants some counseling regarding her stepdaughter, age 18, whom she suspects has bulimia nervosa. You ask her if her stepdaughter exhibits*

A. frequent urinary tract infections (UTIs), dental caries, and bruised or cut hands.

B. dental caries; dizziness; and dry, sparse hair.

C. amenorrhea, weakness, and sleep disturbances.

D. hyperactivity and bizarre behaviors around food.

6-57　*Jill, who is 8 months pregnant, calls you because her father has told her that her mother is gravely ill. Her parents live on the opposite coast of the continental United States from Jill and she would have to take a 4- to 5-hour flight to see her mother. How would you advise Jill?*

A. Tell her that she should not travel at this point in her pregnancy.

B. Evaluate her risk and make your recommendation on the basis of her risk factors and hemoglobin level.

C. Tell her that it is OK for her to make this flight.

D. Evaluate her risk and make your recommendation on the basis of an electrocardiogram.

6-58　*Mary, age 56, has been on antihypertensive medication. You have switched her regimen more than once. On some occasions when you see her for blood pressure checks, her blood pressure is fine; on other occasions, her blood pressure is out of control. She frequently complains about having to take antihypertensives. She feels she doesn't need them. You suspect she is not taking her medication as ordered. You say,*

A. "Mary, you must take your medication as instructed."

B. "Mary, are you taking your blood pressure medication as prescribed?"

C. "Many people find it difficult to remember to take their medication. During the past week, have you missed any of your pills?"

D. "Mary, let's talk about the side effects of your medication."

6-59　*When you plan health programs, a number of factors are important to take into consideration. Which factor is most critical to successful achievement of a health program?*

A. Convenience

B. Content

C. Using visual images

D. Language

6-60　*Coconut oil and cocoa butter are examples of which type of fatty acids?*

A. Saturated fats

B. Monounsaturated fats

C. Polyunsaturated fats

D. Both monounsaturated and polyunsaturated fats

6-61　*Joe, age 76, has peripheral arterial disease (PAD). You know he does not understand your teaching instructions when he says,*

A. "I'll see the podiatrist once a month so he can do my foot care."

B. "I'll soak my feet weekly so my nails will be soft when I trim them."

C. "I'll monitor my BP, and if it really gets out of control, I'll come see you."

D. "I'll cut down on my smoking."

6-62　*As the nurse practitioner in an outpatient clinic, you will be performing a history and physical on Maria, age 15, whose mother comes to the clinic with her. How would you approach the topic of sexuality with Maria?*

A. Ask Maria's mother if you can discuss this issue with Maria.

B. Ask Maria, with her mother present, if it is OK for you to discuss this issue with them both.

C. Ask Maria's mother to leave the room.

D. When you are alone with Maria, tell her that you want to talk to her about this issue and ask her if she wants her mother to be present.

6-63　*Which of the following is a four-item screening tool useful in identifying a client who may have a problem with alcohol abuse?*

A. The AUDIT Test

B. The CAGE questionnaire

C. The Michigan Alcoholism Screening Test

D. The Problem Drinker/Abuser Test

6-64   *Cynthia brings her 15-year-old son, David, into the office. She wants some counseling regarding his behavior problems. David seems "laid back," quiet, and aloof. All of the information is volunteered by Cynthia. What is the first thing you should do?*

A. Test his urine for drugs.

B. Prescribe an antidepressant medication.

C. Refer David to a psychiatrist.

D. Talk to David about what is concerning him.

6-65   *The U.S. Preventive Services Task Force recommends screening which of the following groups for evidence of alcohol dependence, problem drinking, or excessive alcohol consumption?*

A. Individuals whom the provider thinks are abusing alcohol

B. Individuals with altered liver function studies

C. Individuals who have had several recent automobile accidents, regardless of precipitating cause

D. All adult and adolescent clients

6-66   *The U.S. Preventive Services Task Force recommends a variety of strategies for motivating clients to improve exercise strategies. Which strategy is included in its recommendations?*

A. Stressing the increased mortality associated with not exercising

B. Suggesting a running regimen of 5 days a week for maximum benefit and using a personal trainer

C. Meeting with an exercise physiologist and getting a treadmill for home use and setting specific goals for its use

D. Goal setting by the client; writing an exercise prescription with individually tailored recommendations; follow-up

6-67   *Chloe is chronically tired. During a telephone conversation, she asks you for advice. What do you recommend?*

A. To not nap during the day and to establish a routine for sleep at night

B. To add iron to her diet

C. To take a vitamin supplement with iron

D. To make an appointment

6-68   *Mary, who is obese, has started a walking program and wonders how much walking is too much. You tell her she has done too much walking when*

A. her pulse rate increases by 30 beats per minute during the walk.

B. she starts sweating.

C. she still feels fatigued hours after walking.

D. she becomes slightly short of breath.

6-69   *As you speak with Melissa and her mother, you ascertain more signs and symptoms that contribute to a clinical picture of depression. These include*

A. sad, discouraged, irritable mood and feelings of loneliness.

B. going on a spending spree.

C. obsessively exercising.

D. constant hand washing.

6-70   *Which of the following conditions, which may be detected by a complete blood count, has sufficient prevalence to make early detection beneficial?*

A. Anemia

B. Leukocytosis

C. Thrombocytopenia

D. Leukemia

6-71   *Human papillomavirus (HPV) is detectable in 99% of cervical cancers. Recently, a vaccine has been developed to prevent HPV infection and subsequent cervical intraepithelial neoplasia. What is the ideal time/age to administer this vaccine?*

A. At age 3 months

B. At age 2 years

C. Before the initiation of sexual activity

D. Shortly after the initiation of sexual activity

6-72   *Olive has gastroesophageal reflux disease (GERD). She asks for advice as to what she can do to help her condition. You tell her to*

A. take NSAIDs for the discomfort.

B. cut down on smoking.

C. monitor stools for steatorrhea.

D. avoid caffeine and chocolate.

6-73   *In counseling Melissa on dealing with her depression, you are aware of the successful strategies in managing a depressive illness. Apart from pharmacological interventions, some suggested strategies include*

A. an exercise regimen; more exposure to daylight; rethinking one's situation.

B. stressing the importance of rest.

C. doing complete blood work on Melissa and recommending a multivitamin and vitamin E.

D. recommending St. John's wort, an herbal remedy, because Melissa does not want to take antidepressants.

6-74   *Janice is recovering from osteomyelitis of her leg. She asks you for advice as to what she can do to promote healing. You tell her to*

A. put weight on the affected leg more frequently to promote increased circulation, oxygenation, and nutrition to the tissues of the wound area.

B. eat foods high in vitamins and calcium and increase her calorie and protein intake.

C. spend time in the fresh air and expose the wound to fresh air and sunlight.

D. be sure to use strict aseptic technique when changing the dressing, which should be kept wet at all times to improve wound healing.

6-75   *Sidney has diabetes and asks you why exercise is so essential for him. You tell him that*

A. all persons with diabetes are overweight, and therefore exercise is the one tried-and-true method for weight loss.

B. going for a walk or exercising takes the mind off food, so he will not eat as much.

C. after exercising, people tend to be less hungry and thus do not consume as much.

D. exercising lowers blood sugar and helps the body make better use of its food supply.

6-76   *How do you respond to Trisha, who thinks that skipping breakfast is a way of banking calories for later in the day?*

A. "I do the same thing; that way I feel like I can have a bigger lunch."

B. "That's terrible. Didn't your mother always tell you that breakfast is the most important meal of the day?"

C. "Eating breakfast actually gets your metabolism going."

D. "We all need some essential fatty acids that are obtained only from food."

6-77   *Wes, age 60, wants advice regarding what to look for as signs of skin cancer. You tell him to observe any lesions he has and do which of the following?*

A. He should alert you if he observes a lesion with asymmetrical borders, a multicolored lesion, a lesion greater than 6 mm in diameter, or a change in the appearance of a nevus or mole.

B. He should alert you if he observes a new papule that is 2 mm in size.

C. He should have any crusty-appearing lesion evaluated immediately.

D. He should not be concerned if there is no change in any lesion; he does not need formal screening.

6-78   *A smoking cessation program should be initiated when*

A. the client states a readiness to quit.

B. the client is in the hospital.

C. an initial history and physical examination are performed.

D. the client's family convinces the client of the necessity to quit.

6-79   *You see a 3-year-old child in the office for a mild upper respiratory infection without fever. She is behind on her immunizations. What should you do?*

A. Tell the mother to bring her back when her infection is resolved.

B. Give her the killed-virus vaccines and wait to give the live-virus attenuated vaccines.

C. Give her the appropriate immunizations today.

D. Wait until her next scheduled visit.

6-80   *Gary, a gay male client, age 45, arrives in your office with facial bruises. He states that he injured himself opening a door, but he seems nervous. What do you suspect?*

A. He is manifesting early signs of dementia.

B. His injuries are a result of a hate crime or domestic violence.

C. He engaged in self-mutilation.

D. He injured himself as stated.

6-81   *Mark, age 26, has AIDS. He wants to know why you drew a viral load instead of a CD4 count at his last visit. What do you tell him?*

A. A viral load is a more accurate measure of the progression of the disease.

B. CD4 counts do not contribute any information regarding diagnosis and treatment.

C. A viral load and a CD4 count are similar, but a viral load test is less expensive.

D. Once a person has been given a diagnosis of AIDS, the CD4 count does not change.

6-82   *Helen is 24 weeks pregnant and needs to take a trans-Atlantic flight to attend to a sick parent. What recommendation do you make regarding her plane flight?*

A. Tell her to be sure to eat enough while traveling to avoid any drop in blood sugar.

B. Encourage her to decrease her fluid intake because it may be difficult to use the bathroom facilities and her bladder is overdistended as a result of her pregnancy.

C. Tell her to request an aisle seat so that she can ambulate frequently, and advise her to do isometric exercises.

D. She should monitor her blood pressure before and after the flight.

6-83   *Primary prevention measures for sexually transmitted diseases and unwanted pregnancies should be based on an understanding of which of the following psychosocial determinants?*

A. Informing adolescents of disease risk is an essential component of primary prevention.

B. There must be multiple approaches, and these should begin in middle childhood.

C. Working for personality change encourages adolescents to give up destructive behaviors.

D. Handing out latex condoms and showing people how to use them is the best defense against sexually transmitted diseases and unwanted pregnancies.

6-84   *You suspect that a client, age 76, is being physically abused by her husband because she has had unexplainable ecchymotic areas on her face and upper arms in her past two visits to the office. You would like to raise the issue of abuse. Which of the following statements might prompt the best response from the client?*

A. "These bruises are very unusual. Is your husband hurting you?"

B. "How did you get these bruises?"

C. "Would you like to talk about what's going on?"

D. "Do you frequently get a lot of bruises?"

6-85   *Your new client is a woman in her 80s who has a chronic cough that is progressively worsening. As part of your initial assessment, you ask about her occupational history. She states that she was a stay-at-home wife/mother. Why do you ask her about her husband's employment history and his workplace exposures?*

A. Her husband could have been exposed to tobacco smoke at work.

B. Her husband may have had an infectious disease like tuberculosis.

C. Her husband may have retiree benefits that will pay for her health care.

D. Her husband could have brought home contaminated work clothes to which she would have been exposed.

6-86   *You are counseling the parents of a 2-year-old about accidental poisoning. What do you instruct them to administer if their child should accidentally ingest something poisonous?*

A. Burnt toast

B. Tea

C. Ipecac syrup

D. Milk of magnesia

6-87   *Smoking is a risk factor for the top three causes of death. What is your best course of action for dealing with your clients who smoke?*

A. Make your clients aware of the sequelae of smoking.

B. Ask, advise, assess, assist, arrange.

C. Do not bring this topic up unless the client does.

D. Only bring this up if the client has symptoms related to smoking behavior; otherwise, mentioning it is pointless.

6-88   *While examining Marcia, age 12 months, you notice that her teeth are in very poor condition. What is the most appropriate question to ask the parents?*

A. "Does Marcia go to bed with a bottle at night?"

B. "Have you been cleaning Marcia's teeth with a piece of gauze around your finger every day?"

C. "What kinds of foods does Marcia eat?"

D. "Does Marcia chew on her toys?"

6-89   *John is 62 years old and has decided to take up tennis. What are some areas of health counseling that may help prevent injury?*

A. Advising him to eat before playing tennis so he does not become dehydrated

B. Suggesting a narrow grip size for the tennis racket and making sure the strings are tight

C. Suggesting a wide grip and working with a professional to assess how tight the strings should be

D. Discouraging him from beginning a competitive sport like tennis because of the high risk of injury

6-90   *Which of the following most commonly cause(s) intentional, nonoccupational poisoning deaths in adults?*

A. Heroin and cocaine

B. Antidepressants and tranquilizers

C. Motor vehicle exhaust

D. Barbiturates

6-91   *Nina, age 73, has trigeminal neuralgia. She asks you what measures she can take to alleviate some of the nagging problems related to it. You advise her to*

A. chew on the affected side of the mouth to strengthen those muscles.

B. eat and drink hot foods and fluids to help relax the oral mucosa.

C. avoid going to the dentist until the condition is in remission.

D. wear protective sunglasses or goggles when outside.

6-92   *Susan asks you about her husband, who was just told that he has degenerative joint disease (DJD). You know that the most likely joint to be affected by DJD is the*

A. jaw.

B. elbow.

C. hip.

D. ankle.

6-93   *Your 73-year-old newly diagnosed Alzheimer's client comes in for an appointment with her daughter. The daughter asks if there is anything she and her family can do to help the patient. Your best advice is which of the following?*

A. "Try to give your mother several new stimulating skills to perform."

B. "Assist your mother in and monitor her ability to perform activities of daily living (ADLs), and maintain a safe environment."

C. "There is little we can do to slow the progression of this disease."

D. "Your mother should be enrolled in a day-care facility for Alzheimer's patients."

6-94   *Sandra, age 65, had a radical mastectomy 20 years ago and asks you why she still cannot have her blood pressure taken on the affected arm. You tell her that*

A. after 20 years with no problem, she can have her blood pressure taken on that arm.

B. she no longer has to worry about injury or infection to that arm.

C. lymphedema can occur for up to 30 years after a mastectomy; therefore, precautions still need to be taken.

D. although she should not have blood drawn from that arm, she may have her blood pressure taken on that arm.

6-95   A client has incurred a work-related back injury. What can you tell the client about his or her rights under workers' compensation?

A. An employer pays work-related medical expenses only if there is lost time from work.

B. An employer pays for all work-related medical expenses.

C. An employee can sue his or her employer.

D. An employee must prove the employer was negligent before he or she can qualify for workers' compensation benefits.

6-96   An elderly couple comes to your office for their physical exam. The husband is concerned about his wife because she recently tripped on the rug and fell at home. Your best advice to him is,

A. "Be sure that you are available to her at all times so that you can summon someone to help."

B. "Remove or replace any tripping hazards from the home."

C. "Get a home health aide to come in and assist with ADLS."

D. "At this time, a nursing home is probably the best option for your wife."

6-97   Who should have a screening test for skin cancer?

A. All individuals, starting at adolescence, then every 5 years thereafter

B. All individuals every 2 years

C. Individuals with risk factors for skin cancer

D. All individuals during every health examination

6-98   Raymond, age 68, presents with bleeding gums and broken capillaries under his skin. What vitamin deficiency do you suspect he has?

A. Vitamin A

B. Vitamin B_{12}

C. Vitamin C

D. Vitamin D

6-99   Jill states that she cannot tell when her grandmother is dehydrated and that she never seems to drink much fluid. What do you tell her about fluid and electrolyte changes associated with aging?

A. Skin turgor is a reliable measure of body fluid levels.

B. Thirst sensation is the best indicator of body fluid balance.

C. Body weight is the best indicator of body fluid balance.

D. Peripheral edema is a reliable indicator of fluid and electrolyte balance in the older adult.

6-100   Martin is marrying Laura, who has a seizure disorder. He asks for advice regarding her seizures. Which of the following is most important?

A. Encourage Laura to begin jogging with him.

B. Remind Laura to take her anticonvulsant medication when she is experiencing seizures.

C. Do not let Laura drive for several weeks after she has a seizure.

D. Make sure that Laura wears a medical identification bracelet or necklace stating that she has a seizure disorder.

6-101   Your client, Casey, a 69-year-old chronic smoker, has called you to find out the result of his recent chest x-ray, which you ordered because of his increasingly troublesome chronic cough. You have seen a large shadow on the chest x-ray that you suspect is a carcinoma. What should you say to Casey?

A. "I need you to come to the office to discuss your chest x-ray results."

B. "I have seen an area on your chest x-ray that concerns me."

C. "Please let me speak to your wife."

D. "I saw something on your chest x-ray that we need to follow up on, but I am sure it will be all right."

6-102   Your neighbors are building a swimming pool and have two children, ages 2 and 8. What is the best recommendation you could make to them to prevent an accidental drowning of the 2-year-old?

A. Install a fence around the pool.

B. Have the 8-year-old learn cardiopulmonary resuscitation.

C. Never let the children out of your sight.

D. Keep the entrances to the backyard locked at all times.

6-103   *Jim, age 72, states that his ears get plugged up frequently from earwax and asks what he can do. You advise him to*

A. use a cotton-tipped applicator to loosen the wax.

B. flush his ears regularly with water using a bulb syringe.

C. use several drops of mineral oil.

D. irrigate his ears with a commercial preparation and leave it in for 48 hours, using cotton wicks.

6-104   *Smoking cessation strategies are more effective when the health-care educator*

A. stresses the importance of not smoking and the disease sequelae if smoking continues.

B. encourages clients to stop immediately.

C. conducts follow-up reinforcement sessions.

D. involves the entire family in the process.

6-105   *You are conducting a preplacement examination of a female disabled client who has been offered a job as a secretary. You recommend that she request accommodation for her disability under the Americans with Disabilities Act (ADA). Which federal agency has jurisdiction?*

A. Occupational Safety and Health Administration

B. Department of Justice

C. Equal Employment Opportunity Commission

D. Department of Labor

6-106   *Sam, age 73, has lumbar spinal stenosis and asks which exercises he should do to help his condition. You advise him to*

A. do any exercise that results in hyperextension of the lumbar spine.

B. do exercises that encourage lumbar flexion and flattening of the lumbar lordotic curve.

C. refrain from exercising.

D. see a surgeon because surgery is the best treatment option.

6-107   *Susan is a 67-year-old woman with chronic headaches. She has come to you specifically for a referral to a neurologist. She has already seen four neurologists but is not satisfied with the answer that any of them has provided. What should you do?*

A. Explain in an empathic way that there is no need to see another neurologist and that you cannot support another referral.

B. Agree to refer her to another neurologist, and spend as little time with her as possible so that you can focus on clients who have more immediate concerns.

C. Do a complete history and physical, and attempt to find out why the client was dissatisfied with the advice she received from the previous neurological consultations.

D. Rule out any immediate life-threatening problem, and tell the client to return in a few weeks. If at that point she still wants the referral, you will provide it.

6-108   *You see a 19-year-old college student, Melissa, who is listless and speaks in monosyllabic language. Her affect is flat. Her mother has brought her to your primary care office because she is concerned about her. You know that risk factors for depression include which of the following?*

A. Being a college student

B. Believing oneself to be incapable, helpless, a victim, or hopeless

C. Having the summer free from school

D. Not having a car or transportation available

6-109   *Mandy is pregnant with her first baby. She asks you what is the safest drug to use in pregnancy. What do you tell her?*

A. Acetylsalicylic acid (aspirin)

B. Acetaminophen (Tylenol)

C. Erythromycin (E-Mycin, Eryc)

D. Tetracycline (Achromycin, Sumycin)

6-110   *When you are performing a history and physical examination on Jason, age 16, he tells you that although he does not smoke, he uses snuff (smokeless tobacco). He says that he wants the nicotine "high" but does not want it to become a habit like cigarette smoking. What should you tell him about smokeless tobacco?*

A. It may lead to mouth or throat cancer.

B. Smokeless tobacco has no effect on teeth and gums.

C. Smokeless tobacco will increase his appetite.

D. It is less dangerous than cigarette smoking.

6-111   *Martha is concerned because her 6-year-old daughter wets the bed almost every night. Appropriate counseling statements include which of the following?*

A. "Enuresis is a common problem, and it may have a physiological basis. It also may be inherited."

B. "This problem has serious repercussions for the child and must be dealt with on a variety of levels."

C. "Nighttime enuresis is not an inherited problem."

D. "A self-help group for clients may prove helpful in dealing with this recalcitrant behavior."

6-112   *Mr. Kent is a 60-year-old man who has a variety of cardiac risk factors. When you evaluate his risk profile, which of the following should be taken into consideration?*

A. Past surgeries

B. Number of children

C. Temperament

D. Economic advantage

6-113   *A statement that most indicates your 65-year-old client is ready to quit smoking is:*

A. "My wife has been nagging me to quit for years."

B. "I suppose my health would improve if I stopped now."

C. "I tried to quit last week, but when my buddy who still smokes came over, I smoked only one with him."

D. "Can you tell me if there are any Web sites I can visit to get tips on quitting?"

6-114   *What is the best way to promote a personal behavior change in a client?*

A. Write an order for a treatment plan.

B. Stress compliance with your treatment plan.

C. Prescribe a health promotion regimen.

D. Discuss choices with the client and let him or her decide what will work best.

6-115   *Phil, 14 years old, reluctantly tells you that he thinks he has something seriously wrong with him because he has awakened in the morning with a wet sheet around his penis. What do you do?*

A. Perform a test to rule out a sexually transmitted disease.

B. Tell him that this is a normal part of his sexual development.

C. Ask him if he is emptying his bladder before he goes to bed.

D. Tell him that this is abnormal and you want to refer him to a urologist.

6-116   *Your elderly client is on polypharmacy, and you suspect that she may be forgetting or not taking some of her medications. You would like to help her, so you*

A. recommend that she have a friend call and remind her to take her medications.

B. ask her if there is a reason she is not taking her medications.

C. recommend that she use a pill tracker that can be prefilled each week.

D. do nothing because it is common for the elderly to skip their medications sometimes.

6-117   *Susan asks why her husband developed degenerative joint disease (DJD) when there was no family history of it. You tell her that a cause of primary DJD is*

A. trauma.

B. obesity.

C. sepsis.

D. a blood dyscrasia.

6-118   *Mr. Green is a vigorous 70-year-old who comes for early assessment of dementia. He wants to "work" to keep up his mental capacities. You counsel that he should*

A. make sure he gets enough rest because cells need time to regenerate as a result of the stress of the aging process.

B. begin taking a calcium supplement.

C. consider a hobby that challenges his mental capacity, like building model ships or airplanes.

D. play bridge (or any group card game) several times a week.

6-119 *What is one specific intervention that might help Mr. Kent deal with his underlying coronary artery disease (CAD)?*

A. Frequent rest periods

B. Drinking at least one glass of red wine a day

C. Having a pet

D. Practicing relaxation exercises daily

6-120 *Jane, age 72, is very upset about her stress incontinence. She asks you for advice. What do you tell her?*

A. "Unfortunately, stress incontinence is part of the normal aging process."

B. "There are many new pads on the market that provide an efficacious approach to this common problem, thus preventing social isolation."

C. "A diet that incorporates cranberry juice may be effective in curbing this problem."

D. "Kegel exercises may help."

6-121 *You suspect that Ginger, age 6, has parents who smoke. Ginger is being seen in the office for an acute asthma attack. Her mother is present. How do you approach Ginger's mother about this risk factor?*

A. "You know that smoking is detrimental to Ginger's health."

B. "I hope that you don't smoke in front of Ginger."

C. "Is Ginger ever exposed to cigarette smoke?"

D. "I can smell smoke on your clothes. How many packs do you smoke per day?"

6-122 *Alison asks you whether she should do anaerobic or aerobic exercise and what the difference is between them. You tell her that a simple measure of whether or not an exercise activity is aerobic or not is*

A. her heart rate.

B. whether or not she is sweating.

C. her degree of fatigue.

D. whether or not her muscles ache.

6-123 *Henry, age 57, is married and the father of three children. He is overweight and hypertensive and has a sedentary lifestyle. His father died of a myocardial infarction at age 42. Which factor will*

provide the strongest motivation for Henry to change his lifestyle?

A. The fear that he will not live to see his daughter get married

B. Feeling "ownership" of the need to change

C. Feeling guilty that his wife might be left alone to raise the children

D. The desire to enjoy his retirement when the time comes

Answers

6-1   Answer D

For the promotion of personal safety, advise clients to wear wide-base, low-heel shoes with corrugated soles to help prevent slips and falls. Slippers or flimsy or slippery-soled shoes should not be worn. No one should walk around with glasses that are meant only for reading; they should be taken off before moving. Smoking should never take place in bed.

6-2   Answer D

Swimming greatly benefits the heart and lungs but does not help osteoporosis. All caffeine is a risk factor for osteoporosis. Cutting down on coffee is a good first step, but black (regular) tea also contains caffeine. Herbal tea or decaffeinated coffee are better recommendations. Shelley needs an adequate calcium intake, not just a multivitamin. Regular exercise, especially weight-bearing exercise that includes walking and running, is recommended. This is because these types of exercises put the body's weight on the bones, pressing calcium into the bone matrix. Additionally, strengthening the leg muscles helps prevent falls; therefore, simply standing is more beneficial than sitting.

6-3   Answer A

You must investigate the underlying causes of this new change in sexual function and desire. Although testosterone deficiency is a common cause of low desire and is more common in older adults, this change in sexual function is not a natural consequence of aging and should not be treated as such. It is too soon to send this client for sexual counseling, as you must first attempt to ascertain the underlying reason behind the problem. You do not have enough data to presume depression, although depression is a common component of low sexual desire. Also, prescribing serotonin reuptake inhibitors (SSRIs), a type of antidepressant, may create other forms of sexual dysfunction, typically delayed or absent orgasm. You may end up sending this client for counseling and/or prescribing Viagra, but more investigation should be completed first.

6-4   Answer C

When clients are taking NSAIDs, there is always a risk of gastrointestinal tract bleeding, so the clients should be advised to look for signs of this complication. The American Academy of Family Physicians (AAFP) recommends that the smallest possible doses of NSAIDs for the shortest possible duration are best to minimize the incidence of side effects. The AAFP cautions to avoid using NSAIDs in clients taking anticoagulant such as Coumadin, as there may be an additive effect and increased risk of bleeding. Obesity is one of the major contributors to the development of osteoarthritis of the knee. Any weight loss that can occur will remove stress from the client's joints and may improve overall cardiovascular health.

6-5   Answer D

Agriculture continues to rank as the most dangerous industry in the United States. It is important for the health-care provider to provide anticipatory guidance related to farm safety. Various groups such as the National Committee for Childhood Agricultural Injury Prevention (NCAIP) and Farm Safety 4 Just Kids provide resources for farm safety information, including age-appropriate publications such as storybooks and coloring books, as well as a rural health and safety kit that includes games, puzzles, and brochures. Still, farm-related injuries and fatalities continue to occur. Contributing factors include lack of parental supervision, operator fatigue, and children performing tasks inappropriate for age. Education and health counseling is a high priority for all members of the farming family.

6-6   Answer C

Thimerosal is a preservative that contains ethyl mercury 50% by weight. Though the risk of dying from childhood disease is greater than any potential health risks associated with thimerosal, this first answer does not address the parent's concern about thimerosal specifically. The U.S. Food and Drug Administration (FDA) can and does issue

directives to drug manufacturers concerning label warnings; however, to date, the FDA has not issued such a directive about thimerosal because it has not been adequately demonstrated that thimerosal contributes to or causes autism or any other neurodevelopmental disorder. Concerned parents should ensure that all currently used vaccine is thimerosal free, as there may be old stock still in circulation. In the United States, thimerosal is no longer added as a preservative to routinely recommended childhood vaccines, except inactivated influenza vaccine. Concerned parents can request thimerosal-free vaccines. Always address parents' concerns.

6-7   Answer C

If a mother brings in her daughter because she thinks her daughter is sexually active, you should not take as fact the mother's belief. You should find out directly from the daughter. If the daughter admits to being sexually active, you may want to do a vaginal examination and discuss contraception methods or counseling. Notification of a child protective services agency may be warranted if the daughter admits to, or if you suspect, sexual abuse or an incestuous relationship with her father, stepfather, or other male relative given the age of the child and state law on statutory rape, even if sexual activity is consensual and nonfamilial.

6-8   Answer C

A high-carbohydrate diet will increase an athlete's endurance. A fat-and-protein diet provides 95% of total calories from fat and 5% from protein; a normal mixed diet with fat, protein, and carbohydrates provides 55% of total calories from carbohydrates; and a high-carbohydrate diet provides 83% of total calories from carbohydrates. Although fruits and vegetables should be a component of all diets, they should not make up the entire diet. A fruit-and-vegetable diet would not maximize an athlete's endurance time. In a study related to these diets and an athlete's maximum endurance time, a fat-and-protein diet gave 57 minutes of maximum endurance, a normal mixed diet gave 114 minutes, and a high-carbohydrate diet gave 167 minutes.

6-9   Answer D

Grief reactions vary from person to person, and everyone deals differently with their grief. It is not normal, however, to experience extreme feelings of guilt or responsibility for the loved one's loss. If your client is experiencing this or symptoms of prolonged or functional impairment, it may signal that she is experiencing a complicated grief reaction that may require a consultation or further evaluation. It is quite normal for clients to experience waves of depression as well as crying and some loss of appetite.

6-10   Answer C

The most effective interventions available to health-care providers for reducing the incidence and severity of the leading causes of disease and disability in the United States are those counseling interventions that address the personal health practices of clients. This is the first type of clinical preventive service that providers should use, according to the U.S. Preventive Services Task Force. These counseling interventions address use of tobacco, diet, physical activity, sexual practices, and injury prevention. Other interventions that should be used include screening tests, immunizations, and chemoprophylaxis.

6-11   Answer A

To get an accurate result when collecting fecal occult blood samples, the following should be avoided: aspirin or aspirin-containing drugs for 7 days before and during the collection period; red or processed meat and raw fruits and vegetables for 3 days before and during the collection period; and vitamin C or multivitamins containing more than 250 mg of vitamin C per day during the collection period. Clients may have fruit juices and other beverages they normally drink, cooked vegetables or fruits, breads, cereal, fish, chicken, pork, and popcorn. They do not need to avoid shellfish, nor do they need to avoid vigorous exercise.

6-12   Answer D

When teaching clients about gout, include the following information: Although the initial attack of gout causes no permanent damage, recurrent attacks may lead to permanent damage and joint destruction. Kidney stones and kidney damage may result if the gout is not managed adequately. Clients should drink at least 3 quarts of fluid per day to help prevent kidney stones and damage to the kidneys from hyperuricemia, and they should avoid alcohol. Other potential effects of continued hyperuricemia include tophaceous deposits in subcutaneous and other connective tissues.

6-13   Answer C

Researchers in a study on the strength of hearts in men and women found that men's hearts lose 20%–25% of their power from ages 20–70, whereas the power of women's hearts essentially remains unchanged. These researchers found that 70-year-old men who did regular aerobic exercise had the same functioning power of the heart as 20-year-old men. The study helps to illustrate the fact that although men's hearts can, with aging, lose some of their power or strength, aerobic exercise can help to prevent this loss. This is another example of how encouragement of healthy lifestyle choices (e.g., regular aerobic exercise) can enhance or preserve health. Certainly diet and good sleep habits are important, but not as important as exercise for improving overall heart functioning.

6-14   Answer C

Colonoscopy is not a preventive strategy but rather a form of secondary (screening) prevention, as is routine annual testing for fecal occult blood after age 50. Obesity is a weak risk factor for colon and rectal cancer, so weight loss is not the most valuable preventive strategy. No correlation between cigarette smoking and colon and rectal cancer has been discovered. However, the preventive power of regular physical exercise has been established as a protective factor against colon cancer and also against rectal cancer, but to a lesser degree. Likewise, a healthy diet rich in vegetables, fruits, and fiber has been shown to have protective effects against colon and rectal cancer. The effect of regular aspirin use as a protector against colon cancers has been replicated in several studies. Aspirin inhibits the growth of colonic and rectal polyps, perhaps by means of inhibiting prostaglandin synthesis.

6-15   Answer A

To help manage the effects of scleroderma, advise clients to avoid becoming chilled, which could trigger episodes of Raynaud's phenomenon; maintain good skin care; perform physical therapy, particularly of the hands and face, to help maintain mobility; wear loose, warm clothing, gloves, and warm stockings in the winter; and stop smoking altogether (because of the vasoconstrictive effect of nicotine, as well as the respiratory effects of the disease).

6-16   Answer C

Children younger than the age of 7 years often experience frequent ear infections. The eustachian tubes of children this age are horizontal and do not allow the drainage of infecting organisms—viral or bacterial. An infection in the nasopharynx may ascend to a child's horizontal eustachian tube and then into the middle ear by impairing local host defenses or by eustachian tube dysfunction. By age 7, 35% of children experience six or more episodes of acute otitis media. As the child grows, the eustachian tube angles more and is no longer horizontal. If Shirley inserted a foreign body into her ear and it remained in place, occluding the canal, she could develop an infection, but the mother is asking about frequent infections, which are more common than infections induced by foreign bodies. A high-fat diet will not affect cerumen production. The mother cannot be expected to dry her daughter's ears completely after bathing. She should be drying the external canal with a cloth or tissue, nothing smaller.

6-17   Answer C

To encourage physical activity along with parental involvement, advise teachers to assign homework to the students that must be done with their parents and involves physical activity, such as having the parents count how many times in 2 minutes the child can hop on one foot. Recommending play outside may not be safe, depending on the neighborhood. Turning off the TV is a good idea, but children may then substitute some other sedentary method of play, such as computer games.

6-18   Answer A

When delivering bad news, the following framework may prove helpful: (1) preparation (forecast possibility of bad news); (2) setting (give news in person if possible with privacy and adequate time); (3) delivery (give the news clearly but present the hopeful message first and then identify important feelings and concerns); (4) emotional support (remain with client and use empathic statements); (5) information (use clear words and summarize; use handouts as needed); and (6) closure (make a plan for the immediate future and schedule a follow-up appointment). Do not provide false reassurance. Allow time for silence throughout. The specific rationale for providing the hopeful message first is that typically clients remember very little after hearing the distressing news.

6-19   Answer C

If a client is caring for an elderly parent with dementia, recommend that the client get information on home safety and community resources. In this case, Mary should be put in touch with support services for herself and given information about respite care. She should also receive information about resources regarding home safety that can be implemented so that she will not have to worry constantly about her father injuring himself. Mary should be encouraged to keep her father at home as long as possible because changing his environment may tend to worsen his dementia. However, she should not be made to feel guilty if she reaches the decision that she can no longer care for him at home. An elderly person's door should never be locked at night to keep him or her from wandering because there would be no way of escaping in case of a fire.

6-20   Answer A

Screening for hypersensitivity to lung irritants is primary prevention of asthma because you are screening individuals before the development of disease and the commencement of counseling for it. Primary prevention for asthma includes cessation of tobacco smoking and the removal of environmental tobacco smoke left by smokers. The use of newer technologies to precipitate industrial air pollutants before they reach human air space is another emerging strategy. The use of masks has not been shown to be effective as a primary preventive strategy. Screening yearly with pulmonary function tests is secondary prevention, as are chest x-rays.

6-21   Answer A

The best outcomes occur with the immediate use of antivirals such as acyclovir, valacyclovir, and famciclovir, which should be taken until finished. Steroid creams as well as calamine and Burow's solution are helpful and provide relief for some patients but are more supportive. Clients should be instructed to alert their practitioner if they develop any lesions on their face, as ophthalmic lesions can affect the trigeminal nerve and cause blindness—a referral in this case to an ophthalmologist is warranted.

6-22   Answer A

Hazardous chemicals present at hazardous waste sites can leach into groundwater and/or soil and subsequently into drinking water and the food chain. Exposure to pesticides, polychlorinated biphenyls (PCBs), and dioxins has been linked to disruption of the endocrine system. Exposure to these chemicals has not been linked to autism specifically, though it has been linked to neurodevelopment generally. These chemicals are not leukemogenic substances; such substances include solvents such as benzene. For infants, toddlers, and young children, secondary ingestion (hand to mouth) of environmental chemicals is the primary route of entry. As a result, toddlers should not be allowed to play in any area where hazardous environmental chemicals may be present. These chemicals would have to become airborne to be inhaled and play a role in the development of asthma. Insects are potential asthmagens, an exposure that can occur in the home and near a hazardous waste site.

6-23   Answer A

If the hepatitis B vaccine schedule is interrupted, it should be continued. If interrupted after the first dose, the second dose should be given as soon as possible; the third dose can be given 2 months after the second dose and at least 4 months after the first dose. This client's normal schedule would have been a series of three immunizations, with the second and third doses administered 1 month and 6 months, respectively, after the first dose. If a period longer than 6 months has elapsed, a titer must be drawn to evaluate need for further vaccine.

6-24   Answer D

All children will receive approximately 25 vaccines by the time they reach 5 years of age. During early childhood, infants and children are immunized with a wide variety of vaccines, including hepatitis B (hep B); diphtheria, acellular pertussis, and tetanus (DTaP); inactivated polio vaccine (IPV); *Haemophilus influenzae* type b (HIB); measles, mumps, and rubella (MMR); varicella vaccine (VZV); pneumococcal conjugate vaccine (PCV); and influenza, pneumococcal, and meningococcal vaccine. After the age of 5, they will continue to receive a tetanus diphtheria (Td) every 10 years. They may also continue to receive an influenza vaccine yearly depending on their medical history. The immunization schedules change rapidly, so to obtain the most current information, go to http://www.cdc.gov/vaccines/recs/acip/default.htm, which offers current immunization guidelines for children and adults.

6-25   Answer D

Asian food is not associated with an increased risk of DVT. The time difference is immaterial to risk of DVT; jet lag is not associated with DVT. DVT is neither an infectious disease nor an endemic disease. Asia–U.S. flights take more than 8–10 hours; long periods of immobility and dehydration are risk factors for deep vein thrombosis.

6-26   Answer C

High-impact exercise is not recommended with rheumatoid arthritis (RA), as it may increase the damage to joints, but weight loss is a good idea—eating healthy is recommended, and removing excess weight can increase mobility and contribute to a better sense of well-being. Abstaining from exercise altogether is probably not a good idea, as it contributes to increased stiffness and decreases muscle strength needed to support joints. Preservation of joint function and mobility are important for health maintenance for the RA patient. Rest is important, and swollen joints should be rested.

6-27   Answer B

Although you might like to report a gun in the house to the police, especially a gun in a house with a young child, this is not required; the gun may, in fact, be registered. What you do want to do is stress the need to keep the gun in a locked place, where the child has no access to it, with a combination lock on the trigger, and to keep the ammunition and gun in separate places. You might also want to talk about other home safety devices, such as alarms, if the client feels that his or her home is not safe. Unfortunately, your personal bias and views on this situation, as expressed in options C and D, are not pertinent. You should not pass judgment; it is an ineffective strategy for behavioral change. Additionally, you cannot require a meeting with both parents regarding this issue.

6-28   Answer C

Clients with diabetes mellitus should be taught proper foot care, especially the use of a mirror to help them inspect the bottoms (soles) of their feet because peripheral neuropathy may prevent them from feeling any foreign bodies or cuts. Preparations such as alcohol should be avoided because they tend to dry and crack the feet, allowing microorganisms to enter. Soaking the feet in water and use of emollients should also be avoided because they help to keep the feet moist and thus become a good medium for the growth of bacteria.

6-29   Answer A

Foods high in potassium and calcium, such as bananas and milk, help to lower blood pressure. Also, a low-sodium diet is recommended to help reduce the amount of retained water, which, in turn, helps to lower blood pressure. In addition, some diuretics deplete serum potassium, which bananas will help to replace.

6-30   Answer B

A frequently cited model describes five stages in health behavior change: precontemplation, contemplation, preparation, action, and maintenance. Precontemplation is described as the stage in which the individual is not even considering the idea of change; contemplation is the stage when he or she begins to actively think about the health risk but no action is planned; preparation occurs when the individual begins to actively plan and move into early action—for example, by developing a plan or joining a self-help group; action is marked by observable changes in health-related behavior (there may be relapses, but this is part of the process); and maintenance is when the new health action is firmly consolidated as a permanent lifestyle. Prevention of relapse is critical.

6-31   Answer D

Hot showers may transiently exacerbate symptoms. There is no evidence that flying exacerbates multiple sclerosis. Exercise is important to maintain function and flexibility, but it needs to be balanced with rest to avoid excessive fatigue. There is no need to avoid spicy foods, caffeine, and peppermint because of multiple sclerosis.

6-32   Answer D

Although Guillain-Barré syndrome was associated with the use of the "swine flu" vaccine in 1976, studies done every year since have not shown a clear association between influenza vaccination and neurological complications. Tim is a definite candidate for a flu shot because he is older than age 65 and has pulmonary disease. A flu shot is recommended for residents and employees of nursing homes and other chronic care facilities; for clients with diabetes mellitus, renal dysfunction,

hemoglobinopathy, and immunosuppression; and for health-care personnel.

6-33   Answer B

With a client who smokes, it is appropriate to discuss smoking cessation techniques at every visit. Because family practitioners see about 70% of the smokers in the United States during the course of each year, these encounters present excellent opportunities for providers to deliver smoking cessation advice to clients who smoke. This should be done at each visit, regardless of the reason the client is being seen. *Healthy People 2010* includes an objective to increase to at least 75% the proportion of health-care providers who routinely advise their clients who smoke to quit.

6-34   Answer C

Self-tanning lotions or creams are a safe alternative to tanning from natural sunlight, tanning beds, or lamps. These substances contain dihydroxyacetone, a substance approved by the Food and Drug Administration, which binds to the epidermis and chemically produces a skin color resembling a sunlight-induced tan. Self-tanning does not affect melanocytes or melanogenesis, does not increase melanin levels, and does not depend on ultraviolet light. However, it is unrealistic to think that young women will take your advice and avoid the sun completely. While recommending a self-tanning lotion to Melanie, you should also stress that if she insists on getting a tan naturally, she should have brief tanning periods using a sunscreen with a skin protection factor (SPF) of 15 or higher.

6-35   Answer D

When counseling clients about diet and exercise, advise them, regardless of their blood sugar level, that they should eat within an hour after exercising. If they are not able to eat a full meal, they should have a high-carbohydrate snack, such as 6 oz of fruit juice or half a bagel. If more intensive exercise is planned, they should consume a little more, such as half a meat sandwich and a cup of low-fat milk. Advise clients to avoid exercise when their blood sugar is consistently high and ketones are present in the urine. Exercise should be avoided at the peak action time of insulin—for example, 2–4 hours for short-acting insulin, 12 hours for intermediate-acting insulin, and 16 hours for long-acting insulin. In addition, insulin should never be injected into parts of the body that are being used during exercise, such as the arms for tennis players or the legs for joggers, because it will be absorbed into the bloodstream too quickly.

6-36   Answer B

Falls are the most common cause of injuries, the leading cause of hospital admissions for trauma, and the second-most common cause of injury-related deaths for all age groups (about 12,000 annually). About 1 out of 20 persons receives emergency department care for injuries sustained in falls. Children typically fall from buildings or other elevated structures, whereas older adults are more likely to fall during normal household activities. Adult falls are usually a result of gait instability, decreased proprioception and muscle strength, or vision problems. Falls cause nearly 90% of all fractures among older adults. Motor vehicle and bicycle accidents are a cause of death in 1 out of 6 school-age children.

6-37   Answer C

Instructing Marvin on self-monitoring of his blood sugar makes him an active participant in his own health care, which, in turn, will improve his adherence to the plan of care. Although you may want him to call a nutritionist, he may choose not to or may be in denial. Initially you will have Marvin come in frequently for a urinalysis and will monitor glycohemoglobin levels every 3 months, but making him a participant in his care is one way to encourage ownership of the problem, which leads to an active approach.

6-38   Answer D

When counseling clients, practice the "art of the possible." Your goal is not to increase the client's knowledge but to effect behavioral change. Be realistic. For example, a client should not be asked to stop all intercourse. Clients who are not adequately helped the first time will be back again and again. It is practically impossible to counsel clients in this area adequately in one session. Personal connection, repeated messages, praise of progress, and negotiation are the name of the game. Even commercial sex workers, for example, might learn to be more restrictive by insisting on practicing only safe sex or by avoiding high-risk situations such as working with belligerent or drugged clients.

6-39   Answer C

The appropriate response to a client who is concerned about gaining weight after smoking cessation is to suggest several strategies that the client might use to prevent weight gain. Many clients who have stopped smoking and gain weight resume smoking. Therefore, this is an important area to address when the client is considering smoking cessation so that it can be dealt with before the weight is gained. The average amount of weight gained after smoking cessation is about 5 lb. Two strategies to be used are avoiding high-calorie foods (while keeping low-calorie foods available to satisfy the urge to eat) and increasing exercise.

6-40   Answer D

Carbohydrate loading tricks muscles into storing extra glycogen before a competition. In training, a high-carbohydrate diet should be eaten regularly. During the first 4 days of the week before the competition, the individual should train moderately hard (1–2 hours per day) and eat a diet moderate in carbohydrates. During the 3 days before the competition, the individual should cut back on activity and eat a diet very high in carbohydrates. This practice can benefit an athlete who must keep going for 90 minutes or longer.

6-41   Answer B

To adequately address the client's questions, specific and accurate information is required. The client should request a material safety data sheet (MSDS) from his or her employer. Today, many manufacturers have MSDSs for their products online and publicly available. Regardless, employees and health-care professionals have the legal right to request an MSDS from (their clients') employers per OSHA Hazard Communication Standard 29CFR1910.1200 (published by Occupational Safety and Health Administration in 1999). Additionally, health-care professionals have the legal right to access trade secret information if necessary. If the employer refuses, contact the local Occupational Safety and Health Administration (OSHA) office. It is premature and may be unnecessary to request/obtain a chemical sample for laboratory analysis. To recommend terminating employment is unwarranted at this time. The local fire department has chemical-related information for emergency planning and response purposes.

6-42   Answer C

Epidemiologists have identified three stages of the disease process at which preventive actions can be effective: primary prevention, secondary prevention, and tertiary prevention. Health promotion programs usually begin at the primary prevention level, which aims at keeping a disease from beginning or a trauma from occurring. Primary prevention programs aim to reach the widest possible population group that is or might be at risk for a given health problem. Immunization is an example of primary prevention. Health promotion programs aimed at increasing exercise are another example of primary prevention of problems; their goal is to avert problems such as coronary artery disease and diabetes mellitus.

Secondary prevention involves early detection and early intervention against disease before it fully develops. Screening for potential disorders is considered secondary prevention. Mammography is an example of a strategy to detect breast cancer in its early stages. Pap smears are another example of secondary prevention, aimed at detecting cervical cancer in its early stages.

Tertiary prevention takes place after a disease or injury has occurred. Cardiac rehabilitation programs are an example of tertiary prevention. These programs are aimed at improving heart function and reducing the risk of subsequent damage to the heart.

6-43   Answer A

Polyunsaturated fats ("good fats"), such as soybean oil, are liquid at room temperature and come from vegetables. Saturated fats ("bad fats"), such as coconut and palm oils and cocoa butter, harden at room temperature and are found in meat and dairy products made from whole milk or cream as well as in solid and hydrogenated shortening.

6-44   Answer C

The cheapest and easiest remedy for pediculosis (head lice) is to apply mayonnaise or White Rain conditioner to the scalp and hair. The solution smothers the live lice and loosens nits to facilitate their removal from the hair shaft. Although petroleum jelly (Vaseline) also works, it is extremely difficult to remove from the hair. Cutting the hair very short or shaving it should not be necessary.

6-45   Answer A

The Environmental Protection Agency/Food and Drug Administration (EPA/FDA) recommends that pregnant women not eat swordfish, tilefish, shark, or king mackerel and no more than 6 oz per week of albacore tuna because of moderate to high levels of methyl mercury found in these fish. All seafood contains some amount of this environmental contaminant. Light white tuna, salmon, haddock, halibut, shrimp, and pollock have much lower amounts of methyl mercury. These fish are excellent sources of protein and contribute to healthy fetal neurodevelopment. Women should be encouraged to eat these types of fish.

6-46   Answer D

The U.S. Preventive Services Task Force recommends the following for all pregnant women: screening for *Chlamydia*, syphilis, hepatitis B, and asymptomatic bacteriuria; interventions to reduce alcohol abuse with screening and behavioral counseling; counseling to prevent tobacco use and tobacco-caused disease; blood typing and assessment for Rh(D) incompatibility; and behavioral interventions to promote breastfeeding.

6-47   Answer B

Understanding that the pain and fatigue of fibromyalgia are real will enable the client, family, and friends to work with the health-care provider to offer support and education that might assist the couple in dealing with this chronic condition. The couple should be seen together so that they may be counseled about the chronicity of the syndrome and how it may be managed. Support groups and educational classes are a source of help for clients with fibromyalgia.

6-48   Answer B

The best recommendation when counseling an obese client to lose weight is to advise the client to increase activity. Because obese persons usually eat more and exercise less than nonobese persons, simply increasing energy expenditure may result in weight loss. Diet histories from obese persons have shown that their intakes are similar to, or even less than, those of nonobese persons. Although a diet history may not be totally accurate, it will show the types of food the person is eating. Heredity does play a major factor; if both parents are obese, there is an 80% chance that the children will be obese. However, most experts conclude that overweight persons simply eat more and exercise less than nonobese persons.

6-49   Answer A

Delay pregnancy for 3 months following vaccines for measles, mumps, and rubella (MMR); yellow fever; or varicella. These are all live attenuated vaccines. The others are not.

6-50   Answer B

Sensory changes and resulting problems can be a major contributing factor for loss of independence and change in lifestyle to the elderly. Loss of hearing can put your elderly client at risk for accidents and can create social isolation. Assisting your elderly client with referrals and the utilization of assistive devices is an important service to your client.

6-51   Answer A

You should recommend biological monitoring of the firefighter's exposure to carbon monoxide. This particular situation states the firefighter came directly from fighting the fire (fire suppression). By-products of combustion include carbon dioxide (CO_2) and carbon monoxide (CO). Carbon dioxide is a simple asphyxiate (displaces oxygen in a room); carbon monoxide is a chemical asphyxiate (structurally binds with hemoglobin). CO poisoning it not readily reversible and can result in myocardial infarction and death. Diagnosis of CO poisoning is determined by analyzing a blood sample. Often during fire overhaul—that is, after the fire is "out" when firefighters continue to look for "hidden fire" inside attics, walls, and so on— they typically do not wear respiratory protection. As a result, they may be exposed to other dangerous gases, including hydrogen cyanide (HCN). If the firefighter came from the scene after the fire was out, HCN poisoning should be considered. Methane is an explosive gas and could have been the cause of the fire.

6-52   Answer C

Encourage the client with arthritis to rest frequently throughout the day to help alleviate discomfort and pain. Other interventions include applying heat to painful joints, usually in the form of warm packs or warm baths; applying splints to the affected joint to help maintain the joint in correct alignment; using good body mechanics and proper posture to reduce the stress on the affected joints; and losing weight (if overweight) to take stress off the affected joint.

6-53   Answer C

A weight gain of 3–5 pounds in a week should be reported to the clinician. As heart failure progresses, it is not abnormal to have increased dyspnea, especially with exertion that can occur with stair climbing. Loss of appetite may be related to a feeling of fullness and associated with excess fluid or ascites. Peripheral edema is a hallmark of heart failure.

6-54   Answer A

There are many reasons that health-care professionals give inadequate counseling for behavioral change in the primary care setting. The primary reason is a lack of motivation because facilitating behavioral change in clients may be difficult and frustrating. Another reason is that health-care providers are skeptical about the benefits of counseling: Do clients really listen, or are they present only to receive treatment of their chief complaint? The fact that providers are not used to discussing risk factors and health promotion behaviors and counseling regarding self-care activities is another reason information is withheld. The U.S. Preventive Services Task Force examined more than 200 clinical preventive services and suggested health counseling and self-care activities that providers can recommend to their clients.

6-55   Answer D

The patient should be advised that wearing hearing protection whenever exposed to loud noise, whether work related or not, can prevent further hearing loss. Noise-induced hearing loss is irreversible because it destroys the nerve receptors in the inner ear.

6-56   Answer A

Signs and symptoms of bulimia nervosa include frequent urinary tract infections, which usually result from fluid and electrolyte imbalance; more than the average number of dental caries for the person's age and erosion of the teeth, usually as a result of vomiting, which can also cause irritation and infection of the pharynx, esophagus, and salivary glands; bruised or cut hands, which usually result from contact with the teeth when inducing vomiting; and injury to the lower intestinal tract from frequent use of strong laxatives. Bizarre behavior around food; hyperactivity; amenorrhea; and dry, sparse hair are all more typical of anorexia nervosa than bulimia.

6-57 Answer B

Most airlines do not allow pregnant women to travel if they are at more than 35–36 weeks' gestation without a letter from their physician or health-care provider. Commercial aircraft cruising at high altitude are able to pressurize only up to 5,000–8,000 ft above sea level. Women with moderate anemia (hemoglobin less than 8.5 g/dL) or with compromised oxygen saturation may need oxygen supplementation. Women with sickle cell disease may experience a crisis during the desaturation. Other medical risk factors include congenital or acquired heart disease, history of thromboembolic disease, hemoglobin less than 8.5 g/dL, chronic lung disease such as asthma, and medical disease requiring ongoing assessment and medication.

Obstetric risk factors include history of miscarriage, threatened abortion or vaginal bleeding during the present pregnancy, history of ectopic pregnancy (rule out with ultrasound before flying), primigravida older than 35 or younger than 15 years of age, history of diabetes with pregnancy, hypertension, toxemia, multiple gestation in present pregnancy, incompetent cervix, history of infertility, or difficulty becoming pregnant. An electrocardiogram would be indicated only related to a specific risk factor, whereas it would be essential to check the hemoglobin level in making your decision. Even those with sickle cell trait may experience hematuria or renal microthrombosis during desaturation. The fetal circulation and fetal hemoglobin protect the fetus against desaturation during flight.

6-58 Answer C

When asked, approximately 50% of nonadherent clients will admit to not taking their medication as ordered. Clients who admit to missing medication generally overestimate the amount of medication they do take. Although the direct approach may be effective, it is often more productive to inquire in such a way as to allow the client to save face. Any questioning should be done in a nonthreatening and nonjudgmental manner.

6-59 Answer A

Health programs must be convenient if they are to be effective. This includes convenience in location—someplace easily accessible, for example—convenience in times, and convenience and comfort in participating in the program.

A friendly, culturally appropriate, "user-friendly" style is critical. Although the content, language, and visual images of the health information presented are important, nothing is more important than getting the participants to the program. No matter how excellent the content, if no one is there to participate, it is meaningless.

6-60 Answer A

Coconut oil, cocoa butter, and palm and palm kernel oils are all examples of saturated fat, a type of fatty acid. Olive oil is an example of a monounsaturated fatty acid. Corn, cottonseed, soybean, and safflower oils are all types of polyunsaturated fatty acids. There are no combinations of monounsaturated and polyunsaturated fats.

6-61 Answer D

Clients who have been diagnosed with PAD or chronic venous insufficiency should be counseled about the modification of risk factors. Clients need to stop smoking completely, not merely cut down. Stating that "I'll cut down on my smoking" means that Joe has not understood your teaching instructions. It is essential to control hypertension and diabetes, if present. Dietary control must include limitation of fat and salt intake. Clients must be taught to do meticulous daily foot care that includes inspecting feet daily for sores, ulcers, and abrasions, including the use of a mirror to check the soles of the feet. Clients should not walk barefoot and should wear well-fitting supportive shoes. They should not soak their feet and should be careful trimming their nails. All clients should be taught to watch for the signs and symptoms that might indicate progressive ischemia, such as increased pain, increased pallor or cyanosis, and rest pain.

6-62 Answer D

The U.S. Preventive Services Task Force and other groups advise health-care providers to take a complete sexual history on all adolescent and adult clients. Because of the sensitive nature of the topic, the provider needs to emphasize its importance to the client and state the relevance to a total history and physical. The client who is present with another in the room needs to be asked in private if he or she would be more comfortable addressing this topic alone or with the other person present.

6-63   Answer B

The CAGE questionnaire is a four-item screening tool that is useful in identifying a client who may have a problem with alcohol abuse. C stands for "Have you ever felt you ought to cut down on your drinking?"; A for "Have people annoyed you by criticizing your drinking?"; G for "Have you ever felt guilty or bad about your drinking?"; and E for "Have you ever had a drink first thing in the morning (eye opener) to steady your nerves or get rid of a hangover?" The AUDIT test and the Michigan Alcoholism Screening Test are also useful in identifying a client who may have a problem with alcohol abuse, but they are not quite as short and easy to remember or administer. There is no Problem Drinker/Abuser Test.

6-64   Answer D

When an adolescent appears "laid back," quiet, and aloof, measures must be taken to ascertain from the teen what is concerning him or her. It may be appropriate to do a drug test, but first you should share that information with the client and ask if a urine test is necessary—is he or she, in fact, taking recreational drugs, or is there something else going on? You may still want to do a urine test if you do not think the client is credible, but certainly give the client the opportunity to talk. Eventually, the client may need to be referred to a counselor or psychiatrist or started on antidepressant medication, but this should not be the initial action.

6-65   Answer D

The U.S. Preventive Services Task Force recommends screening all adult and adolescent clients for evidence of alcohol dependence, problem drinking, or excessive alcohol consumption. A client's self-report of the quantity and frequency of alcohol use does not usually provide accurate information. Responses such as "I only drink socially" need to be explored. By screening all adult and adolescent clients, you will screen the other individuals mentioned in answers A, B, and C as well.

6-66   Answer D

The U.S. Preventive Services Task Force recommends goal setting by clients, individually tailored physical activity regimens, and telephone follow-up by specially trained staff for motivating clients to improve their exercise habits.

6-67   Answer D

A person who is chronically tired should see a health-care provider rather than self-prescribe. Many self-diagnose iron-deficiency anemia and self-prescribe an iron supplement, which will relieve tiredness only if the cause of the tiredness is iron-deficiency anemia. If the cause is a folate deficiency, taking iron will prolong the tiredness. Taking a vitamin supplement with iron may cure a vitamin deficiency. However, the symptoms of fatigue may have a nonnutritional cause. If the cause of the tiredness is actually a hidden blood loss because of cancer, the diagnosis may not be picked up as early as it could be. When tiredness is caused by a lack of sleep, no nutrient or combination of nutrients can replace a good night's sleep. If nutritional causes and blood loss or other disease process is ruled out as the cause of the fatigue, then a nursing measure that may be beneficial is a discussion of sleep-promoting behaviors.

6-68   Answer C

Fatigue for hours after exercising or feeling sore and stiff means the exercise has either been done for too long or incorrectly. A person should never feel exhausted after the cool-down period of exercising. If that happens, the person should slow down and take it easier next time.

6-69   Answer A

Signs and symptoms of depression include sad mood, crying spells, loss of interest in activities and people, slowed movements, disturbed sleep cycle, trouble concentrating, and thinking about death. There may be an increase in alcohol or drug use. Comorbidity is common, with anxiety symptoms accompanying depression in perhaps 70% of episodes (this percentage differs in different cultural groups). This may bring on restlessness, fidgeting, worrying, and the inability to relax. Going on a spending spree is more indicative of a manic-depressive mood disorder; obsessively exercising is more consistent with anorexia nervosa; and obsessive hand washing is more typical of an obsessive-compulsive disorder.

6-70   Answer A

Anemia, which may be detected by a complete blood count (CBC), is sufficiently prevalent to justify screening, and it is a condition for which early detection may be beneficial. A CBC is often ordered as a routine screening test. It can detect anemia, leukocytosis, thrombocytopenia, and leukemia, as well as other hematological disorders. Anemia is the only condition with sufficient prevalence for which early detection may be beneficial. Anemia is present in nearly 4 million Americans. Iron-deficiency anemia is easily treated and may be harmful in certain populations, such as young children and pregnant women.

6-71   Answer C

To achieve optimum protection, vaccination should ideally occur before the initiation of sexual activity. An estimated 33% of high school freshmen and 62% of seniors engage in sexual intercourse. An estimated 7.4% of students engage in sexual intercourse for the first time before age 13 years. Currently there is controversy over the age at which this vaccine should be administered.

6-72   Answer D

Clients with gastroesophageal reflux disease should avoid caffeine and chocolate, as well as mints, citrus products, alcohol, aspirin, and other NSAIDs. They should discontinue smoking altogether because it interferes with the action and effectiveness of H_2-receptor antagonists and be advised to report worsening of symptoms, such as tarry stools, fever, sore throat, or hallucinations.

6-73   Answer A

Physical exercise, more daylight, and rethinking one's situation ("cognitive restructuring") are all important interventions for depression. Rest will not help, and although having a nutritionally sound diet is recommended, it is not as important as the other suggested strategies. St. John's wort, initially heralded as an important adjuvant treatment of depression, has in later studies proved to be virtually ineffective for depression.

6-74   Answer B

To help Janice recover from osteomyelitis and promote healing, advise her to do the following: Do range-of-motion and strengthening exercises; eat foods high in vitamins and calcium; and increase caloric and protein intake, as well as fluid intake, which helps minimize the risks of kidney damage, yeast infections, and adverse gastrointestinal effects. You do not have enough history in the stem of the question to determine if the client should bear weight. Likewise, it is unclear if exposing the wound

to open air would be helpful or if wet dressings should be applied.

6-75   Answer D

Exercise provides several benefits for persons with diabetes. The most significant benefit is that exercise usually lowers blood sugar and helps the body to use its food supply better. Exercise also helps insulin work better; lowers cholesterol and triglyceride levels; improves blood flow through small vessels; increases the heart's ability to pump; helps burn excess calories; and relieves tension, anxiety, and depression.

6-76   Answer C

Eating breakfast and eating at regular intervals are elements of a successful weight-loss program that can be as important as the content of the meals. Eating breakfast actually gets the metabolism going so that individuals can digest all the essential nutrients. Saying "We all need some essential fatty acids that are obtained only from food" is unrelated to the fact that Trisha skips breakfast. The other responses are inappropriate and critical.

6-77   Answer A

When advising clients what to look for in skin cancer and melanoma, tell them to look for the ABCDs: A for asymmetrical border, B for border irregularity, C for color variations, and D for diameter greater than 6 mm. A papule that is 2 mm in size sounds harmless, depending on the border and color. A crusty-appearing lesion may be an actinic keratosis and is not a medical emergency that needs to be seen immediately. It is overbroad to say that the absence of change in any lesion will negate the need for follow-up.

6-78   Answer A

A smoking cessation program should be initiated when the client states a readiness to quit. Any smoking cessation program will have limited success when used to treat a highly dependent smoker who is not interested in smoking cessation. Therefore, the first crucial step is to assess a client's readiness to quit before initiating a smoking cessation program.

6-79   Answer C

Even though a child has a mild upper respiratory infection, if the child does not have a fever, immunizations should be administered. Missed opportunities for immunizations are lost forever. The contraindications for administering immunizations include anaphylactic reactions to egg ingestion (for live vaccines) and a moderate to severe infection with a fever.

6-80   Answer B

There is no reason to suspect dementia related to the data presented in the question. Self-mutilation is not likely; this behavior usually manifests itself at a younger age, and there would be a pattern of this behavior and usually concurrent behavioral problems. It is possible that the injuries are a result of the stated injury, but Gary's "nervousness" should cause you to consider domestic violence, alcohol or drug abuse, and Gary being the victim of a "hate crime." Contrary to some popular beliefs, battery of lesbians and gay men by their partners exists, although the prevalence is not known. Gay men may find it more difficult to find services related to battery. All gay and lesbian clients should be screened for domestic violence, and just as with heterosexuals, this should be openly discussed. When clients present with nervousness and anxiety or symptoms of depression, you should consider violence, including hate crimes, as possible correlates. Perpetrators of hate crimes may include family members and community authorities. The incidence of alcohol and drug abuse among homosexuals is reported to be slightly higher than among their heterosexual counterparts. Substance abuse should therefore also be explored in a client presenting with Gary's symptoms.

6-81   Answer A

For clients with AIDS, a viral load test is a more accurate measure of the progression of the disease than a CD4 count. The CD4 count is a surrogate marker that provides important, but indirect, measures of the state of a client's HIV disease and immunosuppression. The prognostic information it provides is useful, but incomplete, because the CD4 count can fluctuate depending on the status of the immune system, such as when the client has a cold, or as a result of dietary intake. A CD4 count is still recommended every 6 months, but a viral load test is more accurate.

6-82   Answer C

An alteration in clotting factors and venous dilation during pregnancy may predispose pregnant women to superficial and deep venous thrombosis, or "economy class syndrome." Pregnant women have a rate of acute iliofemoral venous thrombosis that is six times greater than that of nonpregnant women. The pregnant traveler should request an aisle seat and should walk in the aisles at least once an hour during long airplane flights whenever it is safe to do so. General stretching and isometric leg exercises should be encouraged on long flights. Pregnant women should also be encouraged to drink nonalcoholic beverages to maintain hydration and to wear seat belts low around the pelvis throughout the entire flight. They should avoid heavy eating because intestinal gas expansion can be particularly uncomfortable for the pregnant traveler. Monitoring of blood pressure is not essential unless there is an identified underlying risk factor.

6-83   Answer B

Although many sources cite the condom as the most essential form of primary prevention against sexually transmitted diseases and unwanted pregnancies, in reality the best prevention tool is the brain. For this reason, an adequate understanding of psychosocial and cultural determinants underlying sexual behaviors is essential to individualize counseling approaches depending on the client. Teaching should begin before puberty. Middle childhood is a "rationale period" for children. Sex education has vocal opposition in many subcultures. However, preventive teaching and participatory discussion need not focus on sex specifically. Teaching can be centered on making positive future choices and impulse control. This teaching should address girls in particular because of the lifelong consequences of unintended pregnancy and sexually transmitted diseases in women. Although sharing disease-specific information may help, it is only one prong of what should be a multipronged approach to prevention. Likewise, your job as a health counselor is not to change your client's personality or world view nor to solve their deep conflicts; rather, you should offer better and healthier ways for clients to get what they want.

6-84   Answer A

Although stating, "These bruises are very unusual. Is your husband hurting you?" sounds very forthright, studies have shown that such a statement is what the client needs and is willing to respond to. Most clients who have been abused have been waiting to be confronted in a matter-of-fact manner rather than an accusatory tone or one that makes the client seem like the victim. If asked, "How did you get these bruises?" or "Would you like to talk about what's going on?" a client will usually continue the silence, denial, and victimization. Another common approach is to link the question to information that the client has already provided in the encounter, such as, "You said that one bad thing about working opposite shifts is that you frequently argue about child rearing. Does your husband ever hurt you during these arguments?" Another approach is to normalize the problem, such as, "Many of my clients have told me that their husbands hit them; they complain of being abused. Is this how it is for you?"

6-85   Answer D

Her husband could have brought home work clothes that were contaminated with harmful chemicals, including lead, asbestos, and pesticides. As a result, she would have been exposed to these contaminants. After a long latency period, these hazardous substances are known to be a significant contributing factor to lung diseases and cancers. Secondhand smoke can also contribute to lung disease. However, there is no direct mechanism for her being exposed to secondhand smoke unless either her husband and/or someone who resided with her smoked. Tuberculosis is a potential contributing factor to lung disease, and coughing is a symptom of TB. However, an occupational history addresses exposures to a broader range of hazards associated with pneumoconiosis than just tuberculosis. Retiree health-care benefits are inconsequential to this question about the origin of the client's cough.

6-86   Answer C

When counseling parents about accidental poisonings in children, instruct the parents to administer ipecac syrup to induce vomiting if their child accidentally ingests something poisonous. In some instances, however, inducing vomiting is harmful because the chemical ingested may be irritating to the gastrointestinal mucosa as it ascends. When in doubt about inducing vomiting, advise the parents to contact their local emergency department, which will put them in contact with the poison control hotline. If the parent is unable to get to a telephone, less damage will be done by administering ipecac syrup and inducing vomiting than by waiting. Of all poisoning cases, 85% involve children, and 70% of those children are younger than 5 years of age. Families should have a bottle of ipecac syrup to administer on the way to the hospital because many toxins are absorbed rapidly. Burnt toast, tea, and milk of magnesia are old-fashioned home remedies that should be replaced with ipecac syrup.

6-87   Answer B

Although the development of physiological symptoms related to smoking behavior may provide a "teachable moment," and although the client indeed will *not* stop smoking until ready, it is your job to assist that process. Simply informing your client of the dangers of smoking and the health-related consequences is not enough. The Agency for Healthcare Research and Quality (AHRQ) recommends the following five A's. (1) Ask: At every visit, ask about tobacco use. (2) Advise to quit *now* through clear, personalized messages. (3) Assess willingness to quit. (4) Assist: If a client is ready to quit, ask him or her to set a "quit date" and provide self-help materials and possibly pharmacological intervention. If a client is not ready to quit, provide motivational readings, discuss the dangers of exposing others to secondhand smoke, and indicate willingness to help when he or she is ready to quit. (5) Arrange follow-up visits. Make a follow-up appointment for 1 week after the quit date and assess smoking status; explore reasons for not stopping if the client has not been successful. Congratulate those who are successful, identify high-risk situations that they may encounter in the future, and provide coping strategies for those situations.

6-88   Answer A

Baby bottle tooth decay (BBTD) can occur when a child goes to bed with a bottle containing anything but water. Some parents use milk sweetened with sugar, sugared water, fruit juices, or carbonated or noncarbonated beverages. Even milk-based baby formula, because of its lactose content, is a potential promoter of BBTD. Some parents may use a sweetened pacifier at night, and this is also a contributing factor in BBTD. The child should be switched to a plain water bottle or weaned from the practice altogether.

6-89   Answer C

Technological changes have made tennis rackets lighter, creating racket head speed and velocity. To compensate for this, suggest a wide grip, which may distribute forces more evenly to the forearm and elbow. Extremely tight strings accelerate velocity. For a new player, this may be dangerous and can increase the amount of force and impact transmitted to the forearm, elbow, and shoulder. An experienced racket professional may be best suited to assist a new player in making the best selection and equipment adjustments. You should not discourage John from taking up this sport because physical activity is good.

6-90   Answer C

The most common agent of intentional, nonoccupational poisoning deaths in adults is motor vehicle exhaust (25%), followed by cocaine and heroin (11%), antidepressants and tranquilizers (10%), and barbiturates (2%).

6-91   Answer D

Clients with trigeminal neuralgia should always wear protective sunglasses or goggles when outside, working in dusty areas, mowing the lawn, or using any type of spray material. They should also use artificial tears and an eye patch at night. Clients should be counseled to chew on the unaffected side of the mouth and avoid eating or drinking hot foods or fluids. They should also have regular dental examinations because they will not be able to feel pain associated with gum infection or tooth decay.

6-92   Answer C

Degenerative joint disease (DJD), also called osteoarthritis, is characterized by the degeneration and loss of articular cartilage in synovial joints. The joint most likely to be affected is the hip. DJD is the leading cause of disability in the older adult, affecting 20 million to 40 million adults in the United States. By age 40, almost 90% of adults show changes characteristic of DJD in the weight-bearing joints, particularly the hips. Other joints affected include the knees, lumbar and cervical vertebrae, proximal and distal interphalangeal joints of the fingers, first carpometacarpal joint of the wrist, and first metatarsophalangeal (big toe) joint of the foot.

6-93   Answer B

Maintaining safety and preserving the ability to perform ADLs are paramount in the patient with cognitive issues. Because this client has already been diagnosed, and because it is known that memory loss is one of the first signs of Alzheimer's

disease, teaching new skills could be overwhelming and contribute to the sense of frustration that these patients often feel. Some interventions that can slow the progression include medications such as Aricept in the early stages of the disease, ADL training, and therapeutic recreational activities. There are excellent day-care facilities for Alzheimer's patients, which *may*—not necessarily *should*—be considered in the future as a form of respite and assistance to clients as needed.

6-94   Answer C

Lymphedema, a lifelong potential complication of breast and axillary node surgery and radiation, has been documented up to 30 years after surgery. Practicing good limb care is essential for managing and preventing lymphedema. You should advise the client of the following measures to prevent lymphedema: Protect the affected arm from extreme heat and burns (including sunburn), avoid constriction of the affected arm (including by blood pressure cuffs), avoid carrying heavy purses on the affected side, avoid injury and infection of the affected arm (venipunctures are contraindicated), wear gloves when gardening and cleaning, care for minor injuries on the affected arm promptly, and keep regular appointments for follow-up care.

6-95   Answer B

Under state workers' compensation laws, an employer must pay all medical expenses for a work-related injury/illness. In addition to medical expenses, if an employee is out of work as a result of work-related injury or illness, employers must pay for lost wages if the work absence exceeds a specified waiting period (usually a few days). Under these statutes, an employee forfeits his or her right to sue the employer. Workers' compensation is a "no-fault" insurance; the negligence of employer and/or employee is not at issue with respect to a worker's right to receive benefits under these statutes.

6-96   Answer B

Safety is a high-priority concern in the elderly. The first order of concern is to maintain a safe environment in the home. Of course, any other reasons for tripping or falling should always be assessed as well. Maintaining independence is important, and the provider should assist the elderly who want to stay in their home environment if it is feasible. The spouse may want to be available every waking moment, which may not be a realistic request. If it is determined the client needs extensive assistance with self-care activities and ADLs, a home care assistant consult may be necessary.

6-97   Answer C

Individuals with risk factors for skin cancer should have a screening test for skin cancer. Although the U.S. Preventive Services Task Force has not found sufficient evidence to recommend for or against routine screening by primary care providers, other groups, such as the Canadian Task Force on the Periodic Health Examination and the American Academy of Family Physicians, recommend complete skin examinations of adolescents and adults who have risk factors for skin cancer. These risk factors include a personal or family history of skin cancer; clinical evidence of precursor lesions, such as dysplastic nevi, actinic keratoses, or certain congenital nevi; and increased occupational or recreational exposure to sunlight.

6-98   Answer C

Two of the most notable signs of a vitamin C deficiency are bleeding gums and broken capillaries under the skin that occur spontaneously and produce pinpoint hemorrhages. Other signs of vitamin C deficiency include failure to promote normal collagen synthesis, which causes further hemorrhaging; degeneration of muscles, including the heart muscle; rough, brown, scaly, and dry skin; and wounds that fail to heal because scar tissue will not form. Signs of vitamin A deficiency do not appear until after stores are depleted, which takes 1–2 years or less in a growing child. A deficiency of vitamin A affects the bones and teeth, with cessation of bone growth and painful joints; affects the blood with anemia; affects the eyes with night blindness; and affects the skin by plugging hair follicles with keratin, which forms white lumps (hyperkeratosis). Most vitamin B_{12} deficiencies reflect inadequate absorption, not poor intake. Inadequate absorption typically occurs for one of two reasons: a lack of hydrochloric acid or a lack of intrinsic factor. Many people older than age 60 develop atrophic gastritis, a condition characterized by inadequate hydrochloric acid. In vitamin D deficiency, production of the calcium-binding protein in the intestinal cells slows so that even when calcium is adequate in the diet, it passes through the gastrointestinal tract unabsorbed, leaving the bones undersupplied. The symptoms of a vitamin D deficiency are those of calcium deficiency: rickets and osteomalacia.

6-99   Answer C

In older adults, there is a decline in all parameters of renal function, including decreased renal concentrating capacity, impaired sodium conservation, decreased glomerular filtration rate, altered acid-base regulation (decreased ammonia production), and reduced response to antidiuretic hormone. Skin turgor is poor in older adults, so it is not a reliable measure of body fluids. Older adults are usually not thirsty, and edema in an older adult does not necessarily indicate pathology or fluid and electrolyte imbalance. The best indicator of body fluid balance is body weight. In older adults, there is a decrease in the amount of total body water. This is attributable to an increase in body fat relative to a decline in lean body mass as intracellular water decreases.

6-100   Answer D

Martin should make sure that Laura is wearing a medical identification bracelet or necklace, such as those made by MedicAlert, stating that she has a seizure disorder. This will alert others in case she is not responsive. If a person has a seizure disorder, alcoholic beverages should be avoided completely and caffeine intake should be limited. The importance of continuing to take anticonvulsant medications should be stressed even when no seizures are experienced. State and local laws differ regarding persons with seizure disorders. Usually, driving a motor vehicle is prohibited for 6 months to 2 years after a seizure episode.

6-101   Answer B

Although it is always best to give bad news in person, if the client asks for the news over the telephone, it is best not to lie. Instead, begin a dialogue that provides basic information. News should always be conveyed directly to the client and not through a family member. False reassurance, even if bad news is still premature, never builds trust in the long run.

6-102   Answer B

Studies have shown that siblings are usually present when a brother or sister becomes a drowning victim. To help prevent an accidental drowning, young children (even as young as 8 years old) can learn cardiopulmonary resuscitation (CPR). A large number of swimming pool drowning deaths could have been prevented by immediate CPR. Children are very creative and can unlock doors and climb or go around fences. It is impractical to keep the backyard entrances locked at all times because the 8-year-old could certainly unlock them. It is almost impossible for a parent to keep a child in view 24 hours a day. Parents should learn CPR.

6-103   Answer C

Several drops of mineral oil can be used to soften earwax. The adage of "never insert anything smaller than your elbow in your ear" still applies, even with cotton-tipped applicators. Flushing the ears using a bulb syringe should be avoided because the vacuum pressure may be excessive and rupture the tympanic membrane. Commercial preparations can be used to irrigate, but they should never be left in longer than directed because they can cause local irritation.

6-104   Answer C

The health counselor must work with the client because smoking cessation will not be effective unless the smoker is ready to quit. Follow-up reinforcement sessions are essential. The client should be followed first weekly, then monthly, and then quarterly for a year. Treatment for smoking cessation is most effective when the health-care counselor is perceived as being understanding and when the expression of feelings and concerns is encouraged. If a client is smoking more than 20–30 cigarettes per day, he or she should be encouraged to start a tapering-off program; persons who smoke fewer than 20 cigarettes per day should be encouraged to set a "quit date." The client should announce the quit date to family and friends and all should provide additional support during this time. It is not necessary for the health counselor to meet with family, although strategies may be shared if the family requests.

6-105   Answer C

The Equal Employment Opportunity Commission (EEOC) has jurisdiction over the enforcement of the Americans with Disabilities Act (ADA). The Occupational Safety and Health Administration (OSHA) has jurisdiction over workplace safety and health. OSHA is under the umbrella of the Department of Labor. State workers' compensation laws are under the jurisdiction of the states' Department of Justice.

6-106   Answer B

For the client with lumbar spinal stenosis, exercises that encourage lumbar flexion and flattening of the lumbar lordotic curve are particularly helpful. Also, exercises that strengthen the abdominal muscles and promote mobility of the lumbar paraspinal muscles can help minimize lordosis of the lumbar spine. Lumbar extension worsens the radiculopathy by increasing the laxity of the ligamentum. Any exercise that results in hyperextension of the lumbar spine should be avoided. Swimming and walking against the resistance of the water in a swimming pool promote healthful cardiovascular function while maintaining lumbar flexion. Surgery may be necessary for clients who have severe neurological dysfunction and pain.

6-107   Answer C

The correct course of action is to do a complete history and physical examination and try to determine the cause of the client's discontent with the neurology consults. It may be that what this client needs is someone to listen to her and help her deal with her chronic headaches in a different manner. Conversely, there may still be some other underlying, undiscovered cause of her chronic headaches. Requests for repeated referrals are not uncommon.

6-108   Answer B

Although being a college student and lacking structure and transportation over a summer break might contribute to an ongoing depression, they are not risk factors in and of themselves. Believing oneself to be incapable, however, is a risk factor for depression. Other risk factors include being female, living in poverty or a powerless social position, having a severe physical illness, experiencing a severe stressor such as death or loss of a close person, and having a first-degree biological relative with a depressive mood disorder.

6-109   Answer C

Erythromycin (E-Mycin, Eryc) has been found to be the safest drug to use in pregnancy because it has no teratogenic effects on the fetus. Acetylsalicylic acid (aspirin) alters platelet function and can cause maternal and newborn bleeding; acetaminophen (Tylenol) can be toxic to the liver; and tetracycline (Achromycin, Sumycin), if given to a pregnant mother between the fourth month of pregnancy and delivery, will cause abnormalities in tooth development, including brown spotting and unusual shape.

6-110   Answer A

Almost 20% of teenage boys in the United States use smokeless tobacco. It is more common in rural areas than in urban settings. Long-term use is addictive; may lead to mouth or throat cancer; and can cause gum recession, which can lead to the loss of teeth. Smokeless tobacco does not affect appetite. All clients who use tobacco in any form should be counseled to stop because of the risks to oral and general health.

6-111   Answer A

Usually no serious physical problem is present with nighttime enuresis, although the child may have a small or immature bladder. When counseling the parents of a child with nighttime enuresis, tell them that it is a common problem that is often inherited. Stress the idea that the parents are not at fault. A family plan for dealing with the wet bed may include deciding who strips the bed and where the sheets should go. The child needs to play a major role in this plan, and positive reinforcement should be given when the child remains dry through the night.

6-112   Answer C

Past surgeries and number of children are not documented risk factors for coronary artery disease (CAD). Economic disadvantage, rather than economic advantage, is a risk factor. Temperament, however, is a risk factor. Studies from several industrialized nations suggest that people experiencing stressful situations who show their emotions are less likely to develop sustained high blood pressure, although their blood pressure may temporarily rise during the stressor. Social disadvantage, such as race, is another often-overlooked documented risk factor. Those who are discriminated against or who are poor face uncertain life situations and must constantly be vigilant. Both of these are risk factors for CAD. There are five documented psychosocial risk factors for CAD: uncertain life situation, lack of experience to learn which behavioral response will solve a given problem, the possibility of serious harm, the fact that flight-or-fight reactions are unlikely to help, and

the need for sustained mental vigilance. Air traffic controllers, for example, experience all of the above except for lack of experience. These risk factors, as well as temperament, are often overlooked.

6-113   Answer D

Clients who make statements that acknowledge others' displeasure with their negative health behaviors are precontemplative. They are only considering the possibility of making a change. Readiness requires some action that is taken on the part of the patient, as this patient is asking for help and taking that first step to make the change.

6-114   Answer D

The best way to promote a personal behavior change in a client is to discuss choices with the client and let him or her decide what will work best. Because medicine is moving away from the paternalistic model, health-care providers are changing their way of thinking and are involving clients in a shared decision-making model that results in a discourse between providers and clients. Under this shared decision-making model, clients—because of a vested interest in their health and the way information is expressed—tend to listen to the information, make informed choices, and actually practice improved health promotion activities. Providers should use the words *choices* rather than *orders*, *client initiative* rather than *compliance*, and *partnership* rather than *prescription*.

6-115   Answer B

If an adolescent boy tells you he thinks he has something seriously wrong with him because he has awakened in the morning with a wet sheet around his penis, tell him that this a normal progression in his sexual development. In this case, Phil may be embarrassed to ask his friends about this and not realize that "wet dreams" are a normal progression in sexual development. Ejaculation occurs in the early morning hours during an erection while sleeping and is referred to as a nocturnal emission. Phil should be assured that this is perfectly normal.

6-116   Answer B

Nonadherence to taking medications has many reasons. One of them is that there may be side effects that are undesirable or that the medications are costly. The client may not have a reliable means to get refills on a prescription as well. Health-care providers should not assume that the client is forgetful or otherwise stigmatize the elderly client. A first course of action would be to determine why the client is not taking the medications, and if it is simply a matter of forgetting, then a pill tracker or help from a friend may be implemented to assist the patient in remembering.

6-117   Answer B

A primary cause of degenerative joint disease (DJD) is obesity. Repetitive mechanical joint overuse is also a risk factor for DJD and can be seen in athletes such as tennis players and baseball pitchers. Arthritis also occurs in joints that have previously been operated on or injured. The etiology of the primary form of the disease is unknown, although genetic and immunological factors appear to play a role in its development.

6-118   Answer D

Regular interaction with others exercises social and language skills, and playing a card game like bridge reinforces memory, providing a form of cognitive "exercise." Along those same lines, doing crossword puzzles and jigsaw puzzles helps exercise the mind. The benefits of video games and simulations are being researched at present. Although working on model ships or airplanes may provide some stimulation, the solitary nature of these hobbies over time makes them not as beneficial as an activity like card playing that demands social interaction in addition to mental effort. Engaging in rigorous physical activity, not resting, is considered protective of mental abilities. An older adult would do better to take a daily multivitamin, not just calcium, as a mental protective strategy. Research has also shown that a longer education as a youth is a protective factor. Maintaining a sense of self-efficacy—the belief, faith, and action that "I can do it"—and a "use it or lose it" approach are keys to effective mental functioning in older age.

6-119   Answer D

Various relaxation exercises and yoga practices have been shown to lower blood pressure both acutely and chronically. If exercise and/or yoga reduces blood pressure, the client taking antihypertensive drugs may be able to lower the dosage and experience fewer side effects. Although rest may be important, physical activity is even more important, and rest, if not of a relaxed nature, may create a more sedentary lifestyle, which is counterproductive. Although some studies have shown a glass of red wine every day to be cardioprotective, the evidence is not unequivocal, and in the case of a client who has a tendency to drink more alcohol than recommended, this practice is not advisable. Likewise, some studies have shown that a pet can reduce blood pressure, but the evidence is less conclusive than the evidence supporting relaxation practices.

6-120   Answer D

Stress urinary incontinence is not a normal part of the aging process. It may be controlled or alleviated in many women. The diagnosis must be confirmed first to rule out other causes of incontinence. Nonsurgical treatment options include drug therapy with estrogen vaginal cream, pelvic floor electrical stimulation, imipramine, Kegel exercises with biofeedback, pessaries, and occlusive devices. Very often, a combination of several of these will benefit the client. Surgery may be indicated, depending on which structure needs repairing. For example, if a cystocele is producing the symptoms, repair of the anterior vaginal wall prolapse is indicated. Pads may prove helpful, but the underlying causes must first be investigated. There is no evidence that cranberry juice helps curb stress incontinence.

6-121   Answer C

Asking "Is Ginger ever exposed to cigarette smoke?" is less threatening to a parent who may interpret the other questions as indictments of his or her parenting skills. Most parents know they should not smoke around a person with a respiratory problem, and making them feel guilty does not address the problem of how they can stop smoking or how the risk factor can be eliminated from their child's environment.

6-122   Answer A

A simple measure of whether an exercise activity is aerobic is the client's heart rate. If the pulse reaches or exceeds a level of 60% of the maximum normal pulse, the exercise is considered aerobic. This only roughly measures the true degree of increased oxygen uptake by the muscles and is more accurate for measuring the intensity of exercise in beginners than in conditioned athletes. The formula to use is 220 minus the person's age times 0.6 (or 60% of the theoretical maximum normal pulse). This means that for a person 63 years old to have aerobic exercise, the heart rate must reach at least 94 bpm (220 − 63 = 157; 157 × 0.6 = 94). One can usually assume that exercise is aerobic if breathing is deep and sweating occurs in mild to cold temperatures, but this is not as reliable a measure as heart rate. For exercise to be beneficial in reducing the long-term risk for coronary artery disease, it must be aerobic, although any exercise is beneficial for weight loss.

6-123   Answer B

To change behaviors successfully, clients need to feel "ownership in" the need for change. Internal motivation has been shown to be predictive of successful treatment programs. To recognize that a change needs to take place and actually make the move to initiate a change, most clients need to feel that there is more to gain than to lose. The pleasure, comfort, or other gains the client receives from overeating, smoking, and other undesirable behaviors need to be outweighed by the gains the client values and believes are attainable. Although Henry wants to attend his daughter's wedding in the future and be able to enjoy his retirement when the time comes, they are temporary motivators that may not give him the needed impetus because they are far in the future. He needs to take ownership of the problem and start today to make changes that will enable him to enjoy his future.

Bibliography

Albohm, MJ: Getting the right fit. *Healthy Aging*, 31–34, January/February 2007.

Armour, S: Exposing family members to toxins. *USA Today*, October 5, 2000. http://www.usatoday.com/money/bighits/toxin3.htm, accessed December 15, 2007.

Armour, S: Workplace toxins can kill at home. *USA Today*, October 11, 2000. http://www.usatoday.com/money/bighits/toxin1.htm, accessed December 15, 2007.

Centers for Disease Control and Prevention: http://www.cdc.gov/od/science/iso/concerns/thimerisol.htm, Mercury in vaccines, October 23, 2007, accessed December 15, 2007.

Centers for Disease Control and Prevention: http://www.cdc.gov/vaccines/recs/acip/, accessed December 20, 2011.

Conway, AE: Down on the farm: Preventing farm accidents in children. *Pediatric Nursing* 1(33):45–48, 2007.

Dunphy, LM, et al: *Primary Care: The Art and Science of Advanced Practice Nursing*, ed 3. FA Davis, Philadelphia, 2011.

Guirguis-Blake, J, and Yawn, BP: The United States Preventive Services Task Force: Putting recommendations into practice. *The Female Patient*, 34–44, May 2006.

Job Accommodation Network: http://www.jan.wvu.edu/links/adalinks.htm, ADA Hot Links and Document Center, May 21, 2007, accessed December 15, 2007.

Miles-Richardson, S: Endocrine disruption: Is there cause for concern? *Hazardous Substances & Public Health* 12(2), Summer 2002. http://www.atsdr.cdc.gov/HEC/HSPH/v12n2-2.html#endocrine, accessed December 15, 2007.

National Institute of Environmental Health Sciences: http://www.niehs.nih.gov/health/topics/agents/endocrine/index.cfm, Endocrine disruptors, July 27, 2007, accessed December 15, 2007.

National Institute for Occupational Safety and Health: http://www.cdc.gov/niosh/docs/2007-133/pdfs/2007-133.pdf, *Preventing Fire Fighter Fatalities Due to Heart Attacks and Other Sudden Cardiovascular Events*, June 2007, accessed December 15, 2007.

National Travel Health Network and Centre: http://www.nathnac.org/pro/factsheets/documents/Travellersthrombosisrevised April2007.pdf, *Travel Related Deep Vein Thrombosis*, April 2007, accessed December 15, 2007.

Occupational Safety and Health Administration: http://www.osha.gov/pls/oshaweb/owadisp.show_document?p_table=INTERPRETATIONS&p_id=22830, Employee access to MSDSs required by 1910. 1200 vs. 1910.1020, December 7, 1999, accessed December 15, 2007.

Occupational Safety and Health Administration: http://www.osha.gov/pls/oshaweb/owadisp.show_document?p_table=INTERPRETATIONS&p_id=22377, Employee safety and the laundering of contaminated clothing, April 1, 1997, accessed December 15, 2007.

Occupational Safety and Health Administration: http://www.osha.gov/Publications/osha3074.pdf, *Hearing Conservation*, 2002, accessed December 15, 2007.

Rabinowitz, PM: Determining when hearing loss is work related. *Update* 17(3), Fall 2005. http://www.caohc.org/updatearticles/fall05.pdf, accessed December 15, 2007.

Stellar, MA: Universal human papillomavirus vaccination. In the hot seat. *The Female Patient* 32:47–48, May 2007.

Swanson, K, and Phenning, S: The nurse practitioner's role in the management of rheumatoid arthritis. *Journal of Nurse Practitioners* 7(10):858–862.

Thunder, T: Hearing conservation in the U.S.—A road less traveled. Update 17(2), Summer 2005. http://www.caohc.org/updatearticles/summer05.pdf, accessed December 15, 2007.

U.S. Department of Labor, Office of Workers' Compensation Programs, Division of Federal Employees' Compensation Web site: http://www.dol.gov/esa/regs/compliance/owcp/fecacont.htm, accessed December 15, 2007.

U.S. Environmental Protection Agency: http://www.epa.gov/waterscience/fish/, Fish advisories, October 14, 2007, accessed December 15, 2007.

U.S. Environmental Protection Agency: http://www.epa.gov/waterscience/fish/files/MethylmercuryBrochure.pdf, *What You Need to Know About Mercury in Fish and Shellfish*, 2004, accessed December 15, 2007.

U.S. Equal Employment Opportunity Commission: http://www.eeoc.gov/policy/ada.html, *The Americans with Disabilities Act of 1990 (Pub. L. 101-336), Titles I and V*, accessed December 15, 2007.

U.S. Food and Drug Administration: http://www.fda.gov/cber/vaccine/thimerosal.htm, Thimerosal in vaccines, September 6, 2007, accessed December 15, 2007.

U.S. Preventive Services Task Force: *The Guide to Clinical Preventive Services 2006: Recommendations of the U.S. Preventive Services Task Force* (AHRQ Publication No. 06-0588). Agency for Healthcare Research and Quality, Silver Spring, MD.

How well did you do?

85% and above, congratulations! This score shows application of test-taking principles and adequate content knowledge.

75%–85%, keep working! Review test-taking principles and try again.

65%–75%, hang in there! Spend some time reviewing concepts and test-taking principles and then try the test again.

ASSESSMENT AND MANAGEMENT OF CLIENT ILLNESS

Chapter 7: *Neurological Problems*

Jill E. Winland-Brown
Lisa Bedard

Questions

7-1 *Which of the following drugs used for parkinsonism mimics dopamine?*

A. Anticholinergics
B. Levodopa (l-dopa)
C. Bromocriptine
D. Tolcapone

7-2 *How often does the Agency for Healthcare Research and Quality (AHRQ) recommend that providers ask clients about their tobacco-use status?*

A. At every visit
B. At least every 6 months
C. Once a year
D. At the initial history and physical examination

7-3 *What is the most common cause of cerebellar disease?*

A. Hypothyroidism
B. Use of drugs such as 5-fluorouracil or phenytoin
C. Cerebellar neoplasm
D. Alcoholism

7-4 *Current pharmacological therapy for relapsing-remitting multiple sclerosis involves*

A. high-dose steroids.
B. baclofen (Lioresal) or diazepam (Valium).
C. interferon B (Betaseron).
D. benzodiazepines.

7-5 *Julie, age 58, has had several transient ischemic attacks. After a diagnostic evaluation, what medication would you start her on?*

A. Ticlopidine (Ticlid)
B. Clopidogrel (Plavix)
C. Warfarin (Coumadin)
D. Nitroglycerin (Nitro-Dur)

7-6 *Bob, age 49, is complaining of recurrent, intrusive dreams since returning from his Marine combat training. You suspect*

A. depersonalization.
B. schizophrenia.
C. post-traumatic stress disorder.
D. anxiety.

7-7 *Jessie, age 29, sees flashing lights 20 minutes before experiencing severe headaches. How would you describe her headache?*

A. Migraine without aura.
B. Classic migraine.
C. Tension headache.
D. Cluster headache.

7-8 *Marian, age 39, has multiple sclerosis (MS). She tells you that she heard that the majority of people with MS have the chronic-relapsing type of disease and that she has nothing to live for. How do you respond?*

A. "The majority of people have this response to MS."
B. "There are many different clinical courses of MS, and the chronic-relapsing type is only one of them."
C. "The chronic-relapsing type of MS is in the minority."
D. "There is an even chance that you have this type."

7-9 *Deficiency of which nutritional source usually presents with an insidious onset of paresthesias of the hands and feet that are usually painful?*

A. Thiamine
B. Vitamin B_{12}
C. Folic acid
D. Vitamin K

7-10   *Dan, age 82, recently lost his wife to breast cancer. He presents with weight loss, fatigue, and difficulty sleeping. What should your first response be?*

A. "Do you have a history of thyroid problems in your family?"

B. "Do you think a sleeping pill might help you sleep at night?"

C. "Things might look up if you added nutritional supplements to your diet."

D. "Have you thought of suicide?"

7-11   *Decreased facial strength indicates a lesion of which cranial nerve?*

A. Cranial nerve III.

B. Cranial nerve V.

C. Cranial nerve VII.

D. Cranial nerve VIII.

7-12   *The use of tricyclic antidepressants in the elderly increases the risk of*

A. suicide.

B. cardiac arrhythmias.

C. reactive depression.

D. shortness of breath.

7-13   *Some providers have successfully induced remission in clients with multiple sclerosis by using adrenocorticotropic hormone therapy or other pharmacological therapy along with*

A. chelation therapy.

B. plasmapheresis.

C. bone marrow transplantation.

D. intravenous lipids.

7-14   *Sam, age 29, has lost his sense of smell. You would document this as*

A. hyposmia.

B. anosmia.

C. ageusia.

D. agnosia.

7-15   *In the depressed client, antidepressants are most effective in alleviating*

A. suicidal feelings.

B. interpersonal problems.

C. sleep disturbances.

D. anxiety disorders.

7-16   *In the stages of Elisabeth Kübler-Ross's anticipatory grieving, which stage follows that of anger?*

A. Denial

B. Bargaining

C. Depression

D. Acceptance

7-17   *If you suspect that your client abuses alcohol, the most appropriate action would be to*

A. confront the client.

B. obtain further confirmatory information.

C. consult with family members.

D. suggest Alcoholics Anonymous (AA).

7-18   *Which seizure type involves alteration of consciousness?*

A. Myoclonic seizures

B. Absence seizures

C. Clonic seizures

D. Atonic seizures

7-19   *You are performing some neurological assessment tests on Daniel. When you ask Daniel to lie supine and flex his head to his chest, what are you assessing?*

A. Brudzinski sign

B. Kernig's sign

C. Decorticate posturing

D. Decerebrate posturing

7-20   *Jim, age 45, has two small children. He states that his wife made him come to this appointment because she thinks he has been impossible to live with lately. He admits to being stressed and depressed because he is working two jobs, and he says he sometimes takes his stress out on his family. About twice a week he complains of palpitations along with nervous energy. What is the most important question to ask him at this time?*

A. "How is your wife handling stress?"

B. "Have you thought about committing suicide?"

C. "Do you and your wife spend time alone together?"

D. "Tell me more about what you think is causing this."

7-21   Generalized absence seizures usually occur in which age group?

A. Children

B. Adolescents

C. Middle-aged adults

D. Older adults

7-22   What is the leading cause of bacterial meningitis in adults?

A. *Haemophilus influenzae*

B. Meningococcal

C. *Streptococcus pneumoniae*

D. Gram-negative pneumonia.

7-23   Which medication should be avoided in clients with Alzheimer's disease who have concurrent vascular dementia or vascular risk factors?

A. Acetycholinesterase inhibitors like donepezil (Aricept)

B. *N*-methyl-D-aspartate (NMDA) receptor antagonists

C. Anxiolytics like bupirone (Buspar)

D. Atypical antipsychotics like risperidone (Risperdal)

7-24   Dave, age 76, is brought in by his wife, who states that within the past 2 days Dave has become agitated and restless, has had few lucid moments, slept very poorly last night, and can remember only recent events. Of the following differential diagnoses, which seems the most logical from this brief history?

A. Depression

B. Dementia

C. Delirium

D. Schizophrenia

7-25   Which of the following gaits in older adults includes brusqueness of the movements of the leg and stamping of the feet?

A. Gait of sensory ataxia

B. Parkinsonian gait

C. Antalgic gait

D. Cerebellar gait

7-26   Of the four types of strokes, which one is the most common and has a gradual onset?

A. Thrombotic

B. Embolic

C. Lacunar

D. Hemorrhagic

7-27   Barbara, age 36, presents with episodic attacks of severe vertigo, usually with associated ear fullness. Her attacks usually last several hours and she feels well before and after the attacks. To what might you attribute these symptoms?

A. Ménière's disease

B. Vestibular neuronitis

C. Benign paroxysmal positional vertigo

D. Otosclerosis

7-28   Which appropriate test for the initial assessment of Alzheimer's disease provides performance ratings on 10 complex, higher-order activities?

A. MMSE

B. CAGE questionnaire

C. FAQ

D. Holmes and Rahe Social Readjustment Scale

7-29   Herpes simplex encephalitis is characterized by which of the following?

A. Parietal lobe location

B. Temporal lobe location

C. Absence of CSF lymphocytes

D. Decreased CSF protein levels

7-30   Which type of meningitis is a more benign, self-limited syndrome caused primarily by viruses?

A. Aseptic

B. Bacterial

C. Chronic

D. Inflammatory

7-31   Herbert, age 58, has just been diagnosed with Bell's palsy. He is understandably upset and has questions about the prognosis. Your response should be

A. "Although most of the symptoms will disappear, some will remain but can usually be camouflaged by altering your hairstyle or growing a beard or mustache."

B. "Unfortunately, there is no cure, but you have a mild case."

C. "The condition is self-limiting, and most likely complete recovery will occur."

D. "With suppressive drug therapy, you can minimize the symptoms."

7-32   In teaching a client with multiple sclerosis, the provider should emphasize all of the following points except

A. taking a daily hot shower to relax.

B. exercising to maintain mobility.

C. getting plenty of rest.

D. seeking psychological and emotional support.

7-33   Which of the following objective data are associated with significantly better long-term outcomes in children born with open spina bifida?

A. A higher APGAR score

B. Presence of Babinski's reflex

C. Perineal sensation

D. A higher score on the Glasgow Coma Scale

7-34   Diane, age 35, presents with weakness and numbness of the left arm, diplopia, and some bowel and bladder changes for the past week. She states that the same thing happened last year and lasted for several weeks. What diagnosis is a strong possibility?

A. Multiple sclerosis

B. Subdural hematoma

C. Pituitary tumor

D. Myasthenia gravis

7-35   Which of the following conditions is most responsible for developmental delays in children?

A. Cerebral palsy

B. Fetal alcohol syndrome

C. Down syndrome

D. Meningomyelocele

7-36   What is the medication of choice for obsessive-compulsive disorders?

A. Alprazolam (Xanax)

B. Carbamazepine (Tegretol)

C. Clomipramine (Anafranil)

D. Buspirone (Buspar)

7-37   When you move a client's head to the left and the eyes move to the right in relation to the head, this is referred to as

A. extraocular eye movements.

B. oculomotor degeneration.

C. doll's eyes.

D. decerebrate posturing.

7-38   What is a common factor in patients with nonepileptiform seizures?

A. Stress

B. Anxiety

C. Sexual abuse

D. Malingering

7-39   Urine drug screening tests, often performed in the workplace, are frequently effective in finding a person who smokes marijuana because a urine test will be positive for marijuana for up to how long after a person stops smoking the drug?

A. 24 hours

B. 1 week

C. 2 weeks

D. 30 days

7-40   The Hallpike maneuver is performed to elicit

A. a seizure.

B. vertigo.

C. syncope.

D. a headache.

7-41   Which headache preparation has gastrointestinal distress as a side effect?

A. Sumatriptan (Imitrex)

B. Nadolol (Corgard)

C. Naproxen sodium (Anaprox DS)

D. Ergot preparations (Cafergot)

7-42   Sigrid, age 83, has postherpetic neuralgia from a bout of herpes zoster last year. She has been having daily painful episodes and would like to start some kind of therapy. What do you recommend?

A. A tricyclic antidepressant

B. A beta blocker

C. A systemic steroid

D. An NSAID

7-43   Which of the following screening instruments is quick and easy to use and has a high level of diagnostic accuracy to detect alcohol abuse?

A. The CAGE questionnaire

B. The HEAT instrument

C. The DRINK tool

D. MMSE

7-44   Sandra has a ruptured intervertebral disk and is not responding to conservative management. She is requesting surgery for relief of her pain. She is going to have an enlargement of the opening between the disk and the facet joint to remove the bony overgrowth compressing the nerve. This describes which surgical procedure?

A. Laminectomy

B. Diskectomy

C. Foraminotomy

D. Chemonucleolysis

7-45   Susan has a slipped lumbar disk. When assessing her Achilles tendon, what would you expect her reflex score to be?

A. 1

B. 2

C. 3

D. 4

7-46   In the Physicians' Health Study, middle-aged men who suffer from migraine headaches are 42% more likely to have which condition when compared with nonsufferers?

A. Congestive heart failure

B. Peripheral vascular disease

C. Abdominal aortic aneurysm

D. Myocardial infarction

7-47   When you ask a client to walk a straight line placing heel to toe, you are assessing

A. sensory function.

B. cerebellar function.

C. cranial nerve function.

D. the proprioceptive system.

7-48   Janice, age 14, is markedly obese and has a poor self-image. How do you differentiate between compulsive eating and bulimia?

A. Bulimia results in irregular menstruation.

B. A compulsive eater does not induce vomiting.

C. A compulsive eater has tooth and gum erosion.

D. A compulsive eater does compulsive exercising.

7-49   Clients with senile dementia of the Alzheimer's type often die of

A. pneumonia.

B. suicide.

C. pressure sores.

D. malnutrition.

7-50   Which type of encephalitis is the most common?

A. Microbial

B. Herpes simplex virus

C. Viral

D. Pneumococcal

7-51   What is the first symptom seen in the majority of clients with Parkinson's disease?

A. Rigidity

B. Bradykinesia

C. Rest tremor

D. Flexed posture

7-52   Morrison exhibits extrapyramidal side effects of antipsychotic medications. Which of the following symptoms would lead you to look for another diagnosis?

A. Akathisia

B. Dystonia

C. Parkinsonism

D. Hallucinations

7-53   *How is cranial nerve XI tested?*

A. Ask the client to say "ah."

B. Have the client shrug his or her shoulders while you resist the movement.

C. Have the client stick out his or her tongue and move it from side to side.

D. Touch the pharynx with a cotton-tipped applicator.

7-54   *During a mental status exam, which question would be the most helpful to assess remote memory?*

A. "How long have you been here?"

B. "What time did you get here today?"

C. "What did you eat for breakfast?"

D. "What was your mother's maiden name?"

7-55   *Jonas, age 62, experienced a temporary loss of consciousness that was associated with an increased rate of respiration, tachycardia, pallor, perspiration, and coolness of the skin. How would you describe this?*

A. Lethargy

B. Delirium

C. Syncope

D. A fugue state

7-56   *Naloxone (Narcan) is the antidote for an overdose of*

A. acetaminophen.

B. benzodiazepines.

C. narcotics.

D. phenothiazines.

7-57   *When assessing a client's deep tendon reflexes, you note they are more brisk than normal. You document them as*

A. 3.

B. 2.

C. 1.

D. 0.

7-58   *Which of the following is an unusual side effect of tricyclic antidepressants?*

A. Dry mouth

B. Itching

C. Constipation

D. Drowsiness

7-59   *Sarah comes into the office with a severe headache, fever, delirium, nausea, vomiting, and a stiff neck. Which physical maneuver will you perform to help determine a diagnosis?*

A. Kernig's sign

B. Hoover's sign

C. Hoffman's sign

D. Babinski's reflex

7-60   *Which of the following may immediately follow a stroke in the older adult and be the body's attempt to maintain perfusion?*

A. Bradycardia

B. Tachycardia

C. Hypotension

D. Hypertension

7-61   *Gary, age 5, has a diagnosis of encopresis. After the diagnosis, what would be your next action?*

A. Order extensive lab work.

B. Send Gary to a psychologist.

C. Rule out a neurological disorder.

D. Bring Gary's parents in for counseling.

7-62   *The older adult with delirium would present with which of the following behaviors?*

A. Fatigue, apathy, and occasional agitation

B. Agitation, apathy, and wandering behavior

C. Agitation and restlessness

D. Slowness and absence of purpose

7-63   *Karen Ann, age 52, has four children and a very stressful job. After you perform her physical, which was normal, she tells you she has insomnia. You make several suggestions for lifestyle changes that might assist in promoting helpful sleep. You know she misunderstands when she states which of the following?*

A. "I'll wind down before bedtime by taking a warm bath or by reading for 10 minutes."

B. "I'll try some valerian extract from the health food store."

C. "I'll exercise in the evening to tire myself out before bed."

D. "I won't read or watch television while in bed."

7-64 *What does a carotid bruit heard on auscultation indicate?*

A. A normal finding in adults recovering from a carotid endarterectomy

B. An evolving embolus

C. A narrowing of the carotid artery because of atherosclerosis of the vessel

D. A complete occlusion of the carotid artery

7-65 *Mary, age 82, appears without an appointment. She is complaining of a new, unilateral headache; fever; and muscle aches. She denies any precipitating event. On further examination, you note that her erythrocyte sedimentation rate is over 100 mm/min. What do you suspect?*

A. Temporal arteritis

B. Meningitis

C. Subarachnoid hemorrhage

D. Intracerebral hemorrhage

7-66 *What is the most sensitive indicator of increased intracranial pressure and the first symptom to change as the pressure rises?*

A. Dilation of the pupil

B. Hyperventilation

C. Altered mental status

D. Development of focal neurological signs such as hemiparesis

7-67 *When you place a key in the hand of a client whose eyes are closed and ask him to identify the object, what are you assessing?*

A. Stereognosis

B. Graphesthesia

C. Two-point discrimination

D. Position sense

7-68 *George, age 52, has a recurring headache every Monday morning. What do you plan to order?*

A. An EEG

B. A CT scan

C. An MRI

D. An NSAID

7-69 *Lynne, age 72, presents for the first time with her daughter. Her daughter describes some recent disturbing facts about her mother. How can you differentiate between depression and dementia?*

A. You might be able to pinpoint the onset of dementia, but the onset of depression is difficult to identify.

B. A depressed person has wide mood swings, whereas a person with dementia demonstrates apathetic behavior.

C. The person with dementia tries to hide problems concerning his or her memory, whereas the person with depression complains about memory.

D. The person with dementia has a poor self-image, whereas the person with depression does not have a change in self-image.

7-70 *Grace, age 82, has Alzheimer's disease. Her daughter states that she is agitated, has time disorientation, and wanders during the afternoon and evening hours. How do you describe this behavior?*

A. Alzheimer's dementia

B. Sundowning

C. Deficits of the Alzheimer's type

D. Senile dementia

7-71 *Julie, age 15, is 5 ft tall and weighs 85 lb. You suspect anorexia and know that the best initial approach is to*

A. discuss proper nutrition.

B. tell Julie what she should weigh for her height and suggest a balanced diet.

C. speak to her parents before going any further.

D. confront Julie with the fact that you suspect an eating disorder.

7-72 *A thymectomy is usually recommended in the early treatment of which disease?*

A. Parkinson's disease

B. Multiple sclerosis

C. Myasthenia gravis

D. Huntington's chorea

7-73 *Obsessive-compulsive disorder symptoms usually occur*

A. before age 15.

B. during midlife crises.

C. during late adolescence and early adulthood.

D. in later life.

7-74 *Jim, a 45-year-old postal worker, presents for the first time with a sudden onset of intense apprehension, fear, dyspnea, palpitations, and a choking sensation. What is your initial diagnosis?*

A. Anxiety

B. Panic attack

C. Depression

D. Agoraphobia

7-75 *Which of the following antiepileptic drugs are associated with spina bifida?*

A. Dilantin

B. Lamictal

C. Depakote

D. Keppra

7-76 *Mark, age 29, tells you that he has thought about suicide. Which should you say next?*

A. "How long have you felt this way?"

B. "Tell me more about it."

C. "Do you have a plan?"

D. "Have you told anyone else?"

7-77 *The typical perpetrator in a domestic violence situation is one who*

A. has a history of being a victim of abuse.

B. has a criminal record.

C. is involved in a new relationship.

D. is on a lower socioeconomic scale.

7-78 *Which of the following interventions can significantly slow the decline in performing activities of daily living (ADLs) in clients with Alzheimer's disease living in a nursing home?*

A. A simple exercise program

B. *Ginkgo biloba*

C. Doing crossword puzzles

D. Improving nutritional state

7-79 *Which of the following risk factors for a stroke can be eliminated?*

A. Hypertension

B. Carotid artery stenosis

C. Smoking

D. Hyperlipidemia

7-80 *June, age 79, comes to your office with a recent onset of depression. She is taking several medications. Which medication is safe for her to take because depression is not one of the side effects?*

A. Antiparkinsonian agents

B. Hormones

C. Cholesterol-lowering agents

D. Antihypertensive agents

7-81 *Mattie, age 52, has a ruptured vertebral disk with the following symptoms: pain in the midgluteal region, as well as the posterior thigh and calf-to-heel area; paresthesias in the posterior calf and lateral heel, foot, and toes; and difficulty walking on her toes. Which intervertebral disks are involved?*

A. L4–L5

B. L5–S1

C. C5–C6

D. C7–T1

7-82 *What is the main overall goal of therapy for the client with Parkinson's disease?*

A. To halt the progression of the disease

B. To keep the client functioning independently as long as possible

C. To control the symptoms of the disease

D. To ease the depression associated with the disease

7-83 *Ed, age 50, has a chronic, episodic headache. He states that it can wake him up at night, lasts 15 minutes to 3 hours, and has occurred daily over a period of 4–8 weeks. You suspect a*

A. tension headache.

B. migraine headache.

C. cluster headache.

D. potential brain tumor.

7-84   *Which drug has been shown to be an effective aid to smoking cessation?*

A. Oxazepam (Serax)

B. Clorazepate dipotassium (Tranxene)

C. Varenicline (Chantix)

D. Alprazolam (Xanax)

7-85   *Diana, 55, complains of ear pain, right facial weakness, and loss of taste. What diagnosis would you consider?*

A. Lyme disease

B. Stroke

C. Ear infection

D. Brain tumor

7-86   *Which of the following symptoms related to memory indicates depression rather than delirium or dementia in the older adult?*

A. Inability to concentrate, with psychomotor agitation or retardation

B. Impaired memory, especially of recent events

C. Inability to learn new material

D. Difficulty with long-term memory

7-87   *Which statement is accurate regarding a client who is at highest risk for an eating disorder?*

A. The client is male

B. The client is usually 25–35 years of age

C. The client has low self-esteem

D. The client has a bipolar personality

7-88   *You assess for cogwheel rigidity in Sophia, age 76. What is cogwheel rigidity a manifestation of?*

A. Alzheimer's disease

B. Parkinson's disease

C. Brain attack

D. Degenerative joint disease

7-89   *Sally, age 52, presents with a rapidly progressive weakness of her legs that is moving up the trunk. She also has absent reflexes and no sensory change. What do you suspect?*

A. Peripheral neuropathy

B. Guillain-Barré syndrome

C. Myasthenia gravis

D. Radiculopathy

7-90   *With which of the following movements might a client with a cerebellar problem have difficulty?*

A. Inserting a key into the narrow slot of a lock

B. Driving a car with a standard shift

C. Walking up stairs

D. Eating

7-91   *Jessica, a retired nurse, is contemplating surgery for severe sciatica and asks you for your opinion. How do you respond?*

A. "If you continue with conservative treatment for a while, your pain will be relieved faster."

B. "If you have surgery early, rather than continue with conservative therapy, your rate of pain relief and recovery will be faster."

C. "The 1-year outcomes related to pain relief and recovery are the same for both early surgery and conservative therapy."

D. "What has your doctor told you?"

7-92   *Which type of intracranial hematoma is the most common and has the clinical manifestations of headache, drowsiness, agitation, slowed thinking, and confusion?*

A. Epidural

B. Subdural

C. Intracerebral

D. Meningeal

7-93   *Which assessment tool rates the level of consciousness by assigning a numerical score to the behavioral components of eye opening, verbal response, and motor response?*

A. Mini-Mental State Examination

B. Brudzinski sign

C. Glasgow Coma Scale

D. CAGE questionnaire

7-94 *Jeff, age 12, injured his spinal cord by diving into a shallow lake. He is in a wheelchair but can self-transfer. He can use his shoulder and extend his wrist but has no finger control. At what level of the spinal cord was the damage?*

A. C4

B. C5

C. C6

D. C7

7-95 *Which peripheral nervous system disorder usually follows a viral respiratory or gastrointestinal infection?*

A. Cytomegalovirus

B. Herpes zoster

C. Guillain-Barré syndrome

D. Trigeminal neuralgia

7-96 *Don, age 62, calls to complain of a severe headache. Which of his following statements most concerns you?*

A. "It hurts whenever I turn my head a specific way."

B. "It's the worst headache I've ever had."

C. "Nothing I do seems to help this constant ache."

D. "I'm so worried. Can you do a CT scan?"

7-97 *During a mental status exam, which question might you ask to assess abstraction ability?*

A. "What does 'a rolling stone gathers no moss' mean?"

B. "Start with 100 and keep subtracting 7."

C. "What do you think is the best treatment for your problem?"

D. "What would you do if you were in a restaurant and a fire broke out?"

7-98 *When a client is in the precontemplation stage of smoking cessation, which question should the health-care provider ask?*

A. "What would it take for you to consider quitting?"

B. "What would it take for you to quit now?"

C. "What technique do you think will work best for you?"

D. "What do you think will be your biggest challenge to quitting?"

7-99 *Alternately touching the nose with the index finger of each hand and repeating the motion faster and faster with the eyes closed tests*

A. cranial nerve X.

B. cranial nerve XI.

C. cranial nerve XII.

D. cerebellar function.

7-100 *Sophie is 82 and scores 25 on the Mini-Mental State Examination (MMSE). What is your initial thought?*

A. Normal for age

B. Depression

C. Early Alzheimer's disease

D. Late Alzheimer's disease

7-101 *Which of the following complications is the leading cause of death shortly after a stroke?*

A. Septicemia

B. Pneumonia

C. Pulmonary embolus

D. Ischemic heart disease

7-102 *In which syndrome does the client often undergo multiple invasive procedures with negative findings?*

A. Masochist syndrome

B. Malingering syndrome

C. Munchausen syndrome by proxy

D. Munchausen syndrome

7-103 *Marie, age 17, was raped when she was 13. She is now experiencing sleeping problems, flashbacks, and depression. What is your initial diagnosis?*

A. Depression

B. Panic disorder

C. Anxiety

D. Post-traumatic stress disorder

7-104   What is the most sensitive diagnostic test for identifying an alcoholic client?

A. Aspartate transaminase (AST, also called serum glutamic-oxaloacetic transaminase [SGOT])
B. Mean corpuscular volume
C. Alkaline phosphatase
D. γ-glutamyltransferase (GGT)

7-105   Which of the following lab results would indicate a specific infection in the central nervous system?

A. Cerebrospinal fluid (CSF) glucose of 35 mg/dL
B. A CSF pressure of 250 mm of water
C. A CSF red blood cell count of $25/mm^3$
D. A serum white blood cell count of $12,000/mm^3$

7-106   Clients with spinal cord injuries often have bowel incontinence and need to have a bowel program instituted. What is the most effective way to stimulate the rectum to evacuate in the quadriplegic client?

A. Administer stool softeners every night.
B. Insert a rectal suppository and then eventually perform digital stimulation.
C. Administer laxatives every other night.
D. Administer enemas on a regular basis.

7-107   Bell's palsy affects which cranial nerve?

A. Cranial nerve V
B. Cranial nerve VI
C. Cranial nerve VII
D. Cranial nerve VIII

7-108   Major depression occurs most often in which of the following conditions?

A. Parkinson's disease
B. Alzheimer's disease
C. Myocardial infarction
D. Stroke

7-109   Compression of the optic chiasm by a pituitary tumor will cause what type of vision changes?

A. Bitemporal hemianopsia
B. No visual changes
C. Eye floaters
D. Cloudy vision

7-110   The persistent and irrational fear of a specific object, activity, or situation that results in a compelling desire to avoid the dreaded object, activity, or situation is defined as

A. depression.
B. obsession-compulsion.
C. agoraphobia.
D. phobia.

7-111   Which of the following is characteristic of a manic episode?

A. Weight loss or gain
B. Insomnia or hypersomnia
C. Diminished ability to think or concentrate
D. Grandiose delusions

7-112   What are the two most common causes of dementia in older adults?

A. Polypharmacy and nutritional disorders
B. Alzheimer's disease and vascular disorders
C. Metabolic disorders and space-occupying lesions
D. Infections affecting the brain and polypharmacy

7-113   The most common central nervous system side effect of mumps in children is

A. Diplopia.
B. Ataxia.
C. Decreased hearing.
D. Reduced IQ.

7-114   Which of the following tests is highly specific and fairly sensitive for myasthenia gravis?

A. Electromyography nerve conduction tests
B. Magnetic resonance imaging scan of the brain and brainstem
C. Serum acetylcholine receptor antibody level
D. Lumbar puncture

7-115   Which of the following cardiac drugs is used to treat migraine headaches?

A. Beta blockers
B. Nitrates
C. Angiotensin-converting enzyme inhibitors
D. Alpha-adrenergic blockers

Answers

7-1 Answer C

Bromocriptine and pergolide mimic dopamine. The other mechanisms of antiparkinsonian treatments are as follows: anticholinergics restore acetylcholine-dopamine balance; levodopa restores striatal dopamine; and tolcapone and entacapone reduce systemic degradation of oral dopamine.

7-2 Answer A

The Agency for Healthcare Research and Quality (AHRQ) recommends in its smoking cessation clinical practice guideline that providers ask and record the tobacco-use status of every client at every visit.

7-3 Answer D

Alcoholism is the most common cause of cerebellar disease. Hypothyroidism, use of drugs such as 5-fluorouracil and phenytoin, cerebellar neoplasms, hemorrhages, and infarcts also cause cerebellar disease, but alcoholism is the most frequent offender.

7-4 Answer C

Interferon B (Betaseron) is used for the treatment of multiple sclerosis because it decreases the frequency of exacerbations in clients with the relapsing-remitting type of multiple sclerosis. Before the early 1990s, high-dose steroids were used for acute exacerbations, and baclofen (Lioresal) or diazepam (Valium) was used for excessive spasticity and spasms. Benzodiazepines are ordered in a small dosage for anxiety.

7-5 Answer B

Clopidogrel (Plavix), an antiplatelet drug used to reduce blood clot formation by preventing the smallest blood cells (platelets) from sticking together and forming blood clots, should be ordered. The safety of clopidogrel is comparable to that of aspirin, and it has clear advantages over ticlopidine. As with ticlopidine, diarrhea and rash are more frequent than with aspirin, but gastrointestinal symptoms and hemorrhages are less frequent. For patients intolerant to aspirin because of allergy or gastrointestinal side effects, clopidogrel is an appropriate choice.

The benefit of aspirin in women has not been clearly proved. Aspirin also has more side effects than ticlopidine. The desired effect is decreased platelet aggregation rather than anticoagulation, which warfarin would accomplish. Nitroglycerin has no effect on platelets.

7-6 Answer C

Although Bob is experiencing anxiety with his unpleasant dreams, they are a component of post-traumatic stress disorder (PTSD). One of the specific diagnostic criteria of PTSD is reexperiencing the traumatic event in recurrent, intrusive, and distressing images, thoughts, or perceptions. Depersonalization can be seen in depression and schizophrenia but not in PTSD. With schizophrenia, there may or may not be a history of a major disruption in the person's life, but eventually gross psychotic deterioration is evident.

7-7 Answer B

A classic migraine (20% of all migraines) is preceded by either a visual aura, a sensory aura, unilateral weakness, or a speech disturbance. Tension headaches are not accompanied by nausea, vomiting, photophobia, or phonophobia. Cluster headaches occur more often in middle-aged men; cause severe unilateral orbital, supraorbital, or temporal pain; and occur in clusters on a seasonal basis, with 3- to 18-month periods of no headaches.

7-8 Answer B

It is expected that Marian might be depressed because of her multiple sclerosis (MS). Focusing more on what she has "going for her" rather than the type of MS she has should be the first response. At least partial recovery from acute exacerbations can reasonably be expected, although further relapses can occur. Some disability is likely to result eventually, but usually half of all clients live well without significant disability, even 10 years after the onset of symptoms.

There are many different clinical courses of MS. The chronic-relapsing type is only one type; however, it occurs in the highest percentage (40%) of all cases. In the chronic-relapsing clinical type, remissions are fewer and symptoms more disabling and cumulative between exacerbations compared with the exacerbating-remitting form. More symptoms are evident with each exacerbation. The other types of clinical courses, in descending frequency, are exacerbating-remitting (25%), in which attacks are more frequent and begin earlier, remissions are marked by less clearing of manifestations compared with the benign course, and the remissions last longer with stable manifestations between; benign (20%), in which there are minimum deficits from few mild exacerbations to total or nearly total return to the previous functioning; and chronic-progressive (15%) in which the onset is insidious, there are no remissions, and the disabilities become steadily more severe. It is slower in its progression than the chronic-relapsing type.

7-9   Answer B

Deficiency of vitamin B_{12} usually presents with an insidious onset of paresthesias of the hands and feet that are usually painful. A thiamine deficiency, commonly seen with chronic severe alcoholism or malabsorption, results in Wernicke-Korsakoff syndrome, which manifests as confusion, involuntary eye movements, and gait instability or ataxia. A folic acid deficiency results in neural tube defects in the fetus. A vitamin K deficiency results in coagulation disorders.

7-10   Answer D

Direct confrontation should be used when suspecting depression and the possibility of suicide. Fatigue, loss of weight, and insomnia, in combination with the client's history of the death of his spouse, should point in the direction of depression with a suicidal potential. The provider should ask about suicidal ideation and plans, as well as about the availability of companionship and support. Older white men have the highest incidence of suicide among the entire adult population.

7-11   Answer C

Decreased facial strength indicates a lesion of cranial nerve (CN) VII. A CN III lesion would cause diplopia, a CN V lesion would cause decreased facial sensation, and a CN VIII lesion would cause dizziness and deafness.

7-12   Answer B

A study by the Heart and Lung Institute of the National Institute of Health in the mid-1980s showed that class 1 antiarrhythmic drugs given to patients with ventricular arrhythmias following myocardial infarction, instead of preventing deaths, actually increased the number of patients dying. Since then, a series of studies has consistently confirmed this original observation. Because tricyclic antidepressant (TCA) drugs are also class 1

antiarrhythmics, there is every reason to believe that a similar increased risk of death would exist with the TCAs. All antidepressants (not just TCAs) carry warnings about suicide risk. Shortness of breath is not increased with TCAs. Reactive depression, an inappropriate state of depression precipitated by events in the person's life, such as the loss of a home in a fire, does not increase with the use of TCAs.

7-13   Answer B

Plasmapheresis, or plasma exchange, when used with adrenocorticotropic hormone therapy or other pharmacological therapy, has successfully induced remission in some clients with multiple sclerosis. Plasmapheresis is a procedure that removes the plasma component from whole blood, with the goal being to remove inflammatory agents, such as T lymphocytes, through exchanging plasma while suppressing the immune response and inflammation.

7-14   Answer B

Anosmia is the inability to smell. Hyposmia is a diminished sense of smell. Ageusia is the loss of the sensation of taste or the ability to discriminate sweet, sour, salty, and bitter tastes. Agnosia is the inability to discriminate sensory stimuli.

7-15   Answer C

In the depressed client, antidepressants are most effective in alleviating sleep and appetite disturbances. Psychotherapy is most effective in dealing with suicidal feelings and interpersonal problems.

7-16   Answer B

Elisabeth Kübler-Ross's stages of anticipatory grieving are shock, denial, anger, bargaining, depression, and acceptance. Each person goes through each stage at his or her own rate, but the stages vary little from person to person.

7-17   Answer A

If you suspect that your client abuses alcohol, the most appropriate action would be to confront the client. The first confrontation may be met with one of many responses, but it "keeps the door open" for further conversations. The overall goal of all types of confrontation is to help the client understand the need for abstinence. Then the provider should discuss interventions to assist with attaining this goal.

When the client denies alcoholism, one intervention is to have family and friends confront the client at the same time with reflections of how the client's alcohol problem has affected them personally.

7-18   Answer B

Absence seizures occur suddenly with impaired responsiveness, minimal motor movement, and last less than 30 seconds. Absence seizures are most common in children. Myoclonic seizures are sudden shock-like muscle contractions that often manifest in the extremities or the face but may also be generalized. Clonic seizures involve abnormal neuromuscular activity of the entire body involving repetitive muscle contraction and relaxation. Atonic seizures involve loss of muscle tone and strength. If unsupported, the person will fall but will not become unconscious.

7-19   Answer A

When the client is supine and you ask him to flex his head to his chest, you are assessing for the Brudzinski sign. Pain, resistance, and flexion of the hips and knees constitute a positive Brudzinski sign and indicate meningeal irritation. A positive Kernig's sign, which also tests for meningeal irritation, occurs when there is excessive pain or resistance assessed when the client lies supine, with hips and knees flexed, and then the knee is straightened. Decorticate and decerebrate posturing are two positions that reflect neurological lesions. In decorticate posturing, the client is rigid with flexed arms, clenched fists, and extended legs. This posturing is characteristic of a lesion at or above the brainstem. In decerebrate posturing, there is rigid extension of the arms and legs, downward pointing of the toes, and backward arching of the head. This posturing is characteristic of a lesion of the midbrain, pons, or diencephalon.

7-20   Answer B

Although all the questions are important, suicidal ideation is an emergency situation, and if it is present, the client needs immediate admission, preferably to a psychiatric hospital. The next most appropriate question would be to ask him what he thinks is causing the problem, but certainly assessing suicide risk takes priority.

7-21   Answer A

Generalized absence seizures (petit mal seizures) almost always occur in children. With generalized absence seizures, there is usually no aura or postictal state. The seizure usually lasts just a few seconds and consists of staring, accompanied by an altered mental state.

7-22   Answer C

Meningitis is usually caused by one of a number of bacteria. However, the most common bacteria in adults is *Streptococcus pneumoniae*. *Haemophilus influenzae* has become less common in adults because children now receive the Hib vaccine in infancy. Meningitis is less likely caused by a meningococcal or Gram-negative bacillus.

7-23   Answer D

Atypical antipsychotics such as risperidone should be avoided in clients with Alzheimer's disease who also have vascular risk factors because they may increase the risk of stroke. All the other medications listed may be ordered for clients with AD.

7-24   Answer C

The key phrase is the time of onset of the symptoms. Dave's wife stated that her husband's complaints occurred within the past few days, which is characteristic of delirium. In a depressive state, the onset may be weeks to months, whereas with dementia, the onset is usually insidious and gradual.

7-25   Answer A

The gait of sensory ataxia includes brusqueness of movements of the leg and stamping of the feet. A parkinsonian gait involves the trunk bent forward, arms slightly flexed, with an unsteady gait, particularly with turning. The legs are stiff and bent at the knees and hips. The client shuffles forward with an accelerating gait known as festination. An antalgic gait occurs with osteoarthritis of the hip, which causes functional shortening of the leg and produces a characteristic limp. A cerebellar gait is unsteady, with a wide-based stride and an irregular swinging of the trunk. It is more prominent when rising from a chair or turning suddenly.

7-26   Answer A

Thrombotic strokes comprise 40% of all strokes, followed by embolic strokes (30%), lacunar strokes (20%), and hemorrhagic strokes (10%). Thrombotic and lacunar strokes usually have a gradual onset, whereas embolic and hemorrhagic strokes usually have a sudden onset.

7-27   Answer A

A client with Ménière's disease presents with episodic attacks of severe vertigo, usually with associated ear fullness or hearing loss. The duration of the attacks is usually several hours, and the client is well before and after the attack unless hearing loss progresses and persists. The diagnosis is based on a typical history with recurrences. Treatment involves a low-sodium diet, diuretics, and possibly surgery. Vestibular neuronitis has an acute onset with severe vertigo and sometimes follows a viral respiratory infection. Benign paroxysmal positional vertigo is paroxysmal, brief, and purely positional vertigo. Otosclerosis involves progressive hearing loss, sometimes with intermittent vertigo.

7-28   Answer C

The FAQ (Functional Activities Questionnaire) is a measure of functional activities. There are 10 complex, higher-order activities that are appropriate for the initial assessment of Alzheimer's disease. The MMSE (Mini-Mental State Examination) is a test of cognition. The CAGE questionnaire is a screening tool for alcoholism. The Holmes and Rahe Social Readjustment Scale measures major life changes for identifying the impact of stress on an individual.

7-29   Answer B

In adults and children older than 3, herpes simplex encephalitis (HSE) is often localized in the temporal and frontal lobes and is caused by herpes simplex virus type 1 (HSC-1). Cerebral spinal studies show a presence of lymphocytes and increased protein and red blood cell levels in herpes simplex encephalitis.

7-30   Answer A

Aseptic or viral meningitis is a more benign, self-limited syndrome caused primarily by viruses. Bacterial or purulent meningitis has a rapid onset hours or days after exposure. Chronic or subacute meningitis has symptoms that develop over months, and clients are less acutely ill. There is no category titled inflammatory meningitis.

7-31   Answer C

The peripheral facial palsy of Bell's palsy is self-limiting, and complete recovery usually occurs in several weeks or months in the majority of cases. To cope with self-esteem, clients may be encouraged to change their hairstyle, and men may also be encouraged to grow a beard or mustache. There is

no suppressive drug therapy. A course of acyclovir may be ordered. Taking prednisone for 10 days has been found to shorten the recovery period and help with symptoms. Long-term therapy is not warranted because the condition is self-limiting.

7-32   Answer A

Hot showers may exacerbate the symptoms of multiple sclerosis. For the same reason, fevers should be controlled. Teaching points would include avoiding hot showers, controlling fevers, exercising and getting plenty of rest, and seeking psychological and emotional support.

7-33   Answer C

In infants with open spina bifida, the presence of perineal sensation is associated with significantly better long-term outcomes. In several studies, children with perineal sensation as determined by the response to a pinprick in at least one dermatome on one side of the saddle area were continent of urine and feces, never had pressure sores, and were able to walk more than 50 m.

7-34   Answer A

The diagnosis of multiple sclerosis (MS) is often difficult given the large variety of symptoms, but it is a strong possibility in this case. Generally, it occurs in clients ages 20–40. For a diagnosis of MS to be made, two or more parts of the CNS must be involved. In addition, there are several patterns that are diagnostic. A pattern of two or more episodes of exacerbations, separated by 1 month or longer and lasting more than 24 hours, with subsequent recovery, is one of the patterns exhibited here. The most common symptoms of MS include focal weakness, optic neuritis, focal numbness, cerebellar ataxia, diplopia, nystagmus, and bowel and bladder changes.

7-35   Answer B

Fetal alcohol syndrome is most often responsible for developmental delays in children. In descending order, the others are cerebral palsy, Down syndrome, and meningomyelocele.

7-36   Answer C

The medication of choice for obsessive-compulsive disorders is clomipramine (Anafranil), a tricyclic antidepressant. It seems to have a much better effect than alprazolam (Xanax), an antianxiety agent;

carbamazepine (Tegretol), an anticonvulsant; or buspirone (Buspar), a nonbenzodiazepine anxiolytic.

7-37 Answer C

When you move a client's head to the left and the eyes move to the right in relation to the head, the client has doll's eyes. This is the normal response to passive head movement and is an indicator of brainstem function. Doll's eyes are absent when the eyes fail to turn together and eventually remain fixed in the midposition as the head is turned to the side.

7-38 Answer C

In recent research there is an elevated frequency of childhood abuse, especially in those with motor involvement nonepileptiform seizures. Stress, anxiety, and malingering are less frequent.

7-39 Answer D

Marijuana tests positive in the urine for up to 30 days after a person stops smoking the drug.

7-40 Answer B

The Hallpike maneuver is performed to elicit vertigo. It evaluates the effect of head position on the elicitation of vertigo. The client sits with the head to one side with eyes open. The examiner grasps the head and quickly assists the client to a supine position with the head hanging below the level of the table. After 30 seconds, the client is quickly assisted back to the sitting position, the head is rotated to the other side, and the maneuver repeated. Vertigo will be apparent in clients with a peripheral, but not central, cause of vertigo.

7-41 Answer C

Naproxen sodium (Anaprox DS) is an NSAID that can cause gastrointestinal (GI) distress and must be taken with food. Ergot preparations such as Cafergot may cause nausea and vomiting, but not the GI distress caused by an NSAID. Sumatriptan may cause fatigue and drowsiness, and nadolol may cause hypotension and bradycardia, but neither causes GI distress.

7-42 Answer A

Although systemic steroids have been shown to possibly prevent the development of postherpetic neuralgia if given early in the course of herpes zoster, once postherpetic neuralgia is present, tricyclic antidepressants such as amitriptyline (Elavil) have been shown to be effective in relieving the pain. Beta blockers and NSAIDs offer minimal relief.

7-43 Answer A

The CAGE instrument is a widely used questionnaire that has a high degree of accuracy for identifying clients who abuse alcohol. CAGE is an acronym for four questions: the C stands for "Have you ever felt you should cut down on drinking?"; the A for "Have people annoyed you by criticizing your drinking"; the G for "Have you felt bad or guilty about your drinking"; and the E for "Have you had a drink first thing in the morning (an "eye opener") to steady your nerves or to get rid of a hangover?" There are no such measurements as the HEAT instrument or the DRINK tool. The MMSE is the Mini-Mental State Examination, which can help determine the degree of confusion and therefore help to isolate possible causes.

7-44 Answer C

A foraminotomy is an enlargement of the opening between the disk and the facet joint to remove bony overgrowth compressing the nerve. A laminectomy is the removal of a part of the vertebral lamina. It relieves pressure on the nerves. A diskectomy is the removal of the nucleus pulposus of an intervertebral disk. Chemonucleolysis is the injection of the enzyme chymopapain into the nucleus pulposus. It hydrolyzes the nucleus pulposus, thus decreasing the size of the protruding herniation.

7-45 Answer A

A hypoactive or weaker-than-normal reflex is scored as 1. It is present with lower motor neuron involvement, as in a slipped lumbar disk or spinal cord injuries. Hyperactive reflexes, scored as 3 or 4, are present with lesions of upper motor neurons, such as a cerebrovascular accident. A normal reflex is scored as 2.

7-46 Answer D

Middle-aged men who suffer from migraine headaches are 42% more likely to have a myocardial infarction when compared with nonsufferers, according to the Physicians' Health Study involving 20,084 men. Although the exact causation is not known, the president of the American Heart Association believes it is because the blood vessels are very reactive and the cerebral blood flow constricts, resulting in migraine headaches.

When occurring systemically, there may be a constriction of coronary vessels, thus potentially leading to a myocardial infarction.

7-47 Answer D

When you ask a client to walk a straight line placing heel to toe, you are assessing the proprioceptive aspect of the nervous system, which controls posture, balance, and coordination. Assessing dermatomes and the major peripheral nerves tests sensory function. The cerebellum is one of the neural structures involved in proprioception and can be assessed by coordination functions. Cranial nerves are assessed in many ways, but not by walking.

7-48 Answer B

A compulsive eater engages in uncontrolled eating, like the client with bulimia, but does not purge (induce vomiting). Clients with anorexia have an absence of or irregular menstruation. Clients with bulimia have tooth and gum erosion from frequent exposure to gastric enzymes through vomiting. Clients with anorexia and bulimia have compulsive exercising habits; compulsive eaters do not. It is important to distinguish among the types of eating disorders because their treatment differs.

7-49 Answer A

Clients with senile dementia of the Alzheimer's type (SDAT) commonly die of pneumonia (the most common cause of death of clients with Alzheimer's disease). Clients with late-stage Alzheimer's disease have problems related to immobility and usually develop pressure sores. They also have a poor nutritional status and may develop malnutrition. Depressed clients are at more risk for suicide than are demented clients.

7-50 Answer C

Viral encephalitis is the most common type of encephalitis. It is characterized by a progressive altered level of consciousness, seizures, motor weakness, and headache. Herpes simplex virus and microbial encephalitis are other major types of encephalitis. Pneumococcal is a type of meningitis, not encephalitis.

7-51 Answer C

Although rigidity, bradykinesia, and flexed posture are associated with Parkinson's disease, rest tremor is usually the first symptom seen. Rest tremor

disappears with action but recurs when the limbs maintain a posture.

7-52 Answer D

Hallucinations are not extrapyramidal symptoms. Extrapyramidal side effects of antipsychotic medications include akathisia (continuous restlessness and fidgeting); dystonia (involuntary muscular movements or spasms of the face, arms, legs, and neck); and parkinsonism (tremors, shuffling gait, drooling, and rigidity, all characteristic of Parkinson's disease).

7-53 Answer B

Cranial nerve XI is the accessory nerve. It is tested by having the client shrug his or her shoulders while you resist the movement. Having the client say "ah" tests CN X, the vagus nerve. Having the client stick out his or her tongue and move it from side to side tests CN XII, the hypoglossal nerve. Touching the pharynx with a cotton-tipped applicator tests CN IX, the glossopharyngeal nerve.

7-54 Answer D

Remote memory is verbalized after hours, days, or years and may be assessed by asking a client his or her mother's maiden name. Asking questions about things that happened today, such as how long the client has been at your office, what time the client arrived, and what he or she ate for breakfast, tests recent memory.

7-55 Answer C

Syncope is a temporary loss of consciousness associated with an increased rate of respiration, tachycardia, pallor, perspiration, and coolness of the skin. Lethargy is drowsiness from which the client may be aroused; the client responds appropriately but then may immediately fall asleep again. Delirium is confusion, with disordered perception and a decreased attention span. Delirium may also involve motor and sensory excitement, inappropriate reactions to stimuli, and marked anxiety. A fugue state is a dysfunction of consciousness in which the individual carries on purposeful activity that he or she does not remember afterward.

7-56 Answer C

Naloxone (Narcan) is the antidote for an overdose of narcotics. It is given at a dose of 0.4–2.0 mg IV and may be repeated every 2–3 minutes.

For an acetaminophen overdose, a loading dose of acetylcysteine, 140 mg/kg, followed by 70 mg/kg every 4 hours for 72 hours, is given. Flumazenil (Romazicon) is the antidote for an overdose of benzodiazepines. Activated charcoal is the antidote for phenothiazine overdose.

7-57　Answer A

A grade of 3 for deep tendon reflexes indicates that the reflexes are brisker than normal, but this is not necessarily indicative of disease. A grade of 4 is brisk and hyperactive, with clonus of the tendon, and is associated with disease. A grade of 2 is normal. A grade of 1 is low normal, indicating a slightly diminished response. A grade of zero indicates that there is no reflex response.

7-58　Answer B

Dry mouth, constipation, and drowsiness are common side effects of tricyclic antidepressants. Itching is not a common side effect.

7-59　Answer A

Sarah is demonstrating signs of meningeal irritation. Kernig's sign can indicate subarachnoid hemorrhage or meningitis. This is a positive sign when flexing the patient's hip 90 degrees and then extending the patient's knee, which elicits pain. Hoover's sign is when someone lying supine is asked to raise one leg; he or she will involuntarily create counter pressure with the heel of the other leg, for example, in a paralyzed leg. Hoffman's sign causes pain in the trigeminal nerve area in response to mild mechanical stimulation. Babinski's reflex is dorsiflexion of the big toe on stimulation of the sole, indicating a lesion of the pyramidal tract.

7-60　Answer D

In the majority of cases of stroke in older adults, hypertension is the body's attempt to maintain perfusion. More than two-thirds of these clients become normotensive without any intervention within several days after the stroke. If they had been treated, they would have become hypotensive. If the systolic blood pressure is greater than 220 mm Hg in a client with an ischemic stroke, treatment should be considered.

7-61　Answer C

When a diagnosis of encopresis is made, a physical examination should rule out a neurological disorder affecting the lumbosacral spinal cord. Encopresis, repeated involuntary defecation into the clothing, is more common in boys, usually over 4 years of age. Almost half of the children with this condition have abnormal or prolonged external anal sphincter contraction while straining to defecate.

7-62　Answer C

The older adult with delirium would present with agitated and restless behavior. The older adult with depression would be fatigued, apathetic, and occasionally agitated, whereas the person with dementia would be agitated and apathetic and exhibit wandering behavior. Slow and purposeless behavior may indicate either depression or dementia.

7-63　Answer C

Suggestions for making lifestyle changes that might assist a client in promoting helpful sleep include advising the client to wind down before bedtime by taking a warm bath or by reading for 10 minutes, to try some valerian extract (obtainable from a health food store), and not to read or watch television while in bed. Exercising before going to bed is stimulating, but evidence suggests that an afternoon workout improves sleep quantity and quality. In a large study, people fell asleep twice as fast and slept an extra hour once they began going for brisk walks in the afternoon. Bed should be a place for sleep and sex only. In a recent study of valerian extract, it was found to help troubled sleepers drop off faster and stay asleep longer.

7-64　Answer C

A carotid bruit heard on auscultation indicates a narrowing of the carotid artery as a result of atherosclerosis of the vessel. Bruits and heart murmurs have similar characteristics and are both caused by turbulent blood flow; however, they arise from different causes. In this case, the turbulent flow is heard as a bruit because the vessel is narrowed as a result of atherosclerotic changes. Auscultation alone cannot diagnose an evolving embolus. If a complete occlusion of the carotid artery were present, no sound would be heard.

7-65　Answer A

Temporal arteritis, also called giant cell arteritis, presents as a systemic illness with generalized symptoms such as fever, myalgia, arthralgia, anemia, and elevated liver function tests. The headache is a new, throbbing headache on one side of the head or back of the head. The erythrocyte sedimentation rate, which can be used as a screening tool, is usually very elevated (greater than 100 mm/min) with temporal arteritis, and a temporal artery biopsy shows granulomatous arteritis. A client with meningitis would show signs of irritation of the brain and meninges, such as a stiff neck. The client with subarachnoid and intracerebral hemorrhage would have an altered mental status.

7-66   Answer C

Altered mental status is the most sensitive indicator of increased intracranial pressure and is the first symptom to change as the pressure rises. As the pressure continues to rise, brainstem herniation occurs, along with dilation of the pupil, hyperventilation, and focal neurological signs such as hemiparesis.

7-67   Answer A

When you place a key in a client's hand while the client's eyes are closed and ask him or her to identify it, you are assessing stereognosis. Stereognosis is the ability to recognize objects by touching and manipulating them. Graphesthesia is the ability to identify letters or numbers written on each palm with a blunt point. Two-point discrimination is the ability to sense whether one or two areas of the skin are being touched at the same time. Position sense (kinesthetic sensation) is the ability to recognize what position parts of the body are in when the eyes are closed; it is tested by actions such as moving a digit.

7-68   Answer D

An electroencephalogram (EEG) is not useful in the routine evaluation of George's headache. His headache is most likely a tension headache because it is a weekly occurrence. A CT scan or MRI study is recommended only if the headache pattern is atypical, has changed in pattern, or is accompanied by other symptoms. The nurse practitioner should discuss with George strategies to avoid possible triggers, how to abort an attack, how to obtain relief from pain, and how to decrease the frequency and severity of attacks. The initial focus should be on the use of NSAIDs, cool compresses, and stress reduction techniques.

7-69   Answer C

To help differentiate between depression and dementia, keep in mind that the person with dementia tries to hide problems concerning memory, whereas the person with depression complains about memory and discusses the fact that there is a problem with memory. Also, with depression there is usually a time-specific onset, and affected clients tend to be apathetic and withdrawn and have a poor self-image.

7-70   Answer B

Sundowning is a common behavioral change in clients with Alzheimer's disease. It is characterized by increased agitation, time disorientation, and wandering behaviors during the afternoon and evening hours. It is frequently worse on overcast days.

7-71   Answer D

If you suspect anorexia, the best initial approach is to confront Julie with the fact that you suspect an eating disorder. Clients are usually aware that a problem exists but need the extra "push" that confrontation provides. Once they accept the diagnosis, proven treatments include medical monitoring; nutritional counseling; psychotherapy, including behavioral therapy, family counseling, and stress-reduction techniques; medications; and support group participation.

7-72   Answer C

A thymectomy is performed in approximately 75% of clients with myasthenia gravis because of dysplasia of the thymus gland. It is usually recommended within 2 years after diagnosis. The thymus gland is usually inactive after puberty, but in about 75% of clients with myasthenia gravis, the gland continues to produce antibodies because of hyperplasia of the gland or tumors. The thymus is a source of autoantigen that triggers an autoimmune response in clients with myasthenia gravis.

7-73   Answer A

Obsessive-compulsive disorder symptoms usually occur before age 15. Young people in their early teens with obsessive-compulsive disorder are inflexible, lack spontaneity, are ambivalent, and are in a constant state of conflict while harboring hostile feelings. The condition is manifested in this age group when parents of these individuals expect their children to live up to their expectations and condemn them if they fail to achieve the imposed standards of conduct.

7-74   Answer B

A panic attack is characterized by its episodic nature. It is manifested by the sudden onset of intense apprehension, fear, or terror and the abrupt development of some of the following symptoms: dyspnea, palpitations, chest pain or discomfort, choking or smothering sensations, dizziness, a feeling of being detached, diaphoresis, trembling, and nausea. All of these peak within 10 minutes. Anxiety is manifested for longer periods of time. Although depression may involve some psychomotor agitation—either irritability or anxiety—usually there is decreased energy, lack of motivation, fatigue in the morning, and depressed affect. Agoraphobia is fear of leaving the house because of the association of panic attacks with associated environmental cues.

7-75   Answer C

Mothers who have taken Depakote during pregnancy have given birth to babies with spina bifida. Safer medications during pregnancy include Keppra and Lamictal, but they are still considered pregnancy-risk category C. The benefit from their use may be acceptable despite the risks.

7-76   Answer C

A client's intent or commitment to the act of suicide by means of a plan suggests a high risk of actually committing the act. A client is at high risk if he or she has a definite plan, considers using more than one method at a time, and has made preparations for death. Also at high risk is the client who is impulsive, psychotic, or frequently intoxicated.

7-77   Answer A

The typical perpetrator in a domestic violence situation is one who has a history of being a victim of abuse. Domestic violence abusers may or may not have a criminal record, are typically in a long-term relationship, and are from all socioeconomic backgrounds.

7-78   Answer A

A simple exercise program, 1 hour twice a week, has been shown to significantly slow the decline in performing ADLs in persons living in a nursing home. Taking *Ginkgo biloba* and doing crossword puzzles may affect the decline of brain function but don't affect ADLs. Improving nutritional status has not been shown to slow the decline in the ability to perform ADLs.

7-79   Answer C

The best way to prevent a stroke is to identify at-risk clients and control as many risk factors as possible. Some risk factors, such as smoking, may be eliminated and others, such as hypertension, carotid artery stenosis, and hyperlipidemia, can be controlled or treated to reduce the risk of stroke.

7-80   Answer C

The diagnosis of depression in an older adult is especially difficult when a medical illness is present. Antiparkinsonian agents, hormones, and antihypertensive drugs all have depression as a possible side effect. Cholesterol-lowering agents do not cause depression. Other drugs that also have depression as a possible side effect include analgesics, anti-inflammatory drugs, antianxiety agents, anticonvulsants, antihistamines, antimicrobials, antipsychotics, cytotoxic agents, and immunosuppressants.

7-81   Answer B

A ruptured intervertebral disk at the L5–S1 level affects the first sacral nerve root. The client would have pain in the midgluteal region, as well as the posterior thigh and calf to heel area; paresthesias in the posterior calf and lateral heel, foot, and toes; and difficulty walking on the toes. When the L4–L5 level (fifth lumbar nerve root) is affected, it manifests as pain in the hip, lower back, posterolateral thigh, anterior leg, dorsal surface of the foot, and great toe. In addition, there would be muscle spasms, paresthesia over the lateral leg and web of the great toe, and decreased or absent ankle reflexes. When the C5–C6 level is affected (sixth cervical nerve root), there is pain in the neck, shoulder, anterior upper arm, and radial area of the forearm and thumb; paresthesias of the forearm, thumb, forefinger, and lateral arm; a decreased biceps and supinator reflex; and a triceps reflex that is normal to hyperactive. When the C7–T1 level is affected, there is pain and numbness in the medial two fingers and the ulnar border of the hand and forearm.

7-82   Answer B

The main overall goal of therapy for the client with Parkinson's disease is to keep the client functioning independently as long as possible. There is no drug or surgical approach that will prevent the progression of the disease. Treatment is aimed at controlling symptoms. Depression occurs in more than 50% of clients with Parkinson's disease, and it is undetermined whether it is a reaction to the illness or a part of the illness itself.

7-83   Answer C

Middle-aged men get cluster headaches more frequently than women. Ed's presentation (a chronic, episodic headache that can wake up the client at night; lasts 15 minutes to 3 hours; and occurs daily over a period of 4–8 weeks) is a classic instance of a cluster headache. A tension headache may also be chronic and episodic, but it usually lasts from 30 minutes to 7 days. A migraine headache may last from 4–72 hours. Organic disease, such as a brain tumor, would be ruled out once the practitioner looked for signs or symptoms of organic disease, such as abnormal vital signs, altered consciousness, unequal pupils, weakness, and reflex asymmetry. The headache pain in a person with a brain tumor is constant because of increased intracranial pressure.

7-84   Answer C

Varenicline (Chantix) has been proven to be more effective than bupropion (Zyban) for smoking cessation. They are both nonnicotine medications. Wellbutrin is the same as Zyban; it is also used for depression. Oxazepam (Serax), clorazepatedipotassium (Tranxene), and alprazolam (Xanax) are all benzodiazepines that are helpful with anxiety.

7-85   Answer A

Some Lyme disease cases involve the nervous system, causing paralysis of facial muscles, pain in the ear, and loss of taste due to swelling of the auricular nerve. Stroke does not cause loss of taste and seldom causes ear pain. Ear infections often cause ear pain and loss of appetite but not loss of taste or facial weakness. Brain tumors seldom cause loss of taste and ear pain but may cause facial weakness.

7-86   Answer A

The prevalence of depression (5%–10%) does not change with age, but depression is often overlooked in the older adult. The diagnosis requires a depressed mood for 2 straight weeks and at least four of the following eight signs (which can be remembered using the mnemonic SIG E CAPS [like prescribing energy caps]): S for sleep disturbance, I for lack of interest, G for feelings of guilt, E for decreased energy, C for decreased concentration, A for decreased appetite, P for psychomotor agitation or retardation, and S for suicidal ideation.

Dementia and delirium often coexist with depression. Delirium is a confusional state characterized by inattention, rapid onset, and a fluctuating course that may persist for months if untreated. The person with delirium has memory impairment, such as the inability to learn new material or to remember past events. With dementia, there is a cognitive deterioration with little or no disturbance of consciousness or perception; attention span and short-term memory are impaired, along with judgment, insight, spatial perception, abstract reasoning, and thought process and content.

7-87   Answer C

Clients with eating disorders tend to have low self-esteem. Other factors that appear to increase the risk for an eating disorder include female gender, young age, perfectionist personality, family history of eating disorders, attempts to diet, depression, and living in cultures in which thinness is a standard of beauty.

7-88   Answer B

Clients with Parkinson's disease may exhibit "cogwheel rigidity," a condition in which there is an increased resistance in muscle tone when the nurse practitioner moves the client's neck, trunk, or limbs. The muscle is stiff and difficult to move. There is a ratchetlike, rhythmic contraction on passive stretching, particularly in the hands.

7-89   Answer B

The diagnosis of Guillain-Barré syndrome is confirmed by a rapidly progressive weakness, usually in an ascending pattern from the legs up to the trunk and then to the arms and face. There is no significant sensory loss, and the reflexes are usually hyporeflexive or absent.

Guillain-Barré syndrome is a form of peripheral neuropathy. Peripheral neuropathy, which usually involves the distal extremities, does not have the ascending pattern just described. Peripheral neuropathy is also caused by diabetes, alcohol abuse, nutritional deficiencies, trauma, and syphilis. Myasthenia gravis is an autoimmune neuromuscular junction disease in which the client produces antibodies that destroy the acetylcholine receptors on muscle. Radiculopathies are usually caused by mechanical compression and cause neck and low back pain.

7-90　Answer A

Although the client with a cerebellar problem may have difficulty driving a car with a standard shift, walking up stairs, and eating, inserting a key into the narrow slot of a lock requires the most finely coordinated movement and therefore would be the most difficult.

7-91　Answer B

The rates of pain relief and of perceived recovery were faster for clients assigned to early surgery for severe sciatica than those receiving conservative treatment in one large study. Clients are more likely to choose surgery if they are not able to cope with leg pain, find the natural course of recovery from sciatica unacceptably slow, and want to minimize the time to recovery from pain. Clients whose pain is controlled by pain medication may decide to postpone surgery. This does not reduce their chances for complete recovery at 12 months.

7-92　Answer B

A subdural hematoma is the most common of the intracranial hematomas, occurring in 10%–15% of all head injuries. Clients present with headache, drowsiness, agitation, slowed thinking, and confusion. Epidural hematomas occur in 2%–3% of all head injuries. The client usually has a momentary loss of consciousness followed by a lucid period lasting from a few hours to 1–2 days. There is then a rapid deterioration in the level of consciousness. An intracerebral hematoma occurs in 2%–3% of all head injuries. The client presents with a headache, consciousness deteriorating to deep coma, and hemiplegia on the contralateral side. The meninges are the three layers around the brain and spinal cord—the dura mater, arachnoid, and pia mater. A tumor of the nerve tissue is a meningioma.

7-93　Answer C

The Glasgow Coma Scale is an assessment tool that rates the level of consciousness by assigning a numerical score to the behavioral components of eye opening, verbal response, and motor response. The Mini-Mental State Examination (MMSE) tests orientation, registration, attention and calculation, recall, and language. The Brudzinski sign tests nuchal rigidity, which indicates meningeal irritation. The CAGE questionnaire is a screening tool for alcoholism.

7-94　Answer C

A spinal cord injury at the level of C6 allows clients to self-transfer to a wheelchair. Clients can use their shoulders and extend their wrists but have no finger control. An injury at the level of C4 would involve some sensation in the head and neck and some control of the neck and diaphragm, but mobility is restricted. An injury at the level of C5 would allow clients to control their head, neck, and shoulders and flex their elbows, but they would not be able to self-transfer from the wheelchair to the bed. An injury at C7–C8 would allow clients to extend their elbows, flex their wrists, and have some use of their fingers. They would be able to use a manual wheelchair.

7-95　Answer C

Guillain-Barré syndrome (GBS) is an acute demyelinating disorder. It is a peripheral nervous system disorder that usually follows a viral respiratory or gastrointestinal infection. Cytomegalovirus, herpes zoster, and sometimes general anesthesia have been associated with the development of GBS. Trigeminal neuralgia is a chronic disease of the trigeminal cranial nerve.

7-96　Answer B

When a client states, "It's the worst headache I've ever had," it is noteworthy. Other findings suggestive of serious underlying causes of headaches include advanced age, onset with exertion, decreased alertness or cognition, radiation of the pain to between the shoulder blades (suggesting spinal arachnoid irritation), nuchal rigidity, any historical or physical abnormality suggesting infection, and worsening under observation.

7-97　Answer A

Asking the client the meaning of a familiar proverb assesses abstraction ability. It must be kept in mind that many proverbs are culturally derived, and the client may not have heard them before. Asking the client to subtract numbers tests computational ability. Asking clients what they think is the best treatment for their problem elicits information about their mental representation or beliefs about the illness. Asking clients what they would do if a fire broke out in a restaurant assesses their judgment.

7-98   Answer A

In a study on behavioral change related to cigarette smoking, the first stage is the precontemplation phase, during which the client should not be confronted with actually quitting but should be asked the safe question, "What would it take for you to consider quitting?" In the next stage, the contemplation stage, it would be appropriate to ask, "What would it take for you to quit now?" In the preparation stage, one might ask, "What technique do you think will work best for you?" In the action phase, the health-care provider might ask, "What do you think will be your biggest challenge to quitting?" In the maintenance stage, when the client has stopped smoking for more than 6 months, it is appropriate to ask, "What have you learned about people, places, events, and emotions that made you want to smoke?"

7-99   Answer D

Alternately touching the nose with the index finger of each hand and repeating the motion faster and faster with the eyes closed tests cerebellar function, which integrates muscle contractions to maintain posture. Cranial nerve (CN) X is assessed by eliciting the gag reflex and observing for uvula movement, CN XI by checking for the strength of the trapezius muscles, and CN XII by assessing tongue movement.

7-100   Answer A

The total possible score on the MMSE is 30. The median score for persons ages 18–59 is 29. For persons ages 80 and older, the median score is 25. A score of 20–25 indicates early Alzheimer's disease; a score of 10–19 indicates middle-stage Alzheimer's disease. Someone with late-stage Alzheimer's disease may score below 10.

7-101   Answer B

The leading cause of death after a stroke is pneumonia as a complication. The second- and third-most common causes of death, respectively, are pulmonary embolus and ischemic heart disease.

Pulmonary embolus results from immobilization, and ischemic heart disease is present because atherosclerosis affects the coronary arteries, as well as the cerebral vasculature. Septicemia does not usually occur after a stroke.

7-102   Answer D

Munchausen syndrome, named after a fictional German baron and storyteller, is a psychiatric condition, occurring more frequently in women, in which the history often includes multiple invasive procedures with negative findings. When the client is someone other than the person requesting the procedure or causing the problem, it is called Munchausen syndrome by proxy. Malingering is a conscious intent to deceive. There is no masochist syndrome.

7-103   Answer D

Clients with post-traumatic stress disorder (PTSD) have experienced some severe catastrophic event (in this case, rape) and reexperience the event by having recurrent, often intrusive images of the trauma and recurrent dreams or nightmares of the event. Clients frequently have combinations of symptoms of PTSD, panic disorder, and major depression, all relating to the initial traumatic stress event.

7-104   Answer D

The most sensitive diagnostic test for identifying an alcoholic client is the γ-glutamyltransferase (GGT) test. GGT is an enzyme produced in the liver after consumption of five or more drinks daily. A GGT of more than 40 units indicates alcoholism. The assay is 70% sensitive and has a similar specificity. The aspartate transaminase, mean corpuscular volume, and alkaline phosphatase levels are all increased in clients who are alcoholics, but the level of sensitivity and specificity is not as impressive as the GGT.

7-105   Answer A

A low cerebrospinal fluid (CSF) glucose level may indicate a specific central nervous system infection such as meningitis. The normal CSF glucose level is 45–80 mg/dL, which is about 20 mg/dL less than the serum glucose level. An elevated CSF pressure may be the result of several problems, not specifically a central nervous system (CNS) infection. A few red blood cells in the CSF may be a result of the procedure of the lumbar puncture. Elevated white blood cell levels may be the result of any number of infections, not specifically one in the CNS.

7-106   Answer B

With the quadriplegic client, the most effective program to stimulate the rectum to evacuate is to insert a rectal suppository and then eventually perform digital stimulation. The rectum will expel a rectal suppository along with the contents of the sigmoid colon. The bowel can be trained by using this stimulus and eventually all that will be needed will be a digital stimulus. Occasionally, digital evacuation may be necessary. Increasing fluids and roughage in the diet are also part of a bowel program, along with occasional stool softeners or laxatives and, rarely, an enema.

7-107   Answer C

Bell's palsy, a demyelinating viral inflammatory disease, affects cranial nerve VII (the facial nerve) and results in a unilateral loss of facial expression with difficulty in chewing and diminished taste.

7-108   Answer D

Sixty percent of clients suffer major depression during their first year after a stroke. Other depressive symptoms, as well as major depression, may also occur, although usually less often, with thyroid disorders, Parkinson's disease, heart disease, and dementia.

7-109   Answer A

Optic nerve compression occurs when a formation around the brain—such as a tumor or bony structure—presses on the optic nerve and affects its performance. Over time, optic nerve compression may lead to bilateral hemianopsia or optic nerve death. Visual change is expected, eye floaters and cloudy vision are not signs of optic chiasm compression.

7-110   Answer D

A phobia is the persistent and irrational fear of a specific object, activity, or situation that results in the compelling desire to avoid the dreaded object, activity, or situation. A depressed person has feelings of hopelessness and helplessness and has no energy to "fight off" the cause of the fear. An obsession is a recurrent and persistent thought or desire, whereas a compulsion is an uncontrollable urge to perform some repetitive and stereotyped action. Agoraphobia is fear of leaving the house or of open spaces.

7-111   Answer D

Grandiose delusions are exaggerated beliefs of one's importance or identity, one of the criteria for a manic episode. Criteria for a major depressive episode include weight loss or gain, insomnia or hypersomnia, and diminished ability to think or concentrate. Others may include feelings of worthlessness, excessive or inappropriate feelings of guilt, indecisiveness, recurrent thoughts of death, and suicidal ideation.

7-112   Answer B

The two most common causes of dementia in older adults are dementia of the Alzheimer type (Alzheimer's disease) and vascular disorders such as hypertension, atherosclerosis, vasculitis, embolic disease, and cardiac disease. Polypharmacy, nutritional disorders, metabolic disorders, space-occupying lesions, and infections affecting the brain are all additional causes of dementia that can be removed or reversed.

7-113   Answer B

The virus affects the cerebellum, which causes temporary ataxia. Because of childhood vaccinations, decreased hearing is less common.

7-114   Answer C

Of clients with generalized myasthenia gravis, 80%–90% have antibodies to acetylcholine receptors. Electromyography nerve conduction tests are a way to categorize peripheral neuropathies as being demyelinating or axonal. A magnetic resonance imaging scan of the brain and brainstem is useful in helping to diagnose amyotrophic lateral sclerosis. A lumbar puncture is crucial in diagnosing suspected bacterial meningitis.

7-115   Answer A

Beta blockers and calcium channel blockers may be used in the treatment of migraine headaches. Beta blockers, by blocking beta receptors, prevent arterial dilation. Propranolol (Inderal) is the most frequently prescribed of the beta blockers. Calcium channel blockers inhibit arterial vasospasm and block the release of serotonin platelets. They also affect cerebral blood flow, neurotransmission, and neuroreceptor blockade to assist in preventing migraines. Verapamil (Calan) is probably the best known of the calcium channel blockers used for this purpose.

Bibliography

Bader, MK, and Littlejohns, LR: *AANN Core Curriculum for Neuroscience Nursing*, ed 5, American Association of Neuroscience Nurses, Glenview, IL, 2010.

Douglas, D: Perineal sensation in open spina bifida predicts outcome. *Archives of Disabled Children* 92(1):67–70, 2007.

Dunphy, LM, et al: *Primary Care: The Art and Science of Advanced Practice Nursing*, ed 3. FA Davis, Philadelphia, 2011.

Furie, KL, et al: Guidelines for the prevention of stroke in patients with stroke or transient ischemic attack: A guideline for healthcare professionals from the American Heart Association/American Stroke Association. *Stroke* 42(1):227–276, 2011.

Laino, C: Men's migraines up heart attack risk. From the American Heart Association's Scientific Sessions 2006, Chicago, November 12–15. http://www.medscape.com/viewarticle/547915, accessed June 4, 2007.

Panayiotopoulos, CP: *A Clinical Guide to Epileptic Syndromes and Their Treatment*, ed 2. Springer, London, 2010.

Reuben, DB, et al: *2007–2008 Geriatrics at Your Fingertips*, ed 9. American Geriatrics Society, New York, 2007.

Rolland, Y: Exercise program for nursing home residents with Alzheimer's disease: A 1-year randomized, controlled trial. *Journal of the American Geriatrics Society* 55(2):158–165, 2007.

Snyder, PJ, Cooper, DS, and Martin, KA: Clinical manifestations and diagnosis of gonadotroph and other clinically nonfunctioning adenomas. CD-ROM, UpToDate, Inc., 2011.

Wilco, C, et al: Surgery versus prolonged conservative treatment for sciatica. New England Journal of Medicine 356, 22452256, 2007.

How well did you do?

85% and above, congratulations! This score shows application of test-taking principles and adequate content knowledge.

75%–85%, keep working! Review test-taking principles and try again.

65%–75%, hang in there! Spend some time reviewing concepts and test-taking principles and then try the test again.

Chapter 8: *Integumentary Problems*

Jill E. Winland-Brown
Sandra L. Allen

Questions

8-1 A biopsy of a small, yellow-orange papulonodule on the eyelid will probably show

A. fragmented, calcified elastic tissue.

B. mature sebaceous glands.

C. lipid-laden cells.

D. endothelial swelling and an infiltrate rich in plasma cells.

8-2 Justin, an obese 42-year-old, cut his right leg 3 days ago while climbing a ladder. Today his right lower leg is warm, reddened, and painful without a sharply demarcated border. What do you suspect?

A. Diabetic neuropathy

B. Cellulitis

C. Peripheral vascular disease

D. A beginning stasis ulcer

8-3 Balanitis is associated with

A. diabetes.

B. macular degeneration.

C. *Candida* infection of the penis.

D. measles.

8-4 Sophie brings in her husband, Nathan, age 72, who is in a wheelchair. On his sacral area he has a deep crater with full-thickness skin loss involving necrosis of subcutaneous tissue that extends down to the underlying fascia. Which pressure ulcer stage is this?

A. Stage I

B. Stage II

C. Stage III

D. Stage IV

8-5 Which treatment would you order for anogenital pruritus?

A. Suppositories for pain

B. Antifungal cream for itching

C. A high-fiber diet for constipation

D. Zinc oxide ointment

8-6 *Tinea unguium is also known as*

A. tinea capitis.

B. pityriasis versicolor.

C. tinea manuum.

D. onychomycosis.

8-7 Which of the following types of cellulitis is referred to as "flesh-eating bacteria"?

A. Erysipelas

B. Necrotizing fasciitis

C. Periorbital cellulitis

D. Peripheral vascular cellulitis

8-8 Jennifer, age 32, is pregnant and has genital warts (condylomata) and would like to have them treated. What should you order?

A. Benzoyl peroxide

B. Podophyllin

C. Trichloroacetic acid

D. Corticosteroids

8-9 Steve, age 29, has a carbuncle on his neck. After an incision and drainage (I&D), an antibiotic is ordered. What is the most common organism involved?

A. *Streptococcus*

B. *Moraxella catarrhalis*

C. *Staphylococcus aureus*

D. *Klebsiella*

8-10   *Which type of wart has fingerlike, flesh-colored projections emanating from a narrow or broad base?*

A. Common warts

B. Flat warts (verruca plana)

C. Filiform warts

D. Plantar warts

8-11   *The "herald patch" is present in almost all cases of*

A. pityriasis rosea.

B. psoriasis.

C. impetigo.

D. rubella.

8-12   *Tanisha, a 24-year-old African American mother of four young children, presents in the clinic today with varicella. She states that three of her children also have it and that her eruption started less than 24 hours ago. Which action may shorten the course of the disease in Tanisha?*

A. Calamine lotion

B. Cool baths

C. Acyclovir (Zovirax)

D. Corticosteroids

8-13   *You're teaching Mitch, age 18, about his tinea pedis. You know he doesn't understand your directions when he tells you which of the following?*

A. "I should dry between my toes every day."

B. "I should wash my socks with bleach."

C. "I should use an antifungal powder twice a day."

D. "I should wear rubber shoes in the shower to prevent transmission to others."

8-14   *The ABCDEs of melanoma identification include which of the following?*

A. Asymmetry: One half does not match the other half.

B. Border: The borders are regular; they are not ragged, notched, or blurred.

C. Color (pigmentation) is uniform.

D. Diameter: The diameter is 5 mm.

8-15   *Which skin lesion is morphologically classified as pustular?*

A. A wart

B. Impetigo

C. Herpes simplex

D. Acne rosacea

8-16   *Permethrin (Elimite) applied over the body overnight from the neck down is the preferred treatment for*

A. scabies.

B. eczema.

C. herpes simplex.

D. psoriasis.

8-17   *Zinc oxide, magnesium silicate, ferric chloride, and kaolin are examples of*

A. chemical sunscreens.

B. physical sunscreens.

C. agents used in tanning booths.

D. emollients.

8-18   *Pastia lines are present in which disease?*

A. Toxic shock syndrome

B. Rocky Mountain spotted fever

C. Scarlet fever

D. Meningococcemia

8-19   *What is the drug of choice for acute anaphylaxis?*

A. Diphenhydramine (Benadryl) 25–100 mg PO qid for adults

B. Epinephrine 1:1,000 subcutaneously (0.3–0.5 mL) for adults

C. Prednisone (2 mg/kg q 24 hours) PO in one initial daily dose, tapered off over 1–2 weeks

D. Amlodipine besylate (Norvasc) 5 mg qid for 4 weeks

8-20   *Sidney, age 72, has just been diagnosed with temporal arteritis. What do you prescribe?*

A. Systemic corticosteroids

B. Topical corticosteroids

C. Antibiotics

D. Antifungal preparations

8-21   Johnnie, age 52, presents with pruritus with no rash present. He has hypertension, diabetes, and end-stage renal disease (ESRD). One of the differential diagnoses would be

A. uremia from chronic renal disease.

B. contact dermatitis.

C. lichen planus.

D. psoriasis.

8-22   Thin, spoon-shaped nails are usually seen in

A. trauma.

B. a fungal infection.

C. anemia.

D. psoriasis.

8-23   A mother complains that her newborn infant lying on his or her side may appear red on the dependent side of the body while appearing pale on the upper side. When she picks up the baby, this coloring disappears. You explain to her about

A. a temporary hemangioma.

B. hyperbilirubinemia.

C. harlequin sign.

D. mongolian spots.

8-24   A darkfield microscopic examination is used to diagnose

A. scabies.

B. leprosy.

C. syphilis.

D. infections.

8-25   What is the most effective treatment for urticaria?

A. An oral antihistamine

B. Dietary management

C. Avoidance of the offending agent

D. A glucocorticosteroid

8-26   What is the connection between the surface of the skin and an underlying structure called?

A. An ulcer

B. A sinus

C. An erosion

D. An abscess

8-27   What is the initial emergency measure to limit burn severity?

A. Stabilize the client's condition.

B. Identify the type of burn.

C. Prevent heat loss.

D. Eliminate the heat source.

8-28   Sandra, age 69, is complaining of dry skin. What do you advise her to do?

A. Bathe every day.

B. Use tepid water and a mild cleansing cream.

C. Use a dehumidifier.

D. Decrease the oral intake of fluids.

8-29   Which assessment system for a malignant melanoma is used to determine the thickness of a lesion and help in determining prognosis?

A. Clark's

B. Breslow's

C. Brown's

D. Dermatoscope's

8-30   Which of the following statements about malignant melanomas is true?

A. They usually occur in older adult males.

B. The client has no family history of melanoma.

C. They are common in blacks.

D. The prognosis is directly related to the thickness of the lesions.

8-31   Jamie, age 6, was bitten by a dog. Her mother asks you if the child needs antirabies treatment. You tell her,

A. "If the dog was a domestic pet that had been vaccinated, the wound should be cleaned and irrigated."

B. "Antirabies treatment must be started immediately."

C. "Rabies can be contracted only through the bites of wild animals."

D. "Wait until you have observed the animal for 2 weeks to determine if it is rabid."

8-32   A 70-year-old client with herpes zoster has a vesicle on the tip of the nose. This may indicate

A. ophthalmic zoster.
B. herpes simplex.
C. Kaposi's sarcoma.
D. orf and milker's nodules.

8-33   Treatment for a stage I pressure ulcer may include

A. an enzymatic preparation.
B. systemic antibiotics.
C. surgical treatment with muscle flaps.
D. a transparent, semipermeable membrane dressing.

8-34   Janine, age 29, has numerous transient lesions that come and go, and she is diagnosed with urticaria. What do you order?

A. Aspirin
B. NSAIDs
C. Opioids
D. Antihistamines

8-35   A thinning of skin that appears white or translucent is defined as

A. a scale.
B. a cyst.
C. a fissure.
D. atrophy.

8-36   Which lesion results in scales or shedding flakes of greasy, keratinized skin tissue?

A. Eczema
B. Impetigo
C. Psoriasis
D. Herpes

8-37   Why is ultraviolet light therapy used to treat psoriasis?

A. To dry the lesions
B. To kill the bacteria
C. To decrease the growth rate of epidermal cells
D. To kill the fungi

8-38   Nevi arise from

A. plugged follicles.
B. melanocytes.
C. capillary occlusion.
D. epithelium.

8-39   John, age 58, is a farmer. He presents with a painful finger ulcer and a palpable olecranal lymph node. Suspecting an orf skin ulcer, you ask him if he works with

A. sheep and goats.
B. horses.
C. metals.
D. tile.

8-40   Gouty pain in the great toe is

A. toe gout.
B. hyperuricemia of the toe.
C. podagra.
D. tophus.

8-41   Which of the following is a predisposing condition for furunculosis?

A. Diabetes mellitus
B. Hypertension
C. Peripheral vascular disease
D. Chronic fatigue syndrome

8-42   The majority of malignant melanomas are

A. superficially spreading.
B. lentigo maligna.
C. acral-lentiginous.
D. nodular.

8-43   Which type of hemangioma in a newborn occurs on the nape of the neck and is usually not noticeable when it becomes covered by hair?

A. Nevus flammeus (port-wine stain)
B. Stork's beak mark
C. Strawberry hemangioma
D. Cavernous hemangioma

8-44 The purpose of a transparent dressing such as Tegaderm applied over a pressure ulcer is to

A. toughen intact skin and preserve skin integrity.

B. prevent skin breakdown and the entrance of moisture and bacteria but allow permeability of oxygen and moisture vapor.

C. allow necrotic material to soften.

D. use the proteolytic enzymes in the dressing to serve as a debriding agent.

8-45 Your 24-year-old client, whose varicella rash just erupted yesterday, asks you when she can go back to work. What do you tell her?

A. "Once all the vesicles are crusted over."

B. "When the rash is entirely gone."

C. "Once you have been on medication for at least 48 hours."

D. "Now, as long as you stay away from children and pregnant women."

8-46 A linear arrangement along a nerve distribution is a description of which type of skin lesion?

A. Annular

B. Zosteriform

C. Keratotic

D. Linear

8-47 The morphology of which lesion begins as an inflammatory papule that develops within several days into a painless, hemorrhagic, and necrotic abscess, eventually with a dense, black, necrotic eschar forming over the initial lesion?

A. Furuncle-carbuncle

B. Hidradenitis suppurativa

C. Anthrax

D. Cellulitis

8-48 An eczematous skin reaction may result from

A. penicillin.

B. allopurinol (Zyloprim).

C. an oral contraceptive.

D. phenytoin (Dilantin).

8-49 Shelby has a blister filled with clear fluid on her arm. It is the result of contact with a hot iron. How do you document this?

A. Bulla

B. Wheal

C. Cyst

D. Pustule

8-50 Which treatment is considered the gold standard in tissue-conservative skin cancer removal?

A. Cryosurgery

B. Simple excision

C. Photodynamic treatment

D. Mohs' micrographic surgery

8-51 What is the most common rosacea trigger?

A. Alcohol

B. Cold weather

C. Skin care products

D. Sun exposure

8-52 Marie asks what she can do for Sarah, her 90-year-old mother, who has extremely dry skin. You respond,

A. "After bathing every day, use a generous supply of moisturizers."

B. "Use a special moisturizing soap every day."

C. "Your mother does not need a bath every day."

D. "Increase your mother's intake of fluids."

8-53 Which agent is ineffective against psoriasis?

A. Topical antifungals

B. Systemic medications

C. Phototherapy

D. Topical corticosteroids

8-54 What is the most important thing a woman can do to have youthful, attractive skin?

A. Keep well hydrated.

B. Use sunscreen with an SPF of at least 45.

C. Avoid smoking.

D. Use mild defatted or glycerin soaps.

8-55   A differential diagnosis of scarring alopecia may be

A. bacterial infection of the scalp.

B. Addison's disease.

C. drug-induced hair loss.

D. androgenetic baldness.

8-56   Stephen, age 18, presents with a pruritic rash on his upper trunk and shoulders. You observe flat to slightly elevated brown papules and plaques that scale when they are rubbed. You also note areas of hypopigmentation. What is your initial diagnosis?

A. Lentigo syndrome

B. Tinea versicolor

C. Localized brown macules

D. Ochronosis

8-57   Which form of acne is more common in the middle-aged to older adult and causes changes in skin color, enlarged pores, and thickening of the soft tissues of the nose?

A. Acne vulgaris

B. Acne rosacea

C. Acne conglobata

D. Nodulocystic acne

8-58   A Gram stain of which lesion reveals large, square-ended, gram-positive rods that grow easily on blood agar?

A. Dermatophyte infection

B. Tuberculosis (scrofuloderma)

C. Sarcoidosis

D. Anthrax

8-59   Where is the epitrochlear lymph node located?

A. In front of the ear

B. Halfway between the angle and the tip of the mandible

C. In the posterior triangle along the edge of the trapezius muscle

D. In the inner condyle of the humerus

8-60   Johnny, age 12, just started taking amoxicillin for otitis media. His mother said that he woke up this morning with a rash on his trunk. What is your first action?

A. Prescribe systemic antihistamines.

B. Prescribe a short course of systemic steroids.

C. Stop the amoxicillin.

D. Continue the drug; this reaction on the first day is normal.

8-61   Susie asks you about the "blackheads" on her face. You tell her these are referred to as

A. open comedones.

B. closed comedones.

C. papules.

D. pustules.

8-62   Silas, age 82, comes to your office with a fairly new colostomy. Around the stoma he has a papular rash with satellite lesions. What does this indicate?

A. A fungal infection, usually Candida albicans

B. An allergic reaction to the appliance

C. A normal reaction to fecal drainage

D. A fluid volume deficit

8-63   Client teaching is an integral part of successfully treating pediculosis. Which of the following statements would you incorporate in your teaching plan?

A. "It's OK to resume sharing combs, headsets, and so on, after being lice free for 1 month."

B. "Soak your combs and brushes in rubbing alcohol for 8 hours."

C. "Itching may continue after successful treatment for up to a week."

D. "Spraying of pesticides in the immediate environment is essential to prevent recurrence."

8-64   Harry uses a high-potency corticosteroid cream for his dermatoses. You tell him the following:

A. "You must use this for an extended period of time for it to be effective."

B. "It will work better if you occlude the lesion."

C. "It may exacerbate your concurrent condition of tinea corporis."

D. "Be sure to use it daily."

8-65　*The viral exanthem of Koplik's spots is present in*

A. rubeola.

B. rubella.

C. fifth disease.

D. varicella.

8-66　*Which disease usually starts on the cheeks and spreads to the arms and trunk?*

A. Erythema infectiosum (fifth disease)

B. Rocky Mountain spotted fever

C. Rubeola

D. Rubella

8-67　*Jack, age 59, has a nevus on his shoulder that has recently changed from brown to bluish black. You advise him to*

A. have an excisional biopsy.

B. monitor the nevus for a change at the end of 1 month.

C. apply benzoyl peroxide solution.

D. apply hydrocortisone 1% cream.

8-68　*Buddy, age 12, presents with annular lesions with a scaly border and central clearing on his trunk. What do you suspect?*

A. Psoriasis

B. Erythema multiforme

C. Tinea corporis

D. Syphilis

8-69　*Suzanne has a 7-year-old daughter who has had two recent infestations of lice. She asks you what she can do to prevent this. You respond,*

A. "After two days of no head lice, her bedding is lice free."

B. "Boys are more susceptible, so watch out for her brother also."

C. "After several infestations, she is now immune and is no longer susceptible."

D. "Don't let her share hats, combs, or brushes with anyone."

8-70　*Elizabeth, age 83, presents with a 3-day history of pain and burning in the left forehead. This morning she noticed a rash with erythematous papules in that site. What do you suspect?*

A. Varicella

B. Herpes zoster

C. Syphilis

D. Rubella

8-71　*Mary just came from visiting her husband, Sam, age 82, who recently had an ileostomy resulting in a stoma. She did not think that Sam's stoma looked "right." You tell her that the color of the stoma should be*

A. pale pink.

B. beefy red.

C. dark red or purple.

D. flesh colored.

8-72　*Amy, age 36, is planning to go skiing with her fiancé. He has warned her about frostbite, and she is wondering what to do if frostbite should occur. You know she's misunderstood the directions when she tells you which of the following?*

A. "I should remove wet footwear if my feet are frostbitten."

B. "I should rub the area with snow."

C. "I should apply firm pressure with a warm hand to the area."

D. "I should place my hands in my axillae if my hands are frostbitten."

8-73　*Abe, age 57, has just been given a diagnosis of herpes zoster. He asks you about exposure to others. You tell him that*

A. once he has been on the medication for a full 24 hours, he is no longer contagious.

B. he should stay away from children and pregnant women who have not had chickenpox.

C. he should wait until the rash is completely gone before going out in crowds.

D. he should be isolated from all persons except his wife.

8-74 A Wood's light is especially useful in diagnosing which of the following?

A. Tinea versicolor

B. Herpes zoster

C. A decubitus ulcer

D. A melanoma

8-75 What is the treatment for thrush?

A. Nystatin oral suspension for 2 weeks, 2–3 mL in each side of the mouth, held as long as possible

B. Clotrimazole oral troches (10 mg) two times per day for 7 days

C. Fluconazole (100 mg) twice daily for 1 week

D. Antiseptic mouth rinses after each meal

8-76 Adverse effects from prolonged or high-potency topical corticosteroid use on an open lesion may include

A. epidermal proliferation.

B. striae.

C. vitiligo.

D. easy bruisability.

8-77 In a burn trauma, which blood measurement rises as a secondary result of hemoconcentration when fluid shifts from the intravascular compartment?

A. Hemoglobin

B. Sodium

C. Hematocrit

D. Blood urea nitrogen (BUN)

8-78 Debbie, age 29, has a high fever and red, warm, sharply marginated plaques on the right side of her face that are indurated and painful. You diagnose erysipelas. What treatment do you begin?

A. Systemic steroids

B. Topical steroids

C. Systemic antibiotics

D. NSAIDs

8-79 Candidiasis may occur in many parts of the body. James, age 29, has it in the glans of his penis. What is your diagnosis?

A. Balanitis

B. Thrush

C. Candidal paronychia

D. Subungual

8-80 Jane is the 26-year-old Asian mother of Alysia, age 2 months. She is concerned about the large blue spot covering her infant's entire right lower leg. Jane tells you that Alysia was born with the spot. You tell her that

A. when the infant reaches her adult height, the macule can be surgically removed.

B. she should take the infant immediately to a plastic surgeon because this is a rare cancerous lesion.

C. this is a mongolian spot. It is common in Asians and blacks, and no treatment is necessary because it will fade with age.

D. she should always keep the spot covered because sunlight will aggravate it.

8-81 Jim, age 59, presents with recurrent, sharply circumscribed red papules and plaques with a powdery white scale on the extensor aspect of his elbows and knees. What do you suspect?

A. Actinic keratosis

B. Eczema

C. Psoriasis

D. Seborrheic dermatitis

8-82 Psoriasis may occur after months of using

A. vitamins.

B. hormone replacement therapy.

C. NSAIDs.

D. antihistamine nasal sprays.

8-83 Large, flaccid bullae with honey-colored crusts around the mouth and nose are characteristic of

A. a burn.

B. Rocky Mountain spotted fever.

C. measles.

D. impetigo.

8-84 What is the name of the acquired disorder characterized by complete loss of pigment of the involved skin?

A. Tinea versicolor

B. Vitiligo

C. Tuberous sclerosis

D. Pityriasis alba

8-85 *A basal cell carcinoma is*

A. an epithelial tumor that originates from either the basal layer of the epidermis or cells in the surrounding dermal structures.

B. a malignant tumor of the squamous epithelium of the skin or mucous membranes.

C. an overgrowth and thickening of the cornified epithelium.

D. lined with epithelium and contains fluid or a semisolid material.

8-86 *Which of the following warts (human papillomavirus [HPV]) looks like a cauliflower and is usually found in the anogenital region?*

A. Plantar warts

B. Filiform and digitate warts

C. Condyloma acuminata

D. Verruca plana

8-87 *Margaret, age 32, comes into the clinic. She has painful joints and a distinctive rash in a butterfly distribution on her face. The rash has red papules and plaques with a fine scale. What do you suspect?*

A. Lymphocytoma cutis

B. Relapsing polychondritis

C. Systemic lupus erythematosus

D. An allergic reaction

8-88 *Which of the following therapeutic modalities is useful for severe uncontrollable atopic dermatitis?*

A. Emollients

B. Compresses

C. Ultraviolet light

D. Tars

8-89 *Which skin lesions are directly related to chronic sun exposure and photodamage?*

A. Skin tags

B. Seborrheic keratoses

C. Actinic keratoses

D. Angiomas

8-90 *You are teaching Harvey about the warts on his hands. What is included in your teaching?*

A. Treatment is usually effective, and most warts will not recur afterward.

B. Because warts have roots, it is difficult to remove them surgically.

C. Warts are caused by the human papillomavirus.

D. Shaving the wart may prevent its recurrence.

8-91 *A client with a platelet abnormality may present with*

A. red to blue macular plaques.

B. multiple frecklelike macular lesions in sun-exposed areas.

C. numerous small, brown, nonscaly macules that become more prominent with sun exposure.

D. red, flat, nonblanchable petechiae.

8-92 *Dry, itchy skin in older adults results from*

A. the reduction of sweat and oil glands.

B. loss of subcutaneous tissue.

C. dermal thinning.

D. decreased elasticity.

8-93 *What is a safe and effective treatment for mild psoriasis?*

A. Coal tar preparations

B. Systemic steroids

C. Topical antibiotics

D. Systemic antihistamines

8-94 *In burn trauma, silver sulfadiazine (Silvadene), a sulfonamide, is the most commonly used topical agent. What is its mechanism of action?*

A. It is a synthetic antibiotic that appears to interfere with the metabolism of bacterial cells.

B. It is a bacteriostatic agent that inhibits a wide variety of gram-positive and gram-negative organisms by altering the microbial cell wall and membrane.

C. It is a bactericidal agent that acts on the cell membrane and cell wall of susceptible bacteria and binds to cellular DNA.

D. It is a protective covering that prevents light, air, and invading organisms from penetrating its surface.

8-95 *Jerry, age 52, has gout. What do you suggest?*

A. Using salicylates for an acute attack
B. Limiting consumption of purine-rich foods
C. Testing his uric acid level every 6 months
D. Decreasing fluid intake

8-96 *Susan, a new mother, states that when she pushes her index finger on one of her baby's skull bones, it presses in and then returns to normal when she removes her finger. She is concerned about this. You tell her that it is common and is called*

A. craniotabes.
B. molding.
C. caput succedaneum.
D. cephalhematoma.

8-97 *Which of the following secondary skin lesions usually results from chronic scratching or rubbing?*

A. Crusts
B. Scales
C. Lichenification
D. Atrophy

8-98 *Janice states that her son is allergic to eggs, and she heard that he should not receive the flu vaccine. How do you respond?*

A. "Although measles, mumps, rubella, and influenza vaccines contain a minute amount of egg, most egg-allergic individuals can tolerate these vaccines without any problems."
B. "Most of the allergic reactions are caused by the actual vaccinations; therefore, a skin test should be done first."
C. "You're right. We should not give this vaccination to your son."
D. "He should not have a skin test done if he has this allergy because a serious cellulitis may occur at the testing site."

8-99 *Persons with which skin phototype (SPT) sunburn easily after 30 minutes in the sun but never tan?*

A. SPT I
B. SPT II
C. SPT III
D. SPT IV

8-100 *Clubbing is defined as*

A. elongation of the toes.
B. broadening of each thumb.
C. a birth deformity of the feet.
D. a thickening and broadening of the ends of the fingers.

8-101 *Which of the following is a secondary skin lesion?*

A. Acne nodule
B. Neoplasm
C. Seborrheic dermatitis
D. Herpes simplex

8-102 *Samantha, age 52, has an acrochordon on her neck. She refers to it as a*

A. nevus.
B. skin tag.
C. lipoma.
D. wart.

8-103 *Which is the drug of choice for tinea capitis?*

A. A topical corticosteroid
B. Oral griseofulvin (Grisactin)
C. A topical antifungal
D. An antibiotic

8-104 *All of the following medications may cause alopecia except*

A. warfarin (Coumadin).
B. minoxidil (Rogaine).
C. levonorgestrel (Norplant).
D. acetylsalicylic acid (aspirin).

8-105 *Your client had a colostomy several weeks ago and is having difficulty finding a permanent appliance that fits. How long do you tell him to wait for the stoma to shrink before buying a permanent appliance?*

A. 2–4 weeks
B. 4–6 weeks

C. 6–8 weeks

D. Just over 2 months

8-106   *Lance, age 50, is complaining of an itchy rash that occurred about a half hour after putting on his leather jacket. He recalls a slightly similar rash last year when he wore his jacket. The annular lesions are on his neck and both arms. They are erythematous, sharply circumscribed, and both flat and elevated. His voice seems a little raspy, although he states that his breathing is normal. What is your first action?*

A. Order a short course of systemic corticosteroids.

B. Determine the need for 0.5 mL 1:1,000 epinephrine subcutaneously.

C. Start daily antihistamines.

D. Tell Lance to get rid of his leather jacket.

8-107   *When palpating the skin over the clavicle of James, age 84, you notice tenting, which is*

A. indicative of dehydration.

B. common in thin older adults.

C. a sign of edema.

D. indicative of scleroderma.

8-108   *What is an excessive amount of collagen that develops during scar formation called?*

A. A keloid

B. A skin tag

C. An angioma

D. A keratosis

8-109   *Susie, age 6 months, has a Candida infection in the diaper area. What do you suggest to the mother?*

A. "Use rubber or plastic pants to contain the infection and prevent it from getting to the thighs."

B. "Keep the area as dry as possible."

C. "Use baby powder with cornstarch."

D. "Keep Susie away from other babies until the infection is cleared up."

8-110   *A darkfield examination is used to cutaneously diagnose which disease?*

A. Syphilis

B. Viral blisters

C. Scabies

D. Candidiasis

8-111   *The total loss of hair on all parts of the female body is referred to as*

A. female pattern alopecia.

B. alopecia areata.

C. alopecia totalis.

D. alopecia universalis.

8-112   *A client with a nutritional deficiency of vitamin C may have*

A. dry skin and loss of skin color.

B. thickened skin that is dry or rough.

C. flaky skin, sores in the mouth, and cracks at the corners of the mouth.

D. bleeding gums and delayed wound healing.

8-113   *Which structure of the skin is responsible for storing melanin?*

A. Epidermis

B. Dermis

C. Sebaceous glands

D. Eccrine sweat glands

8-114   *The five Ps—purple, polygonal, planar, pruritic papules—are present in*

A. ichthyosis.

B. lichen planus.

C. atopic dermatitis.

D. seborrheic dermatitis.

8-115   *Susan states that her fiancé has been frostbitten on the nose while skiing and is fearful that it will happen again. What do you tell her?*

A. "Don't worry—as long as he gets medical help in the first few hours after being frostbitten again, he'll recover."

B. "Once frostbitten, he should not go out skiing again."

C. "If it should happen again, massage the nose with a dry hand."

D. "Infarction and necrosis of the affected tissue can happen with repeated frostbite."

8-116   *Which of the following should be used with all acne medications?*

A. sunscreen

B. oily makeup

C. plain soap

D. nothing should be used with acne medications

8-117   *What is a noninvasive method of treating skin cancer (other than melanoma) that uses liquid nitrogen?*

A. Mohs' micrographic surgery

B. Curettage and electrodesiccation

C. Radiation therapy

D. Cryosurgery

Answers

8-1   Answer C

A biopsy of a small, yellow-orange papulonodule on the eyelid will probably show lipid-laden cells. This is a description of a noneruptive xanthoma of the eyelid (xanthelasma). Fragmented, calcified elastic tissue is diagnostic of pseudoxanthoma elasticum. A biopsy of sebaceous hyperplasia will show large, mature sebaceous glands. A biopsy revealing endothelial swelling and perivascular round-cell infiltrate that is rich in plasma cells is diagnostic of syphilis.

8-2   Answer B

Cellulitis is a spreading infection of the epidermis and subcutaneous tissue that usually begins after a break in the skin. The skin is warm, red, and painful. Although Justin may have diabetic neuropathy, peripheral vascular disease, or a stasis ulcer, the information is not complete enough for you to suspect those conditions. The information and assessment data given fully support a diagnosis of cellulitis.

8-3   Answer C

Balanitis is associated with *Candida* infection of the penis. Candidiasis (moniliasis) may affect the mouth (thrush), penis (balanitis), or vagina (vaginitis).

8-4   Answer C

A stage III pressure ulcer is one that has a deep crater with full-thickness skin loss involving necrosis of subcutaneous tissue extending down to the underlying fascia. Stage I is nonblanchable erythema of intact skin. Stage II is partial-thickness skin loss involving the epidermis and/or dermis. It may appear as an abrasion, blister, or shallow ulcer. Stage IV involves full-thickness skin loss with extensive destruction; tissue necrosis; or damage to muscle, bone, or supporting structures.

8-5   Answer C

Treating constipation, preferably with a high-fiber diet, may help anogenital pruritus. Most cases of anogenital pruritus have no obvious cause and chiefly cause nocturnal itching without pain. Although the condition is benign, it may be persistent and recurrent. Hydrocortisone-pramoxine (Pramosone) 1% or 2.5% cream, lotion, or ointment helps with pruritus. Suppositories are not necessary. Anogenital hygiene needs to be stressed. Potent fluorinated topical corticosteroids and antifungals may lead to atrophy and striae after several days and should be avoided.

8-6   Answer D

Tinea unguium is tinea of the nails, also known as onychomycosis. Tinea capitis is tinea of the scalp; pityriasis versicolor is tinea versicolor; and tinea manuum is tinea of the hands.

8-7   Answer B

Necrotizing fasciitis is the cellulitis that is known as "flesh-eating bacteria." The hallmark of this infection is its rapid progression and the severity of the symptoms. Loss of life or limb is a potential complication.

8-8   Answer C

Genital warts (condylomata) may be treated using podophyllin (contraindicated in pregnant clients), trichloroacetic acid, or liquid nitrogen. Benzoyl peroxide is used for acne.

8-9   Answer C

Treatment for a furuncle (boil) or carbuncle (cluster of boils) may involve systemic antibiotics. The most common offending organism is and as well as are all causative organisms of pneumonia.

8-10   Answer C

Filiform/digitate warts are fingerlike, flesh-colored projections emanating from a narrow or broad base. Common warts are small, hardened growths of keratinized tissue. Flat warts are pink, light brown, or yellow and slightly elevated papules. Plantar warts appear at maximum points of pressure such as the heads of the metatarsal bones or heels or anywhere on the plantar surface.

8-11   Answer A

The "herald patch" is present in almost all cases of pityriasis rosea. Pityriasis rosea is a common, acute, viral, self-limited eruption that usually begins with a solitary oval, pink, scaly plaque, approximately 3–5 cm in diameter, on the trunk or proximal extremities. It is called the herald patch because it has an elevated red border and a central clearing.

8-12   Answer C

Tanisha should take acyclovir (Zovirax). If started within the first 24–48 hours after the rash appears, it may shorten the course of varicella (chickenpox). Acyclovir is not, however, recommended for children under 2 years of age. In those children, treatment of varicella consists of cool baths with Aveeno for pruritus and calamine lotion to dry the lesions.

8-13   Answer D

If a client has tinea pedis, tell the client to dry between the toes every day, wash socks with bleach, and use an antifungal powder twice per day. Rubber- or plastic-soled shoes can harbor the fungus and therefore should not be worn. The shower should be washed with bleach to kill the fungi. Antifungal powder or sprays are preferred over creams, as fungi thrive in warm, moist environments.

8-14   Answer A

One of the warning signs of cancer is a lesion that does not heal or one that changes in appearance. The ABCDEs of melanoma identification should be taught to all clients. The A is for asymmetry: one half does not match the other half. B is for border irregularity: the edges of a melanoma are ragged, notched, or blurred. The C is for color: pigmentation is not uniform; there may be shades of tan, brown, and black, as well as red, white, and blue. The D is for diameter: greater than 6 mm. E is for an evolving lesion, as well as for elevation.

8-15   Answer D

Acne rosacea, acne vulgaris, folliculitis, candidiasis, and miliaria are classified as pustular lesions. Papular lesions include warts, corns, Kaposi's sarcoma, basal cell carcinoma, and scabies. Vesicular lesions include herpes simplex, varicella, and herpes zoster. Erosive lesions include impetigo, lichen planus, and erythema multiforme.

8-16   Answer A

Permethrin (Elimite) applied over the body overnight from the neck down is the preferred treatment for scabies. Lindane (Kwell) is also often effective. Topical corticosteroids or systemic antihistamines are indicated for eczema. Acyclovir (Zovirax) is the treatment for herpes simplex, and coal tar preparations are used to treat psoriasis.

8-17   Answer B

Zinc oxide, magnesium silicate, ferric chloride, and kaolin are examples of physical sunscreens that reflect and scatter ultraviolet light. Chemical sunscreens such as PABA, benzophenones, and salicylates absorb ultraviolet light and act as a radiation filter. Tanning booths should be avoided because ultraviolet (UVA) radiation emitted by tanning booths damages the deep skin layers.

8-18   Answer C

Pastia lines are present in scarlet fever. All of the diseases listed are caused by bacteria. In scarlet fever, there is diffuse erythema with a sandpaper texture and gooseflesh appearance, with accentuation of erythema in the flexural creases referred to as Pastia lines. In toxic shock syndrome, there is a diffuse sunburnlike erythroderma. In Rocky Mountain spotted fever, there is an early maculopapular rash and then petechial or, rarely, purpuric lesions present on the extremities. In meningococcemia, there are erythematous, nonconfluent, discrete papules early in the disease.

8-19   Answer B

The drug of choice for acute anaphylaxis is epinephrine 1:1,000 subcutaneously (0.3–0.5 mL) for adults. Diphenhydramine IV (Benadryl) is a second-line emergency drug; the oral form would work well as an antihistamine. Prednisone is beneficial in severe or refractory urticaria. Calcium channel blockers, such as amlodipine besylate (Norvasc), may be of value in clients with chronic urticaria unresponsive to antihistamines when used for at least 4 weeks.

8-20   Answer A

Treatment for temporal arteritis involves systemic corticosteroids and immunosuppressives. The erythrocyte sedimentation rate is frequently elevated and a biopsy reveals granulomas and giant cells. Antibiotics and antifungal preparations are not indicated.

8-21   Answer A

All of the conditions listed result in pruritus. Only uremia from chronic renal disease, however, results in pruritus with no rash present. The other conditions—contact dermatitis, lichen planus, and psoriasis—all have a rash present.

8-22   Answer C

Thin, spoon-shaped nails are usually seen in anemia. Causes of thick nails include trauma, fungal infections, psoriasis, and decreased peripheral vascular blood supply.

8-23   Answer C

The harlequin sign is a transient phenomenon in a newborn who has been lying on his or her side. The dependent side is red while the upper side is pale, as if a line has been drawn down the middle of the body. This disappears when the infant's position is changed. Hyperbilirubinemia results in jaundice. Hemangiomas and mongolian spots are birthmarks.

8-24   Answer C

A darkfield microscopic examination is used to diagnose syphilis. A darkfield examination, with its special condenser, causes an oblique beam of light to refract off objects too small to be seen by conventional microscopes, such as the narrow organism *Treponema pallidum* that causes syphilis. Application of a special tetracycline solution followed by shining a Wood's light on the skin may accentuate the burrow of scabietic mites, thus helping to diagnose scabies. A direct acid-fast stain is used to diagnose leprosy, and a potassium hydroxide (KOH) stain helps diagnose *Candida* infections.

8-25   Answer C

The most effective treatment for urticaria (hives) is avoidance of the offending agent. Usually the offending antigen is identifiable and exposure is self-limited. Treatment with oral antihistamines is usually effective for symptomatic relief of itching,

swelling, and nasal symptoms. Dietary management may sometimes be helpful if the cause of the problem is a known food, such as shellfish, nuts, fish, eggs, chocolate, or cheese. Glucocorticoids have a minimal role in treating urticaria; a brief trial may be indicated for temporary relief in a difficult case.

8-26   Answer B

The connection between the surface of the skin and an underlying structure is called a sinus. An ulcer is a depressed lesion in which the epidermis and part of the dermis have been lost. An erosion is a moist, red, shiny, circumscribed lesion that lacks the upper layer of the skin. An abscess is a circumscribed collection of pus that involves the deeper layers of the skin.

8-27   Answer D

The first intervention is to eliminate the heat source. Then, stabilize the client's condition, identify the type of burn, prevent heat loss, reduce wound contamination, and prepare for emergency transportation.

8-28   Answer B

If a client is complaining of dry skin, the client should use tepid water and a mild cleansing cream or soap, use a humidifier to humidify the air, and increase the oral intake of fluids to assist in replacing some of the fluids lost from the skin. Advise the client that it is not necessary to take a bath or shower every day because soaps and hot water are drying.

8-29   Answer B

Breslow's guidelines for malignant melanoma have a scale to show the thickness of a lesion and the accompanying excision margins. There is also a table to show the tumor thickness with the approximate 5-year survival rate. Clark's levels show the grade (I–V) with the correlating location in the dermis.

8-30   Answer D

The prognosis for a patient with a malignant melanoma is directly related to the thickness of the lesion. Malignant melanomas usually occur in middle-aged adults of both sexes. The client usually has a family history of melanoma. Melanomas occur rarely in blacks; when they do, the lesions usually develop on the palms and soles and under the nails.

8-31   Answer A

Dogs are responsible for 80%–90% of animal bites to humans. Annually, 10–20 deaths occur from dog bites. Most of these deaths result from the exsanguination associated with head and neck bites in children younger than age 4. If the dog was a domestic pet that had been vaccinated, the wound should be washed thoroughly with soap and water and then treated like any other wound. Because rabies may be contracted from domestic dogs and cats that have not been vaccinated, the animal should be confined for observation. A rabid animal has an initial anxiety stage, followed by a furious stage. Preventive treatment of suspected rabies is based on immunization through a series of vaccine and immune serum injections. Domestic pets that do not appear rabid are assumed to have been vaccinated against rabies; this needs to be confirmed by the owner. Biting animals with an unknown vaccination record that appear healthy should be kept under observation for 7–10 days. Sick or dead animals should be examined for rabies. Because rabies is almost always fatal, when in doubt, treat. The type of immunization determines the timing of the treatment. If immune globulin is given, half of it is infiltrated around the wound and the remainder is administered intramuscularly. Inactivated human diploid cell rabies vaccine (HDCV) is given as a series of five injections beginning immediately and ending on day 28.

8-32   Answer A

Ophthalmic zoster (herpes zoster ophthalmica) involves the ciliary body and may appear clinically as vesicles on the tip of the nose. The client with a herpetic lesion on the nose indicating ophthalmic zoster needs to be referred to an ophthalmologist to preserve the eyesight. Herpes simplex primarily occurs on the perioral, labial, and genital areas of the body. Kaposi's sarcoma in the older adult usually occurs in the lower extremities. Orf and milker's nodules almost always appear on the hands.

8-33   Answer D

Treatment for a stage I pressure ulcer may include a hydrocolloid or transparent semipermeable membrane. An enzymatic preparation is used for a stage IV ulcer, and surgery may possibly be necessary. The use of antibiotics is recommended only for clients with clinical signs of sepsis. Antibiotics are not indicated when signs of infection are localized.

8-34   Answer D

Transient urticaria requires antihistamines on a regular basis. Aspirin, NSAIDs, and opioids are to be avoided.

8-35   Answer D

Atrophy is a thinning of the skin (epidermis and dermis) and may appear white or translucent. A scale is where epithelial cells are shed in variable sizes. A cyst is an elevated encapsulated lesion that is deeper than a pustule, with distinct borders. A fissure is a linear crack extending from the epidermis to the dermis.

8-36   Answer C

Psoriasis results in scales or shedding flakes of greasy, keratinized skin tissue. The color may be white, gray, or silver, and the texture may vary from fine to thick.

The other lesions—eczema, impetigo, and herpes—result in crusts that are dried blood, serum, or pus left on the skin surface when vesicles or pustules burst. They can be red-brown, orange, or yellow.

8-37   Answer C

Ultraviolet light therapy is used to treat psoriasis to decrease the growth rate of epidermal cells. This assists in decreasing the hyperkeratosis. Treatments are given daily and last only for seconds.

8-38   Answer B

Nevi, commonly called moles, are flat or raised macules or papules that arise from melanocytes during early childhood. A nevus flammeus (port-wine stain) is an angioma, a congenital vascular lesion that involves the capillaries.

8-39   Answer A

An orf skin ulcer results from a parapoxvirus infection, which causes a common skin disease of sheep and goats. It is occasionally transmitted to humans.

8-40   Answer C

Podagra is gouty pain in the great toe. Hyperuricemia results in the deposition of uric acid crystals in the joints.

8-41   Answer A

Predisposing conditions for furunculosis or carbuncles include diabetes mellitus, HIV disease, and injection drug use. Furunculosis (boils) and carbuncles are very painful inflammatory swellings of a hair follicle that result in an abscess, caused by coagulase-positive *Staphylococcus aureus*.

8-42   Answer A

The majority (70%) of malignant melanomas are superficially spreading. These have a good prognosis because they tend to spread superficially before invading the tissues. The next most common type (10%) presents as a black nodule; 5% of melanomas present as lentigo maligna, which arise from precursor lesions, and another 5% are acral-lentiginous. These arise on the hands or feet and are the most common type seen in Asians and African Americans.

8-43   Answer B

A stork's beak mark usually occurs on the nape of the neck and blanches on pressure. Although it does not fade, when it is covered by hair it is usually not noticeable. A nevus flammeus (port-wine stain) is deep red to purple, does not blanch on pressure, and does not fade with age. A strawberry hemangioma is the result of dilated capillaries in the entire dermal and subdermal layers of the skin. Although it continues to enlarge after birth, it usually disappears by 10 years of age. A cavernous hemangioma is the result of a communicating network of venules in the subcutaneous tissue and does not fade with age.

8-44   Answer B

A transparent dressing is applied over a pressure ulcer to prevent skin breakdown and the entrance of moisture and bacteria but allow permeability of oxygen and moisture vapor. A liquid preparation such as benzoin is used to toughen intact skin and preserve skin integrity. Wet-to-dry gauze dressings allow necrotic material to soften. They adhere to the gauze, so the wound is debrided. A proteolytic enzyme such as Elase may serve as a debriding agent in inflamed and infected lesions.

8-45   Answer A

A client who has a varicella rash can return to work once all the vesicles are crusted. Varicella is contagious from 48 hours before the onset of the vesicular rash, during the rash formation (usually 4–5 days), and during the several days while the vesicles dry up. The characteristic rash appears 2–3 weeks after exposure. Treatment is effective only if started within the first few days, and then only to shorten the course of the disease. Clients should avoid contact with pregnant women and children who have not been exposed to varicella.

8-46   Answer B

A zosteriform lesion is a linear arrangement along a nerve distribution and typifies herpes zoster. An annular lesion is ring shaped. Linear simply implies that the lesion appears in lines. A keratotic lesion has horny thickenings.

8-47   Answer C

Although cellulitis, furuncle-carbuncles, and hidradenitis suppurativa are all distinctive abscesses, only anthrax has the morphology described. It results in a dense, black, necrotic eschar gradually forming over the initial lesion. A furuncle-carbuncle is a pustular lesion surrounding one or several hair follicles, and a hidradenitis suppurativa lesion results in scarring and fibrotic bands. Cellulitis begins as a tender, warm, erythematous area of the skin and then takes on multiple presentations but not with a dense black necrotic eschar as described here.

8-48   Answer A

Penicillin, neomycin, phenothiazines, and local anesthetics may cause an eczematous type of skin reaction. Allopurinol (Zyloprim) and sulfonamides may cause exfoliative dermatitis, oral contraceptives may cause erythema nodosum, and phenytoin (Dilantin) and procainamide (Pronestyl) may cause drug-related systemic lupus erythematosus.

8-49   Answer A

A bulla is a primary skin lesion filled with fluid that is larger than 1 cm in diameter. It is also known as a vesicle. A wheal is also a primary skin lesion larger than 1 cm in diameter that is transient, elevated, and hivelike, with local edema and inflammation. A cyst is filled with fluid and may occur in a variety of sizes. A pustule is a superficial, elevated lesion filled with purulent fluid.

8-50   Answer D

Mohs' micrographic surgery (MMS) is considered the gold standard in tissue-conservative skin cancer removal. MMS is a specialized type of surgery consisting of the removal of the entire tumor with the smallest possible margin of normal skin. Cryosurgery involves using liquid nitrogen to burn off the lesions. Simple excision uses a scalpel to excise the lesion. Photodynamic therapy may be used with acne.

8-51   Answer D

Clients with rosacea usually have a long history of flushing in response to sun exposure. Alcohol, cold weather, and skin care products may also be triggers, but not nearly as often. Other triggers may include emotional stress, spicy foods, exercise, wind, hot baths, and hot drinks.

8-52   Answer C

Although increasing fluids and a moisturizing cream will help the general problem, Sarah does not need a bath every day because that will exacerbate the dryness of her skin. Plain water should be used rather than special soap.

8-53   Answer A

Antifungal agents are ineffective against psoriasis. The most common form of treatment is corticosteroids applied topically. Systemic treatments are used in more severe cases, and phototherapy, from either natural or artificial light, may also be helpful.

8-54   Answer C

The most important thing a woman can do to have youthful, attractive skin is not smoke. Smokers develop more wrinkles and have elastosis, decreased tissue perfusion and oxygenation, and an adverse exposure to free radicals on elastic tissue. Other important things to promote the health of the skin are use of a sunscreen with a sun protective factor of at least 15 and keeping the skin well hydrated. Although keeping the skin well hydrated promotes skin health, it does not prevent wrinkles. Using mild defatted glycerin soaps maintains texture and hydration but does not help prevent wrinkles.

8-55   Answer A

One of the differentials of scarring alopecia is bacterial infection of the scalp. Addison's disease, drug-induced hair loss, and androgenetic baldness are all differentials of nonscarring alopecia.

8-56   Answer B

If a client presents with a pruritic rash on his upper trunk and shoulders and you observe areas of hypopigmentation and flat to slightly elevated brown papules and plaques that scale when they are rubbed, suspect tinea versicolor. Lentigines are macular tan to black lesions, ranging from 1 mm to 1 cm in size. They do not increase in color with exposure to the sun. One or more lentigines are seen in normal individuals. Multiple ones need to be further assessed. Localized brown macules are freckles. Ochronosis is a condition with poorly circumscribed, blue-black macules.

8-57   Answer B

Acne rosacea is a chronic type of facial acne that occurs in middle-aged to older adults. Over time, the skin changes in color to dark red, pores become enlarged, and the soft tissue of the nose may exhibit rhinophyma, an irregular bullous thickening. Acne vulgaris is the form of acne common in adolescents and young to middle-aged adults. Acne conglobata begins in middle adulthood and causes serious skin lesions such as comedones, papules, pustules, nodules, cysts, and scars, primarily on the back, buttocks, and chest. Severe (nodulocystic) acne consists mostly of nodules and cysts and always results in scar formation.

8-58   Answer D

Anthrax is diagnosed with a Gram stain of the lesion, which reveals large, square-ended gram-positive rods that grow easily on blood agar. A dermatophyte infection is diagnosed with a potassium hydroxide preparation revealing hyphae and spores. In addition, fungal cultures demonstrate different fungi. Tuberculosis (scrofuloderma) is diagnosed with a histologic examination that reveals caseation necrosis and acid-fast bacilli. Sarcoidosis is diagnosed with a biopsy revealing noncaseating granulomas.

8-59   Answer D

The epitrochlear lymph node is located in the inner condyle of the humerus. The preauricular lymph node is located in front of the ear; the submaxillary (submandibular) lymph node is halfway between the angle and the tip of the mandible; and the posterior cervical lymph node is in the posterior triangle along the edge of the trapezius muscle.

8-60   Answer C

If you suspect a drug reaction to amoxicillin, stop the amoxicillin. Symptomatic relief may be obtained by systemic antihistamines and steroids. Systemic steroids may be necessary with severely symptomatic clients, although topical steroids may help clients with the pruritus.

8-61   Answer A

Open comedones are known as blackheads. A person with acne vulgaris may have open comedones, closed comedones (whiteheads), papules, pustules, cysts, and even scars.

8-62   Answer A

A papular rash with satellite lesions around a stoma indicates a fungal infection. It may be a consequence of persistent skin moisture or an adverse effect of antibiotic therapy. If Silas were having an allergic reaction to the appliance, he would have an erythematous vesicular rash limited to the site of the faceplate of the appliance. If the appliance fits properly, fecal drainage should not come in contact with the skin. Fluid and electrolyte imbalances may occur, but the signs and symptoms would be systemic in nature.

8-63   Answer C

Client education is essential when treating pediculosis. Clients should be informed that itching may continue after successful treatment for up to a week because of the slow resolution of the inflammatory reaction caused by the lice infestation. Clients and parents should be instructed not to share hats, combs, scarves, headsets, towels, and bedding. Combs and brushes can be soaked in rubbing alcohol for 1 hour. Excessive decontamination of the environment is not necessary. Environmental spraying of pesticides is not effective and therefore is not recommended. Bedclothes and clothing should be washed in hot, soapy water.

8-64   Answer C

If a client uses a high-potency corticosteroid cream for a dermatosis, tell the client that it may exacerbate concurrent conditions such as tinea corporis and acne. Topical corticosteroids should not be used indiscriminately on all cutaneous eruptions. They should not be used for an extended period of time, and the lesion should not be occluded. Intermittent therapy with high-potency agents, such as every other day, or 3–4 consecutive days per week, may be more effective and cause fewer adverse effects than continuous regimens. This is also true of lower-potency corticosteroids.

8-65   Answer A

The viral exanthem of Koplik's spots is present in rubeola (measles). Koplik's spots are observed on the buccal mucosa before the rash appears. In rubella (German measles), there are variable erythematous macules on the soft palate, and in fifth disease (erythema infectiosum), there is no exanthem. In varicella (chickenpox), there may be sparse lesions on the mucosal surfaces, especially the hard palate.

8-66   Answer A

Erythema infectiosum (fifth disease) usually starts on the cheeks and spreads to the arms and trunk. Rocky Mountain spotted fever, which is associated with a history of tick bites, starts as a maculopapular rash with erythematous borders appearing first on the wrists, ankles, palms, soles, and forearms. Rubeola (measles) starts as a brownish-pink maculopapular rash around the ears, face, and neck and then progresses over the trunk and limbs. Rubella (German measles) starts as a fine, pinkish, macular rash that becomes confluent and pinpoint after 24 hours.

8-67   Answer A

The ABCDEs (asymmetry, border irregularity, color changes, diameter, evolving/elevation) of melanomas should be taught to all clients. A change in the color variation may indicate a melanoma, and an excisional biopsy should be done. Monitoring for a month may enable a melanoma to extend extensively, resulting in death. Benzoyl peroxide and hydrocortisone may be used with folliculitis.

8-68   Answer C

Psoriasis, erythema multiforme, tinea corporis, and syphilis all have lesions with annular configurations. Tinea corporis (ringworm) has ring-shaped lesions with a scaly border and central clearing or scaly patches with a distinct border on exposed skin surfaces or on the trunk. Psoriasis has annular lesions on the elbows, knees, scalp, and nails. Erythema multiforme has annular lesions that are mostly acral in distribution and are often associated with a recent herpes simplex infection. Secondary syphilis lesions are usually on the palmar, plantar, and mucous membrane surfaces.

8-69   Answer D

Head lice may be transmitted by sharing hats, combs, or brushes, so these practices should be discouraged. The louse can survive for more than

2 days off the scalp, so it can still survive in the bed linen. Girls are more susceptible than boys, and lice occur more often in whites. Immunity against head lice is never acquired.

8-70   Answer B

The rash of herpes zoster is characteristic in that it appears on only one side of the body. Herpes zoster begins in a dermatomal distribution, most commonly in the thoracic, cervical, and lumbosacral areas, although it also occurs on the face. Although herpes zoster is caused by the reactivation of latent varicella virus in the distribution of the affected nerve, varicella (chickenpox) presents with a scattered rash on both sides of the body. A client with syphilis would present with sharply circumscribed, ham-colored papules with a slight scale and lesions over the entire body, especially on the palms and soles. Rubella (German measles) occurs in childhood. It begins on the face and rapidly (in hours) spreads down to the trunk.

8-71   Answer B

A normal stoma is moist and beefy red. A pale pink color may indicate a low hemoglobin level. A dark-red or purple stoma may indicate early ischemia. A black stoma is the result of necrosis. Stomas are never flesh colored.

8-72   Answer B

Rubbing or massaging the frostbitten areas, especially with snow, may cause permanent tissue damage. Advise the client to remove wet footwear if the feet are frostbitten; apply firm pressure with a warm hand to the area; and place the hands in the axillae if the hands are frostbitten.

8-73   Answer B

If a client has just been given a diagnosis of herpes zoster, advise the client to stay away from children and pregnant women who have not had chickenpox until crusts have formed over the blistered areas. Herpes zoster is contagious to people who have not had chickenpox.

8-74   Answer A

A Wood's light is especially useful in diagnosing tinea versicolor or other fungal infections. A Wood's light produces a "black light" through long-wave ultraviolet rays. It accentuates minor losses of melanin, which makes it useful in diagnosing tinea versicolor and vitiligo, in which there is hypopigmentation.

8-75   Answer A

One treatment for thrush includes nystatin oral suspension for 2 weeks, 2–3 mL in each side of the mouth, held as long as possible. When clotrimazole oral troches (10 mg) are used, they should be used five times per day for 14 days (not two times per day for 7 days). Fluconazole 100 mg may be given as a single dose (not twice per day for 1 week). Antiseptic mouthwashes are not effective for thrush.

8-76   Answer D

Adverse effects from prolonged or high-potency topical corticosteroid use may include cutaneous atrophy, telangiectases, and easy bruisability, as well as systemic absorption, which may include growth retardation, electrolyte abnormalities, hyperglycemia, hypertension, and increased susceptibility to infection. Vitiligo is caused by loss of melanin. Striae may occur after use of oral corticosteroids or occlusive topical corticosteroid therapy.

8-77   Answer C

In burn trauma, the hematocrit rises as fluid, not blood, shifts from the intravascular compartment. The hemoglobin level decreases secondary to hemolysis; the sodium level decreases secondary to massive fluid shifts into the interstitium; and the blood urea nitrogen level increases secondary to dehydration.

8-78   Answer C

Erysipelas is caused by *Streptococcus hemolyticus* and must be treated with appropriate antibiotics. A 7-day course of therapy is recommended: penicillin VK, dicloxacillin, or a first-generation cephalosporin. In penicillin-allergic clients, either erythromycin or clarithromycin for 7–14 days is a good choice.

8-79   Answer A

Candidiasis of the glans of the penis is balanitis. Thrush is oral candidiasis; candidal paronychia involves the tissue surrounding the nail; and subungual *Candida* is candidiasis under the nail.

8-80   Answer C

Mongolian spots (congenital dermal melanocytosis) are poorly defined, blue to blue-black flat lesions that usually occur on the trunk and buttocks but may occur anywhere. They are present at birth and are asymptomatic. No treatment is necessary because the spots fade with age.

8-81   Answer C

If a client presents with recurrent, sharply circumscribed red papules and plaques with a powdery white scale on the extensor aspect of his elbows and knees, suspect psoriasis. This is a classic presentation of psoriasis. Besides the extensor aspect of the elbows and knees, it occurs frequently in the presacral area and scalp, although lesions may occur anywhere. Actinic keratosis is distributed on sun-exposed areas such as the face, head, neck, and dorsum of the hand and appears as poorly circumscribed, pink to red, slightly scaly lesions. Eczema presents as a group of pinpoint pruritic vesicles and papules on a coin-shaped erythematous base that usually worsens in winter. Seborrheic dermatitis has a symmetric appearance of raised, scaly, red, greasy papules and plaques that may be sharply or poorly circumscribed.

8-82   Answer C

Psoriasis may occur after extended therapy with many medications, including beta blockers, lithium, NSAIDs, gold, antimalarials, and angiotensin-converting enzyme (ACE) inhibitors, and after heavy alcohol intake.

8-83   Answer D

Large, flaccid bullae with honey-colored crusts around the mouth and nose are characteristic of impetigo. These weeping erosions can appear anywhere but usually appear on the face and nose and around the mouth. Hemorrhagic blisters may be present with a burn. Rocky Mountain spotted fever presents with petechiae beginning at the wrist and ankles and going to the palms and soles, then centrally to the face. Measles begins with red macules on the back of the neck, then spreads over the face and upper trunk. The lesions then become papular and may be confluent over the face.

8-84   Answer B

Vitiligo, which usually appears in childhood, is an acquired disorder characterized by complete loss of pigment of the involved skin. Although tinea versicolor does have areas of hypopigmentation, they are scattered and do not have complete loss of pigment. In tuberous sclerosis, ash-leaf spots, which

are hypopigmented macules, about 2–3 cm in size, are present at birth. Pityriasis alba is also an acquired disorder of hypopigmentation characterized by poorly demarcated, slightly scaly, oval hypopigmented macules that vary from 1.5–2 cm in size.

8-85   Answer A

A basal cell carcinoma is an epithelial tumor that originates from either the basal layer of the epidermis or cells in the surrounding dermal structures. A squamous cell carcinoma is malignant and originates in the squamous epithelium. An overgrowth and thickening of the cornified epithelium is a keratosis. A cyst is a benign closed sac in or under the skin surface that is lined with epithelium and contains fluid or a semisolid material.

8-86   Answer C

Condyloma acuminata is a cauliflower-like wart usually found in anogenital regions and is usually sexually transmitted. Plantar warts appear at maximum points of pressure such as the heads of metatarsal bones or heels; filiform or digitate warts are fingerlike, flesh-colored projections emanating from a narrow or broad base, usually in the facial region; and verruca plana are flat warts that are pink, light brown, or yellow with slightly elevated papules that may undergo spontaneous remission.

8-87   Answer C

If a client comes into the clinic complaining of painful joints and has a distinctive rash in a butterfly distribution on the face that has red papules and plaques with a fine scale, suspect systemic lupus erythematosus. Acute lupus erythematosus occurs most often in young adult women and has a classic presentation of a rash in a butterfly distribution. The lesions are red papules and plaques with a fine scale. In the acute phase, the client is febrile and ill. The presence of these skin lesions in a client with neurological disease, arthritis, renal disease, or neuropsychiatric disturbances also supports the diagnosis. Lymphocytoma cutis is also most common on the face and neck. It occurs in both sexes and has smooth, red to yellow-brown papules up to 5 cm in diameter. Relapsing polychondritis occurs in adults with a history of arthritis. It appears as a macular erythema, tenderness, and swelling over the cartilaginous portions of the ear.

8-88   Answer C

Ultraviolet light is useful for severe, uncontrollable atopic dermatitis. Therapeutic modalities useful for the management of acute atopic dermatitis include emollients, compresses, and ultraviolet light. Although tars are useful for chronic, dry, lichenified lesions, they are not helpful for acute dermatitis. Emollients are best applied and most helpful if used immediately after bathing or showering. Compresses are indicated for acute weeping lesions to help cool and dry the skin, which reduces inflammation.

8-89   Answer C

Actinic keratoses, also called senile or solar keratoses, are epidermal skin lesions that are directly related to chronic sun exposure and photodamage. Skin tags occur in middle-aged adults of both genders and may be associated with acromegaly or acanthosis nigricans. Seborrheic keratoses are lesions most often seen in older adults and do not appear to be related to damage from sun exposure. Angiomas are common, small, red to purple papules unrelated to sun exposure.

8-90   Answer C

Warts are caused by the human papillomavirus. One in four people is infected with this virus and, despite treatment, most warts recur. Broken or abraded skin can spread the transport of the virus as well as vigorous rubbing, shaving, nail biting, and sexual intercourse. Warts do not have roots, contrary to popular opinion. The underside of a wart is smooth and round.

8-91   Answer D

A client with a platelet abnormality may present with red, flat, nonblanchable petechiae. Red to blue macular plaques describe ecchymoses; multiple frecklelike macular lesions in sun-exposed areas indicate xeroderma pigmentosum; and numerous small, brown, nonscaly macules that become more prominent with sun exposure are freckles.

8-92   Answer A

Dry, itchy skin in older adults results from the reduction of sweat and oil glands. Loss of subcutaneous tissue, dermal thinning, and decreased elasticity are normal changes associated with aging, and they may cause wrinkles and sagging of the skin.

8-93   Answer A

A safe and effective treatment for mild psoriasis is the use of coal tar preparations. The concentration is increased every few days from 0.5% to a maximum of 10%. A contact period of several hours is required, and the odor is unpleasant. Topical corticosteroids are widely used because they are relatively easy to apply. Topical steroids are appropriate in cases involving 10% or less of body surface. Topical antibiotics are indicated for acne rosacea; and systemic antihistamines are indicated for pityriasis rosea. Some of the chemicals in coal tar may cause cancer but only in very high concentrations as in coal tar used for industrial paving. Any client using coal tar regularly should be aware of the signs and symptoms and have a skin cancer checkup annually. Ongoing treatment for psoriasis may include topical creams and ointments, such as vitamin D compounds like calcipotriene, corticosteroids, retinoids such as tazarotene, and anthralin. These may be used in combination with sunlight (phototherapy). For severe psoriasis, systemic therapy may be required; this includes the use of such medications as retinoids, methotrexate, and cyclosporine, usually in addition to continued topical treatments and exposure to ultraviolet light.

8-94   Answer C

Silver sulfadiazine (Silvadene), the most commonly used topical agent for burn trauma, is a bactericidal agent that acts on the cell membrane and cell wall of susceptible bacteria and binds to cellular DNA. It is effective against a wide variety of both gram-negative and gram-positive organisms. Mafenide acetate (Sulfamylon) is a synthetic antibiotic that interferes with the metabolism of bacterial cells. Approximately 3%–5% of clients develop a hypersensitivity to mafenide. Silver nitrate is a bacteriostatic agent that alters the microbial cell wall and membrane. It has limited penetrating ability and is ineffective if used more than 72 hours after a burn injury.

8-95   Answer B

For the client with gout, the consumption of purine-rich foods, such as organ meats, should be limited to prevent uric acid buildup. Alcohol should also be limited and fluids increased to 2 L per day. Salicylates should be avoided because they block renal excretion of uric acid. An annual testing of the serum uric acid level is sufficient.

8-96   Answer A

Craniotabes is localized softening of the cranial bones that are so soft that they may be indented by the pressure of a finger. When the pressure is removed, the bone returns to its normal position. This condition corrects itself in a matter of months without treatment. Molding is when the vertex of the head is molded to fit the cervix contours during delivery. The head usually returns to its normal shape within a few days. Caput succedaneum is edema of the scalp that is usually absorbed and disappears by the third day of life without treatment. A cephalhematoma is a collection of blood on the skull bone caused by rupture of a periosteum capillary due to the pressure of birth and usually occurs 24 hours after birth and may take weeks to be absorbed.

8-97   Answer C

Lichenification is a thickening of the skin that usually results from chronic scratching or rubbing. Crusts represent dried serum, blood, pus, or exudate. Scales are yellow, white, or brownish flakes on the surface of the skin that represent desquamation of stratum corneum. Atrophy represents loss of substance of the skin.

8-98   Answer A

If a client is allergic to eggs and does not think that he or she should receive the flu vaccine, advise the client that, although measles, mumps, rubella, and influenza vaccines contain a minute amount of egg, most individuals who are allergic to eggs can tolerate these vaccines without any problems; that some of the allergic reactions are caused by the gelatins in the vaccinations and not the actual vaccinations; and that if the client can eat a whole egg with no reaction, he or she should have no problem with the vaccination. If the history of the allergy is questionable, it is safest to perform a skin test using the vaccine in dilute amounts and then administer the vaccine under strict observation, allowing a 2-hour wait to observe for any reaction.

8-99   Answer A

Skin phototyping (SPT) is a risk classification system designed to estimate one's risk for sun damage. SPT ranges from I to VI. A person with SPT I sunburns easily but never tans. Persons with black skin are termed SPT VI. Persons in the middle types tan easily with minimal sunburn.

8-100   Answer D

Clubbing is defined as a thickening and broadening of the ends of the fingers. Clubbing is a bulbous appearance and swelling of the terminal phalanges, increasing the normal 160° angle between the nailbed and the digit to 180°. In adults, it is usually caused by pulmonary disease and the resultant hypoxia.

8-101   Answer C

Primary skin lesions are original lesions arising from previously normal skin. Secondary lesions can originate from primary lesions. Seborrheic dermatitis is a scale and the only secondary lesion listed. The others—acne nodule, tumor (neoplasm), and a vesicle—are primary lesions.

8-102   Answer B

Skin tags (acrochordons) are benign overgrowths of skin, commonly seen after middle age and usually found on the neck, axilla, groin, upper trunk, and eyelid. A nevus is a mole, and a lipoma is a benign subcutaneous tumor that consists of adipose tissue. A wart is a circumscribed elevation due to hypertrophy of the papillae and epidermis.

8-103   Answer B

The drug of choice for tinea capitis is oral griseofulvin (Grisactin), taken for 6–8 weeks. It should be administered with fat-containing foods because fat is required for optimal absorption. Although topical antifungal agents are effective, they take an extremely long time to work. Topical corticosteroids and antibiotics are not effective for fungal lesions.

8-104   Answer B

Minoxidil (Rogaine) is a vasodilator and may stimulate vertex hair growth. Anticoagulants (e.g., warfarin), oral contraceptives, and salicylates (aspirin) may cause alopecia. Other drugs that may also cause alopecia include antithyroid drugs, allopurinol, propranolol, amphetamines, and levodopa.

8-105   Answer C

Stomas shrink within 6–8 weeks after surgery. At that time, it is safe to buy a permanent appliance. Before that, the stoma needs to be measured weekly to find a well-fitting appliance.

8-106 Answer B

Lance has hives. Although all the actions are appropriate, the first step is to determine the need for 0.5 mL 1:1,000 epinephrine subcutaneously (SQ). With Lance's neck involvement, it is most important to determine if respiratory distress is imminent, in which case the epinephrine must be administered.

8-107 Answer B

Tenting, which occurs when pinched skin over the clavicle remains pinched for a few moments before resuming its normal position, is common in thin older adults. Skin turgor is decreased with dehydration and increased with edema and scleroderma.

8-108 Answer A

A keloid is an elevated, irregularly shaped, and progressively enlarging scar that arises from excessive amounts of collagen during scar formation. A skin tag is a soft papule on a pedicle. An angioma is a benign vascular tumor. A keratosis is any skin condition in which there is a benign overgrowth and thickening of the cornified epithelium.

8-109 Answer B

Clients must be taught to decrease favorable environmental conditions for *Candida*, such as moisture, warmth, and poor air circulation. To prevent diaper rash, the infant should be kept dry as much as possible, and the use of rubber or plastic pants should be discouraged. Baby powder with cornstarch should not be used because it will worsen the infection (*Candida* can utilize the cornstarch as food). There is no need to isolate Susie.

8-110 Answer A

A darkfield examination is used to diagnose syphilis cutaneously. Viral blisters can be diagnosed cutaneously by the Tzanck smear; a scraping can be done to look for scabies; and a potassium hydroxide preparation and culture are used to diagnose candidiasis.

8-111 Answer D

Alopecia universalis is the loss of hair on all parts of the body. Female pattern alopecia is progressive thinning and loss of hair over the central part of the scalp. Alopecia areata appears as round or oval bald patches on the scalp and other hairy parts of the body. Alopecia totalis is the loss of all hair on the scalp.

8-112 Answer D

A vitamin C deficiency results in bleeding gums and delayed wound healing. A protein deficiency results in dry skin and loss of skin color. A vitamin A deficiency results in thickened skin that is dry or rough. A vitamin B_6 deficiency results in flaky skin, sores in the mouth, and cracks at the corners of the mouth.

8-113 Answer A

The epidermis stores melanin, which protects tissues from the harmful effects of ultraviolet radiation in sunlight. The epidermis also protects tissues from physical, chemical, and biological damage; prevents water loss; converts cholesterol molecules to vitamin D when exposed to sunlight; and contains phagocytes that prevent bacteria from penetrating the skin. The dermis is the second layer of the skin. Its fibrous connective tissue gives the skin its strength and elasticity. The sebaceous glands are sebum-producing glands that assist in retarding evaporation and water loss from the epidermal cells. The eccrine sweat glands open directly onto the skin's surface and are widely distributed throughout the body in the subcutaneous tissue.

8-114 Answer B

The five Ps—purple, polygonal, planar, pruritic papules—are present in lichen planus. Lichen planus occurs in clients of all ages but is more common in adults. It has a primary skin lesion with the five Ps that looks like a shiny, violaceous, flat-topped papule that is very pruritic. Ichthyosis vulgaris lesions are fine, small, flaky white scales with minimal underlying erythema that can be found anywhere but are more prominent on the extensor aspects of the extremities. Atopic dermatitis (eczema) presents differently at different ages and in persons of different races, but it usually starts as red, weepy, shiny patches. Seborrheic dermatitis presents as dry scales with underlying erythema.

8-115 Answer D

Permanent tissue damage can occur with a second episode of frostbite on the same skin surface. Susan's fiancé should be extremely careful and wear a warm knit mask covering the entire face with only small holes for his orifices if he insists on skiing. With continued exposure, vasoconstriction and increased viscosity of the blood can cause infarction and necrosis of the nose. Massaging a frostbitten nose may cause tissue damage.

8-116   Answer A

Sunscreen should be used with all acne medications. Oily makeup or oily hair conditioners or scalp products should be avoided. The face should be washed gently at least twice per day with an antibacterial soap.

8-117   Answer D

Cryosurgery is a noninvasive method of treating skin cancer other than melanoma in which liquid nitrogen is used to freeze and destroy the tumor tissue. Mohs' micrographic surgery involves shaving thin layers of the tumor tissue horizontally, then taking a frozen section to determine tumor margins. Curettage and electrodesiccation are used to treat basal cell cancers less than 2 cm in diameter and primary squamous cell cancers that are less than 1 cm in diameter. Radiation therapy is used for lesions that are inoperable because of their location.

Bibliography

Huang, WH, and Clark, AR: Actinic keratosis. *Advance for NPs & PAs* 1(4):31–35, 2010.

Lancaster, MH, and Haddow-Liebel, S: Malignant melanoma. *Advance for NPs & PAs* 3(1):39–42, 2012.

Monroe, N, and Gunder, L: Treating giant cell arteritis to avoid complications. *Clinical Advisor* 14(2):33–38, 2011.

Naldi, L: Traditional therapies in the management of moderate to severe chronic plaque psoriasis: An assessment of the benefits and risks. *British Journal of Dermatology* 152(4):597–615, 2005. http://www.medscape.com/viewarticle/503441, accessed June 5, 2007.

Nouri, K, and Rivas, P: A primer of Mohs micrographic surgery: Common indications. *Skinmed* 3(4):191–196, 2004.

Scheinfeld, NS: Skin disorders in older adults: Age-related changes in quality and texture. *Consultant* 51(7): 457–460, 2011.

Scheinfeld, NS: Skin disorders in older adults: Benign growths and neoplasms. *Consultant* 51(9):650–656, 2011.

Winland-Brown, JW, Porter, BO, and Allen, S: Skin problems. Chap. 7 in Dunphy, L, et al, *Primary Care: The Art and Science of Advanced Practice Nursing.* FA Davis, ed 3, Philadelphia, 2011.

How well did you do?

85% and above, congratulations! This score shows application of test-taking principles and adequate content knowledge.

75%–85%, keep working! Review test-taking principles and try again.

65%–75%, hang in there! Spend some time reviewing concepts and test-taking principles and then try the test again.

Chapter 9: *Head and Neck Problems*

Diane Gerzevitz
Lynne M. Dunphy
Karen Rugg

Questions

9-1 *Acute otitis media is diagnosed when there is*

A. fluid in the middle ear without signs or symptoms of an ear infection.

B. a diagnosis of three or more episodes of otitis media within 1 year.

C. fluid in the middle ear accompanied by otalgia and fever.

D. fluid within the middle ear for at least 3 months.

9-2 *A child's central visual acuity is 20/30 by age*

A. 18 months.

B. 2 years.

C. 3 years.

D. 4 years.

9-3 *Nathan, age 19, is a college swimmer. He frequently gets swimmer's ear and asks if there is anything he can do to help prevent it other than wearing earplugs, which don't really work for him. What do you suggest?*

A. Use a cotton-tipped applicator to dry the ears after swimming.

B. Use eardrops made of a solution of equal parts of alcohol and vinegar in each ear after swimming.

C. Use a hair dryer on the highest setting to dry the ears.

D. Tell Nathan he must change his sport.

9-4 *Jill presents with symptoms of hay fever, and you assess the nasal mucosa of her turbinates to be pale. What diagnosis do you suspect?*

A. Allergic rhinitis

B. Viral rhinitis

C. Nasal polyps

D. Nasal vestibulitis from folliculitis

9-5 *Greg, age 72, is brought to the office by his son, who states that his father has been unable to see clearly since last night. Greg reports that his vision is "like looking through a veil." He also sees floaters and flashing lights but is not having any pain. What do you suspect?*

A. Cataracts

B. Glaucoma

C. Retinal detachment

D. Iritis

9-6 *Leah, 4 months old, has both eyes turning inward. What is this called?*

A. Pseudostrabismus

B. Strabismus

C. Esotropia

D. Exotropia

9-7 *A common cause of conductive hearing loss in adults ages 20–40 is*

A. trauma.

B. otitis media.

C. presbycusis.

D. otosclerosis.

9-8 *A client complains of frequent bouts of severe, intense, disabling left-sided facial pain accompanied by excessive left eye lacrimation (tearing) and worsening anxiety. The pain wakes him at night, and he has even contemplated harming himself during these episodes due to the intensity and unrelenting nature of the pain. What kind of headache is he describing?*

A. Classic migraine

B. Tension headache

C. Sinus headache

D. Cluster headache

9-9   Joy, age 36, has a sudden onset of shivering, sweating, headache, aching in the orbits, and general malaise and misery. Her temperature is 102°F. You diagnose influenza (flu). What is your next course of action?

A.   Order amoxicillin (Amoxil) 500 mg every 12 hours for 7 days.

B.   Prescribe rest, fluids, acetaminophen (Tylenol), and possibly a decongestant and an antitussive.

C.   Order a complete blood count.

D.   Consult with your collaborating physician.

9-10   Mattie, age 64, presents with blurred vision in one eye and states that it felt like "a curtain came down over my eye." She doesn't have any pain or redness. What do you suspect?

A.   Retinal detachment

B.   Acute angle-closure glaucoma

C.   Open-angle glaucoma

D.   Cataract

9-11   A 64-year-old woman presents to your clinic with a sudden right-sided headache that is worse in her right eye. She claims her vision seems blurred, and her right pupil is dilated and slow to react. The right conjunctiva is markedly injected, and the eyeball is firm. You screen her vision and find that she is 20/30 OS and 20/30 OD. She most likely has

A.   open-angle glaucoma.

B.   angle-closure glaucoma.

C.   herpetic conjunctivitis.

D.   diabetic retinopathy.

9-12   Your well-nourished 74-year-old patient has come into the office for a physical and states that she recently had two nosebleeds. She does not take any anticoagulants, and you have ruled out any coagulopathies. The most likely cause of these nosebleeds is

A.   sex hormones.

B.   a trauma or inflammation.

C.   a dietary change.

D.   scurvy.

9-13   June, age 50, presents with soft, raised, yellow plaques on her eyelids at the inner canthi. She is concerned that they may be cancerous skin lesions. You tell her that they are probably

A.   xanthelasmas.

B.   pingueculae.

C.   the result of arcus senilis.

D.   actinic keratoses.

9-14   Jessica, an 8-year-old third-grader, is brought to the office by her grandmother, who is the child's babysitter. She has complained of fever and sore throat for the past 2 days. Five other children in her class have been sick with sore throats. She denies difficulty swallowing and has been drinking fluids, but she has no appetite. A review of system (ROS) reveals that she has clear nasal drainage, hoarseness, and a nonproductive cough. She denies vomiting but has had mild diarrhea. On examination she has a temperature of 101.5°F; 3+ erythematous tonsils; and palpable, tender cervical lymph nodes. Based on these findings, what is the most likely diagnosis?

A.   Mono

B.   Sinusitis

C.   Strep pharyngitis

D.   Viral pharyngitis

9-15   Jill states that her 5-year-old daughter continually grinds her teeth at night. You document this as

A.   temporal mandibular joint malocclusion.

B.   bruxism.

C.   a psychosis.

D.   an oropharyngeal lesion.

9-16   Cydney, age 7, is complaining that she feels as though something is stuck in her ear. What action is contraindicated?

A.   Inspecting the ear canal with an otoscope

B.   Using a small suction device to try to remove the object

C.   Flushing the ear with water

D.   Instilling several drops of mineral oil in the ear

9-17   When a practitioner places a vibrating tuning fork in the midline of a client's skull and asks if the tone sounds the same in both ears or is better in one, the examiner is performing

A. the Rinne test.

B. the Weber test.

C. the caloric test.

D. a hearing acuity test.

9-18   You observe a mother showing her infant a toy. You note that the infant can fixate on, briefly follow, and then reach for the toy. You suspect that the infant is

A. 2 months old.

B. 4 months old.

C. 6 months old.

D. 8 months old.

9-19   The most common cause of loss of vision in the adult over 45 is

A. photopsia.

B. presbyopia.

C. age related macular degeneration.

D. myopia.

9-20   Clonazepam (Klonopin) is occasionally ordered for temporal mandibular joint (TMJ) disease. Which of the following statements applies to this medicine?

A. It is ordered for inflammatory pain.

B. It is ordered for neuropathic pain.

C. It is ordered for a short course of therapy for 1–2 weeks only.

D. It is ordered for muscle relaxation.

9-21   Maury, age 52, has throbbing pain in the left eye, an irregular pupil shape, marked photophobia, and redness around the iris. What is your initial diagnosis?

A. Conjunctivitis

B. Iritis

C. Subconjunctival hemorrhage

D. Acute glaucoma

9-22   Harry, age 69, has had Ménière's disease for several years. He has some hearing loss but now has persistent vertigo. What treatment might be instituted to relieve the vertigo?

A. A labyrinthectomy

B. Pharmacological therapy

C. A vestibular neurectomy

D. Wearing an earplug in the ear with the most hearing loss

9-23   Shelley, age 47, is complaining of a red eye. You are trying to decide between a diagnosis of conjunctivitis and iritis. One distinguishing characteristic between the two is

A. eye discomfort.

B. slow progression.

C. a ciliary flush.

D. no change in or slightly blurred vision.

9-24   Mark, age 18, has a persistent sore throat, fever, and malaise not relieved with penicillin therapy. What would you order next?

A. A throat culture

B. A monospot test

C. A rapid antigen test

D. A Thayer-Martin plate test

9-25   Your client is unable to differentiate between sharp and dull stimulation on both sides of her face. You suspect

A. Bell's palsy.

B. a lesion affecting the trigeminal nerve.

C. a stroke.

D. shingles.

9-26   Sara, age 29, states that she has painless, white, slightly raised patches in her mouth. They are probably caused by

A. herpes simplex.

B. aphthous ulcers.

C. candidiasis.

D. oral cancer.

9-27   *What therapy has proved beneficial for long-term symptom relief of tinnitus?*

A. Aspirin

B. Lidocaine

C. Cognitive behavioral therapy

D. Corticosporin otic drops per minute (gtts) prn

9-28   *Your client, a 75-year-old smoker of 50 years, is at the office today for a routine physical. During your inspection of the oral mucosa, you discover a lesion that you suspect to be cancerous. You document your finding as*

A. a vesicular-like lesion.

B. an ulcerated lesion with indurated margins.

C. a denuded patch with a removable white coating.

D. a red raised lesion.

9-29   *The most common cause of a white pupil (leukokoria or leukocoria) in a newborn is*

A. a cataract.

B. retinoblastoma.

C. persistent hyperplastic primary vitreous.

D. retinal detachment.

9-30   *The trachea deviates toward the unaffected side in all of the following conditions except*

A. aortic aneurysm.

B. unilateral thyroid lobe enlargement.

C. large atelectasis.

D. pneumothorax.

9-31   *How would you grade tonsils that touch the uvula?*

A. Grade 1

B. Grade 2

C. Grade 3

D. Grade 4

9-32   *An 80-year-old woman comes in today with complaints of a rash on the left side of her face that is blistered and painful and accompanied by left-sided eye pain. The rash broke out 2 days ago, and she remembers being very tired and feeling feverish for a week before the rash appeared. On examination the rash follows the trigeminal nerve on the left, and she has some scleral injection and tearing. You suspect herpes zoster ophthalmicus. Based on what you know to be complications of this disease, you explain to her that she needs*

A. antibiotics.

B. a biopsy of the rash.

C. immediate hospitalization.

D. ophthalmological consultation.

9-33   *Which cranial nerve (CN) is affected in sensorineural or perceptive hearing loss?*

A. CN II

B. CN IV

C. CN VIII

D. CN XI

9-34   *The most common cause of sensorineural hearing loss is*

A. trauma.

B. tympanic membrane sclerosis and scarring.

C. otosclerosis.

D. presbycusis.

9-35   *Jim, age 49, comes to the office with a rapid-onset complete paralysis of one-half of his face. He is unable to raise his eyebrow, close his eye, whistle, or show his teeth. You suspect a lower motor neuron lesion resulting in cranial nerve VII paralysis. What is your working diagnosis?*

A. Cerebrovascular accident

B. Trigeminal neuralgia

C. Bell's palsy

D. Tic douloureux

9-36   *When Judith, age 15, asks you to explain the 20/50 vision in her right eye, you respond,*

A. "You can see at 20 ft with your left eye what most people can see at 50 ft."

B. "You can see at 20 ft with your right eye what most people can see at 50 ft."

C. "You can see at 50 ft with your right eye what most people can see at 20 ft."

D. "You can see at 50 ft with the left eye what most people can see at 20 ft."

9-37   A client comes in complaining of 1 week of pain in the posterior neck with difficulty turning the head to the right. What additional history is needed?

A. Recent trauma

B. Difficulty swallowing

C. Stiffness in the right shoulder

D. Change in sleeping habits

9-38   What condition occurs in almost all persons beginning around age 42–46?

A. Arcus senilis

B. Presbyopia

C. Cataracts

D. Glaucoma

9-39   John, age 19, has just been given a diagnosis of mononucleosis. Which of the following statements is true?

A. The offending organism is bacteria and should be treated with antibiotics.

B. Convalescence is usually only a few days, and John should be back to normal in a week.

C. Mono is rarely contagious.

D. John should avoid contact sports and heavy lifting.

9-40   Sam, age 4, is brought into the clinic by his father. His tympanic membrane is perforated from otitis media. His father asks about repair of the eardrum. How do you respond?

A. "The eardrum, in most cases, heals within several weeks."

B. "We need to schedule Sam for a surgical repair."

C. "He must absolutely stay out of the water for 3–6 months."

D. "If the eardrum is not healed in several months, it can be surgically repaired."

9-41   Which manifestation is noted with carbon monoxide poisoning?

A. Circumoral pallor of the lips

B. Cherry-red lips

C. Cyanosis of the lips

D. Pale pink lips

9-42   A child's head circumference is routinely measured at each well-child visit until age

A. 12 months.

B. 18 months.

C. 2 years.

D. 5 years.

9-43   Mary, age 82, presents with several eye problems. She states that her eyes are always dry and look "sunken in." What do you suspect?

A. Hypothyroidism

B. Normal age-related changes

C. Cushing's syndrome

D. A detached retina

9-44   While doing a face, head, and neck examination, you note that the palpebral fissures are abnormally narrow. What are you examining?

A. Nasolabial folds

B. The openings between the margins of the upper and lower eyelids

C. The thyroid gland in relation to the trachea

D. The distance between the trigeminal nerve branches

9-45   The most common offending allergens causing allergic rhinitis are

A. pollens of grasses, trees, and weeds.

B. fungi.

C. animal allergens.

D. food sensitivity.

9-46   A 22-year-old client who plays in a rock band complains that he finds it difficult to understand his fellow musicians at the end of a night of performing, a problem that is compounded by the noisy environment of the club. These symptoms are most characteristic of which of the following?

A. Sensorineural loss

B. Conductive loss

C. Tinnitus

D. Vertigo

9-47 Which assessment test is a gross measurement of peripheral vision?

A. The cover test
B. The corneal light reflex test
C. The confrontation test
D. The Snellen eye-chart test

9-48 Microtia refers to the size of the

A. ears.
B. skull.
C. pupils.
D. eyes.

9-49 The leading cause of blindness in persons ages 20–60 in the United States is

A. macular degeneration.
B. glaucoma.
C. diabetic retinopathy.
D. trauma.

9-50 You have determined that your patient, who presented to your office with jaw aching and a popping sound when opening the jaw wide, has TMD (temporomandibular disorder). Your best approach to management would be

A. initiating a diet of liquids only.
B. advising the patient to chew gum to exercise the jaw.
C. advising the patient to eat softer foods and avoid opening the mouth wide.
D. advising the patient to sleep on a firm pillow to support the jaw.

9-51 When you are assessing the internal structure of the eye, absence of a red reflex may indicate

A. a cataract or a hemorrhage into the vitreous humor.
B. acute iritis.
C. nothing; this is a normal finding in older adults.
D. diabetes or long-standing hypertension.

9-52 Marian, age 79, is at a higher risk than a middle-aged client for developing an eye infection because of which age-related change?

A. Increased eyestrain
B. Loss of subcutaneous tissue

C. Change in pupil size
D. A decrease in tear production

9-53 Mattie says she has heard that it is not good to let a baby go to bed with a bottle. She says that she has always done this with her other children and wonders why it is not recommended. How do you respond?

A. "A bottle in the baby's mouth forces the baby to breathe through the nose. If the nose is clogged, the baby will not get enough oxygen."
B. "A nipple, when placed in the mouth for long periods of time, can cause tooth displacement. This will also affect the adult teeth not grown in yet and will necessitate braces in the teen years."
C. "Normal mouth bacteria act on the sugar in the bottle contents to form acids, which will break down the tooth enamel and destroy the teeth even before they come in."
D. "This encourages the baby to continually want to drink at night. When the child is older, it will become a habit, and the child will end up wearing diapers into the preschool years."

9-54 Martin, age 24, presents with an erythematous ear canal, pain, and a recent history of swimming. What do you suspect?

A. Acute otitis media
B. Chronic otitis media
C. External otitis
D. Temporomandibular joint syndrome

9-55 A 65-year-old man presents complaining of left-sided, deep, throbbing headache along with mild fatigue. On examination the client has a tender, tortuous temporal artery. You suspect temporal arteritis. How do you confirm your diagnosis?

A. MRI of the head
B. Erythrocyte sedimentation rate (ESR)
C. EEG
D. Otoscopy

9-56 Your neighbor calls you because her son, age 9, fell on the sidewalk while playing outside and a tooth fell out. She wants to know what she should put the tooth in to transport it to the dentist. You tell her that the best solution to put it in is

A. salt water.
B. saliva.

C. milk.

D. water.

9-57 Which of the following symptom(s) is (are) most indicative of mononucleosis (Epstein-Barr virus)?

A. Rapid onset of anterior cervical adenopathy, fatigue, malaise, and headache

B. Gradual onset of fatigue, posterior cervical adenopathy, fever, and sore throat

C. Gradual and seasonal onset of pharyngeal erythema

D. Rapid onset of cough, congestion, and headache

9-58 Regular ocular pressure testing is indicated for older adults taking

A. high-dose inhaled glucocorticoids.

B. NSAIDs.

C. angiotensin-converting enzyme (ACE) inhibitors.

D. insulin.

9-59 Marnie, who has asthma, has been told that she has nasal polyps. What do you tell her about them?

A. Nasal polyps are usually precancerous.

B. Nasal polyps are benign growths.

C. The majority of nasal polyps are neoplastic.

D. They are probably inflamed turbinates, not polyps, because polyps are infrequent in clients with asthma.

9-60 Purulent matter in the anterior chamber of the eye is called

A. hyphema.

B. hypopyon.

C. anisocoria.

D. pterygium.

9-61 In older adults, the most common cause of decreased visual functioning is

A. cataract formation.

B. glaucoma.

C. macular degeneration.

D. arcus senilis.

9-62 Sylvia has glaucoma and has started taking a medication that acts as a diuretic to reduce the intraocular pressure. Which medication is she taking?

A. A carbonic anhydrase inhibitor

B. A beta-adrenergic receptor blocker

C. A miotic

D. A mydriatic

9-63 You diagnose acute epiglottitis in Sally, age 5, and immediately send her to the local emergency room. Which of the following symptoms would indicate that an airway obstruction is imminent?

A. Reddened face

B. Screaming

C. Grabbing her throat

D. Stridor

9-64 Mavis is 70 years old and wonders if she can donate her corneas when she dies. How do you respond?

A. "As long as you don't have any chronic illness, your corneas may be harvested."

B. "They will use corneas only from persons younger than age 65."

C. "What makes you feel like you are dying?"

D. "Don't think about such terrible things now."

9-65 The immediate goal of myringotomy and tube placement in a child with recurrent episodes of otitis media is to

A. prevent future infections.

B. have an open access to the middle ear for irrigation and instillation of antibiotics.

C. allow removal of suppurative or mucoid material.

D. relieve pain.

9-66 Manny, age 16, was hit in the eye with a baseball. He developed pain in the eye, decreased visual acuity, and injection of the globe. You confirm the diagnosis of hyphema by finding blood in the anterior chamber. What treatment would you recommend while Manny is waiting to see the ophthalmologist?

A. Apply bilateral eye patches.

B. Have Manny lie flat.

C. Refer him to an ophthalmologist within a week.

D. Make sure Manny is able to be awakened every 30 minutes.

9-67   How do you test for near vision?

A. By using the Snellen eye chart

B. By using the Rosenbaum chart

C. By asking the client to read from a magazine or newspaper

D. By testing the cardinal fields

9-68   You have made a diagnosis of acute sinusitis based on Martha's history and the fact that she complains of pain behind her eye. Which sinuses are affected?

A. Maxillary

B. Ethmoid

C. Frontal

D. Sphenoid

9-69   How do you respond when Diane, age 29, asks why she gets sores on her lips every time she sits out in the sun for an extended period of time?

A. "You are allergic to the sun and must wear sunblock on your lips."

B. "Your lips are dry to begin with, and you must keep them moist at all times."

C. "You have herpes simplex that recurs with sunlight exposure."

D. "You're probably allergic to your lip balm."

9-70   Which of the following signs of thyroid dysfunction is a sign of hyperthyroidism?

A. Slow pulse

B. Decreased systolic BP

C. Exophthalmos

D. Dry, coarse, cool skin

9-71   What significant finding(s) in a child with otitis media with effusion would prompt more aggressive treatment?

A. There is a change in the child's hearing threshold to less than or equal to 20 decibels (dB).

B. The child becomes a fussy eater.

C. The child's speech and language skills seem slightly delayed.

D. Persistent rhinitis is present.

9-72   Tara was born with a cleft lip and palate. When should treatment begin for this condition?

A. Immediately after birth

B. At age 3 months

C. At age 6 months

D. When Tara is ready to drink from a cup

9-73   Clients with allergic conjunctivitis have which type of discharge?

A. Purulent

B. Serous or clear

C. Stringy and white

D. Profuse mucoid or mucopurulent

9-74   Ty, age 68, has a hearing problem. He tells you he is ready for a drastic solution to the problem because he likes to play bingo but cannot hear the calls. What can you do for him?

A. Refer him to a hearing aid specialist.

B. Refer him for further testing.

C. Perform a gross hearing test in the office, then repeat it in 6 months to determine if there is any further loss.

D. Nothing. Tell him that a gradual hearing loss is to be expected with aging.

9-75   David, age 32, states that he thinks he has an ear infection because he just flew back from a business trip and feels unusual pressure in his ear. You diagnose barotrauma. What is your next action?

A. Prescribe nasal steroids and oral decongestants.

B. Prescribe antibiotic eardrops.

C. Prescribe systemic antibiotics.

D. Refer David to an ear, nose, and throat specialist.

9-76   Sharon, age 29, is pregnant for the first time. She complains of nasal stuffiness and occasional epistaxis. What do you do?

A. Order lab tests, such as a complete blood count with differential, hemoglobin, and hematocrit.

B. Prescribe an antihistamine.

C. You do nothing except for client teaching.

D. Refer the client to an ear, nose, and throat specialist.

9-77   *The antibiotic of choice for beta-lactamase coverage of otitis media is*

A. amoxicillin (Amoxil).

B. amoxicillin and potassium clavulanate (Augmentin).

C. azithromycin (Zithromax).

D. prednisone (Deltasone).

9-78   *Tee, age 64, presents with a sore throat. Your assessment reveals tonsillar exudate, anterior cervical adenopathy, presence of a fever, and absence of a cough. There is a high probability of which causative agent?*

A. *Haemophilus influenzae*

B. Group A beta-hemolytic streptococcus

C. Epstein-Barr virus

D. Rhinovirus

9-79   *Which is the most common localized infection of one of the glands of the eyelids?*

A. Hordeolum

B. Chalazion

C. Bacterial conjunctivitis

D. Herpes simplex

9-80   *Matthew, age 52, has allergic rhinitis and would like some medicine to relieve his symptoms. He is taking cimetidine (Tagamet) for gastroesophageal reflux disease. Which medication would you not order?*

A. A first-generation antihistamine

B. A second-generation antihistamine

C. A decongestant

D. A topical nasal corticosteroid

9-81   *In a young child, unilateral purulent rhinitis is most often caused by*

A. a foreign body.

B. a viral infection.

C. a bacterial infection.

D. an allergic reaction.

9-82   *Darren, age 26, has AIDS and presents with a painful tongue covered with what looks like creamy-white, curdlike patches overlying erythematous mucosa. You are able to scrape off these "curds" with a tongue depressor, which assists you in making which of the following diagnoses?*

A. Leukoplakia

B. Lichen planus

C. Oral candidiasis

D. Oral cancer

9-83   *If a client presents with a deep aching, red eye and there is no discharge, you should suspect*

A. bacterial conjunctivitis.

B. viral conjunctivitis.

C. allergic conjunctivitis.

D. iritis.

9-84   *Which of the following conditions produces sharp, piercing facial pain that lasts for seconds to minutes?*

A. Trigeminal neuralgia

B. TMJ

C. Goiter

D. Preauricular adenitis

9-85   *The most frequent cause of laryngeal obstruction in an adult is*

A. a piece of meat.

B. a tumor.

C. mucosal swelling from an allergic reaction.

D. inhalation of a carcinogen.

9-86   *Claude, age 78, is being treated with timolol maleate (Timoptic) drops for his chronic open-angle glaucoma. While performing a new client history and physical, you note that he is taking other medications. Which medication would you be most concerned about?*

A. Aspirin therapy as prophylaxis for heart attack

B. Ranitidine (Zantac) for gastroesophageal reflux disease

C. Alprazolam (Xanax), an anxiolytic for anxiety

D. Atenolol (Tenormin), a beta blocker for high blood pressure

9-87 *Signs and symptoms of acute angle-closure glaucoma include*

A. painless redness of the eyes.

B. loss of peripheral vision.

C. translucent corneas.

D. halos around lights.

9-88 *How should Tommy, age 2.5, have his vision screened?*

A. Using a Snellen letter chart

B. Using the Allen test

C. Using a Snellen E chart

D. Using a Rosenbaum chart

9-89 *Cataracts are a common occurrence in the patient over 60 years of age. You counsel your patient that the best cure for cataracts is*

A. medications.

B. dietary supplements.

C. corrective lens surgery.

D. optical devices.

9-90 *The normal ratio of the artery-to-vein width in the retina as viewed through the ophthalmoscope is*

A. 2:3.

B. 3:2.

C. 1:3.

D. 3:1.

9-91 *Mavis has persistent pruritus of the external auditory canal. External otitis and dermatological conditions such as seborrheic dermatitis and psoriasis have been ruled out. What can you advise her to do?*

A. Use a cotton-tipped applicator daily to remove all moisture and potential bacteria.

B. Wash daily with soap and water.

C. Apply mineral oil to counteract dryness.

D. Avoid topical corticosteroids.

9-92 *When the Weber test is performed with a tuning fork to assess hearing and there is no lateralization, this indicates*

A. conductive deafness.

B. perceptive deafness.

C. a normal finding.

D. nerve damage.

9-93 *Which of the following refractive errors in vision is a result of the natural loss of accommodative capacity with age?*

A. Presbyopia

B. Hyperopia

C. Myopia

D. Astigmatism

9-94 *Henry is having difficulty getting rid of a corneal infection. He asks you why. How do you respond?*

A. "We can't determine the causative agent."

B. "Antibiotics have difficulty getting to that area."

C. "Because the infection was painless, it was not treated early enough."

D. "Because the cornea doesn't have a blood supply, an infection can't be fought off as usual."

9-95 *Mandy was given a diagnosis of flu 2 days ago and wants to start on the "new flu medicine" right away. What do you tell her?*

A. "The medication is effective only if started within the first 48 hours after symptoms begin."

B. "If you treat a cold, it goes away in 7 days; if you don't treat it, it goes away in 1 week."

C. "The medicine has not proven its effectiveness."

D. "I'll start you on zanamivir today. It may shorten the course of the disease and perhaps lessen the severity of your symptoms."

9-96 *Samantha, age 12, appears with ear pain. When you begin to assess her ear, you tug on her normal-appearing auricle, eliciting severe pain. This leads you to suspect*

A. otitis media.

B. otitis media with effusion.

C. otitis externa.

D. primary otalgia.

9-97 *Which method can be safely used to remove cerumen in a 12-month-old child's ear?*

A. A size 2 ear curette

B. Irrigation using hot water from a 3-cc syringe

C. A commercial jet tooth cleanser

D. Cerumen should not be removed from a child this young.

9-98 *When assessing Lenore, age 59, who has a sore throat, you note that she has a positive history of diabetes and rheumatic fever. These facts increase the likelihood that which of the following agents caused her sore throat?*

A. Neisseria gonorrhoeae

B. Epstein-Barr virus

C. Haemophilus influenzae

D. Group A beta-hemolytic streptococcus

9-99 *Marvin has sudden eye redness that occurred after a strenuous coughing episode. You diagnose a subconjunctival hemorrhage. Your next step is to*

A. refer him to an ophthalmologist.

B. order antibiotics.

C. do nothing other than provide reassurance.

D. consult with your collaborating physician.

9-100 *Barbara, age 72, states that she was told she had atrophic macular degeneration and asks you if there is any treatment. How do you respond?*

A. "No, but 5 years from the time of the first symptoms, the process usually stops."

B. "Yes, there is a surgical procedure that will cure this."

C. "If we start medications now, they may prevent any further damage."

D. "Unfortunately, there is no effective treatment, but I can refer you to a rehabilitation agency that can help you adjust to the visual loss."

9-101 *The first-line antibiotic therapy for an adult with no known allergies and suspected group A beta-hemolytic streptococcal pharyngitis is*

A. penicillin.

B. erythromycin (E-Mycin).

C. azithromycin (Zithromax).

D. cephalexin (Keflex).

9-102 *Which manifestation of the buccal mucosa is present in a client with mumps?*

A. Pink, smooth, moist appearance with some patchy hyperpigmentation

B. Dappled brown patches

C. The orifice of Stensen's duct appearing red

D. Koplik's spots

9-103 *Sally, age 19, presents with pain and pressure over her cheeks and discolored nasal discharge. You cannot transilluminate the sinuses. You suspect which common sinus to be affected?*

A. Maxillary sinus

B. Ethmoid sinus

C. Temporal sinus

D. Frontal sinus

9-104 *You are performing a physical on your adult patient and she complains that her nose hurts. Upon inspection, you note a small boil in her left nostril that appears swollen and is painful to the touch. You document your finding as a probable*

A. allergic rhinitis.

B. furuncle.

C. nasal polyp.

D. carcinoma.

9-105 *Natasha, age 4, has amblyopia. How do you respond when her mother asks about treatment?*

A. "We'll wait until she's 7 years old before starting treatment."

B. "Treatment needs to be started now. We'll cover her 'bad' eye."

C. "Treatment needs to be started now. We'll cover her 'good' eye."

D. "No treatment is necessary. She'll outgrow this."

9-106 *When you are assessing the corneal light reflex, an abnormal finding indicates*

A. possible use of eye medications.

B. a neurological problem.

C. improper alignment of the eyes.

D. strabismus.

9-107 Marcia, age 4, is brought into the office by her mother. She has a sore throat, difficulty swallowing, copious oral secretions, respiratory difficulty, stridor, and a temperature of 102°F but no pharyngeal erythema or cough. What do you suspect?

A. Epiglottitis

B. Group A beta-hemolytic streptococcal infection pharyngitis

C. Tonsillitis

D. Diphtheria

9-108 With a chronic allergy, a client's nasal mucosa appear

A. swollen and red.

B. swollen, boggy, pale, and gray.

C. hard, pale, and inflamed.

D. bright pink and inflamed.

9-109 A sexual history of oral-genital contact in a client presenting with pharyngitis is significant when which of the following organisms is suspected?

A. Escherichia coli

B. Haemophilus influenzae

C. Neisseria gonorrhoeae

D. Streptococcus pneumoniae

9-110 You note a completely split uvula in Noi, a 42-year-old Asian. What is your next course of action?

A. Do nothing.

B. Refer Noi to a specialist.

C. Perform a throat culture.

D. Order a complete blood count.

9-111 A smooth tongue may indicate

A. a normal finding.

B. alcohol abuse.

C. a vitamin deficiency.

D. nicotine addiction.

9-112 Monique brings her 4-week-old infant into the office because she noticed small, yellow-white, glistening bumps on her infant's gums. She says they look like teeth, but she is worried that they may be cancer. You diagnose these bumps as

A. Bednar's aphthae.

B. Epstein's pearls.

C. buccal tumors.

D. exostosis.

9-113 Sara, age 92, presents with dry eyes, redness, and a scratchy feeling. You note that this is one of the most common disorders, particularly in older women, and diagnose this as

A. viral conjunctivitis.

B. keratoconjunctivitis sicca.

C. allergic eye disease.

D. corneal ulcer.

9-114 Nystatin (Mycostatin) is ordered for Michael, who has an oral fungal infection. What instructions do you give Michael for taking the medication?

A. "Don't swallow the medication because it's irritating to the gastric mucosa."

B. "Take the medication with meals so that it's absorbed better."

C. "Swish and swallow the medication."

D. "Apply the medication only to the lesions."

9-115 A 42-year-old stockbroker comes to your office for evaluation of a pulsating headache over the left temporal region, and he rates the pain as an 8 on a scale of 1–10. The pain has been constant for the past several hours and is accompanied by nausea and sensitivity to light. He has had frequent headaches for many years but not as severe, and they are usually relieved by over-the-counter medicines. He is unclear as to a precipitating event but notes that he has had visual disturbances before each headache and he has been under a lot of stress in his job. Based on this description, what is the most likely diagnosis of this type of headache?

A. Tension

B. Migraine

C. Cluster

D. Temporal arteritis

9-116 How would you describe the cervical lymphadenopathy associated with asymptomatic HIV infection?

A. Movable, discrete, soft, and nontender lymph nodes

B. Enlarged, warm, tender, firm, but freely movable lymph nodes

C. Hard, unilateral, nontender, and fixed lymph nodes

D. Firm but not hard, nontender, and mobile lymph nodes

9-117 *Which of the following is not a normal sensory deficit associated with aging?*

A. Gradual decline in sense of taste

B. Hearing loss of high-frequency tones

C. Decline in sense of proprioception

D. Loss of all peripheral vision

9-118 *A 62-year-old obese woman comes in today complaining of difficulty swallowing for the past 3 weeks. She states that "some foods get stuck" and she has been having "heartburn" at night when she lies down, especially if she has had a heavy meal. Occasionally she awakes at night coughing. She denies weight gain and/ or weight loss, vomiting, or change in bowel movements. She does not drink or smoke. There is no pertinent family history or findings on review of systems (ROS). Physical examination is normal with no abdominal tenderness, and the stool is OB negative. What is the most likely diagnosis?*

A. Esophageal varices

B. Esophageal cancer

C. Gastroesophageal reflux disease (GERD)

D. Peptic ulcer disease (PUD)

9-119 *Maggie, a 56-year-old woman, comes to the office requesting a test for thyroid disease. She has had some weight gain since menopause and she read on the Internet that all women should have a thyroid test. Based on the recommendations from the U.S. Preventive Services Task Force, which one of the following statements should be considered in this woman's care?*

A. All adults should be screened for thyroid disease.

B. Evidence is insufficient for or against routine screening for thyroid disease in asymptomatic adults.

C. All adults older than 50 should be screened for thyroid disease.

D. All perimenopausal women should be screened for thyroid disease.

9-120 *When you examine the tympanic membrane, which of these structures is visible?*

A. Stapes

B. Cochlea

C. Pars flaccida

D. Round window

9-121 *Judy, age 67, complains of a sudden onset of impaired vision, severe eye pain, vomiting, and a headache. You diagnose the following condition and refer for urgent treatment.*

A. Cataracts

B. Macular degeneration

C. Presbyopia

D. Acute glaucoma

9-122 *What is the easiest way to differentiate between otitis externa and otitis media?*

A. With otitis media, tender swelling is usually visible.

B. With otitis media, there is usually bilateral pain in the ears.

C. With otitis media, there is usually tenderness on palpation over the mastoid process.

D. With otitis externa, movement or pressure on the pinna is extremely painful.

9-123 *Risk factors for oral cancers include*

A. a family history, poor dental habits, and use of alcohol.

B. obesity, sedentary lifestyle, and chewing tobacco.

C. a history of diabetes, smoking, and a high fat intake.

D. smoking, use of alcohol, and chewing tobacco.

9-124 *Marty has a hordeolum in his right eye. You suspect that the offending organism is*

A. herpes simplex virus.

B. *Staphylococcus.*

C. *Candida albicans.*

D. *Escherichia coli.*

Answers

9-1   Answer C

Acute otitis media is diagnosed when there is fluid in the middle ear accompanied by signs or symptoms of an ear infection, including fever and otalgia. During the acute stage, acute otitis media is very painful. Inappropriate or ineffective treatment can lead to otitis media with effusion, which is often painless. An acute infection implies a current, not chronic, problem.

9-2   Answer C

A child's central visual acuity is 20/30 by age 3. At birth, an infant can see about 12 in. away, an approximate 20/300 central visual acuity. It improves to 20/40 by age 2, 20/30 by age 3, and 20/20 by age 4.

9-3   Answer B

Using eardrops made of a solution of equal parts of alcohol and vinegar in each ear after swimming is effective in drying the ear canal and maintaining an acidic environment, therefore preventing a favorable medium for the growth of bacteria, the cause of swimmer's ear. The adage "you shouldn't put anything smaller than your elbow in your ear" holds true today. A hair dryer on the lowest setting several inches from the ear may be used to dry the canal.

9-4   Answer A

The symptoms of hay fever, also called allergic rhinitis, are similar to those of viral rhinitis but usually persist and are seasonal in nature. When assessing the nasal mucosa, you will observe that the turbinates are usually pale or violaceous because of venous engorgement with allergic rhinitis. With viral rhinitis, the mucosa is usually erythematous, and with nasal polyps, there are usually yellowish, boggy masses of hypertrophic mucosa. Nasal vestibulitis usually results from folliculitis of the hairs that line the nares.

9-5   Answer C

A client with retinal detachment complains of a sudden change in vision (either blurry vision, flashing lights, or floaters) but has no pain. On ophthalmoscopy, the retina appears pale, opaque, and folds in and undulates freely as the eye moves. Retinal detachment is an emergency and requires immediate surgery, usually scleral buckling, in which an encircling silicon band is used to keep the choroid in contact with the retina to promote attachment. Iritis is characterized by severe pain. Cataracts and most cases of glaucoma usually present as a gradual change in vision, not a sudden change.

9-6   Answer C

Esotropia is the inward turning of the eyes. Exotropia is the outward turning of the eyes. Strabismus, also called tropia, is the constant malalignment of the eye axes. It is likely to cause amblyopia. Pseudostrabismus has the appearance of strabismus because of the presence of epicanthic folds but is normal in young children.

9-7   Answer D

A common cause of conductive hearing loss in adults ages 20–40 is otosclerosis, a gradual hardening of the tympanic membrane that causes the footplate of the stapes to become fixed in the oval window. Presbycusis, a progressive, bilaterally symmetrical perceptive hearing loss arising from structural changes in the hearing organs, usually occurs after age 50. Trauma may result in a conductive hearing loss, but this is certainly not common.

9-8   Answer D

Cluster headaches come in clusters as this client describes, with exquisite pain awakening the client from sleep. Excessive lacrimation and sweating on the affected side is common. Though this client's pain is unilateral, he does not complain of photophobia and has never had an aura, facts that tend to lead away from a diagnosis of classic migraine. Because the pain is at night, tension headache is a less likely diagnosis. Sinus headache would usually be precipitated by allergies or cold symptoms with nasal congestion.

9-9   Answer B

Management of influenza (flu) is generally symptomatic and includes rest, fluids, acetaminophen (Tylenol), and possibly a decongestant and an antitussive. The client should be advised to call in 4 days if symptoms have not resolved.

9-10   Answer A

The classic sign of retinal detachment is a client stating that "a curtain came down over my eye." Typically, the person presents with blurred vision in one eye that becomes progressively worse, with no pain or redness. With acute angle-closure glaucoma, there is a rapid onset in older adults, with severe pain and profound visual loss. The eye is red, with a steamy cornea and a dilated pupil. With open-angle glaucoma, there is an insidious onset in older adults, a gradual loss of peripheral vision over a period of years, and perception of "halos" around lights. With a cataract, there is blurred vision that is progressive over months or years and no pain or redness.

9-11   Answer B

In angle closure glaucoma, the patient presents with a sudden onset of symptoms as described in this case. This client has a marked visual deficit and pain as well as a fullness of the eye. This is a medical emergency and should be referred immediately because blindness can occur within days without intervention. With open angle type, the onset is more insidious. Herpetic conjunctivitis is generally associated with a herpetic rash, and the pain is dull in character.

9-12   Answer B

The most common reason for epistaxis is a local irritation or trauma (90%). It would be helpful to ask if the patient bumped his or her nose or recently had a sinusitis or irritation to the mucosa that may have predisposed the patient to the nosebleed. Nosebleeds and bruising are common with the elderly patient who is taking an anticoagulant or has an underlying coagulopathy associated with a condition such as Hodgkin's or cancer. Scurvy is unlikely in a well-nourished patient.

9-13   Answer A

Xanthelasmas are soft, raised, yellow plaques on the eyelids at the inner eye canthus. They appear most frequently in women, beginning in the 50s. Xanthelasmas occur with both high and normal lipid levels and have no pathological significance. Pingueculae are yellowish, elevated nodules appearing on the sclera. They are caused by a thickening of the bulbar conjunctiva from prolonged exposure to the sun, wind, and dust. Arcus senilis appears as gray-white arcs or circles around the limbus as a result of deposits of lipid material that make the cornea look cloudy. Actinic keratoses are wartlike growths on the skin that occur in middle-aged or older adults and are caused by excessive exposure to the sun.

9-14   Answer D

The symptoms of GABS (group A beta-hemolytic streptococcus) are sudden onset of sore throat, exudative tonsillitis, tender anterior cervical lymph nodes, and history of fever. In this client, the sore throat has been present for 24 hours and did not come on suddenly and there is no exudate on the tonsils. Rhinitis, hoarseness, and dry cough are associated with a viral etiology. At this point, a rapid strep screen is appropriate, and if the result is negative, a strep culture should be done to rule out GABS. This client should not be treated with antibiotics until a positive GABS is reported.

9-15   Answer B

Bruxism is grinding the teeth while sleeping and frequently occurs in young children. Bite blocks will prevent this until the child grows out of it.

9-16   Answer C

Flushing the ear with water is contraindicated when a client has a probable foreign body or insect in it. The water may cause the object to swell, making removal more difficult. Actions that may be taken include inspecting the ear canal with an otoscope, using a small suction device to try to remove the object, or instilling several drops of mineral oil in the ear.

9-17   Answer B

When a practitioner places a vibrating tuning fork in the midline of a client's skull and asks if the tone sounds the same in both ears or is better in one, the examiner is performing the Weber test. The Weber test is valuable when a client states that hearing is better in one ear than the other. The Rinne test compares air conduction and bone conduction sound. The stem of a vibrating tuning fork is placed on the client's mastoid process and the client is asked to signal when the sound disappears. The fork is then quickly inverted so that the vibrating end is near the ear canal, at which time the client should still hear a sound. Normally, sound is heard twice as long by air conduction as by bone conduction. The caloric test, or oculovestibular test, assesses cranial nerves III, VI, and VIII. Ice water is instilled into the ear; if nerve function is normal, the eyes will deviate to that side. A hearing acuity test assesses the client's ability to hear the spoken word.

9-18   Answer B

By age 3–4 months, an infant can fixate on, briefly follow, and then reach for a toy when the toy is placed in the infant's line of vision. At age 2–4 weeks, an infant can fixate on an object. By age 1 month, an infant can fixate on and follow a light or a bright toy. By age 6–10 months, an infant can fixate on and follow a toy in all directions.

9-19   Answer B

Presbyopia is a normal age-related deficit in aging and is the inability to focus on objects in close range. This is common and begins to develop in a person's mid-40s.

Photopsia or seeing flashing lights is a symptom that requires urgent evaluation as it may be associated with a retinal tear of detachment. Myopia or near-sightedness is common with younger people and is not associated with advancing age. Age related macular degeneration is not uncommon and is associated with a loss in central vision.

9-20   Answer C

Benzodiazepines like clonazepam (Klonopin) may be ordered for temporal mandibular joint disorders for a short course of therapy only (1–2 weeks). They may be helpful for acute pain secondary to masticatory muscle spasm or temporomandibular joint pain. Nonopioid analgesics may be ordered for inflammatory pain, anticonvulsants may be ordered for neuropathic pain, and skeletal muscle relaxants may be ordered for muscle relaxation.

9-21   Answer B

If a client has throbbing pain in the eye, an irregular pupil shape, marked photophobia, and redness (a deep, dull, red halo or ciliary flush) around the iris and/or cornea, suspect iritis. An immediate referral is warranted. The client may also have blurred vision. The client with conjunctivitis has redness more prominently at the periphery of the eye, along with tearing and itching. The client may also complain of a scratchy, burning, or gritty sensation but not pain, although photophobia may be present. The client with subconjunctival hemorrhage presents with a sudden onset of a painless, bright-red appearance on the bulbar conjunctiva that usually results from pressure exerted during coughing, sneezing, or Valsalva's maneuver. Other conditions that may result in a subconjunctival hemorrhage include uncontrolled hypertension and the use of anticoagulant medication. The client with acute glaucoma presents with circumcorneal redness, with the redness radiating around the iris, and a dilated pupil.

9-22   Answer C

For a client who has had Ménière's disease for several years with some hearing loss but now has persistent vertigo, treatment by vestibular neurectomy might relieve the vertigo. In vestibular neurectomy, the portion of cranial nerve VIII controlling balance and sensations of vertigo is severed. Vertigo is usually relieved in 90% of the cases. A labyrinthectomy is the surgery of last resort for a client with Ménière's disease because the labyrinth is completely removed and cochlear function destroyed. This procedure is used only when hearing loss is nearly complete. Oral diuretics and a low-sodium diet may aid in maintaining a lower labyrinth pressure, which may help slightly. Wearing an earplug will not help and may aggravate the condition.

9-23   Answer C

When trying to decide between a diagnosis of conjunctivitis and iritis, one of the distinguishing characteristics is a ciliary flush present in iritis. Photophobia is not usually present in conjunctivitis, but it is always present with iritis. Photophobia occurs with corneal inflammation, iritis, and angle-closure glaucoma. Clients with iritis and those with conjunctivitis both complain of eye discomfort, although in iritis the pain is moderately severe with intermittent stabbing. Both conditions generally produce a slowly progressive redness. Vision is normal with conjunctivitis and blurred with iritis.

9-24   Answer B

If a client has a persistent sore throat, fever, and malaise not relieved with penicillin therapy, a monospot test should be performed to rule out mononucleosis (Epstein-Barr virus). A throat culture and rapid antigen test are performed to help diagnose group A beta-hemolytic streptococcal infection. A Thayer-Martin plate test is performed to diagnose a gonococcal infection.

9-25   Answer B

Bell's palsy affects the facial nerve, resulting in weakness or paralysis of one side of the face. A stroke and shingles are unilateral in their presentation as well. A lesion affecting the sensory portion of the trigeminal nerve could be manifested by bilateral symptoms.

9-26   Answer C

Painless, white, slightly raised patches in a client's mouth are probably caused by candidiasis (thrush). Aphthous ulcers (canker sores) are extremely painful. Herpes simplex (a viral infection), canker sores, and cancerous lesions are usually discrete and not spread over a large area.

9-27   Answer C

Most recently, cognitive behavioral therapy has been recognized as an effective treatment for tinnitus. Therapy is focused on reducing the psychological distress associated with tinnitus and developing coping strategies for dealing with the problem. Antidepressants, such as nortriptyline 50 mg at bedtime, have proved to be effective especially if the tinnitus disrupts sleep. High doses of aspirin over a sustained period of time may actually cause tinnitus. Lidocaine given intravenously suppresses tinnitus in some individuals but is not suitable for long-term suppression. Corticosporin eardrops have proved to have no effect.

9-28   Answer B

Cancerous lesions to the buccal/oral mucosa are generally squamous in nature and are characterized by lesions that are painless and firm in consistency. Lymphadenopathy may be present and associated with the lesion and presents as nonmobile, nontender nodes.

9-29   Answer A

The most common cause of a white pupil (leukokoria or leukocoria) in a newborn is a congenital cataract. The incidence may be as high as 1 in every 500–1,000 live births, and there is usually a family history. Some infants require no treatment; however, surgery may be performed on others during the first few weeks of life. Retinoblastoma, a common intraocular malignancy, is detected within the first few weeks of life and is the second-most common cause of white pupil.

Persistent hyperplastic primary vitreous is the third-most common cause of white pupil and is a congenital developmental abnormality. Retinal detachment may occur as a result of trauma or disease and only rarely occurs in infancy.

9-30   Answer C

The trachea deviates toward the unaffected side with an aortic aneurysm, unilateral thyroid lobe enlargement, and pneumothorax. It deviates toward the affected side with a large atelectasis or fibrosis.

9-31   Answer C

Tonsils that touch the uvula are graded 3. Grade 1 indicates that the tonsils are visible; grade 2 indicates that the tonsils are halfway between tonsillar pillars and uvula; and grade 4 indicates that the tonsils touch each other. Tonsils are enlarged to 2, 3, or 4 with an acute infection.

9-32   Answer D

Because the herpes virus in this case seems to be along the ophthalmic branch of cranial nerve V, there is considerable risk that this client could develop permanent damage in that eye, and an ophthalmological consult needs to be arranged promptly to ascertain damage and prevent any further damage.

9-33   Answer C

Cranial nerve (CN) VIII, the vestibulocochlear (acoustic) nerve, is affected by sensorineural or perceptive hearing loss. Both the cochlear and vestibular branches have sensory pathways. CN II, the optic nerve, has sensory pathways. CN IV, the trochlear nerve, has both sensory and motor pathways. CN XI, the accessory nerve, has motor pathways.

9-34   Answer D

The most common cause of sensorineural hearing loss is presbycusis, a gradual decrease in cochlear function that occurs in most persons with advancing age. Otosclerosis (stapes fixation) and tympanic membrane sclerosis and scarring both result in a conductive hearing loss. Trauma would also result in a conductive hearing loss.

9-35   Answer C

Bell's palsy should be suspected if a client presents with a rapid-onset, complete paralysis of one-half of the face and the inability to raise the eyebrow, close the eye, whistle, or show the teeth. Bell's palsy is a lower motor neuron lesion resulting in cranial nerve VII paralysis. It is often a self-limiting condition, lasting a few days or weeks. Occasionally, facial paralysis may result from a tumor or physical trauma compromising the facial nerve. A cerebrovascular accident (CVA) would affect more than just the face. Trigeminal neuralgia, also called tic douloureux, is a painful disorder of the trigeminal nerve. It causes severe pain in the face and forehead on the affected side and is triggered by stimuli such as cold drafts, chewing, and drinking cold liquids.

9-36   Answer B

An explanation of 20/50 vision in a client's right eye would be: "You can see at 20 ft with your right eye what most people can see at 50 ft." Normal visual acuity is 20/20 on a Snellen eye chart. The larger the denominator, the poorer the vision. If vision is greater than 20/30, refer the client to an ophthalmologist or optometrist.

9-37   Answer A

Though a change in sleeping habits (i.e., new bed pillows) is a possibility, in this case the character of the pain should lead the practitioner to inquire about any traumatic event in the past involving her neck, such as a fall or motor vehicle accident or a history of repetitive activity involving the head or neck, such as a change in exercise routine or a new hobby. Spasm of the trapezius will cause difficulty in turning the head to one side or another. Difficulty swallowing, though significant in some clients, doesn't seem related to the presenting complaint.

9-38   Answer B

Presbyopia occurs in almost all persons beginning about the mid-40s. The lens loses elasticity and becomes hard and glasslike, decreasing its ability to change shape to accommodate for near vision. Arcus senilis, a gray-white arc or circle around the limbus from deposition of lipid material, does not affect vision. Cataracts and glaucoma may occur around age 50 or older.

9-39   Answer D

When teaching clients about mononucleosis (Epstein-Barr virus [EBV]), tell them to avoid

contact sports and heavy lifting, because of splenomegaly and a threat of rupture. Also instruct the patient to avoid stress and advise that convalescence may take several weeks. Antibiotic therapy is not indicated for EBV. Bedrest is necessary only in severe cases.

9-40   Answer A

Most perforated tympanic membranes seen with acute otitis media heal within several weeks. If it has not healed within 3–6 months, a surgical repair can be done, but not until age 7–9 years. Sam can swim on the surface with the use of an ear mold but must not dive, jump, or swim under water.

9-41   Answer B

Cherry-red lips are a manifestation of carbon monoxide poisoning. They also occur with acidosis from aspirin poisoning or ketoacidosis. In light-skinned clients, circumoral pallor of the lips occurs with shock and anemia, and cyanosis of the lips occurs with hypoxemia and chilling. Some lips are normally pale pink.

9-42   Answer C

A child's head circumference is measured, using a measuring tape, at each well-child visit until age 2 years. At birth, head circumference measures about 32–38 cm and is 2 cm larger than the chest circumference. At age 2, both the head and chest measurements are equal. During childhood, the chest circumference exceeds the head circumference by 5–7 cm.

9-43   Answer B

Dryness of the eyes and the appearance of "sunken" eyes are normal age-related changes. With hyperthyroidism, the eyes appear to bulge out (exophthalmos), but in hypothyroidism, the eyes do not appear any different. A moon face is apparent with Cushing's syndrome, and this might make the eyes appear to be sunken in, although on close examination, they are not. With a detached retina, the outward appearance is normal, but the client complains of seeing floaters or spots in the visual field and describes the sensation as like a curtain being drawn across the vision.

9-44   Answer B

The palpebral fissures are the openings between the margins of the upper and lower eyelids. Someone who appears to be squinting is said to have narrow palpebral fissures. The nasolabial folds are the skin creases that extend from the angle of the nose to the corner of the mouth.

9-45   Answer A

The most common offending allergens causing allergic rhinitis are, in descending order, pollens of grasses, trees, and weeds; fungi; animal allergens; and dust mites. Rhinitis is the most troublesome allergic problem and affects 20% of the population.

9-46   Answer A

Sensorineural loss comes from exposure to loud noises, inner ear infections, tumors, congenital and familial disorders, and aging. The etiology of conductive loss includes ear infection, presence of a foreign body, perforated drum, and otosclerosis of the ossicles. The results of the Weber and Rinne test will assist in the diagnosis. Tinnitus is ringing in the ears, and vertigo is dizziness associated with inner ear dysfunction. The client does not complain of either of these symptoms.

9-47   Answer C

The confrontation test is a gross measure of peripheral vision. It compares the client's peripheral vision with the practitioner's, assuming that the practitioner has normal peripheral vision. The cover test detects small degrees of deviated alignment by interrupting the fusion reflex that normally keeps both eyes parallel. The corneal light reflex test assesses the parallel alignment of the eye axes. The Snellen eye chart test assesses visual acuity.

9-48   Answer A

Microtia refers to the size of the ears, specifically ears smaller than 4 cm vertically.

9-49   Answer C

The leading cause of blindness in persons ages 20–60 in the United States is diabetic retinopathy, a progressive microangiopathy with small-vessel damage and occlusion. Macular degeneration is the leading cause of blindness in persons older than age 60. Glaucoma may eventually lead to loss of vision, but the symptoms have a slow progression, usually leading the client to eventual surgery to correct the problem. Trauma rarely leads to blindness.

9-50   Answer C

Temporomandibular disorders are fairly common, and some management can often begin in the primary care setting. The objective is to not overtax the joint. Although drinking liquids would rest the jaw, it is not necessary and is an extreme measure. Altering the diet to include foods that are easier to chew and to limit opening the mouth too widely will ease the pain. Ice for pain and heat for chronic pain may be helpful as well. Chewing gum would create a repetitive stress of the TMJ that would aggravate the condition.

9-51   Answer A

When assessing the internal structure of the eye, absence of a red reflex may indicate the total opacity of the pupil because of a cataract or a hemorrhage into the vitreous humor. It may also be a result of improper positioning of the ophthalmoscope. Acute iritis is noted by constriction of the pupil accompanied by pain and circumcorneal redness (ciliary flush). If areas of hemorrhage, exudate, and white patches are present when the internal structure of the eye is assessed, they are usually a result of diabetes or long-standing hypertension.

9-52   Answer D

Older adults are at a higher risk than middle-aged adults for developing an eye infection because of a decrease in tear production, which results in the inability of the tear ducts to wash out infectious organisms.

9-53   Answer C

Baby bottle caries, which occur in older infants and toddlers who take a bottle of milk, juice, or sweetened liquid to bed, destroy the upper deciduous teeth. The liquid pools around the upper front teeth, and the mouth bacteria act on the carbohydrates, especially sucrose, in the drink, forming metabolic acids that break down the tooth enamel and destroy its protein.

9-54   Answer C

With external otitis, there is pain, an erythematous ear canal, and usually a history of recent swimming. Acute otitis media is also painful, is usually a result of cotton swab use or physical trauma, and usually follows an upper respiratory infection. Chronic otitis media is usually not painful, although during an exacerbation the ear may be painful. Ear pain may also be the result of temporomandibular joint dysfunction. It is usually made worse by chewing or grinding the teeth.

9-55   Answer B

An ESR may help confirm the diagnosis. An elevated ESR—anywhere from 50–100—may be seen in temporal arteritis; however, the ESR may also be normal. The temporal artery supplies the optic nerve, and if temporal arteritis is suspected due to the age of the client (50 and older) and the location and character of the pain, it is essential that a referral to a surgeon be made for immediate biopsy of the artery before damage to the optic nerve occurs.

9-56   Answer C

Milk is the best storage and transport solution for avulsed teeth when one is planning on reimplanting them. If milk is not available, other solutions that might be used include saline (salt water), water, and saliva.

9-57   Answer B

Symptoms most indicative of mononucleosis (Epstein-Barr virus) are gradual onset of fatigue, sore throat, fever, posterior cervical adenopathy, palatine petechiae, and hepatosplenomegaly.

9-58   Answer A

Although regular ocular pressure testing is indicated for all older adults on a routine basis, it is especially important for clients taking an extended regimen of high-dose inhaled glucocorticoids because prolonged continuous use increases the risk of ocular hypertension or open-angle glaucoma. NSAIDs and ACE inhibitors do not require ocular pressure monitoring. Older adults taking insulin need to have regular eye examinations because they are diabetic and have a risk of diabetic retinopathy, not because they are taking insulin.

9-59   Answer B

Nasal polyps are benign growths that occur frequently in clients with sinus problems, asthma, and allergic rhinitis. Polyps are neither neoplastic growths nor precancerous, but they do have the potential to affect the flow of air through the nasal passages. Clients who have asthma and have nasal polyps may have an associated allergy to aspirin, a syndrome that is referred to as Samter's triad.

9-60   Answer B

Hypopyon is purulent matter in an inflamed anterior chamber. A hyphema is blood in the anterior chamber, the result of trauma or spontaneous hemorrhage. Anisocoria, common in 5% of the population, refers to unequal pupil size. In 95% of these persons, it indicates central nervous system disease. A pterygium is a painless, unilateral or bilateral, triangle-shaped encroachment onto the conjunctiva that appears on the nasal side and is caused by excessive ultraviolet light exposure.

9-61   Answer A

In older adults, the most common cause of decreased visual functioning is cataract formation (lens opacity), which should be expected by age 70. Glaucoma (increased ocular pressure) is the second-most common cause of decreased visual functioning. It increases from age 46–60, then levels off. Macular degeneration (loss of central vision), which affects 30% of persons older than age 65, affects a person's ability to read fine print and do handiwork. Arcus senilis does not affect vision.

9-62   Answer A

Carbonic anhydrase inhibitors, such as acetazolamide (Diamox), act as diuretics to reduce the intraocular pressure in clients with glaucoma. A miotic causes contraction of the pupil and a mydriatic dilates the pupil. Because of the effect of pupil dilation on aqueous outflow in angle-closure glaucoma, medications such as atropine and other anticholinergics that have a mydriatic effect should be avoided. Miotics such as pilocarpine (Pilocar) may be given to cause contraction of the sphincter of the iris and to contract the ciliary muscle, which promotes accommodation for near vision and facilitates aqueous humor outflow by increasing drainage through the trabecular meshwork in open-angle glaucoma. But the question is asked about diuretics, which pilocarpine is not. It is a cholinergic agent.

9-63   Answer D

In a pediatric client with acute epiglottitis, a number of symptoms can indicate that airway obstruction is imminent: stridor, restlessness, nasal flaring, as well as the use of accessory muscles of respiration. A reddened face does not indicate a lack of oxygenation. Although the child may scream and grab at the throat, these are not primary indicators of impending airway obstruction.

9-64   Answer B

Corneas are harvested from the cadavers of uninfected persons younger than age 65 who die as the result of an acute trauma or illness. The client's question does not necessarily mean that she is thinking about dying, but it is natural for older adults to think about death, and their thoughts and feelings should be explored.

9-65   Answer C

The immediate goal of myringotomy and tube placement in a child with recurrent episodes of otitis media is to allow removal of suppurative and mucoid material, thus releasing the pressure. This also prolongs the period of ventilation, allowing the middle ear mucosa to return to normal. Ventilation of the middle ear must be done to restore hearing and prevent aberrations in growth and development associated with hearing loss.

9-66   Answer A

The treatment for hyphema is strict bedrest, with the head elevated at least 20°. The client needs to see an ophthalmologist within 24 hours. In the meantime, the application of bilateral eye patches to minimize eye movement; the instillation of atropine 1%, two drops twice daily to reduce ciliary spasm; and the administration of appropriate aspirin-free pain medications are indicated.

9-67   Answer B

Test for near vision by using the Rosenbaum chart. Hold it about 12–14 in. from the client's eyes. A gross estimate of near vision may also be assessed by asking the client to read from a magazine or newspaper held about 12–14 in. away from the eyes. The Snellen eye chart tests vision at a distance of 20 ft. Testing the cardinal fields of gaze does not test for vision but rather for extraocular eye movements.

9-68   Answer B

With ethmoid sinus problems, the pain is behind the eye and high on the nose. Maxillary sinus pain is over the cheek and into the upper teeth; frontal sinus pain is over the lower forehead; and sphenoid sinus pain is in the occiput, vertex, or middle of the head.

9-69   Answer C

Herpes simplex is associated with vesicular lesions on the lips and oral mucosa. The virus remains latent and may recur with sunlight exposure, stressful times, fever, trauma, and treatment with immunosuppressive drugs.

9-70   Answer C

In hyperthyroidism the symptoms of rapid pulse, palpitations, and hypertension due to the excess production of T4 and T3 are common, whereas in hypothyroidism the opposite symptom complex is common. Velvety, warm, moist skin is a symptom of hyperthyroidism, whereas dry, coarse skin is a symptom of hypothyroidism. Hyperthyroidism is also characterized by exophthalmos, which is the term for the eyeball protruding forward. When it is bilateral, it may signify infiltrative ophthalmopathy of Graves' disease. There may be associated edema and conjunctival injection as well.

9-71   Answer A

If a child with otitis media with effusion has a change in the hearing threshold to less than or equal to 20 dB and has notable speech and language delays, more aggressive treatment is indicated. When the child's hearing examination reveals a change in the hearing threshold, it is extremely important that the provider evaluate the child's achievement of developmental milestones in speech and language. Any abnormal findings warrant referral.

9-72   Answer A

Treatment for cleft lip and palate needs to be instituted immediately after birth by constructing a palatal obturator to help the infant feed. Cleft lip and palate rehabilitation is an extensive program involving multiple procedures. A cleft lip may be unilateral or bilateral and complete or incomplete. It may also occur with a cleft in the entire palate or just the anterior or posterior palate.

9-73   Answer C

Clients with allergic conjunctivitis have a stringy, white discharge. Clients with bacterial conjunctivitis have a purulent discharge; those with viral conjunctivitis have serous or clear drainage and preauricular lymph node enlargement. A profuse mucoid or mucopurulent discharge is indicative of chlamydial conjunctivitis. Human papillomavirus (HPV) also is a risk factor for certain types of oral cancers.

9-74   Answer B

Approximately 10% of clients with a hearing loss are helped by medical or surgical treatment. If clients are sent for a hearing aid and not correctly identified as having a hearing loss, the underlying problem may not be resolved.

9-75   Answer A

Barotrauma of the auditory canal causing abnormal middle ear pressure may be relieved by the use of nasal steroids and oral decongestants. With barotrauma, there is no infection, just swelling of the airways, which causes the sensation of abnormal pressure; therefore, antibiotics are not indicated. This is certainly within the practitioner's scope of practice, and a referral is not indicated.

9-76   Answer C

Nasal stuffiness and epistaxis may occur during a normal pregnancy because of increased vascularization in the upper respiratory tract. The gums may also be soft and hyperemic and may bleed with normal toothbrushing. Additional laboratory tests are not necessary at this point. No treatment, other than teaching the client what to expect and do, is indicated.

9-77   Answer B

The antibiotic of choice for beta-lactamase coverage of otitis media is amoxicillin and potassium clavulanate (Augmentin). It is the first-line treatment for otitis media because it is effective against a wide range of bacteria, including beta lactamase. Amoxicillin (Amoxil) is not effective against beta lactamase. Azithromycin (Zithromax) for otitis media is usually reserved for more resistant strains of the common bacterial pathogens. Prednisone (Deltasone) is reserved for otitis media with effusion.

9-78   Answer B

When the following four symptoms present as a cluster, there is a high probability (43%) that the infection is caused by group A beta-hemolytic streptococcus: throat pain with tonsillar exudate, anterior cervical adenopathy, presence of fever, and absence of cough.

9-79   Answer A

Hordeolum (stye) is the most common localized infection of one of the glands of the eyelids.

Treatment includes warm compresses for 15 minutes four times a day and topical antibiotics. A chalazion is a chronic swelling of the eyelids not associated with conjunctivitis. Bacterial conjunctivitis does not involve one of the glands of the eyelids. Primary herpes simplex of the eye usually presents as conjunctivitis with a clear, watery discharge; vesicles on the lids; and preauricular lymphadenopathy.

9-80   Answer B

Caution needs to be used when ordering a second-generation antihistamine for a client taking drugs such as cimetidine (Tagamet), erythromycin (E-Mycin), clarithromycin (Biaxin), and ketoconazole (Nizoral) that can block cytochrome P450 metabolism or if the client has serious hepatic impairment.

9-81   Answer A

In a young child, unilateral purulent rhinitis is most often caused by a foreign body. The key word is *unilateral*. Viral and bacterial infections and allergic reactions usually affect both nares.

9-82   Answer C

Oral candidiasis (thrush) is distinctive because of the ability to rub off the white areas on the tongue with a tongue depressor. Leukoplakia cannot be removed by rubbing the mucosal surface; it appears as little white lesions on the tongue. Oral lichen planus is a chronic inflammatory autoimmune disease; it also has white lesions that do not rub off. Oral cancer must be ruled out in any lesion because early detection is the key to successful management and a good prognosis. Thrush may be seen in denture wearers, in debilitated clients, and in those who are immunocompromised or taking corticosteroids or broad-spectrum antibiotics.

9-83   Answer D

With bacterial conjunctivitis, there is purulent, thick discharge; with allergic conjunctivitis, a stringy mucoid discharge; and with viral conjunctivitis, there is usually a watery discharge. In a client with iritis, there is rarely a discharge.

9-84   Answer A

Trigeminal neuralgia is described as a sharp, piercing, shooting facial pain that is severe but usually lasts only a short time. The origin is the trigeminal nerve (CNV). TMJ is associated with pain on opening and closing the mouth and is also associated with crepitus of that joint. A goiter is generally painless. Preauricular adenitis (enlarged and inflamed preauricular nodes) would be sustained until the etiological cause is identified and treated.

9-85   Answer A

The most frequent cause of laryngeal obstruction in an adult is a piece of meat that lodges in the airway. With a tumor, there would be a gradual growth, and treatment would probably be sought before there is a complete obstruction. Mucosal swelling from an allergic reaction may result in an obstruction, but this does not occur as frequently as a laryngeal obstruction from a piece of meat. Inhalation of a carcinogen would result only in an irritation of the mucosa, if anything.

9-86   Answer D

If a client is taking timolol maleate (Timoptic) drops for chronic open-angle glaucoma, you should be most concerned if the client is also taking atenolol (Tenormin), a beta blocker, for high blood pressure. Because timolol maleate drops are beta-adrenergic blockers, additional beta blockers can cause worsening of congestive heart failure or reactive airway disease, as well as acute delirium. Aspirin therapy as prophylaxis for heart attack; ranitidine (Zantac) for gastroesophageal reflux disease; and alprazolam (Xanax), an anxiolytic for anxiety, do not interact adversely with eyedrops for glaucoma.

9-87   Answer D

Signs and symptoms of acute angle-closure glaucoma include seeing halos around lights, severe eye pain and redness, nausea and vomiting, headache, blurred vision, conjunctival injection, cloudy cornea, mid-dilated pupil, and an increased intraocular pressure. Acute angle-closure glaucoma is less common than primary open-angle glaucoma, accounting for about 10% of all glaucoma cases in the United States. Emergency treatment is indicated, so a prompt referral is necessary when these signs and symptoms occur.

9-88   Answer B

Children ages 2.5–3 years should have their vision screened using the Allen test, which uses picture cards. The Snellen E chart is used for preschoolers ages 3–6, whereas the Snellen letter chart is used for school-age and older clients. The Rosenbaum chart is used for a gross assessment of near vision by having the client hold reading material approximately 12–14 in. away.

9-89   Answer C

Cataracts cannot be cured by medications, dietary supplements, or optical devices. No proven pharmaceutical treatment exists to date that can delay, prevent, or reverse the development of cataracts. The definitive management for cataract is a surgical approach, one that removes the defective lens and replaces it with an artificial one.

9-90   Answer A

The normal ratio comparing the artery-to-vein ratio in the retinal vessels is 2:3 or 4:5, with the arterioles being a brighter red than the veins when viewed through the ophthalmoscope. The arterioles have a narrow light reflex from the center line of the vessel. Veins do not normally show a light reflex. Both arterioles and veins show a gradual and regularly diminishing diameter as you look at them from the disc to the periphery. When hypertension is present, the arterioles may be only about one-half the size of the corresponding vein, and they may appear opaque and lighter. With long-standing hypertension, nicking is present. This occurs when the underlying veins are concealed to some degree by the abnormally opaque arteriole wall at the vessel crossings.

9-91   Answer C

Pruritus of the external ear canal is a common problem. In most cases, the pruritus is self-induced from enthusiastic cleaning or excoriation. The protective cerumen covering must be allowed to regenerate and may be helped to do so by application of a small amount of mineral oil, which helps to counteract dryness and reject moisture. The use of soap and water, as well as cotton-tipped swabs, should be avoided. The adage "you shouldn't put anything smaller than your elbow in your ear" holds true today. If an inflammatory component is present, a topical corticosteroid may be applied. Often, isopropyl alcohol may relieve ear canal pruritus.

9-92   Answer C

A Weber test assesses hearing by bone conduction. With normal hearing, sound is heard equally well in both ears, meaning there is no lateralization.

With conductive deafness, sound lateralizes to the defective ear because it is transmitted through bone rather than air. With perceptive deafness, sound lateralizes to the better ear.

9-93   Answer A

Presbyopia is the natural loss of accommodative capacity with age. In the mid-40s, persons note the inability to focus on objects at a normal reading distance. With hyperopia, objects at a distance are not seen clearly unless accommodation is used, and near objects may not be seen. This is corrected with plus or convex lenses. With myopia, the person is able to focus on very near objects without glasses. Far vision is difficult without the aid of corrective minus or concave lenses. With astigmatism, the refractive errors are different in the horizontal and vertical axes.

9-94   Answer D

Because the cornea is an avascular organ, immune defenses have difficulty fighting off infections.

9-95   Answer D

For the client with flu, oseltamivir (Tamiflu) or zanamivir (Relenza) may be given. If the virus causing the flu is type A influenza, the client may benefit from either one of these drugs. They are most effective if started early in the course of the disease (within 48 hours), although reduction of symptoms and shortening the course of illness are still possible even if started 3–5 days after symptoms begin.

9-96   Answer C

When severe pain is elicited by tugging on a normal-appearing auricle, an acute infection of the external ear canal (otitis externa) is suspected. Otitis media, with or without effusion, cannot be diagnosed without examining the tympanic membrane. Otalgia is simply ear pain.

9-97   Answer C

Irrigation with a soft bulb syringe or a commercial jet tooth cleanser may be used to remove cerumen. Irrigation using lukewarm water should be done when the cerumen is dry and hard but not if the tympanic membrane might be perforated. Cerumen can be safely removed from an infant's ear by the practitioner for adequate visualization of the tympanic membrane by using an ear curette through an operating otoscope, or if an operating otoscope is not available, by using a size 00 ear curette through a size 3-mm speculum.

9-98   Answer D

If a client has a sore throat and a history of diabetes or rheumatic fever, it is very likely that the infection is a result of group A beta-hemolytic streptococcus.

9-99   Answer C

There is no treatment for a subconjunctival hemorrhage other than to reassure the client that the blood will be reabsorbed within 2 weeks.

9-100   Answer D

Currently, there is no effective treatment for atrophic macular degeneration. Laser photocoagulation may slow the exudative form of macular degeneration if performed early in the course of the disease. It seals leaking capillaries and stops the exudation. Clients cope with the disease by using large-print books and magazines, magnifying glasses, and high-intensity lighting.

9-101   Answer A

The first-line antibiotic therapy for an adult with no known allergies and suspected group A beta-hemolytic streptococcus pharyngitis is penicillin.

9-102   Answer C

In a client with mumps, the orifice of Stensen's duct appears red. The buccal mucosa in a normal client appears pink, smooth, and moist, although there may be some patchy hyperpigmentation in dark-skinned clients. Dappled brown patches are present with Addison's disease. Koplik's spots are a prodromal sign of measles.

9-103   Answer A

The maxillary sinus is the largest of the paranasal sinuses and is the most commonly affected sinus. There is usually pain and pressure over the cheek. Inability to transilluminate the cavity usually indicates a cavity filled with purulent material. Discolored nasal discharge, as well as a poor response to decongestants, may also indicate sinusitis. The ethmoid sinuses are usually nonpalpable and may not be transilluminated. The frontal sinuses are just below the eyebrows. Frontal sinusitis also includes pain and tenderness of the forehead.

9-104   Answer B

Nasal furuncles are typically painful and should be allowed to drain on their own. Avoid trauma when inspecting the patient. Instructing the patient to apply warm soaks may facilitate healing along with an antibiotic to treat the causative agent which is most often *Staphylococcus*. Nasal polyps and cancers are usually painless.

9-105   Answer C

Treatment of amblyopia ("lazy eye") includes occluding the client's "good" (or better-seeing) eye and treating any underlying conditions such as cataracts or refractive errors. Treatment must be started by age 3 or 4 because amblyopia is irreversible after age 7. Amblyopia occurs in 50% of clients who have strabismus or misalignment of the eye muscles. Adults with strabismus frequently have double vision; however, young children learn to suppress or ignore double vision. As a result, young children have reduced central vision in the crossed eye from lack of use.

9-106   Answer C

When assessing the corneal light reflex, an abnormal finding indicates improper alignment of the eyes. It is noted when the reflections of the light are on different sites on the eyes. Some eye medications may cause unequal dilation, constriction, or inequality of pupil size that may be noted when assessing for direct and consensual pupil response. A neurological problem may be suspected if the pupils are unequal in size. Strabismus is noted during the cover-uncover test.

9-107   Answer A

A symptom cluster of severe throat pain with difficulty swallowing, copious oral secretions, respiratory difficulty and stridor, and fever but without pharyngeal erythema or cough is indicative of epiglottitis. Streptococcal pharyngitis presents with cervical adenitis, petechiae, a beefy-red uvula, and a tonsillar exudate. A mild case of tonsillitis may appear to be only a slight sore throat. A more severe case would involve inflamed, swollen tonsils; a very sore throat; and a high fever. Diphtheria starts with a sore throat, fever, headache, and nausea, then progresses to patches of grayish or dirty-yellowish membranes in the throat that eventually grow into one membrane.

9-108   Answer B

With a chronic allergy, a client's mucosa appears swollen, boggy, pale, and gray. Redness indicates an acute process and the question asks about a chronic allergy.

9-109   Answer C

A sexual history of oral-genital contact in a client presenting with pharyngitis is significant when infection with *Neisseria gonorrhoeae* is suspected. *N. gonorrhoeae* pharyngitis is a common sexually transmitted disease.

9-110   Answer A

Bifid uvula, a condition in which the uvula is either partially or completely split, occurs in 18% of Native Americans and 10% of Asians and is rare in whites and blacks. There is no need for treatment.

9-111   Answer C

A smooth tongue may result from a vitamin deficiency. Normally, the dorsal surface of the tongue is rough because of papillae. The ventral surface near the floor of the mouth is smooth and shows large veins.

9-112   Answer B

Epstein's pearls are a normal finding in newborns and infants. They appear as small, yellow-white, glistening, pearly papules along the median raphe of the hard palate and on the gums. They look like teeth but are small retention cysts that disappear after a few weeks. Bednar's aphthae are traumatic areas or ulcers that appear on the posterior hard palate on either side of the midline. They result from abrasions while sucking. A buccal tumor is a tumor on the inside of the cheek. Exostosis (torus palatinus) is found in the midline of the posterior two-thirds of the hard palate and is benign. It is a smooth, symmetrical bony structure.

9-113   Answer B

Keratoconjunctivitis sicca is dry eyes, a common disorder among older women. It is associated with dryness, redness, or a scratchy feeling in the eyes. On rare, severe occasions, there is marked discomfort and photophobia. Typically, it is caused by subtle abnormalities of the tear film and a reduced volume of tears. In most cases, tears can be replenished with the aqueous component of tears with over-the-counter artificial tears. Occasionally, mucomimetics are indicated when there is mucin deficiency. Viral conjunctivitis is caused by a virus and is associated with pharyngitis, fever, malaise, and preauricular lymph node enlargement. Allergic eye disease is benign and usually occurs in late adolescence or early adulthood. It is usually seasonal, and allergy treatment may be effective. A corneal ulcer is most commonly the result of a bacterial, viral, or fungal infection.

9-114   Answer C

When ordering nystatin (Mycostatin) for an oral fungal infection, tell the client to swish the medication in the mouth to coat all the lesions and then to swallow it.

9-115   Answer B

Migraines classically are preceded by an aura and accompanied by nausea, vomiting sometimes, and photophobia. They are usually unilateral. Tension headaches are not associated with photophobia and are usually bilateral and associated with limited neck range of motion (ROM). Tension headaches are not preceded by an aura. Cluster headaches are unilateral, frequently occur at night, and bear some resemblance to migraines; however, cluster headaches are accompanied by tearing, nasal stuffiness, and sweating on the same side as the headache and they come in clusters. The client is not in the age range (older than 50) for temporal arteritis.

9-116   Answer D

The cervical lymphadenopathy associated with asymptomatic HIV infection may be described as cervical lymph nodes that are firm but not hard, nontender, and mobile. In a healthy person, cervical nodes are often palpable and are movable, discrete, soft, and nontender. In a client with an acute infection, the cervical nodes are bilateral, enlarged, warm, tender, and firm but freely movable. Cancerous nodes are hard, unilateral, nontender, and fixed. In a client with a chronic inflammation, such as tuberculosis, the nodes are clumped.

9-117   Answer D

A narrowed field of vision may be experienced by some older patients, but a complete loss of peripheral vision is not a normal sensory loss in the aging adult. Additional visual deficits common to the aging adult are deficits in reading fine print (presbyopia), an increased sensitivity to light, and decreased night vision.

9-118   Answer C

Though the historical data is incomplete, this client has no obvious risk factors for esophageal varices or esophageal cancer. She is a nondrinker and denies weight loss and changes in bowel function or color of stools, which could be a clue to a gastrointestinal bleed. The fact that her worse symptoms occur at night with regurgitation and heartburn is classic for GERD. Dysphagia is frequently a prominent symptom in GERD. She has no abdominal tenderness, and aside from the nighttime symptoms and dysphagia, she reports no symptoms with food or lack of food. Clients with peptic ulcer disease (PUD) frequently complain of clusters of pain separated by periods of no symptoms.

9-119   Answer B

The U.S. Preventive Services Task Force (USPSTF) found fair evidence that the thyroid-stimulating hormone test (TSH) can detect subclinical thyroid disease in people without symptoms of thyroid dysfunction, but it found poor evidence that treatment improves clinically important outcomes in adults with screen-detected thyroid disease. The USPSTF concluded that the evidence is insufficient to recommend for or against routine screening for thyroid disease in adults.

9-120   Answer C

The ossicles seen on visualization of the tympanic membrane include the handle and short process of the malleus, and in some individuals you can see the incus through the drum. The pars flaccida is clearly visible. The stapes, cochlea, and round window are not visible.

9-121   Answer D

A client with acute glaucoma requires urgent treatment and usually presents with sudden onset of impaired vision, severe eye pain, vomiting, and headache. You may assess injected conjunctiva; steamy corneas; a fixed, partially dilated pupil; and a narrow chamber angle. A client with cataracts may present with decreased vision, and you would see an opacity, a cloudy lens, and a decreased view of the fundus. With macular degeneration, there is decreased central vision, and with presbyopia, there may be blurred vision but with a gradual onset. Only acute-angle glaucoma requires urgent treatment.

9-122   Answer D

The easiest way to differentiate between otitis externa and otitis media is that with otitis externa, movement or pressure on the pinna is extremely painful. With otitis externa, there may also be tender swelling of the outer ear canal. Bilateral pain in the ears is more suggestive of otitis externa. Clients with acute mastoiditis present with severe pain in, and, especially behind, the ear.

9-123   Answer D

Risk factors for oral cancers include age >50, smoking, use of alcohol, and chewing tobacco.

9-124   Answer B

A hordeolum (stye) is an abscess that may occur on the external or internal margin of the eyelid. It is typically caused by *Staphylococcus* bacteria.

Bibliography

American Academy of Family Physicians, American Academy of Otolaryngology-Head and Neck Surgery, and American Academy of Pediatrics Subcommittee on Otitis Media With Effusion: Clinical practice guideline. *Pediatrics* 113(5):1412–1429, May 2005.

Aronson, AA: Pediatrics, otitis media. eMedicine, updated July 29, 2011. http://www.emedicine.com/EMERG/topic393.htm, accessed August 15, 2012.

Bickley, LS: *Bates' Guide to Physical Examination and History Taking*, ed 9. Lippincott Williams & Wilkins, Philadelphia, 2007.

Bruyere, H :*100 Studies in Pathophysiology*. Lippincott Williams & Wilkins, Philadelphia, 2009

Conboy-Ellis, K, and Braker-Shaver, S: Intranasal steroids and allergic rhinitis. *Nurse Practitioner* 32(4):44–49, 2007.

Daugherty, JA: The latest buzz on tinnitus. *Nurse Practitioner* 32(10):42–47, 2007.

Diamond, S, and Feoktistov, A: Woman with short-lasting, strictly unilateral headaches. *Consultant* 47(12):1047–1052, 2007.

Dowdee, A, and Ossege, J: Assessment of childhood allergy for the primary care practitioner. *Journal of the American Academy of Nurse Practitioners* 19:53–62, 2007.

Dunphy, LM, et al: *Primary Care: The Art and Science of Advanced Practice Nursing*, ed 3. FA Davis, Philadelphia, 2011.

Jarvis, J: *Physical Examination and Health Assessment*, ed 6. WB Saunders, Philadelphia, 2011.

Kopes-Kerr, CP, and Alper, BS: Allergic conjunctivitis. *Clinical Advisor* 10(4), April, 2007.

Larkin, GL: Retinal detachment. eMedicine, updated April 7, 2008. http://www.emedicine.com/emerg/topic504.htm, accessed September 2, 2008.

National Guidelines Clearinghouse: Acute pharyngitis. Institute for Clinical Systems Improvement, Bloomington, MN, May 2005. http://www.guideline.gov/, accessed April 10, 2008.

Nootheti, S, and Bielory, L: Risk of cataracts and glaucoma with inhaled steroid use in children. *Comprehensive Ophthalmology Update* 7(11):31–39, 2006.

U.S Preventative Services Task Force. Screening thyroid disease. Recommendation statement. January 2004. http://www.uspreventativeservicestaskforce.rg/3rduspstf/thyroid/thyrrs.htm. Accessed February 1, 2012.

How well did you do?

85% and above, congratulations! This score shows application of test-taking principles and adequate content knowledge.

75%–85%, keep working! Review test-taking principles and try again.

65%–75%, hang in there! Spend some time reviewing concepts and test-taking principles and then try the test again.

Chapter 10: Respiratory Problems

Jill E. Winland-Brown

Questions

10-1   The antibiotic of choice for the treatment of Streptococcus pneumoniae *infection is*

A. dicloxacillin.

B. erythromycin.

C. penicillin.

D. ampicillin clavulanate.

10-2   *What is the most common cause of sudden and unexpected death in infants, accounting for 80% of postneonatal infant mortality with a peak incidence at 6 months?*

A. Choking

B. Shaken baby syndrome

C. Infantile pneumonia

D. Sudden infant death syndrome (SIDS)

10-3   *In inner-city children, an important cause of asthma-related illness and hospitalizations is*

A. heredity and genetics.

B. vitamin deficiencies.

C. cockroaches.

D. playing on asphalt playgrounds.

10-4   *The diagnosis of tuberculosis does not need to be reported when*

A. the client's Mantoux test shows an induration of 15 mm.

B. a case of tuberculosis is only suspected.

C. an asymptomatic client has a positive chest x-ray for pulmonary tuberculosis.

D. the Mantoux test shows a raised injected or red area without induration.

10-5   *When asthma does not respond to traditional therapy, it may be due to another syndrome that mimics asthma, such as*

A. lower airway obstruction.

B. vocal cord dysfunction.

C. COPD.

D. bronchitis.

10-6   *Approximately 50% of children with viral croup have a(n)*

A. aspirated foreign body.

B. tapered symmetric subglottic narrowing on x-ray.

C. concurrent epiglottitis.

D. history of allergic rhinitis.

10-7   *Which statement is true regarding primary spontaneous pneumothorax?*

A. It usually occurs after individuals have recently started an exercise program.

B. It occurs more commonly in thin elderly men.

C. It usually occurs in healthy individuals without preexisting lung disease.

D. It frequently occurs in Marfan's syndrome.

10-8   *Stridor can be heard on auscultation when a client has*

A. atelectasis.

B. asthma.

C. diaphragmatic hernia.

D. acute epiglottitis.

10-9   *Of all the adults who smoke, what percentage who quit are successful in their efforts?*

A. 2.5%

B. 8%

C. 15%

D. 30%

10-10   *Which of the following underlying lung diseases is the most common cause of a secondary spontaneous pneumothorax?*

A. COPD

B. Lung abscess

C. Cystic fibrosis

D. Tuberculosis

10-11 Harvey has severe obstructive sleep apnea and has just been ordered a continuous positive airway pressure (CPAP) machine. What do you tell him about it?

A. "You put it on at night after you've woken up several times."

B. "You must use it at least 5 nights during the week."

C. "You'll want to use it every night, all night long."

D. "We'll discontinue it if you develop nasal dryness or rhinitis."

10-12 The well-established risk factor(s) for a nosocomial pneumonia caused by a multidrug-resistant organism is (are)

A. antibiotic exposure and a hospital stay of more than 1 week.

B. age greater than 65 and having COPD.

C. having outpatient surgery.

D. having allergies to multiple antibiotics.

10-13 The two most predominant organisms constituting the normal flora of the oropharynx are

A. Streptococci and Staphylococci.

B. Streptococci and Moraxella catarrhalis.

C. Staphylococci and Candida albicans.

D. various protozoa and Staphylococci.

10-14 The most common reason for a chronic cough in children is

A. asthma.

B. a postinfection.

C. a postnasal drip.

D. an irritant.

10-15 Hyperresonance on percussion of the chest occurs with

A. emphysema.

B. pneumonia.

C. pleural effusion.

D. lung tumor.

10-16 Susie, age 10, has a cough that characteristically occurs all day long but never during sleep. You suspect

A. a psychogenic cough (or habit).

B. allergic rhinitis.

C. pertussis.

D. postnasal drip.

10-17 A pulmonary function test, such as spirometry, is helpful in the diagnosis of

A. chronic bronchitis.

B. lung cancer.

C. pneumonia.

D. tuberculosis.

10-18 In trying to differentiate between chronic bronchitis and emphysema, you know that chronic bronchitis

A. usually occurs after age 50 and has insidious progressive dyspnea.

B. usually presents with a cough that is mild and with scant, clear sputum, if any.

C. presents with adventitious sounds, wheezing and rhonchi, and a normal percussion note.

D. results in an increased total lung capacity with a markedly increased residual volume.

10-19 Which statement about viral croup is typically true?

A. Children typically present with a high fever.

B. A persistent severe cough is usually present.

C. It is usually preceded by a prodromal period of 12–72 hours.

D. There is usually no complaint of hoarseness.

10-20 What percentage of adults over 65 years of age typically receives the pneumococcus vaccine?

A. 10%

B. 30%

C. 60%

D. 90%

10-21 The nursing diagnosis of "impaired gas exchange" may be demonstrated by

A. clubbing of the fingers.

B. nasal flaring.

C. the use of accessory muscles.

D. a cough.

10-22   *Other than smoking cessation, which of the following slows the progression of COPD in smokers?*

A. Making sure the environment is free of all pollutants

B. Eliminating all pets from the environment

C. Engaging in moderate to high levels of physical activity

D. Remaining indoors with air conditioning as much as possible

10-23   *Cough and congestion result when breathing*

A. carbon monoxide.

B. sulfur dioxide.

C. tear gas.

D. carbon dioxide.

10-24   *Sally, age 49, has had asthma for several years but has never used a peak expiratory flowmeter. Should you now recommend it?*

A. No, she has been managing fine without it.

B. Yes, she might recognize early signs of deterioration.

C. Present the options and let Sally decide.

D. No, at her age it is not recommended.

10-25   *Which statement about chronic obstructive pulmonary disease (COPD) is true?*

A. The prevalence of COPD is directly related to increasing age.

B. The incidence of COPD is about equal in men and in women.

C. Cigar or pipe smoking does not increase the risk of developing COPD.

D. Environmental factors such as smoke do not affect the potential for COPD.

10-26   *Which group is at the highest risk for tuberculosis?*

A. Racial and ethnic minorities

B. Foreign-born individuals

C. Substance abusers

D. Nursing home residents

10-27   *Michael, age 52, has a gradual onset of dry cough, dyspnea, chills, fever, general malaise,*

headache, confusion, anorexia, diarrhea, myalgias, and arthralgias. *Which diagnosis do you suspect?*

A. Bronchopneumonia

B. Legionnaires' disease

C. Primary atypical pneumonia

D. *Pneumocystis jiroveci* pneumonia

10-28   *The CURB-65 criteria may be used to help assess whether a patient needs to be treated in the hospital or can be effectively treated at home. The R in CURB stands for*

A. respiratory rate.

B. rapid pulse rate.

C. Raynaud's syndrome present.

D. Region of the country where the client resides.

10-29   *Which of the following differential diagnoses should be considered with a chronic cough in children ages 1–5 years after the more common causes have been ruled out?*

A. Allergic rhinitis

B. Chronic sinusitis

C. Enlarged adenoids

D. Cystic fibrosis

10-30   *The causative agent of the community-acquired pneumonia seen most often in the client with an alcohol problem is*

A. *Pneumococcus.*

B. *Mycoplasma.*

C. *Legionella.*

D. *Haemophilus influenzae.*

10-31   *Which of the following drugs causes a cough by inducing mucus production (bronchorrhea)?*

A. Tobacco and/or marijuana

B. Beta-adrenergic blockers

C. Aspirin and NSAIDs

D. Cholinesterase inhibitors

10-32   *Unexplained nocturnal cough in an older adult should suggest*

A. allergies.

B. asthma.

C. congestive heart failure.

D. viral syndrome.

10-33 *Which of the following individuals most likely will have a false-negative reaction to the Mantoux test?*

A. Marvin, age 57

B. Jane, who is on a short course of corticosteroid therapy for an acute exacerbation of asthma

C. Jerry, who has lymphoid leukemia

D. Mary, who recently was exposed to someone coughing

10-34 *When you teach clients about using steroid inhalers for asthma or COPD, what information is essential?*

A. Keep the inhaler in the refrigerator.

B. Do not use another inhaler for 10 minutes after the steroid inhaler.

C. Rinse your mouth after using.

D. Be careful not to shake the container before using.

10-35 *Tina, age 49, is on multiple drug therapy for tuberculosis. She asks you how long she needs to take the drugs. You respond,*

A. "6 weeks to 2 months."

B. "4–6 months."

C. "6–9 months."

D. "1 year."

10-36 *Which sympathomimetic agents are the drugs of choice for asthma?*

A. Alpha agonists

B. Beta-1 agonists

C. Beta-2 agonists

D. Alpha antagonists

10-37 *Which of the following medications commonly prescribed for tuberculosis cannot be taken by pregnant women?*

A. Isoniazid (INH)

B. Rifampin (RIF)

C. Pyrazinamide (PZA)

D. Ethambutol (EMB)

10-38 *An infant who has periodic breathing with persistent or prolonged apnea (greater than 20 seconds) may have an increased risk of*

A. pneumonia.

B. left-sided congestive heart failure.

C. sudden infant death syndrome (SIDS).

D. anemia.

10-39 *What would be the 1-minute Apgar score for a newborn in good condition who needs only suctioning of the nose and mouth and otherwise routine care?*

A. 7–10

B. 6–8

C. 3–6

D. 0–2

10-40 *Increased severity of underlying illness, presence of an indwelling urethral catheter, and use of broad-spectrum antibiotics are risk factors predisposing clients to the development of*

A. tuberculosis.

B. decreased mobility.

C. pressure ulcers.

D. nosocomial pneumonia.

10-41 *Which of the following is considered a therapeutic indication for a bronchoscopy?*

A. To evaluate indeterminate lung lesions

B. To stage cancer preoperatively

C. To determine the extent of injury secondary to burns, inhalation, or other trauma

D. To remove a foreign body lodged in the trachea

10-42 *What is the name of the horizontal groove in the rib cage at the level of the diaphragm, extending from the sternum to the midaxillary line that occurs normally in some children as well as in children with rickets?*

A. The sternal groove

B. The rickettsial groove

C. The manubrial groove

D. Harrison's groove

10-43 Which irregular respiratory pattern has a series of three to four normal respirations followed by a period of apnea and is seen with head trauma, brain abscess, heat stroke, spinal meningitis, and encephalitis?

A. Cheyne-Stokes respiration

B. Biot's breathing

C. Kussmaul's respiration

D. Hypoventilation

10-44 What should be considered in all clients with adult-onset asthma or in clients with asthma that worsens in adulthood?

A. Occupational asthma

B. A suppressed immune system

C. Another immunologic disease

D. Concurrent COPD

10-45 Which is the most notable clinical manifestation of glottis (tongue) cancer?

A. Earache

B. Halitosis

C. Hoarseness

D. Frequent swallowing

10-46 When should a rescue course of prednisolone be initiated for an attack of asthma?

A. When the client is in step 1 (intermittent stage)

B. When the client is in step 2 (mild persistent stage)

C. When the client is in step 4 (severe persistent stage)

D. Whenever the client needs it, at any time and at any step

10-47 When teaching smokers about using nicotine gum to aid in smoking cessation, tell them to

A. chew the gum like regular gum.

B. discard the gum after 30 minutes.

C. drink a cup of coffee before chewing the gum because it assists in the nicotine absorption.

D. chew 6–9 pieces daily to help prevent nicotine withdrawal.

10-48 In which age group does respiratory retraction occur more often?

A. Newborn and infant

B. School-age child

C. Young adult

D. Older adult

10-49 Mary, age 69, has COPD. Her oxygen saturation is less than 85%. She is to start on oxygen therapy to relieve her symptoms. How often must she be on oxygen therapy to actually improve her oxygen saturation?

A. On an as-needed basis

B. Continuously

C. 15 hours per day

D. 24 hours per day

10-50 What is the definition of the spirometric assessment of residual volume?

A. The sum of the vital capacity and the residual volume

B. The amount of gas left in the lung after exhaling all that is physically possible

C. The volume that can be maximally exhaled after a passive exhalation

D. The measurement of the maximum flow rate achieved during the forced vital capacity maneuver

10-51 Which of the following statements is true regarding weight and smoking cessation?

A. Smokers weigh 10–20 lb. less than nonsmokers.

B. When smokers quit, 90% of them gain weight.

C. Men gain more weight than women when they quit.

D. Smokers gain weight after smoking cessation because they replace cigarettes with food.

10-52 Which drug category contains the drugs that are the first line of therapy for COPD?

A. Corticosteroids

B. Inhaled beta-2 agonist bronchodilators

C. Inhaled anticholinergic bronchodilators

D. Xanthines

10-53 Mr. Marks, age 54, has COPD. He has recently been experiencing difficulty in breathing. His arterial blood gas screening reveals pH 7.3, Pao_2 57 Hg, $Paco_2$ 54 mm Hg, and oxygen saturation 84%. Mr. Marks has

A. respiratory acidosis.

B. respiratory alkalosis.

C. metabolic acidosis.

D. metabolic alkalosis.

10-54 You are teaching Shawna, age 14, who has asthma, to use a home peak expiratory flowmeter daily to measure gross changes in peak expiratory flow. Which "zone" would rate her expiratory compliance as 50%–80% of her personal best?

A. White zone

B. Green zone

C. Yellow zone

D. Red zone

10-55 Jill, age 49, has daily symptoms of asthma. She uses her inhaled short-acting beta-2 agonist daily. Her exacerbations affect her activities, and they occur at least twice weekly and may last for days. She is affected more than once weekly during the night with an exacerbation. Which category of asthma severity is Jill in?

A. Mild intermittent

B. Mild persistent

C. Moderate persistent

D. Severe persistent

10-56 What do you include in your teaching about Spiriva (tiotropium) when you initially prescribe it for your client with COPD?

A. Use it every time you use your beta-2 agonist.

B. Stop taking all your other COPD medications.

C. Use this once per day.

D. Stop taking Spiriva if you develop the adverse effect of dry mouth.

10-57 Increased tactile fremitus occurs with

A. pleural effusion.

B. lobar pneumonia.

C. pneumothorax.

D. emphysema.

10-58 The following figure shows a method of assessing for digital clubbing called

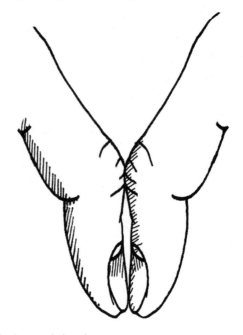

A. phalangeal depth ratio.

B. hyponychial angle.

C. Schamroth sign.

D. the "diamond" test.

10-59 What is the term describing an auscultation sound at the mediastinum in the presence of a mediastinal "crunch" that coincides with cardiac systole and diastole?

A. Homans' sign.

B. Hamman's sign.

C. Manubrium's sign.

D. Louis' sign.

10-60 Which of the following is the most frequent contributor to the incidence of carcinoma of the lung?

A. Chronic pneumonia

B. Exposure to materials such as asbestos, uranium, and radon

C. Chronic interstitial lung diseases

D. Cigarette smoking

10-61   *Marci, age 15, has been given a diagnosis of step 1 (mild intermittent) asthma. What long-term control therapy is indicated?*

A. None

B. A single agent with anti-inflammatory activity

C. An inhaled corticosteroid with the addition of long-acting bronchodilator if needed

D. Multiple long-term control medications with oral corticosteroids if needed

10-62   *Which is the accepted mass screening test for lung cancer?*

A. An annual physical examination

B. A chest x-ray

C. Sputum cytology

D. There is no accepted mass screening test for lung cancer.

10-63   *Sarah has allergic rhinitis and is currently being bothered by nasal congestion. Which of the following meds ordered for allergic rhinitis would be most appropriate?*

A. A decongestant nasal spray

B. An antihistamine intranasal spray

C. Ipratropium

D. Omalizumab

10-64   *What early acid-base disturbance occurs in a teenager admitted for an aspirin overdose?*

A. Respiratory acidosis

B. Respiratory alkalosis

C. Metabolic acidosis

D. Metabolic alkalosis

10-65   *Which of the following statements is true regarding pulmonary tuberculosis?*

A. Manifestations are usually confined to the respiratory system.

B. Dyspnea is usually present in the early stages.

C. Crackles and bronchial breath sounds are usually present in all phases of the disease.

D. Night sweats are often noted as a manifestation of fever.

10-66   *During the history portion of a respiratory assessment, it's particularly important to ask if the client takes which of the following drugs?*

A. Beta-2 agonists

B. Calcium channel blockers

C. Angiotensin-converting enzyme (ACE) inhibitors

D. Birth control pills

10-67   *Persons requiring home oxygen will have an oxygen saturation below*

A. 90%.

B. 85%.

C. 80%.

D. 75%.

10-68   *Which of the following conditions is characterized by intermittent episodes of airway obstruction caused by bronchospasm, excessive bronchial secretion, or edema of bronchial mucosa?*

A. Asthma

B. Atelectasis

C. Acute bronchitis

D. Emphysema

10-69   *Which of the following statements regarding the respiratory status of the pregnant woman is true?*

A. The thoracic cage may appear wider.

B. The costal angle may feel narrower.

C. Respirations may be shallow.

D. Oxygenation is decreased.

10-70   *Jessica, age 9 months, is brought into the clinic by her mother. She has a low-grade fever, stridor with agitation, some retractions, and a cough, but no drooling. You diagnose viral croup. Your next step would be to*

A. hospitalize Jessica.

B. start antibiotic therapy.

C. order supportive treatment.

D. begin treatment with corticosteroids.

10-71   *Theophylline when given for COPD acts*

A. as a bronchodilator.

B. by decreasing and strengthening respirations.

C. to impede mucociliary clearance.

D. with a negative inotropic effect.

10-72 *According to the Committee on Allergic Rhinitis and its Impact on Asthma (ARIA), sinus cleansing should be followed by which of the following as first-line therapy for the treatment of allergic rhinitis?*

A. A leukotriene receptor antagonist

B. An oral or spray decongestant

C. An intranasal corticosteroid spray

D. Sinus cleansing should be sufficient

10-73 *Which of the following medications prescribed for asthma acts to prevent binding of IgE receptors on basophils and mast cells?*

A. Anti-inflammatory agents

B. Bronchodilators

C. Mast cell stabilizers

D. Immunomodulators

10-74 *When teaching a mother who has a child with cystic fibrosis, you emphasize that the most important therapeutic approach to promote the child's pulmonary function is to*

A. continuously administer low-flow oxygen.

B. administer bronchodilators on a regular basis.

C. perform chest physiotherapy with postural drainage, percussion, and vibration.

D. use maintenance antibiotic prophylactic therapy.

10-75 *A cough caused by a postnasal drip related to sinusitis is more prevalent at what time of day?*

A. Continuously throughout the day

B. In the early morning

C. In the afternoon and evening

D. At night

10-76 *Laura, age 36, has an acute onset of dyspnea. Associated symptoms include chest pain, faintness, tachypnea, peripheral cyanosis, low blood pressure, crackles, and some wheezes. Her history reveals that she is taking birth control pills and that she smokes. What do you suspect?*

A. Asthma

B. Bronchitis

C. Pulmonary emboli

D. Pneumothorax

10-77 *Martin, age 76, has just been given a diagnosis of pneumonia. Which of the following is an indication that he should be hospitalized?*

A. Inability to take oral medications and multilobar involvement on chest x-ray

B. Alert and oriented status, slightly high but stable vital signs, and no one to take care of him at home

C. Sputum with gram-positive organisms

D. A complete blood count (CBC) showing leukocytosis

10-78 *What is a common inhaled allergen in allergic asthma (extrinsic asthma)?*

A. Smoke

B. Cold air

C. Strong smells

D. Pet dander

10-79 *Which of the following workers is at risk for developing pneumoconiosis?*

A. Farmers

B. Coal miners

C. Construction workers

D. Potters

10-80 *Harvey is taking theophylline for his COPD. Which of the following increases the clearance rate and might indicate the need for a higher dosage of theophylline to be ordered?*

A. Cigarette smoking

B. Hepatic insufficiency

C. Allopurinol (Zyloprim)

D. Cimetidine (Tagamet)

10-81 *What would the tumor node metastasis (TNM) classification be for a lung tumor that had carcinoma in situ, metastasis to the lymph nodes in the peribronchial or the ipsilateral hilar region, and distant metastasis to the spine?*

A. T1SN1M1

B. T2N0M0

C. T3N1M1

D. T0N1M0

10-82   *Jamie has her asthma well controlled by using only a beta-adrenergic metered-dose inhaler. Lately, however, she has had difficulty breathing during the night and her sleep has been interrupted about three times a week. What do you do?*

A. Prescribe a short course of steroid therapy.

B. Prescribe an inhaled steroid.

C. Prescribe a longer-acting bronchodilator.

D. Prescribe oral theophylline.

10-83   *What is the normal respiratory rate of an 18-month-old child while awake?*

A. 58–75 breaths per minute

B. 30–40 breaths per minute

C. 23–42 breaths per minute

D. 19–36 breaths per minute

10-84   *Coughing up blood or sputum that is streaked or tinged with blood is known as*

A. hemoptysis.

B. regurgitation.

C. bloody sputum.

D. rhinorrhea.

10-85   *What percentage of persons who smoke one pack of cigarettes per day or more have a cough?*

A. 10%–25%

B. 40%–60%

C. 75%

D. 100%

10-86   *Marisa, who is pregnant, has just been given a diagnosis of tuberculosis. What do you do?*

A. Wait until Marisa delivers and then begin therapy immediately.

B. Begin therapy with isoniazid (Nydrazid), rifampin (Rimactane), and pyrazinamide now.

C. Begin therapy with isoniazid, rifampin, and ethambutol (Myambutol) now.

D. Begin therapy with isoniazid now, wait to see how Marisa tolerates it, and then add rifampin, pyrazinamide, or ethambutol.

10-87   *What is the normal ratio of the anteroposterior chest diameter to the transverse chest diameter?*

A. 1:1

B. 1:2

C. 2:3

D. 2:1

10-88   *James, age 12, just moved here from Texas. He presents with a headache, cough, fever, rash on the legs and arms, myalgias, and dysuria. His white blood cell count is 12.9 with 8% bands and 7%–10% eosinophils. Electrolyte levels are normal. Blood cultures are negative. Sputum is not available. A Mantoux skin test so far is negative. What do you suspect?*

A. Pulmonary tuberculosis

B. Lymphoma

C. Asthma

D. Coccidioidomycosis

10-89   *A definitive test for cystic fibrosis is*

A. the sweat test.

B. a sputum culture.

C. a fecal fat test.

D. a Chymex test for pancreatic insufficiency.

10-90   *The definitive test for sleep apnea is*

A. a Holter monitor.

B. a trial period of a continuous positive air pressure (CPAP) appliance.

C. an overnight polysomnogram.

D. an ear, nose, and throat (ENT) specialist confirming an abnormal uvula.

10-91   *What is effective in the treatment of pneumonia, atelectasis, and cystic fibrosis?*

A. Deep breathing

B. Oxygen

C. Inhalers

D. Chest physiotherapy

10-92   Which of the following statements is true when trying to differentiate pulmonary from cardiac causes of dyspnea on exertion?

A. When the cause is pulmonary, the rate of recovery to normal respiration is slow, and dyspnea abates eventually after cessation of exercise.

B. Clients with dyspnea from cardiac causes remain dyspneic much longer after cessation of exercise.

C. In dyspnea arising from cardiac causes, the heart rate will return to preexercise levels within a few minutes after cessation of exercising.

D. Clients with pulmonary dyspnea have minimal dyspnea at rest.

10-93   Evidence-based practice has shown that clients with COPD will benefit the most from which of the following single modalities?

A. Nutritional supplementation

B. Routine use of inspiratory muscle training

C. Pulmonary rehabilitation

D. Psychosocial interventions

10-94   Which of the following statements about sarcoidosis is true?

A. It commonly occurs in persons in their 50s.

B. It is more common in whites than in blacks.

C. Many organs may be involved, but the most involved organ is the lung.

D. It occurs more frequently in men than in women.

10-95   The most common mode of transmission of the common cold in adults is

A. hand-to-hand transmission.

B. persons coughing into the air.

C. environmental pollutants.

D. unclean food utensils.

10-96   In which condition would you assess vesicular breath sounds, moderate vocal resonance, and localized crackles with sibilant wheezes?

A. Bronchiectasis

B. Acute bronchitis

C. Emphysema

D. Asthma

10-97   To ease their breathing, clients with COPD often position themselves in

A. an erect sitting position.

B. a tripod position.

C. a supine position.

D. a prone position.

10-98   After a total laryngectomy for laryngeal cancer, the client will have a

A. permanent tracheostomy.

B. temporary tracheostomy until the internal surgical incision heals.

C. temporary tracheostomy until an implant can be done.

D. patent normal airway.

10-99   Community-acquired bacterial pneumonia is most commonly caused by

A. Streptococcus pneumoniae.

B. Mycoplasma pneumoniae.

C. Haemophilus influenzae.

D. Staphylococcus aureus.

10-100   What is the gold standard for the diagnosis of asthma?

A. Validated quality-of-life questionnaires

B. Client's perception of "clogged" airways

C. Spirometry

D. Bronchoscopy

10-101   A risk factor for pulmonary embolism in women includes which of the following?

A. Extreme thinness

B. Alcohol intake

C. Cigarette smoking

D. Hypotension

10-102   With which voice sound technique do you normally hear a muffled eeee through the stethoscope on auscultating the chest when the client says "eeee"?

A. Bronchophony

B. Egophony

C. Whispered pectoriloquy

D. Tonometry

10-103 Which of the following peripharyngeal upper respiratory tract infections occurs most often in children ages 2–5 years?

A. Peritonsillar abscess

B. Epiglottitis

C. Laryngotracheobronchitis (croup)

D. Bacterial tracheitis

10-104 You've been counseling your client about her asthma. You realize she doesn't understand your suggestions when she tells you that she'll do which of the following?

A. Cover the mattress and pillows in airtight, dustproof covers.

B. Wash the bedding weekly and dry it on a hot setting for 20 minutes.

C. Avoid sleeping on natural fibers such as wool or down.

D. Open the windows and air out the room daily.

10-105 When should well individuals be screened for tuberculosis?

A. Every year

B. Every other year

C. At age 1 year, then again at entry to preschool or kindergarten, and then at some point during adolescence

D. Screening is not necessary

10-106 In which condition would the trachea be deviated toward the nonaffected side?

A. Pleural effusion and thickening

B. Pneumonia

C. Bronchiectasis

D. Pulmonary fibrosis

10-107 Which of the following statements is true regarding the recurrence of a spontaneous pneumothorax?

A. A primary spontaneous pneumothorax is more likely to recur than a secondary one.

B. A secondary spontaneous pneumothorax is more likely to recur than a primary one.

C. Recurrence rates for both primary and secondary spontaneous pneumothorax are similar.

D. Spontaneous pneumothorax rarely recurs.

10-108 Which bacterial agent is the most common pathogen in an acute exacerbation of chronic bronchitis?

A. *Streptococcus pneumoniae*

B. *Haemophilus influenzae*

C. *Branhamella catarrhalis*

D. *Moraxella catarrhalis*

10-109 The inspiratory rate equals the expiratory rate with which breath sound?

A. Bronchial

B. Bronchovesicular

C. Vesicular

D. Tracheal

10-110 Which drug contributes to a decreased response to tuberculin skin testing (TST)?

A. Antibiotics

B. Inhaled allergy medications

C. Corticosteroids

D. Birth control pills

10-111 The classic presentation of a child with epiglottitis shows a triad of the three D's. Which of the following D's does NOT belong?

A. Drooling

B. Dysphagia

C. Dyspnea

D. Distress

10-112 Mark, age 72, has been living in a shelter for 4 months. Today he appears at the clinic complaining of productive cough, weight loss, weakness, anorexia, night sweats, and generalized malaise. These have been bothering him for 8 weeks. What would be one of the first tests you order?

A. Mantoux test

B. Chest x-ray

C. Complete blood work

D. Sputum culture

10-113 *How does pregnancy affect asthma?*

A. During pregnancy, asthma usually improves.

B. During pregnancy, asthma usually worsens.

C. Symptoms in about one-third of pregnant women with asthma improve, about one-third are unchanged, and about one-third worsen.

D. Symptoms in about one-half of pregnant women improve; those of the other half worsen.

10-114 *The most common cause of a persistent cough in children of all ages is*

A. an allergy.

B. recurrent viral bronchitis.

C. asthma.

D. an upper respiratory infection.

10-115 *Which shape of the thorax is normal in an adult?*

A. Elliptical

B. Funnel

C. Pectus carinatum

D. Barrel

Answers

10-1   Answer C

The antibiotic of choice for the treatment of *Streptococcus pneumoniae* pneumonia is penicillin. However, the number of penicillin-resistant pneumococcal infections is increasing. These cases require treatment with more powerful antibiotics. Alternative choices are erythromycin and clindamycin. Dicloxacillin is the antibiotic of choice for infections caused by *Staphylococcus aureus*, erythromycin is the antibiotic of choice for infections caused by *Mycoplasma pneumoniae*, and ampicillin clavulanate is the antibiotic of choice for *Moraxella catarrhalis* infections. Once therapy has been started, the client's respiratory and cardiovascular status should be monitored, along with his or her general overall status, including level of energy, appetite, and temperature. Most clients on the appropriate antibiotic therapy improve within 48–72 hours. Fever that continues more than 24 hours after initiating therapy usually does not indicate failure of the antibiotic; rather, the usual response to therapy is a gradual reduction in the maximum daily temperature.

10-2   Answer D

Sudden infant death syndrome (SIDS) is the most common cause of sudden and unexpected death in infants; 40%–50% of postneonatal infant mortality is caused by SIDS. The peak incidence of SIDS is at ages 2–4 months; 95% of all SIDS deaths occur by age 6 months.

10-3   Answer C

In an inner-city study of 476 children, researchers determined that the combination of cockroach allergy and exposure to the insects is an important cause of asthma-related illness and hospitalizations among that group of children. Levels of cockroach, dust mite, and cat allergens in the children's homes were measured and allergy skin tests were performed on the children. Of these children, 37% were allergic to cockroaches, 35% to dust mites, and 23% to cats. The study then assessed the severity of the children's asthma over 12 months and found that children who were both allergic to cockroaches and exposed to high cockroach allergen levels were hospitalized for their asthma 3.3 times more often than children who were allergic but not exposed to high levels of cockroach allergen, or children who were exposed to high levels of cockroach allergen but who were not allergic.

10-4   Answer D

Tuberculosis is a reportable disease. Every potential case must be reported to the local health department. This includes when the client's Mantoux test shows an induration of 15 mm, when a case of tuberculosis is merely suspected, and when an asymptomatic client has a positive chest x-ray for pulmonary tuberculosis. Screening tests in higher-risk areas with suspected infection that do not have a positive reaction do not need to be reported. These include the appearance of a red area with an induration of less than 10 mm on the first test (less than 5 mm on employees with a yearly screen).

10-5   Answer B

When asthma does not respond to traditional therapy, it may be because the patient has another syndrome that mimics asthma or because he or she has a comorbid condition that complicates it. The two most common syndromes that mimic asthma are vocal cord dysfunction and upper airway obstruction. Both may result in dyspnea and apparent wheezing but not show any response to standard asthma therapy. COPD and bronchitis may be comorbid conditions that may complicate asthma.

10-6   Answer B

Approximately 50% of children with viral croup show a tapered symmetric subglottic narrowing or "steeple" sign on the anteroposterior view on an x-ray. The x-rays do not correlate with the level of disease. Epiglottitis differs clinically from croup by an abrupt onset of severe symptoms, often over a matter of hours.

10-7   Answer C

A primary spontaneous pneumothorax usually occurs in healthy individuals without preexisting lung disease. It occurs more commonly in young, tall, asthenic men and is an accumulation of air in the normally airless pleural space between the lung and chest wall. Persons with Marfan's syndrome are more prone to aortic aneurysms, not to pneumothorax.

10-8   Answer D

Stridor, a high-pitched inspiratory crowing sound, can be heard on auscultation when a client has acute epiglottitis or croup. Persistent fine crackles can be heard with atelectasis, expiratory wheezes with asthma, and persistent peristaltic sounds with diminished breath sounds on the same side with a diaphragmatic hernia.

10-9   Answer B

Nearly 17 million Americans try to quit smoking each year. Only about 1.3 million Americans are able to remain smoke free. Only 8% or so of smokers who quit smoking are successful in their efforts. Although the overall success rate of smoking cessation is disappointing, smoking cessation programs have been extremely helpful. Motivation is the key to a successful effort, along with making every clinical encounter an opportunity to discuss the topic. At the very least, every client should be asked about his or her smoking history. Clinicians should advise smokers to quit, assist them in setting a quitting date, provide self-help materials, and evaluate them for nicotine replacement therapy (patches, nasal spray, or gum) or pharmacological therapies.

10-10   Answer A

Secondary spontaneous pneumothoraces are most often due to underlying emphysematous COPD or HIV-associated *Pneumocystis jiroveci* pneumonia (PCP). Other predisposing conditions include lung abscess, cystic fibrosis, and tuberculosis.

10-11   Answer C

CPAP administered through a nasal mask has become the most common treatment for obstructive sleep apnea (OSA). Depending on the patient's mode of breathing, a larger mask encompassing the mouth may also be used. CPAP dramatically eliminates apneas and hypopneas, improves sleep architecture, and reduces daytime sleepiness, even for those with mild sleep apnea. In order to be effective, the machine must be used all night long, every night. Minor adverse effects of CPAP include feelings of suffocation, nasal drying or rhinitis, ear pain, difficulty in exhaling, mask and mouth leaks, chest and back pain, and conjunctivitis. Most of these can be alleviated.

10-12   Answer A

Treatment of nosocomial pneumonia is complicated by the frequent involvement of multidrug-resistant organisms. Prior exposure to antibiotics and a hospital stay of more than 1 week are well-established risk factors for infection with these organisms.

10-13   Answer A

Streptococci (especially *Streptococcus viridans*) and *Staphylococci* (especially *Staphylococcus aureus*) are the two most predominant types of organisms constituting the normal flora of the oropharynx. They are followed by *Streptococcus pyogenes*, *Streptococcus pneumoniae*, *Moraxella catarrhalis*, *Neisseria* species, and *Lactobacilli*.

10-14   Answer B

The most common reason for a chronic cough in children is a postinfection. The other reasons, in order of frequency, are asthma, a postnasal drip, and irritants. Uncommon causes include other respiratory infections, pertussis, a foreign body, cystic fibrosis, congenital abnormalities, and psychogenic reasons.

10-15   Answer A

Hyperresonance on percussion of the chest is found when too much air is present, such as occurs with emphysema or a pneumothorax. A dull sound on percussion indicates an abnormal density in the lungs, such as occurs with pneumonia, pleural effusion, a lung tumor, or atelectasis.

10-16   Answer A

If a cough characteristically occurs all day long but never during sleep, suspect that it is a psychogenic cough (or habit). Allergic rhinitis results in a cough that is seasonal, pertussis in a cough that is followed by a "whoop," and a postnasal drip results in a throat-clearing cough.

10-17   Answer A

A pulmonary function test, such as spirometry, is helpful in the diagnosis of restrictive lung disease and obstructive lung disease, including chronic bronchitis and asthma. Clients with postinfectious or cough-variant asthma may show mild obstruction, but they often have normal spirometry. A chest x-ray confirms the diagnosis of pneumonia. While spirometry may show a decrease in lung capacity with advanced lung cancer, it is not diagnostic.

10-18   Answer C

In trying to differentiate between chronic bronchitis and emphysema, remember that chronic bronchitis presents with adventitious sounds, wheezing and rhonchi, and a normal percussion note. Chronic bronchitis usually occurs after age 35, with recurrent respiratory infections. There is usually a persistent, productive cough of copious mucopurulent sputum, and pulmonary function studies show normal or decreased total lung capacity with a moderately increased residual volume. In a client with emphysema, the onset is usually after age 50. There is an insidious progressive dyspnea and the cough is usually absent or mild with scant, clear sputum, if any. There are also distant or diminished breath sounds and a hyperresonant percussion note. The pulmonary function studies show an increased total lung capacity with a markedly increased residual volume.

10-19   Answer C

Viral croup is usually preceded by a prodromal period of 12–72 hours. Typically, a low-grade fever is present, along with a hoarse voice, mild cough, and coryza.

10-20   Answer C

Despite widespread endorsement by numerous medical and nursing organizations, the pneumococcal vaccine was administered to 60% of adults over the age of 65 in 2008. Experts from the Advisory Committee on Immunization Practices estimate that as many as 90% of deaths attributed to *Streptococcus pneumoniae* could be prevented if use of the currently available vaccine were more common. Pneumococci account for more deaths than any other vaccine-preventable disease. Healthy People 2020 cites a target of 90% of noninstitutionalized adults over the age of 65 having the vaccine by 2020.

10-21   Answer A

The nursing diagnosis of "impaired gas exchange" may be demonstrated by clubbing of the fingers. Nasal flaring and cough are present if the client has a nursing diagnosis of "ineffective airway clearance" or "ineffective breathing pattern." The use of accessory muscles to assist breathing may indicate a nursing diagnosis of "ineffective breathing pattern."

10-22   Answer C

Research has shown that engaging in moderate to high levels of physical activity slows the decline in smokers' lung function and may help prevent as many as 21% of COPD cases.

10-23   Answer B

Cough and congestion result when breathing sulfur dioxide. Carbon monoxide produces dizziness, headache, and fatigue. Tear gas irritates the conjunctiva and produces a flow of tears. Carbon dioxide produces sleepiness.

10-24   Answer B

Daily peak flow monitoring has long been recommended for clients with asthma. Guidelines from the National Asthma Education and Prevention Program of the National Heart, Lung, and Blood Institute increase the flexibility of this recommendation and suggest that the use of peak flow measurements be individualized. The guidelines recommend that all clients with persistent asthma assess peak flow each morning. Subsequent assessments are necessary during the day when the morning measurement is less than 80% of the client's personal best peak expiratory flow (PEF) measurement. The goal of daily PEF monitoring is to recognize early signs of deterioration in airway function so that corrective steps can be initiated.

10-25   Answer A

The prevalence of chronic obstructive pulmonary disease (COPD) is directly related to increasing age. Men are affected much more often than women because the percentage of men who smoke is greater than that of women. The risk of developing COPD is related to the number of cigarettes smoked and the duration of smoking. Cigar or pipe smoking also increases the risk of developing COPD, but to a lesser extent than does cigarette smoking. Environmental factors, including secondhand smoke, also affect the potential for COPD. The usual client with COPD is one who is older than age 50 and has smoked one pack of cigarettes per day for more than 20 years.

10-26   Answer A

Groups at high risk for tuberculosis include racial and ethnic minorities (70% of all reported cases in the United States); foreign-born individuals (24% of all cases in the United States); substance abusers (5–20 times normal); individuals with HIV infection (40–100 times normal); and residents of prisons, nursing homes, and shelters (2–10 times normal).

10-27   Answer B

If a client has a dry cough, dyspnea, chills, fever, general malaise, headache, confusion, anorexia, diarrhea, myalgias, and arthralgias, suspect Legionnaires' disease. Legionnaires' disease has a gradual onset. Bronchopneumonia has a gradual onset with a cough, scattered crackles, minimal dyspnea and respiratory distress, and a low-grade fever. Primary atypical pneumonia has a gradual onset with a dry, hacking, nonproductive cough; fever; headache; myalgias; and arthralgias. *Pneumocystis jiroveci* pneumonia occurs in clients with AIDS. It has an abrupt onset with a dry cough, tachypnea, shortness of breath, significant respiratory distress, and fever.

10-28   Answer A

The CURB-65 criteria to determine the severity of community acquired pneumonia (CAP) is an objective, easy tool to remember. A point is given for each of the following if present. The C is for confusion (new documentation). The U is for BUN greater than 19 mg per dL. The R is for a respiratory rate equal to or greater than 30 breaths/min. The B is for the BP (systolic less than 90 mm Hg or a

diastolic pressure equal to or less than 60 mm Hg). A point is also given if the patient is 65 years of age or over. A score of 1 is low risk, and the patient may be treated at home. With a score of 2, there should be a short period of hospitalization or closely monitored outpatient treatment. A score of 3 or greater indicates severe pneumonia, and the patient should be hospitalized with consideration of ICU placement.

10-29   Answer D

A chronic cough in children ages 1–5 years should suggest bronchiectasis or cystic fibrosis after the more common causes—allergic rhinitis, chronic sinusitis, and enlarged adenoids—have been ruled out. Although rare, chronic cough in children younger than age 1 should suggest congenital malformations or neonatal infections, including viral and chlamydial pneumonias. Other relatively rare causes of chronic cough in young infants include recurrent aspiration of milk, saliva, or gastric contents.

10-30   Answer A

The community-acquired pneumonia seen most often in the client with or without an alcohol problem is pneumococcal, which is caused by the gram-positive bacteria *Pneumococcus* (also called *Streptococcus pneumoniae*). Alcoholics are at risk for the usual pathogens, but they also have a higher incidence of pneumonia caused by gram-negative organisms (including *Klebsiella pneumoniae*, *Legionella*, and *Haemophilus influenzae*) and anaerobic pneumonia secondary to aspiration than do people who are not alcohol abusers.

10-31   Answer D

Cholinesterase inhibitors cause a cough by inducing mucus production (bronchorrhea). Tobacco and marijuana cause a cough by being direct irritants. Beta-adrenergic blockers, aspirin, and NSAIDs cause a cough by potentiating reactive airway disease.

10-32   Answer C

Unexplained nocturnal cough in an older adult should suggest congestive heart failure. Older adults, whose physical activity may be restricted by arthritis or other associated diseases, may not present with the usual symptom of dyspnea on exertion. The main complaint instead may be a chronic unexplained cough that may occur only at night while the client is recumbent or a cough that may worsen at night.

10-33   Answer C

Individuals predisposed to have a false-negative reaction to the Mantoux test include newborns and those older than age 60; those in an immunosuppressive state, such as persons taking long-term corticosteroids and anticancer agents or those with HIV infection or chronic renal failure; persons with a neoplasm, especially lymphoid leukemia and lymphomas; and persons with an acute infection, such as measles, mumps, chickenpox, typhoid fever, brucellosis, typhus, and pertussis. Tuberculosis had been close to eradication until HIV appeared. Coughing alone is not predictive of TB.

10-34   Answer C

After using a steroid inhaler, the client should always rinse his or her mouth to prevent oral candidiasis ("thrush"). Brushing the teeth will get rid of any bad taste. The inhaler or diskus should be shaken first. If the client is also taking a beta-2 agonist, tell him or her to take that first, as that will open the airway, allowing more of the steroid medication to be administered.

10-35   Answer C

With the use of multiple drug therapy for tuberculosis, the duration of the therapy has shortened from 1 year to a standard of 6–9 months. The current minimal acceptable duration for treatment of all children and adults with culture-positive TB is 6 months. An alternative regimen for persons who cannot take PZA (e.g., pregnant women) consists of a 9-month regimen of INH and RIF. If the client has a drug-resistant organism or is immunodeficient, the precise duration of therapy is uncertain but may extend from 1–2 years in some cases.

10-36   Answer C

The sympathomimetic agents that are the first-line drugs of choice for hyperreactive airway disease—asthma—are the beta-2 agonists. There are different adrenergic receptors in different tissues. Beta-2 adrenergic agents (agonists) are more specific in their action to promote bronchodilation and are less likely to be associated with side effects. In addition to promoting bronchodilation, these agents also increase secretion of electrolytes by the airways and enhance mucociliary activity. Protein kinase A

levels increase within the smooth muscle cells, resulting in inhibition of myosin phosphorylation and smooth muscle cell relaxation. Alpha agonists cause vasoconstriction and beta-1 adrenergic agents (agonists) increase cardiac contractility and heart rate, effects that are undesirable in clients with asthma. Alpha antagonist is not a drug class.

10-37   Answer C

Pyrazinamide (PZA) should not be taken by pregnant women. Active tuberculosis should be treated with isoniazid and ethambutol and continued for at least 18 months to prevent relapse. Two-drug regimens are not recommended if isoniazid resistance is suspected. If a third drug or a more potent drug is necessary due to extensive or severe disease, rifampin could be added. Because of the risk of ototoxicity, streptomycin should not be prescribed. Isoniazid is the safest drug during pregnancy.

10-38   Answer C

An infant who has periodic breathing with persistent or prolonged apnea (greater than 20 seconds) may have an increased risk of sudden infant death syndrome. Rapid respiratory rates accompany pneumonia, anemia, fever, pain, and heart disease. Tachypnea (a very rapid respiratory rate of 50–100 breaths per minute) during sleep may be an early sign of left-sided congestive heart failure.

10-39   Answer A

A 1-minute Apgar score of 7–10 indicates that the newborn is in good condition, needing only suctioning of the nose and mouth and otherwise routine care. A 1-minute Apgar score of 3–6 indicates a moderately depressed newborn requiring more resuscitation and close monitoring. A 1-minute Apgar score of 0–2 indicates a severely depressed newborn requiring full resuscitation, ventilator support, and intensive care. The interpretation of Apgar scores is 7–10, good to excellent; 4–6, fair; and less than 4, poor.

10-40   Answer D

Risk factors predisposing clients to the development of nosocomial (hospital-acquired) pneumonia include increased severity of the underlying illness, presence of an indwelling urethral catheter, use of broad-spectrum antibiotics (which increase the risk of superinfection), previous hospitalization, presence of intravascular catheters, intubation (especially prolonged intubation), and recent thoracic or upper abdominal surgery.

10-41   Answer D

There are both diagnostic and therapeutic indications for a bronchoscopy. The therapeutic uses include removal of mucous plugs, secretions, and foreign bodies; assistance with difficult endotracheal intubations; and treatment of endobronchial neoplasms. Diagnostic uses include evaluation of indeterminate lung lesions (abnormal chest film); preoperative staging of cancer; determination of the extent of injury secondary to burns, inhalation, or other trauma; assessment of airway patency, including problems associated with endotracheal tubes, wheeze, and stridor; investigation of unexplained symptoms (cough, hemoptysis, stridor, and so on) or unexplained findings (recurrent laryngeal nerve paralysis, recent diaphragmatic paralysis); evaluation of suspicious or malignant sputum cytology; bronchoalveolar lavage for interstitial lung disease; and specimen collection for selective cultures or suspected infection. The key word is *therapeutic*.

10-42   Answer D

Harrison's groove is the name of the horizontal groove in the rib cage at the level of the diaphragm, extending from the sternum to the midaxillary line. It occurs normally in some children and also occurs in children with rickets. The other grooves are just listed as distractors.

10-43   Answer B

Biot's breathing is the term for an irregular respiratory pattern of a series of three to four normal respirations followed by a period of apnea. It is seen with head trauma, brain abscess, heat stroke, spinal meningitis, and encephalitis. Cheyne-Stokes respiration is similar, except that the pattern is regular. The most common cause of Cheyne-Stokes respiration is severe congestive heart failure, followed by renal failure, meningitis, drug overdose, and increased intracranial pressure. This regular pattern occurs normally in infants and older adults during sleep. Kussmaul's respiration is hyperventilation with an increase in both the rate and depth of the breaths. Hypoventilation is a reduced rate and depth of breathing that causes an increase in carbon dioxide in the bloodstream.

10-44   Answer A

Occupational asthma should be considered in all clients with adult-onset asthma or in clients with asthma that worsens in adulthood. As many as one in five cases of asthma may be a result of exposure to chemicals in the workplace. Approximately 250 chemicals have been found to cause occupational asthma symptoms, which usually appear soon after a worker is first exposed to the asthma-inducing chemical but sometimes may appear months to years later.

10-45   Answer C

Clinical manifestations of cancer of the larynx include earache, halitosis, hoarseness, change in the voice, painful swallowing, dyspnea, and a palpable lump in the neck. The most notable manifestation of glottic (tongue) cancer is hoarseness or a change in the voice because the tumor prevents complete closure of the glottis during speech.

10-46   Answer D

A rescue course of prednisolone should be initiated for an attack of asthma whenever the client needs it, at any time and at any step. Attempts should be made to use systemic corticosteroids in an acute or rescue fashion: a short burst followed by tapering to the lowest dose possible and preferably discontinued, with inhaled steroids prescribed for chronic or maintenance therapy.

10-47   Answer B

When teaching smokers about using nicotine gum to aid in smoking cessation, tell them to discard the gum after 30 minutes. The gum should not be chewed like regular gum. A piece is chewed only long enough to release the nicotine, which produces a peppery taste, and then "parked" between the gums and buccal mucosa to allow for nicotine absorption. Drinking liquids while the gum is in the mouth should be avoided. Acidic beverages such as coffee should be avoided for 1–2 hours before the use of the gum. The smoker should be instructed to chew 9–12 pieces daily to help prevent nicotine withdrawal.

10-48   Answer A

Retractions occur more often in the newborn and infant than at other ages because the intercostal tissues are weak and underdeveloped. Supraclavicular or suprasternal retractions suggest upper airway obstruction, while retraction of intercostals or subcostal muscles suggests lower airway obstruction.

10-49   Answer C

To decrease mortality in clients with COPD whose oxygen saturations are less than 85%, oxygen must be used at least 15 hours per day to be of more than symptomatic benefit. The oxygen can be either a specific concentration delivered by mask or a flow rate administered through a nasal cannula. It is needed to maintain adequate oxygenation levels during both activity and rest. The goal of therapy is a Pao_2 of 60 mm Hg or Sao_2 of 90%.

10-50   Answer B

The definition of the spirometric assessment of residual volume is the amount of gas left in the lung after exhaling all that is physically possible. This measurement is expressed as a ratio of total lung capacity to vital capacity. The total lung capacity is the sum of the vital capacity and the residual volume. The expiratory reserve volume is the volume that can be maximally exhaled after a passive exhalation. The peak flow is the measurement of the maximum flow rate achieved during the forced vital capacity maneuver.

10-51   Answer D

Smokers weigh 5–10 lb less than nonsmokers of comparable age and height. When smokers quit, 80% of them gain weight; the average weight gain is 5 lb, but about 10% of that 80% who gain weight gain more than 25 lb. On average, women gain more weight than men: 8 lb as compared with 5 lb. Heavy smokers (those who smoke two packs per day or more) gain more weight than light smokers. This weight gain is caused by replacing the habit of smoking cigarettes with eating to satisfy the need for oral gratification.

10-52   Answer B

All the drugs listed may be appropriate for COPD, but inhaled short-acting beta-2 agonist bronchodilators are the first line of therapy in the Global Initiative for Chronic Obstructive Lung Disease (GOLD) in stage 1.

10-53   Answer A

Respiratory acidosis results when the serum $Paco_2$ exceeds 45 mm Hg and the serum pH is less than 7.35. It occurs when there is a reduction in the rate of alveolar ventilation in relation to the rate of carbon dioxide production. The end result is an accumulation of dissolved carbon dioxide or carbonic acid. Mr. Marks's COPD leads to alveolar hypoventilation with an acute retention of carbon dioxide, resulting in acute respiratory acidosis. With respiratory alkalosis, hyperventilation is usually evident, the $Paco_2$ is less than 35 mm Hg, and the pH is greater than 7.45. In metabolic acidosis, the HCO_3 is less than 22 mEq/L and the pH is less than 7.35. In metabolic alkalosis, the HCO_3 is more than 26 mEq/L and the pH is greater than 7.45.

10-54   Answer C

Shawna should perform a peak expiratory flowmeter reading daily during a 2-week period when she feels well. The highest number recorded during this period is her "personal best." A green zone (80%–100% of her personal best) is when no asthma symptoms are present and she should continue with her normal medication regimen. A yellow zone (50%–80% of her personal best) occurs when asthma symptoms may be starting and signals caution. A red zone (below 50% of her personal best) indicates that an asthma attack is occurring and that Shawna should take her inhaled beta-2 agonist and repeat the peak flow assessment. There is no white zone.

10-55   Answer C

Jill has daily symptoms of asthma. She uses her inhaled short-acting beta-2 agonist daily. Her exacerbations affect her activities, and they occur at least twice weekly and may last for days. She is affected more than once weekly during the night with an exacerbation. Jill is in the step 3 (moderate persistent) category of asthma severity. This is because she has daily symptoms along with exacerbations affecting her activity and nocturnal symptoms that occur more than once per week. In step 1 (mild intermittent) asthma, symptoms are no more frequent than twice weekly, and nocturnal symptoms are no more frequent than twice per month. In step 2 (mild persistent) asthma, symptoms are more frequent than twice weekly but less than once a day, exacerbations may affect activity, and nocturnal symptoms are more frequent than twice per month. In step 4 (severe persistent) asthma, the client has continuous symptoms with limited physical activity, frequent exacerbations, and frequent nocturnal symptoms.

10-56   Answer C

Spiriva (tiotropium) is a once-daily, long-acting anticholinergic. It results in improved lung function studies and reduction in the use of rescue medication and in COPD exacerbations. The most frequently reported adverse side effect is that of dry mouth, which is easily remedied with increased hydration.

10-57   Answer B

Increased tactile fremitus occurs with compression or consolidation of lung tissue, such as occurs in conditions like lobar pneumonia. Decreased tactile fremitus occurs when anything obstructs the transmission of vibrations, such as occurs in conditions like pleural effusion, pneumothorax, and emphysema or with an obstructed bronchus.

10-58   Answer C

The Schamroth sign is useful as a quick method of assessing for digital clubbing. The dorsal surfaces of the terminal phalanges of similar fingers are placed together. With clubbing, the normal diamond-shaped window at the bases of the nailbeds disappears and a prominent distal angle forms between the end of the nails. Normally, this angle is minimal or nonexistent. The phalangeal depth ratio measures the ratio of the distal phalangeal depth to the interphalangeal depth. It is normally less than 1 but increases to more than 1 with finger clubbing. *Hyponychial* refers to the nailbed, and there is no such thing as a diamond test.

10-59   Answer B

An auscultation sound at the mediastinum in the presence of a mediastinal "crunch" that coincides with cardiac systole and diastole is known as Hamman's sign, named after the American physician Louis Hamman. It is present with spontaneous mediastinal emphysema or pneumomediastinum. Homans' sign is pain in the calf when the foot is passively dorsiflexed; it is a possible sign of deep vein thrombosis (DVT) in the calf. There is no Manubrium or Louis sign.

10-60   Answer D

The following contribute to the incidence of carcinoma of the lung: cigarette smoking; exposure to materials such as asbestos, uranium, and radon; and chronic interstitial lung diseases such as pulmonary fibrosis arising from scleroderma. It is estimated that approximately 2 million persons will develop carcinoma of the lung in each of the next several years; 85% of all lung carcinomas are secondary to cigarette use.

10-61   Answer A

No long-term control therapy is indicated for all clients with step 1 (mild intermittent) asthma, be they adolescents, children, or adults. Clients with step 1 asthma need only quick relief with a beta-2 agonist as needed. There is no indication for long-term control until they approach step 2 (mild persistent) asthma.

10-62   Answer D

Currently, there is no accepted mass screening test for lung cancer. Because of cost, mass screening for lung cancer in healthy individuals with no risk factors is not recommended. Individuals who are at high risk (those who are cigarette smokers, have been exposed to radon or asbestos, and have a strong family history) should be periodically screened through the use of an annual physical examination, chest x-ray, and possibly sputum cytology. Suspicious chest x-rays should be followed by further diagnostic tests.

10-63   Answer A

For Sarah, with allergic rhinitis, who has nasal congestion, a decongestant nasal spray would be indicated. For rhinorrhea, an antihistamine intranasal spray or ipratropium would be indicated. Omalizumab may be necessary for a grade 4 allergic rhinitis–severe persistent.

10-64   Answer B

Respiratory alkalosis is the early acid-base disturbance that occurs in an aspirin overdose (salicylate intoxication). It results from direct stimulation of the respiratory center in the medulla, which causes an increase in pH and a decrease in $Paco_2$. This leads to metabolic acidosis as the body compensates by renal excretion of bicarbonate to normalize the pH.

10-65   Answer D

In the client with pulmonary tuberculosis, night sweats are often noted as a manifestation of fever. With pulmonary tuberculosis, systemic manifestations are usually present; symptoms are not confined to the respiratory system. Fever occurs in 50%–80% of cases, and symptoms such as malaise and weight loss are frequent. Dyspnea, an ominous feature, usually occurs with widespread advanced disease. Crackles and bronchial breath sounds may be present, but more often there are no abnormal findings, even in well-developed pulmonary disease.

10-66   Answer C

A cough occurs in about 10% of clients who take ACE inhibitors such as captopril (Capoten) and enalapril (Vasotec). A complete history of prescribed and over-the-counter (OTC) drugs, including any herbal preparations, should be taken. Knowing all drugs taken is important, but because of the potential for ACE inhibitors to cause a cough, it is particularly important to ask about this category of drugs when doing a respiratory assessment.

10-67   Answer B

Requirements for home oxygen include (1) a Pao_2 of 55 mm Hg or less or an oxygen saturation (Sa) below 85% and (2) a Pao_2 of 55–59 mm Hg if erythrocytosis (hematocrit of 56% or more) or cor pulmonale (P wave more than 3 mm in leads II and III) is present. Because hypoxia leads to pulmonary hypertension and increases the work of the right ventricle, low-flow oxygen may help prevent or deter development of cor pulmonale. The goal of therapy is a Pao_2 of 60 mm Hg or SaO_2 of 90%, which usually can be accomplished with 1–2 L of oxygen per minute for 15 hours per day.

10-68   Answer A

Asthma is characterized by intermittent episodes of airway obstruction caused by bronchospasm, excessive bronchial secretion, or edema of bronchial mucosa. Atelectasis is a collapse of alveolar lung tissue, and findings reflect the presence of a small, airless lung. It is caused by complete obstruction of a draining bronchus by a tumor, thick secretions, or an aspirated foreign body. Acute bronchitis is an inflammation of the bronchial tree characterized by partial bronchial obstruction and secretions or constrictions. It results in abnormally deflated portions of the lung. Emphysema is a permanent hyperinflation of lung beyond the terminal bronchioles with destruction of the alveolar walls.

10-69   Answer A

In the pregnant woman, the thoracic cage may appear wider and the costal angle may feel wider than in the nonpregnant state. Respirations may be deeper, although this can be quantified only with pulmonary function tests. Oxygenation is not decreased.

10-70   Answer D

A key change in the treatment of croup is the administration of corticosteroids. Prior treatment used to just be supportive. Steroids have potent vasoconstrictive and anti-inflammatory properties. They reduce airway inflammation, vascular permeability, and mucosal edema associated with croup. After U.S. emergency department providers began administering systemic corticosteroids to children presenting with croup symptoms, the need for endotracheal intubation decreased. Mist therapy, oral hydration, and minimal handling are also recommended. The presence of stridor at rest requires hospitalization. Antibiotic therapy is not indicated because this condition is viral.

10-71   Answer A

Theophylline, a methylxanthine derivative, acts as a bronchodilator, decreases dyspnea, improves mucociliary clearance, improves gas exchange, enhances respiratory muscle performance, increases neuroinspiratory drive, and has a positive inotropic effect. The decision to institute theophylline therapy must be individualized and should not be universally made in all clients with COPD. It should be added to the treatment plan in clients who have not achieved an optimal clinical response to beta agonists and ipratropium (Atrovent) metered-dose inhalers.

10-72   Answer C

According to the ARIA guidelines, sinus cleansing should be followed with an intranasal corticosteroid spray as first-line therapy. Intranasal corticosteroid sprays are a primary means of reducing mast cell degranulation and reducing tissue inflammation. All of the other choices are also indicated in the treatment of allergic rhinitis.

10-73   Answer D

Immunomodulators such as omalizumab, a monoclonal antibody, prevents biding of IgE receptors on basophils and mast cells. Mast cell stabilizers stabilize mast cells and interfere with chloride channel function.

10-74   Answer C

Daily performance of chest physiotherapy with postural drainage, percussion, and vibration to remove the abnormally viscous mucus is essential for the client with cystic fibrosis. With cystic fibrosis, the problem lies at the level of the epithelial cells of the small airways, not the bronchi; therefore, bronchodilators do not help. Antibiotics should be administered during an infectious process, not prophylactically. Oxygen therapy may be required for hypoxemia, but not continuously. Recent studies have shown that there is some improvement when using short-term oxygen therapy, which increases the blood oxygen levels and improves sleep and exercise. There are recommendations to follow up with research into the effects of long-term oxygen treatment on sleep quality and exercise in individuals with CF.

10-75   Answer D

Some conditions have a characteristic timing of a cough. A cough caused by a postnasal drip related to sinusitis is more prevalent at night. A cough associated with an acute illness, such as a respiratory infection, is continuous throughout the day. A cough in the early morning is usually caused by chronic bronchial inflammation from habitual smoking. A cough in the afternoon and/or evening may reflect exposure to irritants at work.

10-76   Answer C

If a client presents with an acute onset of dyspnea with associated symptoms of chest pain, faintness, tachypnea, peripheral cyanosis, low blood pressure, crackles, and some wheezes, and has a history of taking birth control pills and smoking, suspect pulmonary emboli. Other signs and symptoms associated with pulmonary emboli include loss of consciousness and a pleural friction rub. Precipitating and aggravating factors include the use of oral contraceptives and prolonged recumbency. Acute dyspnea would also occur with asthma, but the physical findings would include bilateral wheezing; sibilant, whistling sounds; and prolonged expiration. With bronchitis, dyspnea is not necessarily the presenting symptom. A cough precedes the dyspnea, and there would be rhonchi present on auscultation. With a pneumothorax, there is an acute onset of dyspnea, and the physical findings would include decreased or absent breath sounds with a tracheal shift.

10-77   Answer A

For a client diagnosed with pneumonia, the following are indications for hospitalization: inability to take oral medications; multilobar involvement on chest x-ray; acute mental status changes; a severe vital sign abnormality (pulse rate greater than 140 per minute, systolic blood pressure less than 90 mm Hg, or a respiratory rate greater than 30 per minute); a secondary suppurative infection such as empyema, meningitis, or endocarditis; or a severe acute electrolyte, hematological, or metabolic abnormality.

10-78   Answer D

Allergic asthma (extrinsic asthma) is a chronic inflammatory disorder of the airways. The symptoms of allergic and nonallergic asthma are the same, but the triggers are not. Allergic asthma is triggered by inhaled exposure to allergens. The most common of these are dust mites, pet dander, pollens, mold, grass, and ragweed. Nonallergic asthma triggers generally don't cause inflammation but can aggravate airways, especially if they're already inflamed. Nonallergic triggers include smoke, exercise, cold air, strong smells like chemicals and perfume, air pollutants, and intense emotions.

10-79   Answer B

Coal miners are at risk for developing pneumoconiosis. Pneumoconiosis is caused by the inhalation of dust particles and is an occupational hazard in mining and stone cutting. Farmers may be at risk for grain and/or pesticide inhalation. Construction workers handling asbestos may develop asbestosis. Potters, stonecutters, and miners are at risk for silicosis from inhaling silica (quartz) dust. A related respiratory disease, histoplasmosis is a systemic fungal respiratory diseased caused by fungus in the soil with a high organic content and undisturbed bird droppings, such as those around old chicken coops, caves, and so on.

10-80   Answer A

Cigarette smoking increases the clearance rate of theophylline and may result in the need for a larger dose. Hepatic insufficiency, allopurinol (Zyloprim), and cimetidine (Tagamet) all decrease the clearance rate of theophylline and may result in the need for a smaller dose.

10-81　Answer A

A T1SN1M1 indicates that the lung carcinoma is in situ, has metastasis to the lymph nodes in the peribronchial or the ipsilateral hilar region, and has distant metastasis to the spine. Although the TNM system is generalized for all solid tumors, it is often adapted for specific types of cancers. *T* is for the relative tumor size, *N* indicates the presence and extent of lymph node involvement, and *M* denotes distant metastases. For specific lung cancer staging, the *T* may range from 0, with no evidence of primary tumor, to 4, which indicates that the tumor has invaded the mediastinum or involves the heart, great vessels, trachea, esophagus, vertebral body, or carina, and there is presence of malignant pleural effusion. The *N* may range from 0, indicating no regional lymph node metastasis, to 3, indicating metastasis to the contralateral, mediastinal, scalene, or supraclavicular nodes. The *M* is either X, indicating that the presence of distant metastasis cannot be assessed, or 1, meaning that distant metastasis is present.

10-82　Answer B

If a client develops moderate asthma, defined as more than two episodes per week, an inhaled steroid should be prescribed and used in conjunction with the beta-2 adrenergic metered-dose inhaler. With no improvement, a longer-acting bronchodilator, such as salmeterol xinafoate (Serevent), may be added. If the asthma worsens, then a short course of oral steroids may be tried. Theophylline is no longer used except in extremely resistant cases.

10-83　Answer B

The normal respiratory rate of an 18-month-old child (age 1–2 years) while awake is 30–40 breaths per minute. Between ages 6 and 12 months, the awake child breathes between 58 and 75 times per minute. An awake child age 2–4 years breathes between 23 and 42 times per minute; and a child age 4–6 years breathes between 19 and 36 times per minute.

10-84　Answer A

Hemoptysis is defined as expectoration of blood. The client often reports coughing up blood or sputum that is streaked or tinged with blood. In addition, hemoptysis may be manifested as fresh (bright red) or old blood or, in the case of bleeding from an infected lung cavity, it may present as slow oozing or frank bleeding. In cases of profuse hemoptysis, blood clots may be expectorated.

10-85　Answer B

Of persons who smoke one pack of cigarettes per day or more, 40%–60% have a cough. It is defined as chronic bronchitis if the cough has been productive for at least 3 months during each of 2 consecutive years.

10-86　Answer C

Treatment of tuberculosis in pregnant women is essential and should not be delayed; therefore, Marisa's treatment should begin now. The preferred initial treatment is isoniazid (Nydrazid), rifampin (Rimactane), and ethambutol (Myambutol). The teratogenicity of pyrazinamide is undetermined, so it is not wise to use this drug unless resistance to the other drugs is demonstrated or is likely.

10-87　Answer B

The normal anteroposterior diameter of the chest as compared with the transverse diameter is approximately 1:2. An anteroposterior measurement that equals the transverse measurement is defined as a barrel chest, which usually indicates some obstructive lung disease.

10-88　Answer D

Coccidioidomycosis is the leading mycotic (fungal) infection in the southwestern United States, with an annual morbidity estimated at 35,000 cases. Although the majority of those infected recover spontaneously without antibiotic intervention, for immunocompromised persons, the disseminated disease can lead to high morbidity and a greater than 50% mortality rate. Providers should suspect coccidioidomycosis in clients presenting with pulmonary complaints, particularly those who may have recently visited an endemic area. An influenza-like syndrome appears 7–28 days after inhalation of *Coccidioides immitis* in less than half of clients infected. Symptoms, in descending order of frequency, include fever, cough, chest pain, chills, sputum production, sore throat, and hemoptysis. Cutaneous manifestations occur in 10% of clients, particularly younger ones, and present as generalized maculopapular erythematous eruptions. Coccidioidomycosis is readily treatable if recognized at an early stage. For the majority of infected individuals, the prognosis is excellent even without therapy. Systemic antifungal therapy should be considered in infants, older adults, debilitated persons, those with prolonged primary disease, and populations at high risk of dissemination. Intravenous amphotericin B is the mainstay of therapy.

10-89   Answer A

The definitive tests for cystic fibrosis (CF) are the sweat test and DNA analysis. The diagnosis is confirmed by a positive sweat test or by confirming the presence of two of the recognized CF mutations in DNA, one each on the maternally and paternally derived chromosome 7. Sweat testing can be performed at any age. However, newborns in the first few weeks of life may not produce a large enough volume of sweat to analyze, but in those who do, the results will be accurate. Immunoreactive trypsinogen (IRT) levels are elevated in most infants with CF for the first several weeks of life; however, this test has relatively poor specificity because as many as 90% of the positives on the initial screen are false positives. Early diagnosis of CF improves the poor prognosis for untreated CF. If untreated, most clients die by age 1–2 years. With current care, median survival is age 29.

A sputum or throat culture positive for mucoid *Pseudomonas aeruginosa* is suggestive of CF. An abnormal Chymex test for pancreatic insufficiency is a supportive laboratory test to diagnose CF. A fecal fat test, while reliable, is not specific to CF; any condition affected by malabsorption or maldigestion will be associated with increased fecal fat.

10-90   Answer C

The definitive test for sleep apnea is an overnight polysomnogram. This all-night recording of the client's sleep, performed in a sleep center, is the gold standard for identifying the presence, type, and severity of sleep apnea.

10-91   Answer D

Chest physiotherapy is effective in the treatment of pneumonia; atelectasis; and diseases resulting in weak or ineffective coughing, such as cystic fibrosis. This technique uses percussion and postural drainage along with coughing and deep breathing exercises. It is performed by positioning the client so that the involved lobes of the lung are placed in a dependent drainage position and then using a cupped hand or vibrator to percuss the chest wall. Nasotracheal suctioning is quite uncomfortable but still useful in the appropriate clinical setting in the absence of significant coagulopathy.

10-92   Answer B

When trying to differentiate pulmonary from cardiac causes of dyspnea on exertion, it is important to remember that clients with dyspnea from cardiac causes remain dyspneic much longer after cessation of exercise. The heart rate also takes longer to return to preexercise levels. When the cause is pulmonary, the rate of recovery to normal respiration is fast and the dyspnea is gone a few minutes after the cessation of exercise. Clients with pulmonary dyspnea usually do not have dyspnea at rest. Clients with severe cardiac dyspnea demonstrate a volume of respiration that is greater than normal at every level of exercise, and they experience the dyspnea sooner after beginning the exertion.

10-93   Answer C

The Joint American College of Chest Physicians (ACCP) and American Association of Cardiovascular and Pulmonary Rehabilitation (AACVPR) evidence-based clinical practice guidelines for pulmonary rehabilitation offer evidence that pulmonary rehabilitation is beneficial for clients with COPD and those with other chronic lung conditions. Pulmonary rehabilitation improves the symptom of dyspnea, improves the health-related quality of life, reduces the number of hospital days and other measures of health-care utilization, and is cost effective. Evidence is insufficient to support the routine use of nutritional supplementation in pulmonary rehabilitation of clients with COPD. Current practice and expert opinion support including psychosocial interventions as a component of comprehensive pulmonary rehabilitation programs for clients with COPD, but clients benefit the most from pulmonary rehabilitation.

10-94   Answer C

Sarcoidosis is a multisystem disorder of unknown cause that has a prevalence of about 20 cases in 10,000. It usually occurs in clients ages 20–40, but it can occur at any age. Sarcoidosis occurs more frequently in women than in men, and in the United States, it is more common in blacks than in whites (about 10:1). Although many organs may be involved, the most involved organ is the lung (90%).

10-95   Answer A

Hand-to-hand transmission (after handling fomites serving as reservoirs of infection) is the most common mode of transmission of the common cold in adults, underscoring the importance of frequent hand washing in the prevention of new cases. Colds are also caused by viruses spread through direct inhalation of airborne droplet sprays aerosolized by the infected person while speaking, coughing, or sneezing.

10-96   Answer B

In acute bronchitis, the breath sounds are vesicular, vocal resonance is moderate, and the adventitious sounds are localized crackles with sibilant wheezes. In bronchiectasis, the breath sounds are usually vesicular, but vocal resonance is usually muffled and crackles are the adventitious sounds. In emphysema, the breath sounds are of decreased intensity and often with prolonged expiration, vocal resonance is muffled or decreased, and the adventitious sounds are occasional wheezes and often fine crackles in late inspiration. In asthma, the breath sounds are distant, vocal resonance is decreased, and wheezes are the adventitious sounds.

10-97   Answer B

Clients with COPD often sit in a tripod position: leaning forward with their arms braced against their knees, a chair, or a bed. This provides clients with leverage so that their rectus abdominal, intercostal, and accessory neck muscles can all assist with expiration.

10-98   Answer A

After a total laryngectomy for laryngeal cancer, the client will have a permanent tracheostomy because no connection exists between the trachea and the esophagus.

10-99   Answer A

Streptococcus pneumoniae causes 30%–75% of all community-acquired bacterial pneumonia, followed by *Mycoplasma pneumoniae* (5%–35%), *Haemophilus influenzae* (6%–12%), and *Staphylococcus aureus* (3%–10%).

10-100   Answer C

Spirometry remains the gold standard for the diagnosis of asthma as well as for periodic monitoring of the condition. Routine use of validated quality-of-life questionnaires may detect impairment and severity of the disease.

10-101   Answer C

A large prospective study in women showed that obesity, cigarette smoking, and hypertension increased their risk for pulmonary embolism. Alcohol intake does not predispose a woman to pulmonary embolism.

10-102   Answer B

Hearing a muffled (and sometimes nondistinct) *eeee* through the stethoscope when auscultating the chest when the client says "eeee" is known as egophony. When consolidation is present, the *eeee* sound changes to an *aaaaa* sound. With bronchophony, when the client repeats "99-99-99," normally you can hear a soft, muffled, indistinct sound but cannot distinguish what is being said. With whispered pectoriloquy, when the client whispers "1-2-3," a normal response is faint, muffled, and almost inaudible. Tonometry measures intraocular pressure.

10-103   Answer B

The peripharyngeal upper respiratory tract infection that occurs most often in children ages 2–5 years is epiglottitis. Peritonsillar abscess occurs more frequently during the teenage years; laryngotracheobronchitis (croup) in children ages 3 months to 3 years; and bacterial tracheitis in children ages 3–10 years.

10-104   Answer D

To control the common asthma trigger of dust mites, the following measures are recommended: Cover the mattress and pillows in airtight, dustproof covers; wash the bedding weekly and dry it on a hot setting for 20 minutes; avoid sleeping on natural fibers such as wool or down; remove all carpeting from bedrooms; and reduce indoor humidity to less than 50%. Opening the windows daily would allow allergens to enter.

10-105   Answer D

Routine screening for TB no longer is recommended. The current guidelines include some of the following individuals; persons with HIV infection; a resident or employee in a prison or long-term care facility; an employee in a health-care facility; infants, children, and adolescents exposed to adults in high-risk categories; foreign-born persons arriving within 5 years from countries that have high TB incidence or prevalence; and persons on immunosuppressive therapy.

10-106   Answer A

With pleural effusion and thickening, the trachea would be deviated toward the nonaffected side because of fluid displacing the pleural space. The trachea is usually not displaced with pneumonia. With bronchiectasis, the trachea is midline or deviated toward the affected side, and with pulmonary fibrosis, the trachea is deviated to the most affected side.

10-107   Answer C

Recurrence rates for both primary and secondary spontaneous pneumothorax are similar. Recurrence rates range from 10%–50%, and about 60% of those clients will have a third recurrence. After three episodes, the recurrence rate exceeds 85%. Repeated spontaneous pneumothorax should be treated by pleurodesis or surgical intervention, including parietal pleurectomy.

10-108   Answer A

While viral bronchitis requiring only supportive care is the most common etiology of acute exacerbations of chronic bronchitis, bacterial involvement must be considered when there is increased sputum production lasting over a week or new chest x-ray findings. *Streptococcus pneumoniae* is the most common agent, followed by *Haemophilus influenzae* and *Moraxella catarrhalis*, similar to the causative agents of sinusitis and community-acquired pneumonia. *Branhamella catarrhalis* and *M. catarrhalis* are the same organism.

10-109   Answer B

With bronchovesicular breath sounds, the inspiratory rate equals the expiratory rate. With bronchial or tracheal breath sounds, the inspiratory rate is shorter than the expiratory rate, and with vesicular breath sounds, the inspiratory rate is greater than the expiratory rate.

10-110   Answer C

Drugs such as corticosteroids and other immunosuppressive agents contribute to a decreased response to TST. Other factors that may contribute to a decreased response to TST include viral infections (measles, mumps, chickenpox, HIV), bacterial infections (typhoid fever, pertussis), nutritional factors (severe protein depletion), diseases affecting lymphoid organs, and stress (surgery, burns).

10-111   Answer C

Dyspnea does not belong. The clinical triad of the three D's (drooling, dysphagia, and distress) is the classic presentation of epiglottis.

10-112   Answer A

Although all of these tests might be indicated, the first test that should be ordered for a client presenting with productive cough, weight loss, weakness, anorexia, night sweats, and generalized malaise for 8 weeks' duration would be a Mantoux skin test for tuberculosis (TB). The client is at high risk for developing TB because of his residence in a shelter and his low socioeconomic status.

10-113   Answer C

Symptoms in about one-third of pregnant women with asthma will improve during pregnancy; about one-third will be unchanged; and about one-third will worsen. Pregnancy is associated with changes in lung volume. There is an increase in tidal volume and a 20%–50% increase in minute ventilation. The clinical course of asthma during pregnancy may be predicted by the course during the first trimester, and most clients have the same pattern of response with repeated pregnancies. The treatment of asthma during pregnancy follows the same principles as with other clients. Medications not specifically required should not be given in the first trimester, and all medications should be given at their minimal effective dose and frequency.

10-114   Answer B

The most common cause of a persistent cough in children of all ages is recurrent viral bronchitis. Recurrent viral bronchitis is most prevalent in preschool and young school-age children, and there may be a genetically determined host susceptibility to frequently recurring bronchitis. The key words are *persistent cough*. Young clients with recurrent cough often have asthma, but it is not usually persistent. Providers should be suspicious of underlying asthma contributing to a recurrent cough when there is a family history of allergies, atopy, or asthma. Similarly, allergies and an upper respiratory infection do not present with a persistent cough; rather, they present with an intermittent one.

10-115   Answer A

The normal adult has a thorax that has an elliptical shape with an anteroposterior:transverse diameter ratio of 1:2 or 5:7. Funnel breast (pectus excavatum) is a markedly sunken sternum and adjacent cartilages; it is congenital and usually not symptomatic. Pigeon breast (pectus carinatum) is a forward protrusion of the sternum with ribs sloping back at either side and vertical depressions along the costochondral junctions; it is less common than pectus excavatum and requires no treatment. A barrel-shaped chest is present when the anteroposterior and transverse diameters of the chest are equal and the ribs are horizontal instead of in the normal downward slope; it is associated with normal aging and with chronic emphysema and asthma caused by hyperinflation of the lungs.

Bibliography

Dillon, PM: *Nursing Health Assessment—A Critical Thinking, Case Studies Approach*, ed 2. FA Davis, Philadelphia, 2007.

Dunphy, LM, et al: *Primary Care: The Art and Science of Advanced Practice Nursing*, ed 3. FA Davis, Philadelphia, 2011.

Freeman, D, Lee, A, and Price, D: Efficacy and safety of tiotropium in COPD patients in primary care: The SPiRiva Usual CarE (SPRUCE) Study. *Respiratory Research*, 8(1):45, 2007.

Garcia-Aymerich, J, et al: Regular physical activity modifies smoking-related lung function decline and reduces risk of chronic obstructive pulmonary disease: A population cohort study. *American Journal of Respiratory and Critical Care Medicine* 175(5): 458–463, 2007.

Ilowite, JS, and Nair, GB: Asthma: What next when your patient doesn't respond to therapy? *Consultant* 51(5):305–312, 2011.

Lynch, P: Asthma education for children: Basic strategies can make a big difference. *Advance for NPs & PAs* 2(7):18–22, 2011.

Niemiec, LA: Treatment of viral croup: No humidity needed. *Advance for NPs & PAs* 1(4):25–28, 2010.

Rance, K: The asthma-allergy connection. Complex companions. *Advance for Nurse Practitioners* 15(4): 31–33, 2007.

Sanassi, LA: Severe persistent asthma in adults: The rise of omalizumab. *Advance for NPs & PAs* 2(5):19–24, 2011.

Smith, A: Managing allergic rhinitis: Making sense of the options. *Clinician Reviews/Convenient Care* (suppl.), 4–10, Spring 2011.

How well did you do?

85% and above, congratulations! This score shows application of test-taking principles and adequate content knowledge.

75%–85%, keep working! Review test-taking principles and try again.

65%–75%, hang in there! Spend some time reviewing concepts and test-taking principles and try the test again.

Chapter 11: *Cardiovascular Problems*

Jill E. Winland-Brown
Denese Sabatino

Questions

11-1 Harry comes to your office with waxing and waning ischemic symptoms over a period of days and weeks, an increase in angina while at rest, and transient ST changes on his electrocardiogram. This presentation leads you to believe that he is experiencing

A. a stroke.

B. a myocardial infarction.

C. stable angina.

D. unstable angina.

11-2 A newly discharged outpatient surgery client presents with insidious onset of edema and dusky blue discoloration of the head and upper extremities. You know it is a medical emergency and suspect which of the following?

A. Evolving cerebral infarction

B. Impending myocardial infarction

C. Superior vena cava syndrome

D. Temporal arteritis

11-3 Selma has acute peripheral arterial occlusion of a lower extremity. Before you begin your examination, you know that it

A. may present with only complaints of coldness or paresthesia of the extremity.

B. may present as the only disease.

C. always occurs in the lower extremities.

D. will result in an extremity that appears "blue."

11-4 Characteristics of ischemic arterial ulcers include

A. an irregularly shaped border with crusting or scaling at the edges.

B. severe pain.

C. a location anywhere on the leg.

D. a moist ulcer base with ill-defined borders.

11-5 Which of the following statements regarding the Joint National Committee (JNC) on Prevention, Detection, Evaluation, and Treatment of High Blood Pressure category about prehypertension is true?

A. Clients with prehypertension usually remain in that category forever.

B. Clients with a blood pressure (BP) in the range of 130/80 to 139/89 mm Hg are twice as likely to develop hypertension as those with lower values.

C. All clients in this category should be started on diuretics immediately to avoid future end-organ disease.

D. Diastolic BP control should be the focus of treatment.

11-6 Signs of right-sided heart failure include

A. a low cardiac output.

B. signs of fluid retention.

C. dyspnea.

D. elevated pulmonary venous pressure.

11-7 An anterior wall myocardial infarction most likely occurs from occlusion of the

A. left circumflex artery.

B. left main artery.

C. right coronary artery.

D. left anterior descending artery.

11-8 Which resuscitation recommendation was made by the American Heart Association to improve survival rates in clients with a return of spontaneous circulation (ROSC) following a cardiac arrest?

A. Hypothermia

B. Hyperthermia

C. Initiation of intravenous lidocaine

D. A rebreathing mask

11-9   *Ted, age 18, is to have a cardiac screening examination to determine if he can play college basketball. The diagnostic test of choice for detecting hypertrophic cardiomyopathy or idiopathic left ventricular hypertrophy is a(n)*

A. echocardiogram.

B. electrocardiogram.

C. arteriogram.

D. stress test.

11-10   *Which would be the LAST step you would consider in a client with long-term chronic ischemic heart disease?*

A. Use of aspirin

B. Use of beta blockers, calcium channel blockers, and nitrates

C. Risk factor and lifestyle modification

D. A coronary angiogram

11-11   *There are four classifications of heart failure that often are interwoven; they include systolic, diastolic, acute, and/or chronic. Clients who present with JVD, dyspnea with exertion, peripheral edema and abdominal fullness would most likely be experiencing chronic right sided heart failure. A routine diagnostic work up would include all of the following except*

A. BNP.

B. BMP.

C. echocardiogram.

D. CTA.

11-12   *Impaired blood flow to the extremities is caused by which of the following common disorders?*

A. Raynaud's disease

B. Peripheral vascular disease

C. Polycythemia

D. Buerger's disease

11-13   *Liver function tests should be monitored routinely every 4 months in the client on maintenance therapy with all hypolipidemic drugs except*

A. bile acid sequestrants (Questran, Colestid).

B. hydroxymethylglutaryl-coenzyme A reductase inhibitors (statins).

C. nicotinic acid (niacin).

D. fibric acid derivatives (gemfibrozil).

11-14   *When auscultating a client's heart, you note a short, high-frequency click (opening snap) after S_2 during the beginning of diastole. What could this indicate?*

A. Aortic regurgitation

B. Mitral stenosis

C. Mitral regurgitation

D. Nothing; this is normal

11-15   *Which resuscitation recommendation made by the American Heart Association has the highest priority?*

A. Timely delivery of an epinephrine bolus

B. Rapid provision of advanced airway management

C. High quality, uninterrupted chest compression

D. Early electrical therapy

11-16   *An active 68-year-old man under your care has known acquired valvular aortic stenosis and mitral regurgitation. He also has a history of infectious endocarditis. He has recently been told he needs elective replacement of his aortic valve. When he comes in, you discover that he has 10 remaining teeth in poor repair. Your recommendation would be to*

A. defer any further dental work until his valve replacement is completed.

B. instruct the client to have dental extraction done cautiously, having no more than two teeth per visit removed.

C. suggest that he consult with his oral surgeon about removing all the teeth at once and receiving appropriate antibiotic prophylaxis.

D. coordinate with his cardiac and oral surgeons to have the tooth extraction and valve replacement done at the same time to reduce the risk of anesthetic complications.

11-17   *Marvin, age 56, is a smoker with diabetes mellitus. He has just been diagnosed as hypertensive. Which of the following drugs has the potential to cause the development of bronchial asthma and inhibit gluconeogenesis?*

A. Angiotensin-converting enzyme (ACE) inhibitors

B. Beta blockers

C. Calcium channel blockers

D. Diuretics

11-18   *To determine the presence of target organ damage and other risk factors in the client with hypertension, basic diagnostic tests that should be ordered include*

A. chest x-ray, electrocardiogram, urinalysis, complete blood count, chemistry profile, lipid profile, and thyroid-stimulating hormone (TSH) level.

B. renal arteriogram.

C. plasma renin activity and 24-hour urinary sodium.

D. echocardiogram.

11-19   *What is the most important question to ask when a client presents with chest pain?*

A. "What were you doing at the time of onset of chest pain?"

B. "What was the time of the onset of pain?"

C. "Are you a smoker?"

D. "When was the last time you had blood work done?"

11-20   *Which of the following is the most important preventable cause of premature death in women?*

A. Hypertension

B. Obesity

C. Cigarette smoking

D. Alcoholism

11-21   *Mitral valve prolapse is characterized by*

A. elongation of the chordae tendineae and enlarged valve leaflets.

B. ballooning (prolapse) of the cusps into the ventricle during diastole.

C. an early diastolic murmur.

D. an early systolic murmur.

11-22   *At least 75% of clients need two or more antihypertensive agents to reach their blood pressure goal. In choosing combination therapy for a client with stage 2 hypertension (HTN) (SBP greater than 160 and or DBP greater than 100) in a 59-year-old male with a PMH relevant for uncontrolled essential HTN, DM, SOB, DOE, stage 1 diastolic heart failure, with an EF of 55% and a serum creatinine of 0.4, the best initial combination treatment would include*

A. Lasix and a beta blocker.

B. thiazide diuretic and an ACE inhibitor.

C. nitrate and a beta blocker.

D. thiazide and a calcium channel blocker.

11-23   *Pharmacological therapy for mitral valve disease includes*

A. treatment of dyspnea with diuretics to relieve congestion.

B. reduction of fast ventricular rates with digoxin, beta blockers, or calcium channel blockers.

C. preload reduction with antihypertensive agents to decrease regurgitant flow.

D. daily antibiotic use to ward off bacterial infections.

11-24   *A blood pressure of 160/100 mm Hg is classified as*

A. prehypertension.

B. stage 1 hypertension.

C. stage 2 hypertension.

D. stage 3 hypertension.

11-25   *The most common cause of elevated total and low-density lipoprotein cholesterol levels in the United States is*

A. heredity.

B. hypothyroidism.

C. diabetes.

D. a diet high in saturated fat.

11-26   *Which of the following usually indicates hyperlipidemia?*

A. Lipoma

B. Xanthelasma

C. Jaundiced skin

D. Multiple actinic keratoses

11-27   *Which statement is true of hydroxymethylglutaryl-coenzyme A reductase inhibitors (statins)?*

A. They are the first drugs of choice for men younger than age 45.

B. They should be given in the morning after breakfast.

C. They may cause myopathies, especially at higher dosages or in combination with certain drugs.

D. They are contraindicated in clients taking Coumadin.

11-28   *Rona, age 69, has hypertension (HTN), drinks one glass of white wine per day, and is slightly overweight. She asks you if making changes in her life at this age will make any difference. You tell her that lifestyle modifications for the control of HTN*

A. are not as effective in older adults because HTN is an inevitable consequence of aging.

B. require a marked reduction in weight and a very limited choice of foods to achieve any benefit.

C. should include at least three glasses of red wine every day because it improves high-density lipoprotein cholesterol levels, a known cardiovascular risk factor, which may be worsened by HTN.

D. may prevent HTN, lower elevated blood pressure, and reduce the number and dosage of antihypertensive medications needed to manage a condition.

11-29   *Jamie, age 49, who has a history of hyperlipidemia, has symptoms that lead you to suspect unstable angina. Your next action would be to*

A. start aspirin therapy and schedule an exercise stress test at the client's convenience.

B. initiate lipid-lowering agents.

C. hospitalize the client in a monitored setting with pharmacological control of ischemia, arrhythmias, and thrombosis as appropriate.

D. prescribe a Holter monitor and start her on a beta blocker.

11-30   *When indicated, which procedure needs endocarditis prophylaxis?*

A. Vaginal or cesarean deliveries

B. Insertion or removal of intrauterine devices

C. Dental procedures or extractions

D. Body piercings

11-31   *Which of the following statements is true about hypertension (HTN) during pregnancy?*

A. Methyldopa (Aldomet) is the drug of first choice for control of mild to moderate HTN in pregnancy.

B. Beta blockers are safe during the pregnancy.

C. ACE inhibitors (I and II) are safe during all trimesters.

D. Beta blockers are safe only in the first trimester of pregnancy.

11-32   *Which of the following conditions would warrant bacterial endocarditis prophylaxis?*

A. Prosthetic heart valves

B. Surgical repair of atrial septal defect

C. MVP without significant mitral regurgitation

D. Cardiac pacemakers

11-33   *Murmurs are graded according to their intensity (loudness). A murmur that is audible with the stethoscope off the chest is a*

A. grade III murmur.

B. grade IV murmur.

C. grade V murmur.

D. grade VI murmur.

11-34   *Nicotinic acid is an inexpensive drug used to treat serum hyperlipidemia. Which of the following statements is true about nicotinic acid?*

A. Nicotinic acid lowers low-density lipoprotein cholesterol levels, raises high-density lipoprotein cholesterol levels, and decreases triglyceride levels.

B. Nicotinic acid is the drug of choice for individuals with diabetes.

C. Nicotinic acid may decrease the effect of some antihypertensive agents.

D. Rare adverse reactions of nicotinic acid include flushing, pruritus, and gastrointestinal upset.

11-35   *You are managing a client with CHF. The client is presently on Carvedilol 12.5 mg bid, Lisinopril 2.5 mg PO daily, Lasix 80 mg PO daily, and Spironolactone 25 mg PO daily. He is in to see you for a 2-week follow-up and shares he has gained 7 lbs in the last week. He shares he has been faithful to his fluid and dietary restrictions and that his urinary output is somewhat less than it has been. What medication could you add to optimize the response to the loop diuretic?*

A. Bumex

B. Metolazone

C. Demadex

D. Diamox

11-36   *Martin, age 56, has hypertension and has been taking antihypertensive medication for about 10 years. He has been very stable. You have not seen him in about 6 months. His examination today should specifically*

A. include only a blood pressure measurement with the client seated comfortably.

B. include a funduscopic examination.

C. be a focused examination limited to the respiratory and cardiovascular systems.

D. include a discussion of weaning him off his medication.

11-37 *Larry, age 66, is a smoker with hypertension and hyperlipidemia. He is 6 months post MI. To prevent reinfarction, the most important behavior change that he can make is to*

A. quit smoking.

B. maintain aggressive hypertension therapy.

C. stick to a low-fat, low-sodium diet.

D. continue with his exercise program.

11-38 *Which of the following statements is true of auscultation of the aortic valve?*

A. It is best performed using the diaphragm of the stethoscope.

B. It is best heard at the second left intercostal space.

C. Auscultation need only be done at one site.

D. It is best performed using the bell of the stethoscope.

11-39 *During pregnancy, many women develop which cardiovascular change?*

A. Diastolic murmur

B. Hypertension

C. Bradycardia

D. Systolic murmur

11-40 *Which of the following causes coronary valve leaflets to billow into the atrium during ventricular systole and runs in families?*

A. Mitral regurgitation

B. Mitral valve prolapse

C. Aortic regurgitation

D. Aortic stenosis

11-41 *When performing a cardiac assessment, where is the most essential site for assessing edema?*

A. Dependent areas

B. Periorbital areas

C. Upper extremities

D. Cerebral edema

11-42 *Clinical findings associated with aortic regurgitation include*

A. pulsus paradoxus.

B. waterhammer pulses.

C. pulsus alternans.

D. weak, thready pulses.

11-43 *When teaching a client with hypertension about restricting dietary sodium, you would include which of the following instructions?*

A. Sodium restriction can cause serious adverse effects.

B. Diets with markedly reduced intake of sodium may be associated with other beneficial effects beyond blood pressure control.

C. Seventy-five percent of sodium intake is derived from processed food.

D. A goal of 3 g of sodium chloride or 1.2 g of sodium per day is easily achievable.

11-44 *Which classification of antihypertensive drugs is the most effective for treating hypertension in African American clients and older adults?*

A. Diuretics

B. ACE inhibitors

C. Beta blockers

D. Alpha-adrenergic blockers

11-45 *Deep vein thrombosis may result in*

A. generalized edema of the involved extremity.

B. atrophy of leg muscles.

C. loss of sensation in the affected extremity.

D. the release of fat emboli.

11-46 *New recommendations from the American Heart Association suggest that clients older than 80 years maintain a systolic blood pressure at what level when no contraindications exist?*

A. Less than 100

B. Less than 110

C. 120–130

D. 140–145

11-47 *Greg has just been given a diagnosis of congestive heart failure. Which of his medications should be discontinued?*

A. Nifedipine (Procardia XL) for long-term management of his chronic stable angina

B. Hydrochlorothiazide (HydroDIURIL) for his hypertension

C. Enalapril (Vasotec) for his hypertension

D. Butalbital (Esgic) for his headaches

11-48 *Nathan, age 63, comes for his annual physical. He has a history of mild hypertension and hyperlipidemia that he has not been successful in treating by diet and weight loss. His only complaint is a problem with impotence. On physical examination, you note a palpable, pulsatile abdominal mass in the umbilical region; a bruit above the umbilical region; and diminished femoral pulses. You suspect*

A. renal artery stenosis.

B. an abdominal aortic aneurysm.

C. a cardiac tumor.

D. a thoracic aortic aneurysm.

11-49 *Sheila, age 78, presents with a chief complaint of waking up during the night coughing. You examine her and find an S_3 heart sound, pulmonary crackles (rales) that do not clear with coughing, and peripheral edema. What do you suspect?*

A. Asthma

B. Nocturnal allergies

C. Heart failure

D. Valvular disease

11-50 *Many older adults develop postural hypotension with hypertensive drug therapy. What is included in your teaching with these individuals?*

A. Drug therapy will be discontinued as soon as their blood pressure stabilizes to prevent this problem from recurring.

B. Slight dehydration will prevent postural hypotension from occurring.

C. Clients should sleep in a high Fowler's position to prevent this from happening.

D. Clients should be taught to sit on the edge of the bed before standing.

11-51 *Which of the following conditions is the least frequent cause of heart failure?*

A. Hypertension

B. Aortic stenosis

C. Ischemic cardiomyopathy

D. Valvular heart disease (mitral and tricuspid)

11-52 *What is a causative factor in the formation of blood clots causing deep venous thrombosis?*

A. Blood flow turbulence

B. Intact vessels

C. Thin blood

D. Hypercoagulability

11-53 *When a client is getting ready for cardiac catheterization, which question is essential to ask?*

A. "Are you allergic to shellfish?"

B. "Have you ever had a catheterization before?"

C. "Have you completed an advanced directive?"

D. "What current medications are you on?"

11-54 *A client presents with substernal chest pain that is provoked by exertion and relieved by rest and nitroglycerin. What do you suspect?*

A. Stable angina

B. Unstable angina

C. Acute coronary syndrome (ACS)

D. Simple overexertion

11-55 *Which drug may be used to convert atrial fibrillation to sinus rhythm?*

A. Digitalis

B. Lidocaine

C. Amiodarone (Cordarone)

D. Adenosine (Adenocard)

11-56 *What is a common funduscopic change associated with hypertension?*

A. Optic disk swelling

B. Gray lesions

C. Deep intraretinal hemorrhages

D. A cup-disk ratio greater than 1:2

11-57 Which classification of antihypertensive drugs is the first-choice therapy for treating hypertension and angina in clients with known coronary artery disease?

A. Diuretics

B. Beta blockers

C. Calcium channel blockers

D. ACE inhibitors

11-58 Sarah, who is postmenopausal, has controlled asthma, hypertension being effectively treated with medication, and smokes cigarettes. She has a low-density lipoprotein (LDL) cholesterol level of 170 mg/dL and a high-density lipoprotein (HDL) cholesterol level of 40 mg/dL. To reduce Sarah's risk of a coronary event, the treatment plan would focus on

A. lowering her LDL cholesterol level.

B. lowering her HDL cholesterol level.

C. aggressively treating and controlling her hypertension and asthma.

D. getting Sarah to stop smoking.

11-59 Mr. Michaels has a long-standing cardiac problem. His electrocardiogram rhythm strip is shown below. Which medication should he be taking to prevent a pulmonary or cerebral problem?

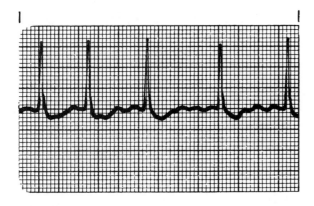

Lead II

A. An ACE inhibitor, such as enalapril (Vasotec)

B. An antiarrhythmic agent, such as procainamide (Procan-SR)

C. An anticoagulant, such as warfarin or dabigatran

D. An anticonvulsant, such as phenytoin (Dilantin)

11-60 Which of the following antihypertensive agents would most likely produce a rebound hypertensive crisis following its abrupt withdrawal?

A. Doxazosin (Cardura)

B. Lisinopril (Prinivil)

C. Losartan (Cozaar)

D. Clonidine (Catapres)

11-61 Sexual activity is a major concern for clients with chronic ischemic heart disease. Which statement is true?

A. The sexual partner should be included in the education process.

B. The physical stress of sexual intercourse is equivalent to running a half mile.

C. Antianginal medication taken just after sexual activity can help prevent symptoms.

D. Sexual activity should be attempted only in the morning when the client is well rested.

11-62 The leading cause of death in women in the United States is

A. trauma.

B. cardiovascular disease.

C. diabetes.

D. cancer.

11-63 Which of the following statements is true concerning auscultation of the typical murmur associated with aortic stenosis?

A. It is a harsh, crescendo-decrescendo ejection type that often radiates to the carotid arteries.

B. It is a diastolic murmur.

C. It is best heard at the apex of the heart.

D. The loudness of the murmur reflects the severity of the lesion.

11-64 The cardinal sign of right-sided heart failure in infants and children is

A. hepatomegaly.

B. edema of the lower extremities.

C. tachypnea.

D. cyanosis.

11-65   Headache, flushing, tachycardia, and peripheral edema are adverse effects associated with which class of antihypertensive agents?

A. Beta blockers

B. Calcium channel blockers

C. ACE inhibitors

D. Diuretics

11-66   Before counseling partners about sexual activity following a myocardial infarction, the provider should consider what factor(s)?

A. Most clients do not want to know how their condition affects their sex life.

B. Spouses are knowledgeable about their partner's condition; therefore, they do not need counseling.

C. Most clients return to the same frequency of sexual intercourse after they have regained their physical strength.

D. Depression, loss of interest, spousal reluctance, and anxiety may interfere with a client's resumption of sexual activities.

11-67   Charles has chronic ischemic heart disease and is taking a beta blocker, which results in

A. an increase in high-density lipoprotein cholesterol.

B. a reduced heart rate.

C. a decreased diastolic filling time.

D. An increase in oxygen demand.

11-68   Which drugs are used to lower blood pressure in a client with coexisting benign prostatic hypertrophy?

A. Beta blockers

B. ACE inhibitors

C. Alpha-adrenergic blockers

D. Calcium channel blockers

11-69   Which of the following is usually the earliest sign or symptom of chronic occlusive arterial disease in the extremities?

A. Loss of hair over the lower extremity

B. Intermittent claudication

C. Painful ulcerations of the toes of the affected extremity

D. Muscle atrophy

11-70   What are the recommendations when treating high triglycerides?

A. Aggressively treat with fenofibrates.

B. Treatment should be with combination therapy with a statin and fenofibrate.

C. Focus on lifestyle changes as initial therapy.

D. Use a bile acid sequestrant.

11-71   While much teaching is needed for your client with congestive heart failure (CHF), the most beneficial thing you can tell him that might prevent rehospitalization may be

A. "Be sure to use two pillows at night."

B. "Weigh yourself every day and if your weight increases by 3 lb in 24 hrs or 5 lb in one week, call me."

C. "Take your pulse daily; if it increases by six beats, call me."

D. "Let me know if you're sleeping more than 10 hours a day and feel depressed."

11-72   Which is the most common symptom of digitalis toxicity?

A. Nausea and vomiting

B. Tingling of the extremities

C. Rash

D. Headache

11-73   Dana has ischemic arterial ulcers. What is your first priority when counseling her?

A. Tell her that increasing coffee intake will stimulate heart rate and circulation.

B. Tell her to decrease water intake slightly to improve blood viscosity.

C. Tell her to reduce risk factors to improve tissue perfusion.

D. Tell her to begin an intense aerobic program.

11-74   Clients with Prinzmetal's angina frequently have a history of Raynaud's disease and which other disorder?

A. Syncope

B. Insomnia

C. Migraine headaches

D. Leg cramps

11-75   Terry, a 42-year-old black man who just moved into the area, comes into the clinic for a new-client visit. He brings his medical records from his previous health-care provider; the records show a blood pressure of 140/104 mm Hg on two separate occasions. Recent laboratory tests (complete blood count, chemistry profile, urinalysis, and thyroid-stimulating hormone) are normal. A recent electrocardiogram shows normal sinus rhythm with left ventricular hypertrophy. He denies any medical problems and tells you he has never been diagnosed with hypertension. He is not taking any medications, does not smoke, and drinks about two beers a day. He is currently unemployed. His blood pressure today is 150/110 mm Hg. Your next step would be to

A. obtain plasma and urine catecholamine measurements.

B. have him keep a food diary for 1 week, then return for a repeat blood pressure reading.

C. begin drug therapy with hydrochlorothiazide (HydroDIURIL) 25 mg.

D. start him on metoprolol (Lopressor) 100 mg twice a day.

11-76   Which of the following statements about hypertension is true?

A. It is frequently caused by pheochromocytoma.

B. It is usually the result of an underlying, correctable problem.

C. The cause is unknown in approximately 95% of cases.

D. It has a higher incidence among adult white men than any other group.

11-77   Which of the following findings are suggestive of renovascular hypertension?

A. Bilateral flank pain on percussion

B. Renal arterial bruits in the abdomen, flanks, or back

C. A palpable mass in the right lower quadrant

D. Decreased urine output

11-78   Cough, loss of taste, and rash are adverse effects associated with which class of antihypertensive agents?

A. Diuretics

B. Beta blockers

C. ACE inhibitors

D. Calcium channel blockers

11-79   To reduce the incidence of coronary events in an individual without coronary artery disease who has two or more risk factors, the goal serum low-density lipoprotein cholesterol level should be

A. 170–190 mg/dL.

B. 150–170 mg/dL.

C. 130–150 mg/dL.

D. less than 130 mg/dL.

11-80   The cholesterol component(s) considered most responsible for atherosclerotic plaque formation is (are)

A. total cholesterol.

B. low-density lipoprotein cholesterol.

C. high-density lipoprotein cholesterol.

D. phospholipids.

11-81   The classic 12-lead electrocardiogram change(s) that indicate(s) an acute coronary syndrome is (are)

A. ST-segment elevation.

B. T-wave inversion.

C. flipped P waves with a prolonged PR interval.

D. deep Q waves.

11-82   Rick is modifying his diet to try to lose weight, but after 3 months, he has not lost any weight, even though he has complied with his diet plan. A follow-up lipid profile reveals the following: total cholesterol, 238 mg/dL; triglycerides, 100 mg/dL; high-density lipoprotein cholesterol, 28 mg/dL; and low-density lipoprotein cholesterol, 190 mg/dL. What would you recommend?

A. Continuing the diet plan for another month

B. Starting an exercise program with a goal of uninterrupted aerobic exercise for 30 minutes 2 days a week

C. Stopping his current diet plan and trying another

D. Starting hypolipidemic drug therapy

11-83   Which of the following drugs should be considered as first-line therapy for a client with hypertension and heart failure?

A. Enalapril (Vasotec)

B. Diltiazem (Cardizem)

C. Atenolol (Tenormin)

D. Metoprolol (Lopressor)

11-84 Janice, age 64, arrives at the office this morning without an appointment. She appears quite anxious and pale and is complaining of an intermittent aching across her sternum and into her jaw and left arm that started about an hour ago and woke her out of a sound sleep. She took an antacid and acetaminophen (Tylenol), but they did not seem to help. Her blood pressure is 160/90 and heart rate is 98. An electrocardiogram shows normal sinus rhythm with 2-mm ST-segment elevations in leads II, III, and AVF. What do you suspect?

A. An acute anterior wall myocardial infarction (MI)
B. An acute inferior wall MI
C. Severe gastrointestinal reflux
D. An anxiety attack

11-85 For the routine management of heart failure, which one of the following medication classes would not be recommended?

A. ACE inhibitor
B. Beta blocker
C. Calcium channel blocker
D. Diuretic

11-86 The prevalence of which of the following conditions is higher in women, and therefore aggressive teaching needs to be done at every visit?

A. Myocardial infarction
B. Angina pectoris
C. Myocardial ischemia
D. Transient ischemic attacks (TIAs)

11-87 During a cardiovascular assessment, why is it important to note funduscopic changes?

A. You may pick up beginning cataracts in this age group.
B. You should note any glaucoma because some medications will be contraindicated.
C. Changes may suggest the possibility of target organ involvement.
D. You may be able to pick up arcus senilis.

11-88 Your post-MI client is allergic to ASA. Which drug should he be on indefinitely?

A. Coumadin
B. Heparin
C. Pentoxifylline (Trental)
D. Clopidogrel (Plavix)

11-89 Many clients with mitral valve prolapse exhibit

A. a slow heart rate.
B. somnolence.
C. a lengthened PR interval on electrocardiogram.
D. fatigue.

11-90 Individuals with clinical evidence of chronic ischemic heart disease (abnormal electrocardiogram, chest pain syndrome, unusual dyspnea, or fatigue) should have a full evaluation done to evaluate their risk for myocardial infarction or sudden death. When initially collecting data for this risk stratification, which would be the last step to be considered if at all?

A. Careful history and physical examination
B. Exercise stress testing with or without nuclide imaging
C. Cardiac catheterization
D. Chest x-ray

11-91 Mort is hypertensive. Which of the following factors influenced your choice of using an alpha blocker as the antihypertensive medication?

A. Mort is black.
B. Mort also has congestive heart failure.
C. Mort has benign prostatic hyperplasia (BPH).
D. Mort has frequent migraine headaches.

11-92 Martha, age 36, presents with a complaint of increasing shortness of breath and fatigue over the past 6 months. She has been trying to lose weight, has been on a walking exercise program for over a year, and had taken the fenfluramine-phentermine (Fen-Phen) combination years ago but stopped when its adverse effects were reported. Your examination reveals a grade II/VI systolic murmur along the apex. What do you do?

A. Obtain pulmonary function tests.
B. Instruct the client about other exercise activities that may not produce her symptoms.
C. Refer the client to a cardiologist for an echocardiogram and cardiovascular work-up.
D. Start endocarditis prophylaxis.

11-93   To reduce the progression of atherosclerotic lesions and occlusions in postcoronary artery bypass graft clients, it is recommended that the low-density lipoprotein cholesterol level be aggressively reduced to

A. 70 mg/dL.
B. 80–100 mg/dL.
C. 101–120 mg/dL.
D. 121–140 mg/dL.

11-94   Jessica is pregnant and is being seen for the first time. She states that she was told that her blood pressure (BP) has been high for a long time, but she never wanted to take medication for it. Today her BP is 172/98, her lungs are clear, and she has no pedal or ankle edema. What medication would you most likely order?

A. Methyldopa (Aldomet)
B. Atenolol (Tenormin)
C. Nifedipine (Adalat, Procardia)
D. Clonidine (Catapres)

11-95   Jim, age 72, has a history of type 2 diabetes mellitus that has been controlled by diet. He has come for a routine examination and reports feeling more tired than usual. On his electrocardiogram (ECG), you notice Q waves in leads II and III, and he is in atrial fibrillation that was not present on his previous ECGs. What do you do?

A. Immediately hospitalize Jim and order a cardiology consultation, start intravenous administration of an anticoagulant and nitrates, and run serial cardiac enzyme tests.
B. You do nothing because you know the normal progression of type 2 diabetes in older adults includes changes in their ECG as a result of neuropathy involving the transmission of electrical impulses.
C. Initiate aspirin therapy and refer Jim to a cardiologist for evaluation of occult ischemic heart disease and left ventricular function as soon as possible. Initiate lipid-lowering therapy because Jim may have had an acute myocardial infarction.
D. Initiate lipid-lowering therapy because Jim may have had an acute myocardial infarction.

11-96   Which of the following cardiac tests is used to identify intermittent ectopy and to match symptoms with underlying rhythms and should be used if the interval between symptom occurrence is greater than 48 hours?

A. 12-lead ECG
B. Holter monitor
C. Event monitor
D. Echocardiogram

11-97   Your client has documented hypertension (blood pressure of 140/92 mm Hg confirmed on multiple visits) and no other medical history. What would you consider low down on the list of priorities?

A. Immediate initiation of antihypertensive drug therapy to prevent any complications
B. Identification of known causes of hypertension
C. Assessment of the presence or absence of target organ damage and the extent of the disease
D. Identification of clinical cardiovascular disease (CVD) and risk factors, as well as other concomitant disorders that may guide prognosis and treatment

11-98   Which statement regarding rheumatic fever in children is true?

A. The peak period of risk is ages 1–5 years.
B. The disease is more common in boys.
C. The disease is more common in whites.
D. Group A beta-hemolytic streptococcal infections of the upper respiratory track remain the primary environmental trigger of rheumatic fever in children.

11-99   Which of the following is usually indicative of an abdominal aortic aneurysm?

A. RUQ tenderness
B. Venous hum in abdomen
C. Ascites
D. Positive bruit or wide, diffuse pulsation in epigastric area

11-100   For clients with known coronary artery disease, it is recommended that the low-density lipoprotein cholesterol be

A. 200 mg/dL or more.
B. 100 mg/dL or less.

C. 101–130 mg/dL.

D. 131–200 mg/dL.

11-101   Which statement about mitral valve prolapse (MVP) is true?

A. MVP occurs in about 10% of the population.

B. MVP is usually detected in older adults.

C. The incidence is equal in men and women younger than age 20.

D. The incidence is more common in women younger than age 20.

11-102   Bob is being seen in the office, and you suspect an acute ischemic syndrome and an acute myocardial infarction. Which would be the last step that you would consider?

A. Prompt admission to a monitored bed with cardiology consultation

B. Initiation of aspirin, intravenous heparin, and anti-ischemic therapy with nitrates or beta blockers

C. Measurement of serum lipid levels to determine risk factors of hyperlipidemia

D. Evaluation for possible angiography with rescue percutaneous transluminal coronary angioplasty or thrombolytic therapy

11-103   When teaching your client with a new diagnosis of aortic stenosis, which of the following statements made by him leads you to believe he needs more teaching?

A. "I will need antibiotic prophylaxis to prevent endocarditis."

B. "You told me I still need aggressive treatment of my hypertension."

C. "I'll continue the use of diuretics and nitrates that my previous doctor gave me."

D. "I'll have a yearly Doppler echocardiography to evaluate the progression of the valve lesion."

11-104   Which of the following statements about aortic stenosis (AS) is true?

A. The disease is typically manifested during midlife.

B. Once symptoms appear, life expectancy without surgery is about 10 years.

C. Right from the early course of the disease, symptoms are bothersome.

D. The cardinal symptoms include dyspnea, angina, and syncope.

11-105   Management of a client with hypertension with an abdominal aortic aneurysm would include

A. computed tomography scan without contrast.

B. changing the client's BP medications.

C. referral to a cardiologist.

D. immediate cardiac catheterization.

11-106   Discriminating between symptoms of occlusive arterial disease and other disorders (such as musculoskeletal or neurological disorders) requires a careful history. Which symptom is noted with occlusive arterial disease?

A. Pain occurring in the calves or thighs when walking, with relief obtained when standing still

B. Pain when standing that is not relieved by sitting or lying down

C. Severe pain at rest that requires the client to raise the legs in the air to obtain relief

D. Redness and pronounced superficial veins

11-107   Which of the following statements is true of mitral regurgitation?

A. It may be noted as a holosystolic murmur.

B. It is caused by stiff, noncompliant leaflets that limit flow from the left atrium to the left ventricle.

C. It occurs only as the result of congenital malformation of the mitral valve, which inhibits contact and closure of the cusps.

D. It results in a prolonged PR interval on electrocardiogram.

11-108   Shirley, age 58, has been a diabetic for 7 years. Her blood pressure is normal. Other than her diabetes medications, what would you prescribe today during her routine office visit?

A. An ACE inhibitor

B. A calcium channel blocker

C. A beta blocker

D. No hypertension medication

11-109 *Sam, age 70, originally had symptoms of syncope and then symptomatic ventricular tachycardia with aborted sudden death. He is now treated pharmacologically. He asks you when he can resume driving. How do you respond?*

A. "You may drive again in 1 month."

B. "You should not drive again for 6 months."

C. "As this may recur, let's wait until you're free of any symptoms for 1 year."

D. "You probably shouldn't drive anymore."

11-110 *Pathological U waves on the ECG are most commonly associated with which disorder?*

A. Hypercalcemia

B. Hypocalcemia

C. Hyperkalemia

D. Hypokalemia

Answers

11-1 Answer D

The clinical presentation of unstable angina may include waxing and waning of ischemic symptoms over a period of days or weeks. It often involves a progressive increase in symptoms in those with previous stable angina, including rest angina, and may include transient ST changes on the electrocardiogram. The differential diagnosis of unstable angina versus ST-segment elevation myocardial infarction (STEMI) versus non-STEMI is confirmed by the elevation of serum troponin. Important to note is the possibility of acute coronary syndrome without the alteration in electrocardiographic display.

11-2 Answer C

Superior vena cava syndrome occurs when there is obstructed venous return from the upper extremities, head, and neck region. Symptoms include edema and dusky blue discoloration of the upper extremities and head. Both the location of the obstruction and the rapidity with which it develops will determine the severity of symptoms. Diagnostic studies include chest radiography, CT, and venography. A CT scan is the most widely used. The most common cause of superior vena cava syndrome is cancer. Primary or metastatic cancer in the upper lobe of the right lung can compress the superior vena cava. Lymphoma or other tumors located in the mediastinum can also cause compression of the superior vena cava. Less often, the superior vena cava can become blocked with a blood clot from within. As more invasive medical procedures are being performed on clients, this cause of superior vena cava syndrome is being seen more frequently. Blood clot (thrombus) formation that causes superior vena cava syndrome is a complication of pacemaker wires, dialysis, and other intravenous catheters that are threaded into the superior vena cava (SVC). Signs and symptoms of SVC Syndrome may include shortness of breath and swelling of the arms and face. The symptoms occur because blood cannot return to the heart. Management of SVC is directed at managing the underlying cause and consists of various measures aimed at decreasing the severity of the obstruction.

11-3 Answer A

The manifestation of acute peripheral arterial occlusion is classically a dramatic one with sudden pain, pallor, paresthesia, paralysis, and pulselessness. However, it may also be more gradual and less dramatic, presenting with only complaints of coldness or paresthesia of the extremity. The occlusion may be caused by previously unknown cardiac disease, a vascular lesion, or an occult systemic disease, such as connective tissue diseases or arteritis, and should serve as a clue to look for other conditions because it rarely occurs by itself. Occlusions can occur in upper or lower extremities.

11-4 Answer B

Characteristics of ischemic arterial ulcers include severe pain and a discrete border (which may have a "punched-out" appearance) with a pale, dry ulcer base and a slightly inflamed "halo" around the border if infected. They are typically located distally and are usually a result of trauma.

11-5 Answer B

The JNC includes a category designated as prehypertension. The range for the systolic pressure is 120–139 and for diastolic pressure is 80–89. Clients with prehypertension are at an increased risk for progression to hypertension. Clients in the 130/80 to 139/89 mm Hg blood pressure (BP) range have twice the risk of developing hypertension as those with lower values. Diagnostic work-up of HTN should includes the following:

Assess risk factors and comorbidities

Reveal identifiable causes of HTN

Assess presence of target organ damage (TOD)

Conduct history and physical exam

Obtain lab studies to include U/A, blood glucose, Hct, lipid panel, serum potassium, creatinine and calcium

Electrocardiogram and echo as presentation dictates

NOTE: Latest studies from AHA and ACC: Hypertension is very common among older adults. Sixty-four percent of older men and 78% of older women have high BP, placing them at heightened risk for heart disease, including heart failure, stroke, coronary artery disease, and atrial fibrillation, as well as chronic kidney disease and diabetes mellitus. Despite its prevalence, rates of BP control remain substantially lower in the elderly than in younger clients. In fact, over age 80, only one in three men and one in four women have adequate control of their BP. Faced with an aging client population and compelling data that confirm the benefits of BP-lowering medications in the elderly (80 or more years), the American College of Cardiology (ACC) and the American Heart Association (AHA) released the first expert consensus document to help clinicians reduce the risks for developing and effectively manage hypertension in older adults.

There has been uncertainty about the appropriate therapeutic target for clients 80 years and older. Levels of less than 140/90 mm Hg in persons 65–79 years and a systolic BP between 140 and 145 mm Hg in persons 80 years and older if tolerated were discussed; hypertension in older adults is usually characterized by an elevated systolic BP and a normal or low diastolic BP due to age-associated stiffening of the large arteries.

Medications should be used as appropriate. Angiotensin converting enzyme (ACE) inhibitors, beta blockers, angiotensin receptor blockers, diuretics, and calcium channel blockers are all effective in lowering BP and reducing cardiovascular outcomes among the elderly; clinicians should select medications based on efficacy, tolerability, specific comorbidities, and cost. For example, a person who has had a heart attack should be started on a beta blocker and an ACE inhibitor.

11-6   Answer B

Signs of right-sided heart failure focus on fluid retention with edema and hepatic congestion, and depending on the extent of the disease, ascites will be evident. Signs of left-sided heart failure focus on a low cardiac output and an elevated pulmonary venous pressure, with dyspnea being the cardinal feature. It should be noted that heart failure may be systolic dysfunction, diastolic dysfunction or a combination of both. Treatment is directed contingent on the classification of heart failure (systolic or diastolic) and by the NY Heart Association Functional Class or the ACC/AHA stage.

11-7   Answer D

Occlusion of the left anterior descending artery results in damage to the anterior septal wall and the left ventricle. Occlusion of the right coronary artery usually results in damage to the inferior wall of the left ventricle, as well as potential damage to the right atrium, right ventricular, SA node, AV node, and papillary muscles of the mitral valve.

When the left circumflex artery (LCX) is the dominant vessel, occlusion can be responsible for damage to the inferior wall of the left ventricle. The LCX normally supplies the lateral wall of the left ventricle, as well as the posterior wall.

11-8   Answer A

Resuscitation Guidelines 2010 from the American Heart Association recommend, for the post–return of spontaneous circulation (ROSC) to the client who remains nonresponsive, that mild hypothermia should be provided to improve survival rates. Studies suggest the mortality rate in clients provided cooling was lower, and there was also an improvement in neurological outcomes.

For clients who remain nonresponsive post-ROSC with no contraindications, rapid cooling to a core temperature of 32–34°C should be initiated. The client should be maintained at this temperature for 12–24 hours at which time slow reversal of the cool state should be initiated. Further recommendations address the management of hemodynamics, electrocardiographics, fluid and electrolytes, and a purposeful assessment to determine the etiology to optimize the outcome.

11-9   Answer A

In athletes younger than age 30, the three most common causes of sudden death are hypertrophic cardiomyopathy, idiopathic left ventricular hypertrophy, and coronary artery anomalies. The diagnostic test that should be employed to detect a potential problem is an echocardiogram, which many colleges are now instituting as part of their screening criteria for athletes. The echocardiogram will detect hypertrophic cardiomyopathy and idiopathic left ventricular hypertrophy. The arteriogram is a reliable test available to detect coronary artery anomalies. An alternative to arteriogram for the diagnosis of CAD is the CT angiogram *coronary computed tomography angiogram*.

- A coronary computed tomography angiogram (CTA) uses advanced CT technology, along with intravenous (IV) contrast material (dye), to obtain high-resolution, three-dimensional pictures of the moving heart and great vessels.

- CTA is also called multislice computed tomography (MSCT), cardiac CT, or cardiac CAT. During CTA, x-rays pass through the body and are picked up by detectors in the scanner, three-dimensional images on a computer screen. These images enable physicians to determine whether plaque or calcium deposits are present in the artery walls.

- CTA is used as a noninvasive method for detecting blockages in the coronary arteries. A CTA can be performed much faster (in less than 1 minute) than a cardiac catheterization, with potentially less risk and discomfort as well as decreased recovery time.

An electrocardiogram will diagnose rhythm disturbances. A stress test will record the effects of stress on the heart.

11-10   Answer D

Long-term secondary prevention for chronic ischemic heart disease includes the use of aspirin, beta blockers, nitrates, and risk factor and lifestyle modification. Further pharmaceutical management may include diuretics, ACE inhibitors and/or angiotensin receptor blockers, spironolactone, and digoxin. Calcium channel blockers for the most part should be avoided. If utilized, the preferred calcium channel blockers include amlodipine or felodipine. To evaluate the progression of the disease, periodic testing should include noninvasive procedures such as exercise stress, stress-echoes, as well as close monitoring of pro-BNP and renal status. Comprehensive lab review likewise includes evaluation of LFTs, TSH, and HgbA1c. Invasive testing, including coronary angiography, should be reserved for clients who have markedly positive stress tests or angina that is refractory to medical treatment.

11-11   Answer D

Diagnostics would include a serum pro-BNP to assess degree of cardiac dysfunction. BNP is a hormone released from the ventricle in response to increased heart workload. It serves as a counterregulatory hormone to counteract innate compensatory mechanism. A BMP would be assessed to determine fluid and electrolyte status as well as renal status. Echocardiography is routinely obtained to monitor myocardial contractility, as well as valvular status. A CTA would not be routinely monitored.

11-12   Answer B

Impaired blood flow to the extremities results in leg aches and is most often caused by peripheral vascular disorders. Peripheral vascular disease (PVD) affects the arteries and veins. When the disease is arterial, it is usually the result of accumulated fatty streaks and fibrous plaques (high levels of low-density lipoproteins). When the disease is venous, problems relate to venous incompetence secondary to valve obstruction, leading to chronic venous insufficiency and varicose veins. All of the other conditions listed are appropriate differential diagnoses, and a thorough history and physical examination must be performed to rule them out. However, the most common cause of leg aches remains peripheral vascular disorders.

11-13   Answer A

Bile acid sequestrants (Questran, Colestid) are not absorbed from the gastrointestinal tract and lack systemic toxicity; therefore, liver function tests do not need to be monitored in clients taking these drugs. Hepatotoxicity is a serious, yet infrequent, adverse effect of hydroxymethylglutaryl-coenzyme A reductase inhibitors (statins), occurring about 1% of the time. Hepatic enzymes should be assessed before initiation and then as indicated secondary to dosage adjustment and/or product labeling. Nicotinic acid (niacin) is contraindicated in clients with active liver disease, peptic ulcer disease and or severe gout. Fibric acid derivatives such as gemfibrozil are contraindicated in clients with severe renal or hepatic disease.

11-14   Answer B

When auscultating the heart, if you note a short, high-frequency click (opening snap) after S_2 during the beginning of diastole, suspect mitral stenosis.

Mitral stenosis occurs with a stiff stenotic valve. The valve opening becomes restricted, impeding forward flow. The stenosis generates increased left atrial pressures, which are necessary to overcome the increased resistance to flow. The "snap" is created when the mitral valve leaflet is rapidly reversed toward the left ventricle in early diastole (as left ventricular pressures are reduced) by the high left atrial pressures.

11-15   Answer C

The American Heart Association and an International Liaison Committee determined in the 2011 guidelines of evidence-based practice that the primary goal in a resuscitation event is the provision of high-quality chest compression. The only other intervention noted to increase survival and neurologic recovery up to 1 year after resuscitation was the timely appropriate provision of hypothermia after return of spontaneous circulation (ROSC).

11-16   Answer C

The client's poor dental status is a probable source of endocarditis. Proper management of his dental work is essential before valve replacement because it will lower the risk for endocarditis. Removing the teeth in a single procedure reduces the repetitive risks of extraction-related bacteremia, as well as the possibility of developing antibiotic resistance from repeating prophylaxis regimens. Performing the extraction concurrently with valve surgery will add stress and risk of bacteremia to the procedure.

11-17   Answer B

Beta blockers should not be ordered for Marvin for two reasons: He smokes and he is a diabetic. The adverse effects of all beta blockers include the potential for developing bronchial asthma and for inhibiting gluconeogenesis, and therefore they may prolong hypoglycemic episodes.

11-18   Answer A

To determine the presence of target organ damage and other risk factors in the client with hypertension, basic diagnostic tests that should be ordered include a chest x-ray, electrocardiogram, urinalysis, complete blood count, chemistry profile, lipid profile, and thyroid-stimulating hormone level. Renal arteriogram, plasma renin activity, 24-hour urinary sodium, and echocardiogram are more expensive tests. They are indicated when hypertension is severe or refractory to treatment or when underlying renal pathology is suspected.

11-19   Answer B

If your client presents with chest pain, be sure to determine the time of onset because this may influence the course of treatment. Thrombolytic agents must be given within 6 hours of onset of pain to be effective.

11-20   Answer C

Cigarette smoking is the most important preventable cause of premature death in women. Cigarette smoking increases cerebrovascular disease (CVD) incidence and mortality. More than 50% of MIs in women younger than age 50 years are related to smoking. Women who smoke and use oral contraceptives increase their risk even more, while smoking cessation can lower their risk of CVD by 33% within 2 years.

11-21   Answer A

Mitral valve prolapse (MVP) is a congenital syndrome characterized by elongation of the chordae tendineae and enlarged valve leaflets. Ballooning of the cusps (prolapse) into the atrium occurs to varying degrees during ventricular systole. MVP is characterized by a midsystolic click and late systolic murmur.

11-22   Answer B

In a client with uncontrolled essential hypertension, the risk of the development of Diastolic heart failure is a concern as the increased workload on the heart has the propensity to cause left ventricular hypertrophy (LVH) and subsequent dysfunction. Thiazide diuretic and an ACE inhibitor in the client described in this scenario is the initial combination therapeutic of choice. Thiazide therapy will assist in the achievement of a stable fluid balance, and an ACE inhibitor in the client with diabetes mellitus is well supported as being efficacious.

While a beta blocker may be considered, studies suggest the choice of a beta blocker should be specific when instituted in the client with heart failure. Coreg (Carvedilol) and metoprolol succinate (Toprol–XL) are noted to be superior in decreasing morbidity and mortality. These may be considered in this client if exquisite blood pressure management is not achieved and added in a further combination therapeutic plan.

11-23   Answer A

Pharmacological therapy for mitral valve disease includes treatment of dyspnea with diuretics to relieve congestion. It also consists of afterload (not preload) reduction with antihypertensive agents to decrease regurgitant flow. Other therapies may include antiarrhythmics for atrial fibrillation because this condition can exacerbate symptoms as a result of ventricular filling. Beta blockers may be prescribed for clients with mitral valve prolapse (MVP) to help control palpitations; however, fatigue is a problem with MVP, and beta blockers may exacerbate the fatigue. *Antibiotic prophylaxis to prevent infective bacterial endocarditis is not indicated because the client with MVP is at no greater risk of developing endocarditis than the general population.* Anticoagulation with acetylsalicylic acid (ASA [aspirin]; 81–325 mg/d) is prescribed for some individuals with MVP who also have a history of transient ischemic attack (TIA), ischemic stroke, or atrial fibrillation.

11-24   Answer C

In the JNC guidelines, hypertension stages 2 and 3 have been combined. A blood pressure of 160 or greater systolic and 100 or greater diastolic is considered to be stage 2 hypertension. Pharmacological therapy is definitely indicated. Several drugs are usually required for management of this stage. Hypertensive clients should have a goal BP of under 140/90 or, if they have diabetes or chronic kidney disease, under 130/80. Choice of appropriate antihypertensives should include a review of client comorbidities. With cardiac disease, the client would most likely benefit from a beta blocker. If the cardiac disease is associated with heart failure, the choice of beta blocker should be narrowed to Coreg or Toprol XL. With heart failure and diastolic dysfunction, exquisite hemodynamics must be achieved to optimize cardiac function, so the addition of hydralazine as well as isosorbide dinitrate (Isordil) and spironolactone (Aldactone) may be considered. If the client has diabetes mellitus or low-grade renal insufficiency and the serum creatinine remains controlled, the choice may be an ACE inhibitor. Calcium channel blockers of the dihydropuridines subcategory (Norvasc) may also be considered.

11-25   Answer D

Although heredity, hypothyroidism, and diabetes contribute to abnormal serum lipid levels, a diet high in saturated fat is the most common cause of elevated total and low-density lipoprotein cholesterol in the United States.

11-26   Answer B

Xanthelasmas (small, yellow, raised plaques on the eyelids) are lipid deposits that may indicate hyperlipidemia.

11-27   Answer C

Hydroxymethylglutaryl-coenzyme A reductase inhibitors (statins) may cause—albeit rarely—myopathies, especially at higher dosages or in combination with certain drugs, such as gemfibrozil (Lopid), nicotinic acid (Nicobid), or erythromycin (E-Mycin). Any reports of muscle pain and weakness should be evaluated. According to National Cholesterol Education Program guidelines, bile acid sequestrants are preferred over statins for primary prevention of coronary events in men younger than age 45 and women younger than age 55. The liver is more active in the production of cholesterol during the evening hours; therefore, the recommendations for all statins (except atorvastatin [Lipitor], which has a longer half-life) is for dosing to be done in the evening or at bedtime. Statins may increase the international normalized ratio and require an adjustment of Coumadin dosage; however, Coumadin use is not a contraindication to use of statins.

11-28   Answer D

Lifestyle modifications are essential for the control of hypertension (HTN). Weight reduction of as little as 4.5 kg (10 lb) reduces blood pressure in a large proportion of overweight persons with HTN. It can also enhance the blood pressure–lowering effect of concurrent antihypertensive agents and reduce cardiovascular risk factors. The Dietary Approaches to Stop Hypertension (DASH) recommendations allow a combination of foods, with a diet rich in fruits, vegetables, and low-fat dairy products, and are not based on excessive calorie restriction. Elevated blood pressure is not an inevitable consequence of aging. Excessive alcohol intake is an important risk factor for HTN because it can cause resistance to antihypertensive therapy. Individuals who drink should be counseled to limit their daily intake to no more than 1 oz of ethanol for average-sized men and 0.5 oz of ethanol for women or lighter-weight individuals (1 oz of ethanol equals 2 oz of whiskey, 24 oz of beer, or 10 oz of wine).

11-29   Answer C

According to the Agency for Healthcare Research and Quality clinical practice guidelines, clients with angina at rest, postinfarction angina, or rapidly progressive unstable angina with electrocardiogram changes should be managed with hospitalization in a monitored setting, bedrest, control of precipitating factors, and initiation of medical therapy. The American Heart Association in concert with an International Liaison Committee recommends percutaneous coronary intervention (PCI) for timely diagnostic and potential revascularization at the point of care.

11-30   Answer C

Dental procedures and extractions require antibiotic prophylaxis against bacterial endocarditis when comorbid conditions exist, such as a prior history of a client who has undergone valvular replacement. The recommendations from cardiologists reflect an analysis of relevant literature regarding procedure-related endocarditis. The recommendations serve only as guidelines. Because endocarditis may occur even with appropriate use of antimicrobials, one must be concerned if fever, night chills, weakness, myalgia, or malaise are reported after procedures.

11-31   Answer A

Evidence-based guidelines from the American Association of Clinical Endocrinologists single out methyldopa and nifedipine as preferable antihypertensive medications in pregnancy, with magnesium sulfate for women with pre-eclampsia who are at high risk for seizures. Methyldopa is the drug of first choice for control of mild to moderate hypertension in pregnancy and is the most widely prescribed antihypertensive for this indication. The wide use of this drug in pregnancy reflects the fact that it has the best documented maternal and fetal safety record, including favorable long-term (4.5–7.5 year) pediatric follow-up data. During long-term use in pregnancy, methyldopa does not alter maternal cardiac output or blood flow to the uterus or kidneys, and for all these reasons, it is generally considered the agent of choice for chronic blood pressure control in pregnancy.

While earlier studies suggested that administration of beta blockers (particularly those without intrinsic sympathomimetic activity) during pregnancy might increase the chance of intrauterine growth retardation, recent studies have been more reassuring on this point. Nevertheless, the available data are insufficient to rule out unrecognized adverse effects of early and prolonged use of beta blockers pregnancy. When used for short periods (less than 6 weeks) during the third trimester, beta blockers are effective and well tolerated provided there are no signs of intrauterine growth impairment. ACE inhibitors and angiotensin receptor blockers (ARBs) have been associated with serious fetal abnormalities.

11-32   Answer A

Bacterial endocarditis prophylaxis is recommended for high-risk clients, including those with prosthetic heart valves, previous bacterial endocarditis, complex cyanotic congenital heart disease, and surgically constructed systemic pulmonary shunts or conduits. Moderate-risk clients requiring this include those with most other congenital cardiac deformities, such as ventricular septal defect (VSD), rheumatic heart disease, and other acquired cardiac defects, like those successfully surgically repaired, hypertrophic cardiomyopathy, and mitral valve prolapse (with valvular regurgitation and/or thickened valves).

11-33   Answer D

The intensity of a murmur is determined by the quantity and velocity of blood flow across the sound-producing area, its distance from the stethoscope, and the type of tissue between the murmur and the stethoscope. A murmur that is audible with the stethoscope off the chest is a grade VI murmur. A grade I murmur is barely heard; grade II is quietly heard and is approximately the same tone level as the S_1–S_2; grade III is heard; grade IV is loud; grade V is very loud; and grade VI is the loudest. A thrill may accompany murmurs of grades IV, V, and VI.

11-34   Answer A

Nicotinic acid lowers low-density lipoprotein cholesterol levels, and is effective in the management of the highly atherogenic lipoprotein. It raises high-density lipoprotein cholesterol levels and decreases triglyceride levels; may potentiate the effect of some antihypertensive agents; and may commonly (not rarely) cause adverse reactions including flushing, pruritus, and gastrointestinal upset. Nicotinic acid is not the drug of choice for individuals with diabetes. A potential adverse effect of nicotinic acid is impairment of glucose intolerance; therefore, it should be used with caution in clients with diabetes. If nicotinic acid is administered, serum glucose and liver function tests should be closely monitored. Nicotinic acid should likewise be avoided in clients with gout and/or peptic ulcer disease.

11-35   Answer B

The addition of metolazone is the appropriate next intervention in the management of congestive heart failure that presents with a decreased sensitivity to loop diuretics and Aldactone combination. The client should be reminded of the importance of strict medication and dietary recommendations. He should likewise be counseled to contact the office if his weight increases by 3 lbs or more in 24 hours or 5 lbs in 1 week. With the addition of metolazone, the client should be reminded of the importance of maintaining a home blood pressure log. In addition, he should contact the office if increasing shortness of breath or dyspnea on exertion occurs or if he experiences abdominal distension, palpitations or syncopal events.

11-36   Answer B

Funduscopic examination for hypertensive retinopathy (arteriovenous nicking, arteriole narrowing, hemorrhages, exudates, and disk edema) should be included in the physical examination of a client with hypertension (HTN). When examining the client with HTN, at least two blood pressure measurements separated by 5 minutes should be performed with the client seated. An additional blood pressure reading taken with the client standing should also be considered for evaluation of "white coat HTN." Further diagnostic work-up should include assessment of risk factors and comorbidities. Assess for identifiable causes of hypertension, some of which may include sleep apnea, drug-induced HTN, chronic kidney disease, diabetes, smoking, and physical inactivity. Physical assessment should include auscultation of heart tones and assessment of apical location to determine left ventricular hypertrophy. A comprehensive work-up should include lab studies, fasting lipid panel, thyroid-stimulating hormone, HgbA1c, and a basic metabolic panel. Urine for microalbuminuria may be indicated. Client education should include discussion of the importance of weight loss, smoking cessation, and reducing alcohol intake as well as

directions for maintaining a heart-healthy low-sodium (Na) diet. Additional discussion should include maintaining an exercise program with a target of exercising most days of the week, with consideration of the client's limitations. Cardiac rehab should be instituted when indicated.

11-37   Answer A

All of these behavior changes are important, but for smokers, quitting is the single-most important change they can make to reduce future risk of MI.

11-38   Answer A

Auscultation of the aortic valve (the second heart sound [S_2], which signifies closure of the aortic and pulmonic valves) is best performed using the diaphragm of the stethoscope because it is a high-pitched sound and is best heard at the second right intercostal space. It should also include auscultation at other locations such as neck, apex, and right parasternal region because important findings are sometimes present in other locations.

11-39   Answer D

Several changes to the cardiovascular system can be seen during pregnancy. The increase in cardiac workload often results in the development of a systolic murmur. A mammary souffle is a murmur that develops from increased blood flow through the mammary artery occurring late in pregnancy or during lactation. As the pregnancy progresses and the diaphragm rises, the heart rises and rotates, displacing the apical impulse. The blood pressure is usually lower during the first and second trimesters, and the heart rate is slightly higher (not slower, as in bradycardia) than in the nonpregnant state.

11-40   Answer B

Mitral valve prolapse causes one or both leaflets to billow into the atrium during ventricular systole and runs in families.

11-41   Answer A

When assessing for edema, check the client's most dependent areas such as the legs, sacrum, and scrotum. Peripheral edema is the accumulation of fluid within the interstitial spaces of the extremities. When the edema involves the lower extremities, it is a symptom of an underlying disorder; it may be caused by cardiac conditions (e.g., heart failure, chronic venous insufficiency, or thrombophlebitis), renal and hepatic disease, or by trauma, tumors, or inflammation. Anasarca is generalized body edema, which may indicate right-sided CHF.

11-42   Answer B

Waterhammer pulses (Corrigan's pulses) are present in a client with aortic regurgitation or aortic insufficiency. The forceful, high-volume left ventricular ejection of blood into the aorta during systole is accompanied by a reflux of blood back into the left ventricle during diastole. *Usually, the peripheral vascular resistance is low in aortic regurgitation*, which maximizes the forward flow of blood into the periphery. As a result of this forceful movement of blood and subsequent backflow, the waveform of peripheral pulses is characterized by a rapid rise and collapse. Other findings resulting from this phenomenon include pistol-shot pulses (Duroziez' murmur), which are audible on auscultation of the femoral artery; alternating flushing and paling of the nailbed capillaries (Quincke's capillary pulsation); and systolic head bobbing as the collapsed neck vessel fills rapidly (Musset's sign).

11-43   Answer C

When teaching a client with hypertension about restricting dietary sodium, it is important to stress that 75% of sodium intake is derived from processed food. Although concern about severe sodium restriction has been raised, there is no evidence that lower levels of sodium intake cause any hazards. A sodium reduction to approximately 6 g of sodium chloride or 2.4 g of sodium a day is recommended for most clients and is easily achievable. The bottom line to stress to the client is that reducing the sodium will reduce water retention, resulting in less burden on the heart.

11-44   Answer A

Diuretics are effective in lowering blood pressure in all clients, especially African Americans and older adults. Numerous studies have shown reductions in morbidity and mortality with these agents. Relative to beta blockers and ACE inhibitors, diuretics are more potent in African Americans, older adults, obese clients, and other subgroups who exhibit increased plasma volume or low plasma renin activity. Alpha-adrenergic blockers may be used effectively if the client has coexisting prostatism.

11-45   Answer A

Deep vein thrombosis (DVT) may result in generalized edema of the involved extremity. DVT usually originates in the pelvis and lower extremities. It is typically asymptomatic. Pulmonary embolus may be the first indication of thrombosis. Thrombus formation may not be clinically apparent because of the large capacity of the venous system and development of collateral circulation around obstructions. Pain is the most common symptom and may be aching or throbbing. Most pulmonary emboli are caused by DVT. There is no atrophy of the leg muscles, and although there is pain, there is not a loss of sensation. DVT may result in a thromboembolism. Other emboli include tumors that have invaded the venous circulation (tumor emboli), amniotic fluid, air, fat, bone marrow, or foreign intravenous material.

11-46   Answer D

A systolic blood pressure (BP) of 140–145 is the target for ages 80 and up. This range is associated with a lower cardiovascular risk than higher levels—and possibly fewer side effects than lower levels. But do not be concerned if clients over 80 are doing well with a systolic BP less than 140 mm Hg and a diastolic BP over 65 mm Hg.

11-47   Answer A

Nifedipine (Procardia XL), a calcium channel blocker, should be discontinued, along with most antiarrhythmic agents, when a client develops congestive heart failure (CHF) because both of these classes of medications are important causes of worsening heart failure. However, amiodarone is an antiarrhythmic used successfully in the treatment of clients with CHF. Diuretics are the most effective means of providing symptomatic relief in clients with CHF, so Greg should stay on his hydrochlorothiazide (HydroDIURIL). ACE inhibitors, such as enalapril (Vasotec), should be the initial treatment, along with diuretics in most symptomatic clients, so Greg can also continue taking this. The barbiturate butalbital (Esgic) is not contraindicated in clients with CHF.

11-48   Answer B

A pulsating abdominal mass in the region of the umbilicus is suggestive of an abdominal aortic aneurysm. Abdominal aortic aneurysms may be asymptomatic or may cause abdominal or back pain as well as impotence or difficulties with digestion. Abdominal aortic aneurysms can also cause chest pain. Thoracic aneurysms must be quite large to produce symptoms and consequently may be discovered incidentally by chest x-ray. The symptoms are caused by expansion and compression of adjacent thoracic structures and may include dysphagia, hoarseness, and edema of the head and arms. Aneurysm rupture is catastrophic and may present with severe chest, abdominal, or back pain; paralysis; or shock. Renal artery stenosis is a common cause of secondary hypertension and presents in the same manner as essential hypertension. Primary cardiac tumors are rare and are usually atrial myxomas. Metastases to the heart from malignant tumors elsewhere in the body are more frequent. The client usually presents with fever, malaise, weight loss, leukocytosis, an elevated erythrocyte sedimentation rate, and peripheral or pulmonary emboli.

11-49   Answer C

The greater the number of symptoms in a client, the more reliable is the diagnosis of heart failure. One of the classic symptoms of heart failure that Sheila has is a nocturnal cough that wakes her up. Other findings indicative of heart failure include an elevated jugular venous pressure, an S_3 heart sound, a laterally displaced apical impulse, pulmonary crackles (rales) that do not clear with coughing, and peripheral edema that is not caused by venous insufficiency. A persistent night cough is often the only symptom seen with some types of asthma, but the cough is dry without any of the other symptoms that Sheila has. Allergies may present as a dry cough at night with a postnasal drip. Valvular heart disease may present with dyspnea, orthopnea, and paroxysmal nocturnal dyspnea but not a cough with crackles (rales).

11-50   Answer D

Because some older adults develop postural hypotension with hypertensive drug therapy, the clinician must insist that these clients change position slowly while on HTN medication and that they sit on the edge of the bed for several minutes before standing. In addition, clients with postural hypotension should be urged to avoid volume depletion by drinking adequate quantities of water. Lifestyle modifications cannot be stressed enough.

11-51   Answer D

Valvular heart disease (mitral and tricuspid) has become the least common cause of heart failure of the conditions listed because of the declining incidence and severity of rheumatic fever. On the other hand, aortic stenosis occurs frequently and is reversible. The most common cause of heart failure is ischemic cardiomyopathy. Systemic hypertension remains a common cause of congestive heart failure.

11-52   Answer D

The causative factors in the formation of blood clots are referred to as Virchow's triad. They include venous stasis, vessel injury, and hypercoagulability.

11-53   Answer A

While all these questions are important, if your client is allergic to shellfish, she or he may be allergic to the dye used for cardiac catheterization. Of note, recent studies suggest that a true allergy to iodine is a medical myth.

Many people are labeled as having an iodine allergy if they have a reaction to iodine-containing foods or drugs, such as seafood and Betadine. They are then sometimes denied radiocontrast dyes or other products that contain iodine, but this precaution is not usually necessary.

Iodine molecules are too small to trigger an antibody-mediated allergic reaction. A reaction to iodine-containing foods or products is usually either caused by an agent other than the iodine or is not a true allergy. *Seafood allergies* are usually due to proteins in the seafood. *Povidone-iodine* (Betadine, etc.) reactions are usually due to irritation or contact dermatitis. *Potassium iodide* (Iosat, ThyroSafe, ThyroShield) reactions are extremely rare, less than one in a million. And it is likely that *iododerma*, an acnelike rash due to the large dose of iodine, is not a true IgE-mediated immune reaction. *Radiocontrast dye* reactions are often caused by the high osmolarity, *not* by the iodine. Explain that the radiologist can use a *low*-osmolarity contrast dye to lower the risk. Help prevent confusion by avoiding the term *iodine allergy*. Instead, refer to the specific reaction, such as seafood allergy, povidone-iodine dermatitis, or contrast-media sensitivity, especially when asking about allergies and making notes in client records.

11-54   Answer A

Substernal chest pain that is provoked by exertion and relieved by rest or nitroglycerin is considered typical or stable angina and carries a high risk for unstable coronary artery disease (CAD). Chest pain radiating to one or both arms, sometimes accompanied by nausea, vomiting, or diaphoresis, is associated with a high risk of acute coronary syndrome. "Anginal equivalents" may include symptoms not typically associated with CAD, such as discomfort radiating to the jaw, neck, or ear, if they are also associated with exertion. New-onset or worsening exertional dyspnea is the most common anginal equivalent in the elderly.

11-55   Answer C

Drugs that convert atrial fibrillation to sinus rhythm are amiodarone (Cordarone), disopyramide (Norpace), flecainide (Tambocor), propafenone (Rythmol), and ibutilide (Corvert). Digoxin is effective only for rate control at best and should be used only as a second-line agent. Lidocaine is used for ventricular dysrhythmias, and adenosine (Adenocard) is the treatment of choice in the case of paroxysmal supraventricular tachycardia (PSVT). Adenocard can serve as a diagnostic tool in PSVT, allowing the provider to assess the electrocardiographic presentation by slowing ventricular response, or it may convert the PSVT to normal sinus rhythm (NSR) contingent on the etiology of the electrical conduction disturbance.

11-56   Answer A

Funduscopic changes associated with hypertension include optic disk swelling, AV nicking, hard exudates, creamy yellow lesions, and soft exudates such as cotton wool (also seen with subacute bacterial endocarditis). Deep intraretinal hemorrhages (dot hemorrhages) are seen with diabetes. A cup-disk ratio greater than 1:2 is seen with open-angle glaucoma.

11-57   Answer B

Beta blockers are the first-choice therapy for treating hypertension and angina in clients with known coronary artery disease because they control angina by decreasing myocardial demand through reduction of heart rate, systolic blood pressure, and contractility. Beta blockers have also been shown to reduce the risk of subsequent myocardial infarctions (MIs) and sudden cardiac death in clients who have had a previous MI.

11-58   Answer A

According to the National Cholesterol Education Program (NCEP) expert panel, Sarah's treatment should focus on lowering her low-density lipoprotein (LDL) cholesterol to less than 100 mg/dL because she has several risk factors for coronary artery disease. Certainly treating her hypertension and asthma and assisting her with a smoking cessation treatment program will also help. Further recommendations may include weight management, encouraging physical activity on most days of the week. The powerhouse medications for the reduction of LDL cholesterol remains the hydroxymethylglutaryl-coenzyme A reductase inhibitors (statins). Note that there is a slight risk of rise in hepatic enzymes with statin usage. Baseline levels should be obtained and levels should be reassessed as per product recommendation.

11-59   Answer C

Mr. Michaels's electrocardiogram rhythm strip shows atrial fibrillation. To prevent continuous release of microemboli into the circulation, resulting in a pulmonary embolism or cerebrovascular accident, Mr. Michaels will probably be taking warfarin or dabigatran.

Dabigatran (Pradaxa) may be ordered instead of warfarin for nonvalvular atrial fibrillation because Dabigatran does not need monitoring. Dabigatran also prevents more strokes than warfarin—about 5 fewer strokes per 1,000 clients per year—with a similar overall bleeding risk. But there are safety concerns. Keep these nuances in mind.

Switching from warfarin to dabigatran. Switch clients with poor international normalized ratio (INR) control or those who cannot be well monitored. To switch, stop warfarin and wait until the INR is below 2, then start dabigatran. There are cases of bleeding when dabigatran is started too soon. Prescribe 150 mg bid or 75 mg bid if creatinine clearance is 15–30 mL/min. Do not routinely switch clients who are doing well on warfarin. Dabigatran causes more gastrointestinal bleeds and may prevent fewer MIs.

Missed doses. Encourage careful adherence to the twice-daily regimen. Dabigatran starts to wear off about 15 hours after the dose is taken. If clients miss a dose, advise taking it as soon as possible unless the next dose is due in less than 6 hours. Tell clients *not* to double up on doses.

Bleeding. Dabigatran does not have any antidote, such as vitamin K. For serious bleeding, stop dabigatran and give fresh frozen plasma or whole blood if necessary.

Surgery. Stop dabigatran at least 1 day before surgery or, for clients with renal insufficiency, 3 days before surgery. Surgeons may stop it sooner for surgeries with a high bleeding risk.

Dyspepsia. Dabigatran capsules contain tartaric acid to improve absorption, so dyspepsia is common. Taking them with food, an H2 blocker, or a proton pump inhibitor might help. PPIs may decrease absorption, but probably not enough to reduce dabigatran's efficacy. If dyspepsia persists, use warfarin instead.

In addition, digitalis (Digoxin) is usually ordered, sometimes in combination with either a beta blocker or a calcium channel blocker. The antiarrhythmic agent procainamide (Procan-SR) is used for ventricular arrhythmias. Anticonvulsants, such as phenytoin, are not indicated.

11-60   Answer D

Abrupt withdrawal of clonidine (Catapres), a central acting alpha agonist, will most likely produce a rebound hypertensive crisis. Blood pressure may return to or even exceed pretreatment levels after withdrawal of clonidine. This response is rarely seen following withdrawal of beta blockers, diuretics, ACE inhibitors (e.g., lisinopril), or calcium channel blockers. The most noticeable symptoms include sweating, palpitations, nervousness, headache, abdominal cramping, and nausea, along with elevated blood pressure. The mechanism for clonidine withdrawal is thought to be catecholamine overproduction.

11-61   Answer A

True statements concerning sexual activity for clients with chronic ischemic heart disease include that the sexual partner should be included in the education process, that antianginal medication taken before sexual activity can help prevent symptoms, and that sexual activity should be attempted when the client is well rested, although morning hours may not always be best. Chronic angina exhibits a circadian rhythm characterized by a propensity toward transient ischemic episodes in the morning hours. The physical stress of sexual intercourse is usually equivalent to that of climbing one flight of stairs at a normal pace or any other activity that induces a heart rate of 120 beats per minute. Clients should be reassured that if they can carry out these activities without symptoms, they can probably engage in sexual activity without symptoms. If symptoms occur, they may be managed with proper precautions such as timing activities more than 2 hours after meals, taking an extra dose of a short-acting beta blocker 1 hour before intercourse, or taking nitroglycerin 15 minutes before intercourse.

11-62   Answer B

The leading cause of death for women in the United States is cardiovascular disease, including heart and cerebrovascular disease. Although the incidence of cardiovascular disease is lower in younger women, it dramatically increases in women older than age 45 and is a major cause of chronic illness and disability in these women. Women often present atypically and subsequently have higher morbidity and mortality rates related to CAD secondary to lost opportunity to treat because the diagnosis of acute coronary syndrome is often missed.

11-63   Answer A

Auscultation of the typical murmur associated with aortic stenosis usually reveals that it is a systolic murmur of a harsh, crescendo-decrescendo ejection type, best heard at the base of the heart. It often radiates to the carotid arteries. In clients with a calcified aortic valve, the murmur is harsh and rasping at the base. As the client's left ventricular dysfunction worsens, the typical harsh murmur becomes quieter and resembles the murmur of mitral regurgitation, which often is a secondary diagnosis due to left ventricular dysfunction. The loudness of the murmur does not reflect the severity of the lesion.

11-64   Answer A

Hepatomegaly is the cardinal sign of right-sided heart failure in infants and children. Edema of the lower extremities is indicative of right ventricular heart failure in older children and adults. Tachypnea is the cardinal sign of left-sided congestive heart failure in children. Cyanosis is a clue to the presence of heart disease but is not specifically a sign of right-sided heart failure.

11-65   Answer B

Headache, flushing, tachycardia, and peripheral edema are adverse effects associated with calcium channel blockers. Calcium channel blockers may antagonize any of several cell membrane calcium entry channel receptors. As a result, some of these agents can express different effects on regional circulation. Although verapamil (Calan) and diltiazem (Cardizem) may reduce sinus rate, dihydropyridine calcium channel blockers may cause more potent peripheral vasodilation and can also cause headache, flushing, and tachycardia. Calcium channel blockers may also cause peripheral edema from reflex postcapillary constriction, which causes an increase in capillary hydrostatic pressure. This leads to movement of intravascular fluid to peripheral tissues and edema that is unassociated with weight gain.

11-66   Answer D

Before counseling partners about sexual activity following a myocardial infarction (MI), the provider should consider that depression, loss of interest, spousal reluctance, and anxiety may interfere with a client's resumption of sexual activities. The diagnosis of heart disease affects the spouse as well as the client. Spouses may display anxiety and depression yet often are not included in the assessment, counseling, and treatment processes. The level of sexual activity reported 1 year after an MI is only about 60% of the level before illness.

11-67   Answer B

Beta blockers reduce the heart rate, which results in a decrease in oxygen demand and an increase in coronary blood flow from the increased diastolic filling time. Studies have also shown that beta blockers reduce mortality in clients who have had acute myocardial infarctions and reinfarction. Adverse effects of all beta blockers include a decrease in high-density lipoprotein cholesterol, bronchospasm, fatigue, sleep disturbance, worsening of congestive heart failure, gastrointestinal disturbances, and impotence.

11-68   Answer C

Alpha-adrenergic blockers are used both to lower blood pressure and to relieve some of the symptoms associated with benign prostatic hypertrophy. They decrease the resistance along the prostatic urethra by relaxing the smooth muscle component of the prostate. Alpha-adrenergic blockers can cause postural hypotension during the initial doses of therapy; therefore, the dosage should "start low and go slow" and then gradually increase depending on the effectiveness. Clients should be advised to take an alpha blocker at bedtime because of the

profound orthostasis associated with it. Further side effects may include dry mouth and sedation. Clients should be advised of the risk of increased sedation when combined with any sedating medication. The Joint National Committee suggests an alpha blocker should never be instituted as initial solo therapy but rather be added to the most appropriate antihypertensive therapy for overall individual client physiologic comorbidities.

11-69   Answer B

The clinical symptoms of chronic occlusive arterial disease occur slowly over a period of years and result primarily from tissue underperfusion and ischemia. Usually, the earliest symptom is intermittent claudication. Later signs and symptoms of chronic occlusive arterial disease in the lower extremities include changes in skin texture, loss of hair, muscle wasting, reduced muscle strength and sensation, and the development of ulcers on the toes or heels.

11-70   Answer C

Based on an algorithm for screening and managing clients with elevated triglycerides, experts have established an optimal level of triglycerides of less than 100 mg/dL and recommend intensive diet and lifestyle changes for clients with borderline elevated triglycerides.

For clients with borderline triglyceride levels of 150–199 mg/dL, experts recommend losing 5% of current body weight and limiting carbohydrates to 50%–60% of daily caloric intake. Weight loss has a beneficial effect on lipids and lipoproteins with a 5%–10% weight reduction resulting in a 20% decrease in triglycerides, an approximate 15% reduction in LDL cholesterol, and an 8%–10% increase in HDL cholesterol. The American Heart Association recommends limiting added sugars to less than 10% of daily caloric intake and provides guidance on fructose consumption, recommending that borderline clients consume less than 100 grams.

For clients with very high triglyceride levels, drug therapy is used to reduce the risk of pancreatitis.

Guidelines suggest using nonfasting triglyceride levels, which simplifies testing for clients and clinicians by eliminating the traditional 12-hour fast. In the United States, 31% of adults have triglyceride levels that exceed 150 mg/dL, and Mexican Americans (36%) are more likely than whites (33%) and blacks (16%) to have high triglycerides.

11-71   Answer B

Despite the technological advances of recent years, including cardiac resynchronization, implantable defibrillators, left ventricular assist devices, and totally implantable artificial hearts, it should be remembered that many clients with chronic heart failure are elderly and have multiple comorbidities. Clients who gain 3 lb in 1 day or 5 lb in 1 week should be seen immediately, which might prevent rehospitalization. Most clients require pillows at night and will probably have a recumbent cough, but the fluid overload characteristic of congestive heart failure (CHF) will be manifested by the weight gain. These clients may be depressed, thus sleeping more, and although treating the depression is important, it will not prevent a rehospitalization due to worsening CHF. Additional symptoms to advise clients to monitor for may include lower extremity edema, abdominal distention, jugular venous distention, palpitations, and increasing dyspnea on exertion. As clients are managed on an outpatient basis, they should be fully educated on interventions that will assist in improving presentation. Some of the educational discussions may include maintaining a low-sodium diet, avoidance of alcohol, daily weights, and daily blood pressure monitoring. Frequencies of visits to a heart failure specialist will be determined on an individual basis because titration of medications requires close assessment to optimize outcomes.

11-72   Answer A

The most common symptom of digitalis toxicity is nausea and vomiting. Other adverse side effects may include, headache, diarrhea, stomach pain, loss of appetite, unusual tiredness or weakness, slow heartbeat, palpitations, irregular heartbeat, drowsiness, confusion, fainting, changes in vision including seeing a halo or light around objects, and disorientation. The symptoms usually occur before any cardiotoxic effects take place and are warning signs that the dosage needs to be adjusted. Tingling of the extremities is not a symptom of digitalis toxicity.

11-73   Answer C

The first priority for managing ischemic arterial ulcers is to improve tissue perfusion. When counseling clients, tell them to decrease their risk of further damage by reducing risk factors. Ways to reduce risk factors include stopping smoking, reducing fat (lipid) intake, avoiding restrictive garments and trauma (mechanical, chemical, and thermal), maintaining adequate hydration, and avoiding caffeinated drinks. Smoking and caffeine can cause vasoconstriction and reduce blood flow. Lipid lowering can restore some of the arterial vessels' ability to vasodilate and "self-regulate" blood flow in response to tissue needs. Adequate hydration reduces blood viscosity, improves blood flow, and reduces chances for microemboli formation. Although an intense aerobics program should not be initiated, Buerger-Allen exercises should be done three to four times per day. The client raises the extremity 45° and then lowers it to a supine position, repeating this five times over a 2-minute period. The changes in position cause the arteries of the legs to refill by gravity.

11-74   Answer C

Prinzmetal's (variant) angina usually has no precipitating factors and occurs at rest as a result of spasms of the coronary artery. Clients with Prinzmetal's angina frequently have a history of migraine headaches and Raynaud's disease.

11-75   Answer C

Pharmacological therapy is indicated for Terry because his blood pressure has been elevated on three separate occasions. Target organ damage to the heart is suggested by the left ventricular hypertrophy noted on his electrocardiogram, which may suggest the need for a two-drug combination. Diuretics such as hydrochlorothiazide (HydroDIURIL) have been proved to reduce hypertensive morbidity and mortality and should be the first drug of choice. In addition to being inexpensive, diuretics, when used as antihypertensive agents in blacks who have low plasma renin activity, are more potent than other antihypertensive drugs. This client may benefit from a second line addition of an ACE inhibitor, an angiotensin receptor blocker, a beta blocker, or a calcium channel blocker.

The client does not report symptoms suggesting pheochromocytoma, and its occurrence is rare, so plasma and urine catecholamine level tests are not indicated at this time. Analyzing the client's food diary, although a necessary intervention, will not sufficiently meet this client's needs as priority intervention.

11-76   Answer C

The cause of hypertension is unknown (idiopathic) in approximately 95% of cases. This form of hypertension is known as primary or essential hypertension. The remaining 5% of cases are secondary to underlying disease processes such as renal disease, renal artery stenosis (RAS), pregnancy, endocrine disorders, pheochromocytoma. Confounding issues to address include obesity, NSAID usage, alcohol usage, and smoking.

The incidence of hypertension is greatest in adult black men and women.

11-77   Answer B

Renal artery bruits, which indicate renal artery stenosis, particularly those of diastolic timing, are a suggestive sign of renovascular hypertension. They are often heard or palpated (as a thrill) in the abdomen, flanks, or back. Systolic bruits are commonly detected, especially in older adults, and may not be associated with renal artery stenosis.

11-78   Answer C

A cough, loss of taste, and a rash are all adverse effects of ACE inhibitors. They all disappear with discontinuance of the medication and may or may not reappear if therapy is resumed with another ACE inhibitor. Some diuretics may cause electrolyte disturbances, fatigue, and, depending on the type, rash and impotence. Beta blockers may cause bronchospasm, increase plasma triglyceride levels, and result in central nervous system disturbances. Calcium channel blockers may cause adverse vasodilatory effects such as headache, flushing, palpitation, and ankle edema.

11-79   Answer D

The National Cholesterol Education Program (NCEP) guidelines recommend a goal serum low-density lipoprotein cholesterol level of less than 130 mg/dL for individuals without coronary artery disease but with two or more risk factors.

11-80   Answer B

The cholesterol component considered most responsible for atherosclerotic plaque formation is an elevated low-density lipoprotein cholesterol level.

11-81   Answer A

The classic 12-lead electrocardiogram (ECG) change that indicates an acute coronary syndrome (ACS) is ST-segment elevation. The American Heart Association, in its therapeutic recommendations, discusses ST-segment elevation myocardial infarction (STEMI) as well as non-ST-segment elevation myocardial infarction (NSTEMI) in defining optimal

therapeutic management of an ACS client. It is important to remember an actively evolving infarction could be present with no electrocardiographic changes appreciated. When assessing a client with a suspected ACS, timely assessment and management is essential. Timely cardiac catheterization and laboratory assessments and possible percutaneous coronary intervention is essential in decreasing mortality and morbidity. Further therapeutics may likewise include but not be limited to aspirin, Plavix, beta blocker and ACE inhibitor, statin therapy, and smoking cessation therapy if indicated.

11-82   Answer D

Because dietary therapy has not resulted in any significant reduction of Rick's low-density lipoprotein (LDL) cholesterol level, starting him on hypolipidemic drug therapy is strongly recommended to help him achieve an LDL cholesterol goal of less than 130 mg/dL. To further help reduce the risk of heart disease, regular physical activity of moderate intensity (the minimal goal is 30 minutes, five times a week), along with lowering blood pressure and reducing weight, is important. No further diagnostic intervention is indicated unless the client begins to complain of symptoms of ischemia, such as chest pain, increasing fatigue, or dyspnea.

11-83   Answer A

ACE inhibitors such as enalapril (Vasotec) should be considered as first-line therapy for a client with hypertension (HTN) and heart failure. Research from the Framingham Heart Study demonstrated that HTN continues to be the major cause of left ventricular failure in the United States. In treating heart failure, ACE inhibitors alone or with a diuretic are effective in reducing morbidity and mortality. Evidence suggest beta blockers, such as carvedilol and metoprolol succinate, are of great value in managing stable systolic dysfunction heart failure and decreasing morbidity and mortality. Alternative medications, such as a nitrate and hydralazine combination, are effective for clients who develop hyperkalemia or renal dysfunction with ACE inhibitors or angiotensin receptor blockers.

Contingent on the etiology of the heart failure (such as systolic versus diastolic dysfunction), additional medications may include metoprolol succinate (Toprol XL) or carvedilol (Coreg) in systolic dysfunction or isosorbide dinitrate (Isordil) and hydralazine (Apresoline) for diastolic dysfunction.

11-84   Answer B

A 12-lead electrocardiogram (ECG) showing 2-mm ST-segment elevations in leads II, III, and AVF indicates an acute inferior wall myocardial infarction (MI). When ST-segment elevation MI (STEMI) in the inferior leads are noted, a right-sided 12-lead ECG should be included because up to 30% of clients with inferior-wall MI have been noted to have right ventricular involvement, which then changes therapeutic management strategies. When a right ventricular involvement is present, the provider should be conservative with the administration of nitroglycerin (NTG) and aggressive fluid offloading. Every attempt to optimize fluid and electrolyte stability should be undertaken, and as in all cases of STEMI, the client should be quickly transported to a percutaneous coronary intervention center for diagnostic work-up. In specific situations intervention may be streamlined. With inferior wall MI, further complications may include disturbances located at the SA node (bradycardia) or AV node (first-degree AV block, second-degree type 1 Mobitz heart block, third-degree heart block), and the health-care provider may auscultate the acute finding of a systolic murmur secondary to papillary muscle involvement of the mitral valve.

Ischemic syndromes often follow a circadian rhythm, with an MI occurring more frequently in the morning hours between 8 a.m. and noon. Ischemic heart disease should always be a consideration in female clients because it causes 23% of all deaths in women and is the leading cause of death in women older than age 50.

In anterior wall MIs, the danger of left ventricular failure and acute-onset pulmonary edema is always a concern. Once again, exquisite management of fluid and electrolytes is necessary.

As it relates to conduction abnormalities, it is not uncommon to note the development of a second-degree type 2 heart block or third-degree heart block. Bundle branch blocks may likewise be noted. In the occurrence of a right bundle branch block, the clinician should always review the axis to assess for the development of a bifascicular block because it may influence therapeutic decisions.

Gastrointestinal reflux may produce pain suggestive of angina but is usually related to a heavy meal, occurs in recumbency or bending over, and is usually relieved by antacids, which Janice's was not. Anxiety attacks do not usually wake someone out of a sound sleep and would not produce an abnormal ECG except for tachycardia.

11-85   Answer C

Calcium channel blockers, with the exception of amlodipine and felodipine, should not be ordered for the routine management of heart failure. The clinician must consider treatments that will decrease the cardiac workload, reduce mortality, and control atrial fibrillation. To reduce mortality, ACEIs should be ordered, which are indicated for all patients with LV systolic dysfunction, unless there are specific contraindications, such as history of intolerance or adverse reactions to these agents, serum K > 5.5 mEq, or symptomatic hypotension. If the patient cannot tolerate ACEIs, ARBs can be used. Vasodilators and nitrates can also be used if ACEIs are not tolerated. Diuretics should be added to this therapy if symptoms persist or volume overload becomes obvious.

11-86   Answer B

The prevalence of angina pectoris is higher in women than in men, but the prevalence of myocardial infarction is higher in men. Although not always recognized by female clients, coronary heart disease (CHD) still remains the single-most common cause of death in women 20 years or older in the United States.

11-87   Answer C

Because hypertension and diabetes are risk factors for coronary artery disease, it is important to note any funduscopic changes early in the progression of the disease.

11-88   Answer D

All clients who have sustained a myocardial infarction (MI) and in whom the therapy is not contraindicated should continue to take ASA (acetylsalicylic acid, or aspirin) indefinitely. For clients who are allergic to or intolerant of aspirin, clopidogrel can be substituted.

Note the following properties of the oral antiplatelet drugs Brilinta, Plavix, and Effient: Brilinta (ticagrelor) competes with Plavix (clopidogrel) and Effient (prasugrel) for acute coronary syndrome or after placement of a stent. Plavix was the first antiplatelet agent approved by the Food and Drug Administration (FDA) and is used most often, but it has a delayed onset and variable response because it has to be activated by cytochrome P_{450} (CYP3A4) enzymes in the liver. Effient is more effective than Plavix but causes more bleeding, so it is not for clients with a prior stroke or transient ischemic attack or those over age 75. Brilinta seems to be more effective than Plavix for acute coronary syndrome and usually does not cause any more major bleeding than Plavix does. For every 1,000 clients with acute coronary syndrome treated for a year, Brilinta prevents 11 more cardiovascular deaths, 11 more MIs, and at least 6 more stent thromboses than does Plavix. But these statistics are affected by the dose of aspirin used with Brilinta. More than 100 mg/d of aspirin makes Brilinta *less* effective. Ensure that clients on Brilinta take only 81 mg/d of aspirin. Brilinta has a faster onset than Plavix and Effient because it is not a prodrug. It also wears off faster because it binds to platelets *reversibly* instead of permanently. This fast offset is an advantage for clients who need coronary artery bypass graft or other surgery. But both Brilinta and Plavix should be stopped 5 days before surgery, and Effient should be stopped at least 7 days beforehand. Brilinta's short duration may be a disadvantage in the long run because it has to be taken twice a day instead of once a day like the others. If a client is on Brilinta, avoid using strong CYP3A4 inhibitors or inducers, such as clarithromycin, ketoconazole, and rifampin. Do not exceed 40 mg/d for simvastatin or lovastatin, and monitor digoxin levels when starting or stopping Brilinta. Keep in mind that Brilinta can cause dyspnea, especially during the first week. Consider switching to Plavix or Effient if needed.

11-89   Answer D

Although many clients with mitral valve prolapse (MVP) are asymptomatic, clients may appear with a variety of symptoms, including what some have described as "MVP syndrome": a characteristic click, fatigue, palpitations, postural hypotension, chest pain, atrial and ventricular arrhythmias, anxiety, and symptoms of autonomic dysfunction (excessive secretion of catecholamines causing vasoconstriction and orthostatic tachycardia).

11-90   Answer C

Cardiac catheterization is not generally performed during initial data collection. Selected individuals may require catheterization for severe or extremely unstable symptoms; however, angiography is generally reserved for those with positive exercise stress tests. The initial history and physical examination should explore severity of symptoms, functional disability, quality of life, and cardiac risk factors. This information assists the provider in identifying high-risk individuals who would benefit from further diagnostic testing. Electrocardiographic stress testing has a high false-positive rate. The use of thallium or sestamibi agents with exercise testing has a lower frequency of false-positive results. Nuclide imaging may be used for initial evaluation of clients or to confirm those with a questionable history and a positive exercise stress test. A chest x-ray can identify any structural abnormalities such as cardiomegaly or aortic aneurysm that suggest underlying cardiovascular pathology.

11-91   Answer C

An alpha blocker is the antihypertensive agent of choice because Mort has benign prostatic hyperplasia (BPH). In addition to lowering the client's blood pressure, an alpha blocker will provide symptomatic relief of his BPH. Calcium channel blockers or diuretics are effective antihypertensive agents in blacks, whereas a beta blocker would be the drug of choice if Mort had migraine headaches in addition to his BPH. Diuretics and ACE inhibitors are the drugs of choice for treating congestive heart failure with accompanying hypertension.

11-92   Answer C

Martha should be referred to a cardiologist for an echocardiogram and cardiovascular work-up because she has taken the fenfluramine-phentermine (fen-phen) combination. The U.S. Department of Health and Human Services issued the following recommendations for individuals who took fenfluramine and dexfenfluramine: Persons who have had the drugs should undergo a careful history and cardiovascular examination by their health-care provider; and individuals with signs or symptoms suggesting valvular disease should have an echocardiogram.

11-93   Answer A

A study by the Post Coronary Artery Bypass Graft Trial investigators found that aggressively lowering the low-density lipoprotein (LDL) cholesterol level to 70 mg/dL in clients who had previously undergone bypass surgery was more effective in reducing the progression of atherosclerotic lesions and occlusions than any other moderate treatment. Maintaining the LDL at 70 may reverse some atherosclerotic lesions. When the LDL is less than 70, studies suggest a degree of plaque reversibility may result.

11-94   Answer A

Methyldopa, an alpha-adrenergic inhibitor, is used to treat chronic hypertension during pregnancy. At low doses, it can be used as monotherapy. At higher doses, it may cause sodium and fluid to accumulate, so diuretic therapy may be required. Blood pressure (BP) drops during normal pregnancy, and no data suggest the use of medication in clients with BP less than 160/100 mm Hg. Jessica, however, has a history of high BP, and today it is high as well. Methyldopa has a pregnancy rating of B, meaning that studies in humans have found no harm to the fetus, but studies in other animals have shown harm to the fetus, or there are no reliable studies in humans. Atenolol (Tenormin) has been associated with mild intrauterine growth restriction when used in randomized trials focusing on the treatment of chronic hypertension during pregnancy. It has a category rating of D (unsafe in pregnancy). Nifedipine (Adalat, Procardia) is used occasionally to treat preterm contractions and is rated as category C (safety for use during pregnancy has not been established). Clonidine (Catapres) is usually a third-line agent if other medications cannot be tolerated. It is rated as category C in pregnancy.

11-95   Answer C

Older adults and clients with diabetes frequently demonstrate defective anginal warning systems—a result of altered cardiac neural pathways (older age, diabetics), physical interruption of nerve pathways (cardiac transplant or bypass surgery), an abnormally high pain perception threshold, or milder degrees of ischemia. Because Jim is an older adult with diabetes, he may have had a silent myocardial infarction (MI), as well as silent ischemia. Neither his electrocardiogram nor his clinical presentation suggests an acute MI, so hospitalization is not indicated. However, aspirin therapy (unless contraindicated for other reasons) is indicated because it has been shown to be an independent factor in reducing the risk of subsequent MI. Work-up for a possible silent MI should include, when clinical status is stable, exercise stress testing

with thallium imaging to determine ischemic burden and changes indicative of MI. Evaluation for left ventricular wall motion abnormalities and ejection fraction with echocardiography may also confirm previous MI or the presence of ischemia. Likewise, the client has a newly developed atrial fibrillation, which has the propensity to alter cardiac output and forward flow with resultant decreases in peripheral perfusion as well as possible subsequent heart failure. An electrophysiology (EP) consult may provide benefit, as a return to normal sinus rhythm and possible cardiac resynchronization therapy (CRT) or cardiac resynchronization therapy defibrillator (CRT-D) may optimize clinical status contingent on the results of the echo and QT interval.

11-96   Answer C

An event monitor is used to identify intermittent ectopy and match symptoms with underlying rhythm and should be used if the interval between symptom occurrence is greater than 48 hours. A 12-lead ECG should be done to evaluate conduction delays, cardiac intervals, and pre-excitation syndromes. A Holter monitor (24 hours) should be ordered to identify frequency of ectopy, evaluate diurnal variations, and match symptoms with underlying rhythm. An echocardiogram should be ordered to evaluate valvular abnormalities and ventricular function.

11-97   Answer A

Treatment of hypertension is dependent on risk stratification. Full evaluation of the client is necessary to determine the presence of target organ damage (TOD), cardiovascular disease (CVD), and major risk factors. Also, those with identifiable causes should have the underlying problem addressed. If the client has no risk factors (except diabetes) and no TOD or CVD, the client would initially be started on lifestyle modification. The Joint National Committee on Prevention, Detection, Evaluation, and Treatment of High Blood Pressure recommends that individuals who have high-normal blood pressure, as well as known renal insufficiency, heart failure, or diabetes mellitus, should be considered for prompt pharmacological therapy and lifestyle modifications.

11-98   Answer D

Group A beta-hemolytic streptococcal infections of the upper respiratory tract remain the primary environmental trigger that acts on predisposed children to cause rheumatic fever and subsequent cardiovascular disease. Although the incidence of the disease has significantly declined over the past half century, there has been a resurgence in several regions of the United States since the mid-1980s. Children between the ages of 5 and 15 are at most risk; blacks are slightly more at risk than whites, and girls are more at risk than boys. In general, once the condition has been diagnosed, antibiotic therapy is indicated.

Penicillins

Penicillin remains the treatment of choice for group A streptococcal upper respiratory tract infections, since it is the only antibiotic that has been evaluated in controlled studies. A single injection of intramuscular benzathine benzylpenicillin is the most effective treatment in eradicating group A streptococci, probably because of its long duration of action. It can also be used for mass prophylaxis.

Oral phenoxymethylpenicillin administration for streptococcal pharyngitis must be continued for 10 days. Other orally administered penicillins include ampicillin, amoxicillin, and the semisynthetic penicillins.

Macrolides

For penicillin-allergic clients, treatment with oral erythromycin for 10 days is often used. Newer macrolides are reported to be associated with fewer adverse effects but are generally more expensive. Short-course therapy with these newer macrolides is effective, but more definitive data are required before use in primary prevention is recommended.

Cephalosporins

First- and second-generation cephalosporins have been used to treat group A streptococcal infections. As a rule, cephalosporins are more expensive than penicillin. Short-course therapy (less than 10 days) with some cephalosporins is also under evaluation.

11-99   Answer D

A positive bruit or wide, diffuse pulsation in the epigastric area is indicative of an abdominal aortic aneurysm. Right upper quadrant tenderness, a venous hum, and ascites are indicative of right-sided congestive heart failure.

11-100   Answer B

According to the National Cholesterol Education Program guidelines, for clients with known coronary artery disease (CAD), it is recommended that the low-density lipoprotein (LDL) cholesterol

level be 100 mg/dL or less. Studies, including the Scandinavian Simvastatin Survival Study and the West of Scotland Coronary Prevention Group Study, reported that lowering LDL cholesterol levels resulted in a significant reduction of vascular events such as myocardial infarction or cerebrovascular accident in individuals with and without CAD. It has likewise been shown that with an LDL level of 100 or lower, further progression of the disease process is arrested, and with LDL of 70 or lower, existing atherosclerotic plaque may actually undergo a degree of revision.

11-101   Answer D

Mitral valve prolapse is more common in women younger than age 20 than in other populations. MVP occurs in about 2%–4% of the population and is usually detected in young adulthood. The incidence is equal in men and women after age 20. Physical assessment findings demonstrate a murmur followed by a midsystolic click. When evaluating the client with a diagnosis of MVP, a review of systems should review any symptoms of heart disease. Clients should be questioned about any development of chest pain, palpitations, or syncope and asked if they have developed any activity intolerance or any recent weight gain, ankle edema, abdominal fullness or distention, or any dyspnea on exertion (DOE).

11-102   Answer C

Regardless of the client's risk factors, individuals demonstrating acute ischemic changes require immediate treatment of symptoms. It is also essential to identify and treat the underlying cause of disruption of blood flow in order to salvage or reduce the size of injury to the myocardium. This is an acute, actively evolving event, and timely revascularization is indicated. Bob should be rapidly transported because percutaneous coronary intervention is a priority.

Evaluating serum lipid levels during an acute event may lead to false results. Serum cholesterol responds to acute stress events with a decrease in both low-density lipoprotein (LDL) cholesterol and high-density lipoprotein (HDL) cholesterol, as well as an increase in triglyceride levels. This change can persist for up to 6 weeks. Lipid profiles drawn during an acute myocardial infarction will generally demonstrate lower total, LDL, and HDL cholesterol levels, resulting in an underestimation of this risk factor.

11-103 Answer C

Clients with aortic stenosis should avoid overuse of diuretics and nitrates because they can reduce preload and result in orthostatic hypotension and syncope. They should also avoid beta blockers and calcium channel blockers because they may further depress left ventricular function and precipitate failure. Treatment of associated conditions such as hypertension, arrhythmias, and heart failure should be maintained, and close follow-up is indicated. It should be understood that therapy has limited effectiveness in terms of improving the functional status; therefore, routine imaging, such as yearly Doppler echocardiography to evaluate the progression of the valve stenosis, myocardial contractility, and ejection fraction, is recommended.

11-104 Answer D

Aortic stenosis (AS) has a classic triad of chest pain, dyspnea on exertion progressing to dyspnea at rest, heart failure, and syncope. In adults, manifestations of reduced cardiac output secondary to AS are usually not present until late in the course of the disease and typically occur between ages 60 and 70. Symptoms of aortic stenosis usually develop gradually after an asymptomatic latent period of 10–20 years. Aortic stenosis may be congenital or acquired and ultimately results in reduction in the opening of the valve area, a diminished stroke volume, and gradual increase in the size of the left ventricle, with concomitant systolic and or diastolic dysfunction, reduced cardiac output, and predictable progression deterioration. Clients with aortic stenosis fall into one of four categories of severity: mild, moderate, severe, or critical. [See Table 11-1]

TABLE 11-1. CLASSIFICATION OF AORTIC STENOSIS SEVERITY

SEVERITY	VALVE AREA (cm²)	MAXIMUM AORTIC VELOCITY (m/sec)	MEAN PRESSURE GRADIENT (mm Hg)
Mild	1.5–2.0	2.5–3.0	<25
Moderate	1.0–1.5	3.0–4.0	25–40
Severe	0.6–1.0	>4.0	>40
Critical	<0.6	—	—

11-105 Answer C

Management of a client with hypertension who also has an abdominal aortic aneurysm would include an abdominal aortic ultrasound or computed tomography (CT) scan with contrast, aggressive management of the client's hypertension, and referral to a cardiologist. Because most arterial aneurysms are atherosclerotic in origin, coronary artery disease (CAD) and arterial disease are frequent comorbid conditions. The client should be evaluated for occult CAD. Determining the size of the aneurysm is essential so that decisions can be made about whether to treat medically with close monitoring or to refer for surgical intervention. In a good-risk client with an abdominal aortic aneurysm in the range of 4.5–5 cm, elective surgical treatment is advisable. Serial observation with ultrasound every 3–4 months is appropriate for asymptomatic abdominal aortic aneurysms smaller than 4.5 cm and for larger asymptomatic aneurysms in poor-risk clients. If the aneurysm becomes symptomatic or enlarges, then elective surgery is appropriate. Control of hypertension is essential to reduce stress on the aneurysm and slow its progression. A cardiac catheterization will show the size/condition of the cardiac arteries, not the abdominal arteries.

11-106 Answer A

Symptoms of occlusive arterial disease include pain occurring in the calves or thighs when walking, with relief obtained when standing still, and severe pain at rest that requires the client to hang the leg over the side of the bed to obtain relief. True intermittent claudication occurs with walking and is relieved by standing. With the progression of occlusive disease, ischemic symptoms worsen. Pain, usually in the foot or toes, can occur at rest and is typically worse at night. Assuming a dependent position with the extremity off the side of the bed can afford some relief (rest pain indicates 90% occlusion). Pseudoclaudication may be caused by lumbar spinal stenosis, which causes lower-extremity symptoms with any erect posture (standing as well as walking) and is not relieved by standing still; instead, the client must sit or lie down to obtain relief of symptoms. Pallor or mottling of the extremities due to collapsed superficial veins may also occur with occlusive arterial disease.

Initial treatment goals of claudication are achieved through medical therapy. Surgery is reserved for severe cases.

- Medical management goals are to impede the progression of peripheral arterial occlusive disease (PAOD).

- Exquisite management of hypertension and diabetes and tight control of cholesterol and triglycerides are a foundation of therapy in the client who abuses tobacco:

- The most expedient way to impede the progress of PAOD is to stop tobacco use.

- Improved walking distance and ankle pressure have been attributed to smoking cessation.

- In clients with claudication, exercise plays a vital role in medical management. Clients with PAOD reduce their activity and daily walking because of claudication pain and fear of further damage. This decrease in activity leads to an increasingly sedentary lifestyle that is even more detrimental.

- Regular walking programs result in substantial improvement in most clients with claudication. Improvements have ranged from 80%–234% in controlled studies.

- Studies suggest a daily walking program of 45–60 minutes. The client is instructed to walk until claudication pain occurs, rest until the pain subsides, and repeat the cycle.

- While the exact mechanism for improvement in walking distance with exercise remains unknown, regular exercise is thought to condition muscles to work more efficiently (more extraction of blood) and increase collateral vessel formation.

11-107   Answer A

Mitral regurgitation may be noted as a holosystolic murmur. Because ventricular pressure exceeds atrial pressure at the beginning of systole, regurgitant backflow begins with the first heart sound (S_1). The ensuing regurgitant murmur persists up to the second heart sound (S_2), provided that the ventricular pressure at the end of systole still exceeds the atrial pressure. The direction of regurgitant flow (intra-arterial jet) may be noted on auscultation. If the direction of the jet is medial against the atrial septum near the base of the aorta, the murmur radiates from the apex to the second left intercostal space and even into the neck. If the jet is directed posterolaterally within the left atrial cavity, the murmur can be noted into the axilla, to the left scapula, and occasionally to the vertebral column. Mitral regurgitation is caused by shrunken, deformed cusps or shortened, fused chordae tendineae, which prevent closure of the leaflets.

11-108   Answer A

ACE inhibitors have been found to postpone progression of microalbuminuria and ultimately nephropathy in clients with diabetes. They have few adverse effects, and because of their renoprotective properties, they are suggested as part of the initial therapy for normotensive diabetic clients. Their use is contraindicated in women who are pregnant, and they should be used with caution in women of childbearing age. ACE inhibitors may also exacerbate hyperkalemia in clients with advanced renal insufficiency or hyporeninemic hypoaldosteronism. Older adults with advanced renal disease and clients with renal artery stenosis may experience a decline in renal function with ACE inhibitors. If a client does not tolerate the use of ACE inhibitors, angiotensin receptor blockers (ARBs) can be used. Some studies suggest that ACE inhibitors and ARBs—which act by different mechanisms—be used together in all diabetic clients because of their benefit in preventing or slowing the progression of nephropathy. In addition to the preceding pharmacologic recommendations, it is equally important to maintain stable serum cholesterol levels. It is not unreasonable to institute statin therapy when no contraindications exist.

Statin therapy has been associated with a 19%–55% reduction in cardiovascular disease events in clients with diabetes with and without known vascular disease. There are also data to suggest that statins may have benefits on the rate of development of diabetes. Statins may reduce the rate of progression of microvascular complications, including diabetic retinopathy, nephropathy, and neuropathy.

11-109   Answer B

An important management concern in clients who have experienced syncope, symptomatic ventricular tachycardia, or aborted sudden death is to provide recommendations concerning automobile driving. Most states have driving restrictions concerning clients with seizures but not with cardiac problems, even though they may be at high risk. Clients with syncope or aborted sudden death thought to have been due to temporary factors (acute MI, bradyarrhythmias subsequently treated with permanent pacing, drug effect, electrolyte imbalance) should be strongly advised after recovery not to drive for at least 1 month. Other clients, like Sam, with symptomatic ventricular tachycardia or aborted sudden death, whether treated pharmacologically, with antitachycardia devices, or with ablation therapy, should not drive for at least 6 months. Longer restrictions are warranted in these clients if spontaneous arrhythmias persist. Clinicians should be aware of local regulations.

11-110   Answer D

Pathological U waves on an ECG are most commonly associated with hypokalemia. Low serum potassium levels affect the transmembrane gradient across the cardiac cells. The finding is readily apparent in the precordial leads. Other ECG findings associated with low serum potassium levels include flattened or inverted T waves, ST-segment depression, and in severe cases, ventricular dysrhythmias.

Bibliography

Carbone, I, and Friedrich, MG: Myocardial edema imaging by cardiovascular magnetic resonance: Current status and future potential. *Current Cardiology Report* 14(1):1–6, 2012.

Chamorrow, C, et al: Anesthesia and analgesia protocol during therapeutic hypothermia after cardiac arrest: A systematic review. *Anesthesia Analogue* 110(5): 1328–1335, 2010.

Chobanian, AV, et al: The seventh report of the Joint National Committee on Prevention, Detection, Evaluation, and Treatment of High Blood Pressure—The JNC 7 report. *Journal of the American Medical Association* 289:2560–2570, 2003.

Dunphy, LM, et al: *Primary Care: The Art and Science of Advanced Practice Nursing*, ed 3, FA Davis, Philadelphia, 2011.

Franklin, BA, and Vanhecke, TC: Preventing reinfarction: Changing behavior after the MI, part 1. *Consultant* 47(6):517–522, May 2007.

Franklin, BA, and Vanhecke, TC: Preventing reinfarction: Changing behavior after the MI, part 2. *Consultant* 47(6):569–574, May 2007.

Gibson, P, and Carson, MP: Hypertension and pregnancy. eMedicine, updated December 13, 2007. http://www.emedicine.com/med/topic3250.htm, accessed February 21, 2008.

Healthy People 2020. Centers for Disease Control and Prevention. http://www.cdc.gov/nchs/healthy_people.htm, accessed September 7, 2012.

IOM (Institute of Medicine). *The Future of Nursing: Leading Change, Advancing Health*. National Academies Press, Washington, DC, 2011.

Lamendoia, C: Highlights of the Preventive Cardiovascular Nurses Association 13th annual symposium. Medscape Nurses. http://www.medscape.com/viewarticle/557957, accessed July 18, 2007.

Loscalzo, J, Libby, P, and Braunwalk, E: Cardiovascular disorders. In A. Fauci et al (Eds), *Harrison's Principles of Internal Medicine*, ed 17, 1635–1681. McGraw Hill, New York, 2008.

Pyle, K, et al: Keeping cardiac arrest patients alive with therapeutic hypothermia. *American Nurse Today* 2(7):32–36, July 2007.

Trost, J, and Hillis, D: Intra-aortic balloon counterpulsation. *American Journal of Cardiology* 97(99): 1391–1398, 2006.

Yaakob, W, and Schabel, S: Photo quiz—Upper extremity swelling in a smoker. *Consultant* 47(4):381–388, April 2007.

How well did you do?

85% and above, congratulations! This score shows application of test-taking principles and adequate content knowledge.

75%–85%, keep working! Review test-taking principles and try again.

65%–75%, hang in there! Spend some time reviewing concepts and test-taking principles and try the test again.

Chapter 12: *Abdominal Problems*

Jill E. Winland-Brown

Questions

12-1 *Lipids are broken down in which area of the gastrointestinal tract?*

A. Esophagus

B. Stomach

C. Small intestine

D. Large intestine

12-2 *Marvin, a known alcoholic with cirrhosis, is frequently admitted for coagulopathies and occasionally receives blood transfusions. His wife asks you why he has bleeding problems. How do you respond?*

A. "Occasionally he accumulates blood in the gut."

B. "There is an interruption of the normal clotting mechanisms."

C. "Long-term alcohol abuse has made his vessels very friable."

D. "His bone marrow has been affected."

12-3 *Jonas, age 34, had a Billroth II (hemigastrectomy and gastrojejunostomy with vagotomy) performed 1 week ago and just started eating a bland diet. What do you suspect when he complains of epigastric fullness, distention, discomfort, abdominal cramping, nausea, and flatus after eating?*

A. Obstruction

B. Dumping syndrome

C. Metabolic acidosis

D. Infectious colitis

12-4 *A common complication of viral gastroenteritis in children is*

A. dehydration.

B. gastrointestinal bleeding.

C. peritonitis.

D. bacterial sepsis.

12-5 *The most important diagnostic test for celiac disease is*

A. confirming malabsorption by laboratory tests.

B. a barium enema.

C. a peroral biopsy of the duodenum.

D. a gluten-free diet trial with an accompanying improvement in mucosal histological response.

12-6 *What is the most common cause of melena?*

A. Colon cancer

B. Upper gastrointestinal bleeding

C. Drug abuse

D. Smoking

12-7 *Which physical examination maneuver for diagnosing appendicitis is done by deep palpation over the left lower quadrant (LLQ) with resultant pain in the right lower quadrant (RLQ)?*

A. Rovsing's sign

B. Psoas sign

C. Obturator sign

D. McBurney's sign

12-8 *Sam has ulcerative colitis and is on a low-residue diet. Which foods do you recommend that Sam avoid?*

A. Potato skins, potato chips, and brown rice

B. Vegetable juices and cooked and canned vegetables

C. Ground beef, veal, pork, and lamb

D. White rice and pasta

12-9 *Which of the following treatments for ulcerative colitis is contraindicated?*

A. A high-calorie, nonspicy, caffeine-free diet that is low in high-residue foods and milk products

B. Corticosteroids in the acute phase

C. Antidiarrheal agents

D. Colectomy with permanent ileostomy in severe cases

12-10 *Olive has an acute exacerbation of Crohn's disease. Which laboratory test value(s) would you expect to be decreased?*

A. Sedimentation rate

B. Liver enzyme levels

C. Vitamins A, B complex, and C levels

D. Bilirubin level

12-11 *You suspect that Harry has a peptic ulcer and tell him that it has been found to be strongly associated with*

A. anxiety and panic attacks.

B. long-term use of NSAIDs.

C. infection by *Helicobacter pylori*.

D. a family history of peptic ulcers.

12-12 *You are doing routine teaching with a patient who has a family history of colorectal cancer. You know she misunderstands the teaching when she tells you she will*

A. decrease her fat intake.

B. increase her fiber intake.

C. continue her daily use of aspirin.

D. increase her fluid intake.

12-13 *The proper order of assessing the abdomen is*

A. palpation, percussion, auscultation, inspection.

B. inspection, palpation, auscultation, percussion.

C. inspection, auscultation, percussion, palpation.

D. percussion, auscultation, inspection, palpation.

12-14 *Which of the following antibiotics causes more episodes of nausea and/or vomiting than the others?*

A. Azithromycin

B. Erythromycin

C. Penicillin

D. Tetracycline

12-15 *Melva presents with an exacerbation of acute pancreatitis and you are going to admit her to the hospital. Which is the most important factor in determining a negative long-term outcome for her?*

A. Age

B. Infection

C. Pain

D. Length of time between exacerbations

12-16 *One of the alarm signs or symptoms of irritable bowel syndrome that requires prompt investigation is*

A. blood or pus in the stool.

B. weight gain.

C. hyperkalemia.

D. first onset in the teen years.

12-17 *In a 2-month-old infant with vomiting and diarrhea, the most effective way of determining a fluid deficit is to check for*

A. decreased peripheral perfusion.

B. hyperventilation.

C. irritability.

D. hyperthermia.

12-18 *By what age do abdominal respirations cease in a child?*

A. 2 years

B. 5 years

C. 7 years

D. 13 years

12-19 *An infant who is ruminating should be diagnosed and treated for*

A. cystic fibrosis.

B. esophagitis.

C. Meckel's diverticulum.

D. intussusception.

12-20 *In counseling Maria, age 24, who is healthy, you advise her to limit her intake of sugar to prevent*

A. dental caries.

B. obesity.

C. diabetes.

D. hyperactivity.

12-21 *Rose has gastroesophageal reflux disease. You know she misunderstands your teaching when she tells you that she will*

A. avoid coffee, alcohol, chocolate, peppermint, and spicy foods.

B. eat smaller meals.

C. have a snack before retiring so that the esophagus and stomach are not empty at bedtime.

D. stop smoking.

12-22   When percussing the abdomen, hyperresonance is present

A. when there is gaseous distention.

B. over a distended bladder.

C. over adipose tissue.

D. over fluid or a mass.

12-23   Which protozoal infection is the most common intestinal infection in the United States that also occurs worldwide?

A. Salmonellosis

B. Giardiasis

C. Botulism

D. Shigellosis

12-24   When George tells you that his feces are foul smelling, you suspect which of the following?

A. Blood in the stool

B. Ingestion of a low-fat diet

C. Prostate cancer

D. Appendicitis

12-25   Ruby has a colostomy and complains that her stools are too loose. What food(s) do you suggest to help thicken the stools?

A. Cheese

B. Leafy green vegetables

C. Raw fruits and vegetables

D. Dried beans

12-26   Which laxative is safe for long-term use?

A. Mineral oil

B. Bisacodyl (Dulcolax)

C. Methylcellulose (Citrucel)

D. Magnesium hydroxide (milk of magnesia)

12-27   Stacy, a nursing student, is to begin her series of hepatitis B vaccinations. You test her for a serological marker and the results show

hepatitis B surface antibodies (HBsAb). You tell Stacy that she

A. needs to begin the hepatitis B series as soon as possible.

B. needs to be tested again because one reading is not indicative of immunity.

C. is permanently immune to hepatitis B.

D. has an acute hepatitis B infection.

12-28   You elicit costovertebral angle tenderness in Gordon, age 29. Which condition do you suspect?

A. Cirrhosis

B. Inflammation of the kidney

C. Inflammation of the spleen

D. Peritonitis

12-29   While you are obtaining Henry's history, he tells you that he had a portacaval shunt done in the past. What does this imply?

A. A history of liver cancer

B. A history of alcohol abuse

C. A congenital biliary problem

D. Heavy tobacco use

12-30   In the ABCs of irritable bowel syndrome, the B stands for

A. bloody stool.

B. bad odor to stool.

C. bloating or visible distention.

D. bowel attack.

12-31   Cydney has been given a diagnosis of ascariasis. Which symptoms would you expect to see?

A. Low-grade fever, productive cough with blood-tinged sputum, wheezing, and dyspnea

B. Nocturnal perianal and perineal pruritus

C. Diarrhea, cramps, and malaise

D. Ascites and facial and extremity edema

12-32   You are trying to differentiate between functional (acquired) constipation and Hirschsprung's disease in a neonate. Distinguishing features of Hirschsprung's disease includes which of the following?

A. Small ribbonlike stools

B. Obvious abdominal pain

C. Female gender

D. Small weight gain

12-33 *The metabolism of which drug is not affected in Marsha, age 74?*

A. Alcohol

B. Anticonvulsants

C. Psychotropics

D. Oral anticoagulants

12-34 *Rebound tenderness may indicate*

A. peritoneal inflammation.

B. a ventral hernia.

C. portal hypertension.

D. Crohn's disease.

12-35 *Shelby has recently been diagnosed with pancreatitis. Which of the following objective findings, also known as Grey Turner's sign, can result from the pancreatic inflammatory process that you might find on a rare occasion?*

A. Left-sided pleural effusion

B. Bluish discoloration over the flanks

C. Bluish discoloration over the umbilicus

D. Jaundice

12-36 *Marisa, age 42, has celiac disease. She is prone to osteopenic bone disease as a result of impaired calcium absorption because of*

A. increased calcium absorption by the small intestine.

B. increased absorption of the fat-soluble vitamin D.

C. the binding of calcium and magnesium in the intestinal lumen by unabsorbed dietary fatty acids.

D. decreased magnesium absorption.

12-37 *Sandra has celiac disease. You place her on which diet?*

A. A low-fat diet

B. A low-residue diet

C. A gluten-free diet

D. A high-protein diet

12-38 *Martin has had an ileostomy for ulcerative colitis. Which self-care measures do you teach him to relieve food blockage?*

A. Lie in a supine position.

B. Massage the peristomal area.

C. Take a hot shower or tub bath.

D. Drink cold fluids.

12-39 *You suspect that Nikki has a gastroduodenal ulcer caused by Helicobacter pylori and plan to treat her empirically. What medications should you order?*

A. Bismuth subsalicylate (Pepto-Bismol), tetracycline (Tetracap) or amoxicillin (Amoxil), and metronidazole (Flagyl)

B. Bismuth subsalicylate (Pepto-Bismol) and omeprazole (Prilosec)

C. Amoxicillin (Amoxil) and omeprazole (Prilosec)

D. Clarithromycin (Biaxin) and metronidazole (Flagyl)

12-40 *Marian, age 52, is obese. She complains of a rapid onset of severe right upper quadrant abdominal cramping pain, nausea, and vomiting. Your differential diagnosis might be*

A. appendicitis.

B. irritable bowel syndrome.

C. cholecystitis.

D. Crohn's disease.

12-41 *Mona is breastfeeding her 5-day-old daughter, who has just been found to have physiological jaundice with a bilirubin level of more than 20 mg/dL. You should tell Mona that she*

A. should stop breastfeeding altogether.

B. can continue breastfeeding.

C. should discontinue breastfeeding for 24 hours.

D. should alternate breast milk with formula for every other feeding.

12-42 *The most common causes of upper gastrointestinal hemorrhage are*

A. esophagitis and carcinomas.

B. erosive gastritis and peptic ulcer disease.

C. peptic ulcer disease and esophageal varices.

D. carcinomas and arteriovenous malformations.

12-43   *Sandy, age 52, presents with jaundice, dark urine, and light-colored stools, stating that she is slightly improved over last week's symptoms. Which stage of viral hepatitis do you suspect?*

A. Incubation

B. Prodromal

C. Icteric

D. Convalescent

12-44   *Lucy, age 49, has pain in both the left and right lower quadrants. What might you suspect?*

A. A gastric ulcer

B. Gastritis

C. Pelvic inflammatory disease

D. Pancreatitis

12-45   *Duodenal and gastric ulcers have many of the same manifestations. Which is more common with gastric ulcers rather than duodenal ulcers?*

A. Epigastric or abdominal pain

B. Vomiting

C. Possibility of perforation

D. Obstruction of the gastrointestinal tract

12-46   *Which procedure enlarges the opening between the stomach and duodenum to improve gastric emptying?*

A. Billroth I

B. Total gastrectomy

C. Pyloroplasty

D. Vagotomy

12-47   *Zena just had a hemorrhoidectomy. You know she hasn't understood your teaching when she tells you that she'll*

A. take a sitz bath after each bowel movement for 1–2 weeks after surgery.

B. drink at least 2,000 mL of fluids per day.

C. decrease her dietary fiber for 1 month.

D. take stool softeners as prescribed.

12-48   *The most common viral infection causing diarrhea in the United States is*

A. enteric adenovirus.

B. a Norwalk-like virus.

C. rotavirus.

D. *Giardia lamblia.*

12-49   *Martha has a Cushing's ulcer. What might have precipitated this?*

A. Her house burned down when she was not at home.

B. She was in a bad auto accident in which she sustained a head injury.

C. She spent the weekend deep-sea diving.

D. She was on an overseas airline flight that lasted more than 24 hours.

12-50   *Anson tells you that he thinks his antacids are causing his diarrhea. You respond,*

A. "Antacids contain fructose that may not be totally absorbed and results in fluid being drawn into the bowel."

B. "Antacids contain sorbitol or mannitol, sugars that aren't absorbed and can cause fluid to be drawn into the bowel."

C. "Antacids contain caffeine, which decreases bowel transit time."

D. "Antacids may contain magnesium, which decreases bowel transit time and may contain poorly absorbed salts that draw fluid into the bowel."

12-51   *Which of the following is a hospital-based nosocomial infection that has seen a serious rise in the past decade?*

A. Pneumonia

B. Hepatitis B

C. Staphylococcus infection

D. *Clostridium difficile* colitis

12-52   *The American Cancer Society recommends a flexible sigmoidoscopy for colorectal cancer screening in persons at average risk every*

A. 3 years, beginning at age 40.

B. other year.

C. 2 years, beginning at age 45.

D. 5 years, beginning at age 50

12-53   *Striae most commonly occur with*

A. pregnancy.

B. excessive weight gain.

C. diabetes.

D. ascites.

12-54   Which of the following pharmacologic agents used to treat constipation may cause flatulence and bloating and requires adequate fluid intake?

A. Stool softeners

B. Saline laxatives

C. Lubricants

D. Bulking agents

12-55   Samantha is 100 lb. overweight and wants to have a gastroplasty performed. In discussing this with her, you explain that by having this procedure she may

A. develop diarrhea.

B. lose too much weight.

C. develop hemorrhoids.

D. vomit after she eats.

12-56   Which modality(ies) is(are) the most effective in patients with metabolic syndrome?

A. Specific vitamin and mineral supplements

B. Diet and exercise

C. Specific pharmacological therapy

D. Eliminating alcohol and smoking from their lifestyle

12-57   Susan, age 59, has no specific complaints when she comes in for her annual examination. She does, however, have type 2 diabetes, slight hypertension, dyslipidemia, and central obesity. You diagnose her as having

A. a cardiovascular emergency.

B. a glycemic event.

C. metabolic syndrome.

D. multiple organ dysfunction.

12-58   Timothy, age 68, complains of an abrupt change in his defecation pattern. You evaluate him for

A. constipation.

B. colorectal cancer.

C. irritable bowel syndrome.

D. acute appendicitis.

12-59   Once gastric cancer has been diagnosed, which test should be ordered to accurately determine the correct staging?

A. Computed tomography

B. Magnetic resonance imaging

C. Endoscopic ultrasound

D. Ranson's test

12-60   Sally had an ileostomy performed for inflammatory bowel disease. What type of fecal output can Sally expect?

A. Hard, formed stool

B. Semisoft stool

C. Semisoft to very soft stool

D. A continuous, soft-to-watery effluent

12-61   Tina has a chronic hepatitis C infection. She asks you how to prevent its transmission. You respond,

A. "Do not donate blood until 1 year after diagnosis."

B. "A vaccine is available to prevent transmission."

C. "There is no possibility of transmission through razors or toothbrushes."

D. "Abstain from sex during your period."

12-62   Sylvia, age 59, has acute hepatitis. You're told it's from a drug overdose. Which drug do you suspect?

A. Flagyl

B. Acetaminophen

C. Sumatriptan

D. Hydrocortisone

12-63   Which type of hernia usually occurs at a previous surgical incision site?

A. Umbilical

B. Congenital

C. Hiatal

D. Ventral

12-64   Bobby, age 6, has constant periumbilical pain shifting to the right lower quadrant, vomiting, a small volume of diarrhea, absence of headache, a mild elevation of the white blood cell count with an early left shift, and white blood cells in the urine. You suspect

A. appendicitis.

B. gastroenteritis.

C. acute pancreatitis.

D. Rocky Mountain spotted fever.

12-65   How do you respond when Andrea, who is taking her newborn home from the hospital, asks you when her baby's umbilical cord stump will fall off?

A. "Within 7 days."

B. "In 10–14 days."

C. "In 14–21 days."

D. "In 21–30 days."

12-66   The most common cause of mechanical bowel obstruction in all ages is

A. volvulus.

B. intussusception.

C. cancer.

D. a hernia.

12-67   Rose, your client with gastroesophageal reflux disease, has many other concurrent conditions. She wants to know if there are any medications she should NOT take. You tell her to avoid

A. antibiotics.

B. NSAIDs.

C. oral contraceptives.

D. antifungals.

12-68   Hyperactive bowel sounds (borborygmi) are present in which of the following conditions?

A. Cirrhosis

B. Laxative use

C. Late mechanical bowel obstruction

D. Pancreatic cancer

12-69   To differentiate among the different diagnoses of inflammatory bowel diseases, you look at the client's histological, culture, and radiological features. Mary has transmural inflammation, granulomas, focal involvement of the colon with some skipped areas, and sparing of the rectal mucosa. What do you suspect?

A. Crohn's disease

B. Ulcerative colitis

C. Infectious colitis

D. Ischemic colitis

12-70   Simon states that he is worried because he has a bowel movement only every third day. You respond,

A. "You should have two to three stools per day."

B. "You should defecate once a day."

C. "You should have at least three stools per week."

D. "There is no such thing as a 'normal' pattern of defecation."

12-71   Dottie brings in her infant who has gastrointestinal reflux. What do you tell her about positioning her infant?

A. Always position infants on their back to prevent sudden infant death syndrome.

B. Rotate your infant between lying on the back and on the stomach.

C. The infant should be placed on the left side.

D. Place the infant in whatever position the infant remains quiet.

12-72   Which of the following signs or symptoms indicates biliary obstruction with liver disease?

A. Pruritus

B. Increased abdominal girth

C. Right upper quadrant pain

D. Easy bruising

12-73   A second-generation cephalosporin, cefmetazole is to be given to your patient undergoing colorectal surgery. You know that the dosing recommendation to prevent an incisional surgical site infection (SSI) is

A. three doses prior to surgery.

B. one dose prior to surgery.

C. a weekly course of therapy.

D. therapy beginning after surgery.

12-74   Marcie just returned from Central America with traveler's diarrhea. Which is the best treatment?

A. Metronidazole (Flagyl)

B. Supportive care

C. Quinolone antibiotics

D. Gastric lavage

12-75   Which type of hepatitis is transmitted by the fecal-oral route, sewage, contaminated water, shellfish, and possibly blood?

A. Hepatitis A (HAV)

B. Hepatitis B (HBV)

C. Hepatitis C (HCV)

D. Hepatitis D (HDV)

12-76   Treatment for achalasia may include

A. balloon dilation of the lower esophageal sphincter.

B. beta blockers.

C. a fundoplication.

D. an esophagogastrectomy.

12-77   Sally, age 21, is to undergo a tonsillectomy. She has heard that when this surgery is performed in adults, it is extremely difficult. She's heard about taste changes after a tonsillectomy. What do you tell her?

A. "As the tongue is responsible for sweet, sour, salty, and bitter taste abilities, they will all be affected somewhat."

B. "You will have some alterations, but we'll have to wait and see how you are affected personally."

C. "You may notice a slight difference initially, but there are no lasting changes in taste."

D. "About half of the patients have some permanent alterations in the sense of taste."

12-78   Clients with sprue usually have

A. a large-in-stature appearance.

B. accelerated maturity.

C. polycythemia.

D. steatorrhea.

12-79   Sara is taking polyethylene glycol (GoLYTELY) in preparation for a barium enema. What do you teach her about the medication?

A. Drink the solution at room temperature.

B. Take the medication with food so that it will be absorbed better.

C. Take the medication in the early evening so as not to interfere with sleep.

D. Drink all of the solution in one sitting.

12-80   Rebound tenderness at McBurney's point would alert you to

A. appendicitis.

B. peritonitis.

C. a spleen injury.

D. irritable bowel syndrome.

12-81   A concern with older patients having abdominal surgery is

A. older patients have an increased peristalsis, and bowel sounds must be checked very frequently.

B. older adults have a diminished response to painful stimuli that may mask abdominal health problems.

C. because older adults are prone to diarrhea after surgery, you must be vigilant about skin breakdown.

D. because of liver enlargement, postoperative medications are processed faster.

12-82   A mother is bringing in her 4-year-old child, whom she states has acute abdominal pain and a rash. Which of the following do you initially rule out?

A. Rocky Mountain spotted fever

B. Measles

C. Appendicitis

D. A food allergy

12-83   Maura had a less than 7% value on her Schilling test. What medication do you anticipate that Maura might need?

A. Folic acid

B. Vitamin B_{12}

C. Thyroid medication

D. Hormone replacement therapy

12-84   Which of the following statements about cirrhosis is true?

A. Biliary cirrhosis is the most common type of cirrhosis in the United States.

B. Alcoholic cirrhosis occurs only in malnourished alcoholics.

C. Cirrhosis is reversible if diagnosed and treated at an early stage.

D. Women tend to develop cirrhosis more quickly with less alcohol intake than men.

12-85 *For an uncomplicated* Salmonella *infection, the antibiotic of choice is*

A. ampicillin (Polycillin).

B. amoxicillin (Amoxil).

C. trimethoprim-sulfamethoxazole (Bactrim).

D. No antibiotic is indicated.

12-86 *Margie, age 52, has an extremely stressful job and was just given a diagnosis of gastric ulcer. She tells you that she is sure it is going to be malignant. How do you respond?*

A. "Don't worry, gastric ulcers are not cancerous."

B. "About 95% of gastric ulcers are benign."

C. "You have about a 50:50 chance of having gastric cancer from your ulcer."

D. "Even if it is cancer, surgery is 100% successful."

12-87 *You assess for Cullen's sign in Dan, age 62, after surgery. Cullen's sign may indicate*

A. intra-abdominal bleeding.

B. a ventral hernia.

C. appendicitis.

D. jaundice.

12-88 *Sidney has ulcerative colitis and asks you about a Koch pouch. You respond,*

A. "It's a method of bowel training for clients with chronic diarrhea."

B. "It's a name for a continent ileostomy."

C. "It's a packet of daily pills to take to relieve diarrhea."

D. "It's like a sanitary pad and it's used to contain any rectal leakage."

12-89 *Tenesmus refers to*

A. projectile vomiting.

B. severe lower abdominal pain.

C. constipation.

D. a persistent desire to empty the bowel or bladder.

12-90 *Steve, age 79, has gastroesophageal reflux disease (GERD). When teaching him how to reduce his lower esophageal sphincter pressure, which substances do you recommend that he avoid?*

A. Apples

B. Peppermint

C. Cucumbers

D. Popsicles

12-91 *Which is the most common presenting symptom of gastric cancer?*

A. Weight loss

B. Dysphagia

C. Hematemesis

D. Gastrointestinal bleeding

12-92 *After treating a patient for Helicobacter* pylori *infection, what test do you order to see if it has been cured?*

A. An enzyme-linked immunosorbent assay titer

B. A urea breath test

C. A rapid urease test (*Campylobacter*-like organism)

D. A repeat endoscopy

12-93 *Which area(s) of Jill's gastrointestinal tract may be affected by her Crohn's disease?*

A. All areas from the mouth to the anus

B. The colon

C. The sigmoid colon

D. The small intestine

12-94 *How do diphenoxylate (Lomotil) and loperamide (Imodium) help relieve diarrhea?*

A. They reduce bowel spasticity and acid secretion in the stomach.

B. They decrease the motility of the ileum and colon, slowing the transit time and promoting more water absorption.

C. They increase motility to assist in removing all of the stool.

D. By decreasing the sensations of the gastric nerves, they send a message to the brain to slow down peristalsis.

12-95 *Which organ structure produces and secretes bile to emulsify fats?*

A. Salivary glands

B. Pancreas

C. Liver

D. Gallbladder

12-96   *The majority of the population of the United States has antibodies against which type of hepatitis?*

A. Hepatitis A

B. Hepatitis B

C. Hepatitis C

D. Hepatitis D

12-97   *Which laboratory value would you expect to be increased in the presence of significant diarrhea?*

A. Serum potassium

B. Serum sodium

C. Serum chloride

D. Bicarbonate

12-98   *Harvey just came back from Mexico. Which pathogen do you suspect is responsible for his diarrhea?*

A. *Enterococci*

B. *Escherichia coli*

C. *Klebsiella*

D. *Staphylococci*

12-99   *Marty, age 52, notices a bulge in his midline every time he rises from bed in the morning. You tell him it's a ventral hernia, also known as*

A. inguinal hernia.

B. epigastric hernia.

C. umbilical hernia.

D. incisional hernia.

12-100   *Which of the following findings is NOT associated with diverticulitis?*

A. Left lower quadrant abdominal pain

B. A history of irritable bowel syndrome

C. A tender mass in the left lower quadrant

D. An elevated temperature

12-101   *When Sammy asks you what he can do to help his wife, who has dumping syndrome, what do you suggest he encourage her to do?*

A. Eat foods higher in carbohydrates.

B. Eat three large meals plus three snacks per day.

C. Eat foods with a moderate fat and protein content.

D. Drink fluids with each meal.

12-102   *Sigrid, age 82, has irritable bowel, chronic constipation, and diverticulitis. Which pharmacological agent do you recommend?*

A. Bulking agents

B. Stool softeners

C. Laxatives

D. Lubricants

12-103   *Patients with irritable bowel syndrome (IBS) are more likely to have which of the following organic gastrointestinal disease?*

A. Thyroid dysfunction

B. Colorectal cancer

C. Celiac sprue

D. Lactose malabsorption

12-104   *Ellie, age 42, has a seizure disorder and has been taking phenytoin (Dilantin) for years. Which supplement should she also be taking if no other problems exist?*

A. Vitamin B_{12}

B. Iron

C. Folic acid

D. Calcium

12-105   *Tom has just been diagnosed with celiac disease. Which of the following might you tell him?*

A. There is a new pharmaceutical cure for celiac disease.

B. A strict gluten-free diet is the only treatment for celiac disease.

C. Your children will not be at a higher risk for developing this disease.

D. The presence of celiac disease is decreasing dramatically in the United States.

12-106   *All of the following medications are used for the control of nausea and vomiting. Which medication works by affecting the chemoreceptor trigger zone, thereby stimulating upper gastrointestinal motility and increasing lower esophageal sphincter pressure?*

A. Anticholinergics such as scopolamine (Donnatal)

B. Antidopaminergic agents such as prochlorperazine (Compazine)

C. Antidopaminergic and cholinergic agents such as metoclopramide (Reglan)

D. Tetrahydrocannabinols such as dronabinol (Marinol)

12-107 *You are counseling Lillian, who is lactose intolerant, about foods to avoid. You know she misunderstands the teaching when she tells you she can have*

A. yogurt.

B. foods containing whey.

C. prehydrolyzed milk.

D. oranges.

12-108 *Nausea is difficult to discern in a young child. What question might you ask to determine if the child has nausea?*

A. "Are you sick to your tummy?"

B. "Are you hungry?"

C. "Are you eating the way you normally eat?"

D. "Are you nauseous?"

12-109 *You auscultate Julie's abdomen and hear a peritoneal friction rub. Which condition do you rule out?*

A. Peritonitis

B. A liver or spleen abscess

C. A liver or spleen metastatic tumor

D. Irritable bowel syndrome

12-110 *You suspect appendicitis in Andrew, who is 18. With his right hip and knee flexed, you slowly rotate his right leg internally to stretch a muscle. He states that it is painful over his right lower quadrant. Which sign did you elicit?*

A. Rovsing's sign

B. Psoas sign

C. Obturator sign

D. McBurney's sign

12-111 *A palpable spleen 2 cm or less below the left costal margin in a 2-year-old child is*

A. indicative of splenomegaly.

B. a sign of internal hemorrhaging.

C. normal.

D. a sign of infection.

12-112 *The most common cause of elevated liver function tests is*

A. hepatitis.

B. biliary tract obstruction.

C. chronic alcohol abuse.

D. a drug-induced injury.

12-113 *Your client's 2-month-old daughter is admitted with gastroenteritis and dehydration after 2 days of vomiting and diarrhea. When she asks you what is causing the diarrhea, how do you respond?*

A. "She must be lactose intolerant from the formula, and this alters the fluid balance."

B. "Her body's telling you that it's time to initiate some solids into her system."

C. "The virus is causing irritation of the gastrointestinal lining, which causes an increase in gastrointestinal motility."

D. "The infectious agent invaded the gastrointestinal mucosa and affected the balance of water and electrolytes."

12-114 *Which oral medication might be used to treat a client with chronic cholelithiasis who is a poor candidate for surgery?*

A. Ursodiol (Actigall)

B. Ibuprofen (Advil)

C. Prednisone (Deltasone)

D. Surgery is the only answer.

12-115 *Martina, age 34, has AIDS and currently suffers from diarrhea. You suspect that she has which protozoal infection of the bowel?*

A. Giardiasis

B. Amebiasis

C. Cryptosporidiosis

D. *Escherichia coli*

12-116 *A false-positive result with the fecal occult blood test can result from*

A. ingestion of large amounts of vitamin C.

B. a high dietary intake of rare-cooked beef.

C. a colonic neoplasm that is not bleeding.

D. stool that has been stored before testing.

12-117   *Nora, age 78, has terminal cancer and is wasting away. What should you order to stimulate her appetite?*

A. Megestrol (Megace)

B. Sertraline (Zoloft)

C. Vitamin C

D. Alprazolam (Xanax)

12-118   *Matt, age 26, recently returned from a camping trip and has gastroenteritis. He says that he has been eating only canned food. Which of the following pathogens do you suspect?*

A. *Campylobacter jejuni*

B. *Clostridium botulinum*

C. *Clostridium perfringens*

D. *Staphylococcus*

Answers

12-1   Answer C

Lipids are broken down in the small intestine by the pancreatic lipases. Carbohydrates, proteins, and nucleic acids are also broken down in the small intestines by various enzymes.

12-2   Answer B

Because of Marvin's alcoholism and his resulting dietary insufficiencies, there is an inadequate amount of vitamin K in the liver for the thrombin to convert fibrinogen to fibrin; thus, the sequence of coagulation is disrupted.

12-3   Answer B

Dumping syndrome may occur 1–3 weeks after gastric surgery when the client starts to consume larger meals. Food enters the intestine faster and in larger quantities than before the surgery, causing the client to experience epigastric fullness, distention, discomfort, abdominal cramping, nausea, and increased flatus.

12-4   Answer A

Dehydration is the most common complication of viral gastroenteritis in children. Gastrointestinal bleeding is uncommon. Peritonitis and bacterial sepsis are other causes of diarrhea.

12-5   Answer D

The diagnosis of celiac disease is classically established by a trial period of a gluten-free diet with an accompanying improvement in the mucosal histological response. Laboratory tests may confirm malabsorption, but they are not diagnostic of celiac disease. A barium enema may show dilation of the small intestine, but in mild celiac disease, the enema results may be normal. A peroral biopsy showing the gross absence of duodenal folds on endoscopy is a clue to the presence of celiac disease, but it is not diagnostic because this symptom may also occur in tropical sprue, intestinal lymphoma, Zollinger-Ellison syndrome, and other diseases.

12-6   Answer B

Melena is defined as black, tarry stools that test positive for occult blood. The most common cause of melena is upper gastrointestinal (GI) bleeding, but bleeding in the small bowel or the right colon can also produce melena. It is the action of gastric acid and intestinal secretions that reduces bright red blood to black, tarry stools. To produce melena, about 100–200 mL of blood must be present. Because of GI transit time, it is possible for melena to continue for several days, after the acute bleeding has stopped.

12-7   Answer A

All these are physical examination maneuvers for diagnosing appendicitis. If pain is elicited during the examination, appendicitis is suspected. Rovsing's sign is deep palpation over the LLQ with sudden, unexpected pain in the right lower quadrant. Psoas sign is pain when the patient is instructed to try to lift the right leg against gentle pressure applied by the examiner or pain when the client is placed in the left lateral decubitus position and the right leg is extended at the hip. The obturator sign occurs when the client with the right hip and knee flexed experiences pain when the examiner slowly rotates the right leg internally, which stretches the obturator muscle. McBurney's sign is pain elicited when pressure is applied to McBurney's point, which is located halfway between the umbilicus and the anterior spine of the ilium.

12-8   Answer A

Potato skins, potato chips, fried potatoes, brown rice, and whole-grain pasta products should be avoided if a client with ulcerative colitis is on a low-residue diet that was ordered to reduce intestinal motility and allow the bowel to rest.

12-9   Answer C

Antidiarrheal agents are contraindicated in the presence of ulcerative colitis because they may precipitate colonic dilation. Sulfasalazine (Azulfidine) is often prescribed for its antibiotic and inflammatory effects; however, it interferes with folate metabolism, and therefore folate supplements may be required. A high-calorie, nonspicy, caffeine-free diet that is low in high-residue foods and milk products; corticosteroids in the acute phase; and a colectomy with permanent ileostomy in severe cases are all treatments for ulcerative colitis.

12-10   Answer C

Folic acid and serum levels of most vitamins, including A, B complex, C, and the fat-soluble vitamins, are decreased in Crohn's disease as a result of malabsorption. The sedimentation rate, liver enzymes, and bilirubin levels are all increased.

12-11   Answer C

Although stress-related conditions such as anxiety and panic attacks and long-term use of NSAIDs may contribute to and aggravate peptic ulcer disease, about 90% of the cases of peptic ulcers have been found to be caused by infection with the bacteria *Helicobacter pylori*.

12-12   Answer D

Increasing fluid intake has not been shown to decrease the risk of colorectal cancer. Current recommendations to aid in preventing colorectal cancer include decreased fat and increased fiber consumption and the daily use of aspirin. The daily use of aspirin has been shown to decrease the incidence of colorectal cancer, as well as dramatically decrease the incidence of metastasis.

12-13   Answer C

The proper order of assessing the abdomen is inspection, auscultation, percussion, and palpation. It is important to inspect the abdomen first before percussion or palpation to avoid causing any discomfort that might alter the client's position. Auscultation is important before percussion and palpation because both of these techniques can increase peristalsis, which would give a false interpretation of bowel sounds on auscultation.

12-14   Answer B

Erythromycin is the antibiotic that causes the most cases of gastrointestinal upset such as nausea or vomiting. Other medications that commonly cause nausea and vomiting are opiates, estrogen, ipecac, digitalis, chemotherapy, and theophylline.

12-15   Answer B

The most important factor in determining long-term negative outcomes for pancreatitis is the presence of infection. Despite best practices, mortality associated with severe acute pancreatitis remains approximately 25% because of systemic complications.

12-16   Answer A

One of the alarm signs or symptoms of irritable bowel syndrome that requires prompt attention is blood or pus in the stool. Other warning signs and symptoms are first onset in a person over 50, weight loss, progressive dysphagia, dehydration, evidence of steatorrhea, recurrent vomiting, fever, anemia, hypokalemia, and a strong family history of colon cancer.

12-17   Answer A

In a 2-month-old infant with vomiting and diarrhea, the most effective way of determining a fluid deficit is to check for decreased peripheral perfusion, dry oral mucous membranes, and sunken fontanels. The body compensates for loss of fluid by shifting the interstitial fluid into the intravascular space, thereby maintaining perfusion of vital organs. If the fluid loss continues, circulating volume is diminished, and vasoconstriction occurs in the peripheral vessels, resulting in decreased perfusion.

12-18   Answer C

Abdominal respirations cease by age 7 years. The absence of abdominal respirations in children younger than age 7 indicates peritoneal inflammation.

12-19   Answer B

In the process of rumination, food is regurgitated, mouthed, or chewed, and then reswallowed. It may be psychogenic or self-stimulated. In some cases when there is an attempt to stimulate the gag reflex in infants, esophagitis has been shown to be present and the rumination is in response to the pain in the throat.

12-20 Answer A

Reducing sugar intake is one of the preventive measures to take against dental caries. Other measures include regular brushing and flossing. Sugar has not been correlated with hyperactivity, and simple sugars do not cause diabetes. Dietary fat, rather than sugar, is the culprit in obesity.

12-21 Answer C

She should not have a snack before retiring. Clients with gastroesophageal reflux disease should be instructed to avoid coffee, alcohol, chocolate, peppermint, and spicy foods; eat smaller meals; stop smoking; remain upright for 2 hours after meals; elevate the head of the bed on 6–8 in. blocks; and refrain from eating for 3 hours before retiring.

12-22 Answer A

Hyperresonance is present when there is gaseous distention. Dullness occurs over a distended bladder or adipose tissue and when there is fluid or a mass present.

12-23 Answer B

Giardiasis, a protozoal infection of the upper small intestine, is caused by *Giardia lamblia*. It is the most common intestinal protozoal infection in the United States that also occurs worldwide. *Clostridium botulinum*, which causes botulism, is an enterotoxin, whereas *Salmonella*, causing salmonellosis, and *Shigella*, causing shigellosis, are both bacteria.

12-24 Answer A

A distinct foul odor to the stool may indicate blood in the stool, ingestion of a high-fat diet, or colon cancer.

12-25 Answer A

Cheese, bread, pasta, rice, pretzels, and yogurt all help to thicken stools. Leafy green vegetables, raw fruits and vegetables, and dried beans may all loosen stools.

12-26 Answer C

Bulk-forming agents such as methylcellulose (Citrucel) are the only laxatives that are safe for long-term use. They contain natural vegetable fiber that is not absorbed. This creates bulk and draws water into the intestine, thus softening the stool. Mineral oil reduces the absorption of the fat-soluble vitamins A, D, E, and K and may cause damage to the liver and spleen because of systemic absorption. Irritant or stimulant laxatives, such as bisacodyl (Dulcolax), work by stimulating the motility and secretion of the intestinal mucosa. Osmotic and saline laxatives and cathartics, such as magnesium hydroxide (milk of magnesia), when used over the long term, may suppress normal bowel reflexes.

12-27 Answer C

The marker for permanent immunity, hepatitis B surface antibodies in the serum will be present 4–10 months after exposure and immunity to hepatitis B. Hepatitis B surface antigen is the earliest indicator of the presence of an acute infection and is present 4–12 weeks after exposure. This marker is also indicative of a chronic infection.

12-28 Answer B

Costovertebral angle tenderness occurs when one hand is "thumped" with the ulnar edge of the other fist over the 12th rib at the costovertebral angle on the back and tenderness or sharp pain occurs. It indicates inflammation of the kidney.

12-29 Answer B

A portacaval shunt is the surgery often performed for bleeding esophageal varices. They are associated with alcoholic cirrhosis and portal hypertension, commonly the result of a history of alcohol abuse. Bleeding esophageal varices occur when the small esophageal veins become distended and rupture from increased pressure in the portal system.

12-30 Answer C

In the ABCs of irritable bowel syndrome, the A is for abdominal pain or discomfort—typically in the lower abdomen but could be anywhere; the B is for bloating or visible distention; the C is for constipation—hard, difficult to evacuate, or infrequent stools; the D is for diarrhea—loose, watery, or frequent stools; and the E is for extrabowel symptoms such as fatigue, headache, backache, muscle pain, urinary frequency, and sleep disturbance.

12-31 Answer A

Ascariasis is the most common of the intestinal helminths (parasitic worms). It causes pulmonary manifestations such as low-grade fever, productive cough with blood-tinged sputum, wheezing, and dyspnea because the larvae are transmitted to the lungs from the vascular system. The larvae burrow through alveolar walls, migrating up the bronchial tree to the pharynx, and then down the esophagus back to the intestines. Nocturnal perianal and perineal pruritus occur with enterobiasis (pinworm infection). Diarrhea, cramps, and malaise are common with trichinosis. Ascites and facial and extremity edema are common with trichuriasis.

12-32   Answer A

Hirschsprung's disease is common in male infants, results in small ribbonlike stools, usually has no accompanying abdominal pain unless there is obstruction, and may be accompanied by failure to thrive. The infant with functional (acquired) constipation is usually male and has very large stools and abdominal pain, but failure to thrive is uncommon.

12-33   Answer A

Although drug metabolism by the liver is usually impaired in older adults, the metabolism of alcohol is unchanged.

12-34   Answer A

Rebound tenderness is present when there is pain on release of pressure to the abdomen and is a reliable indicator of peritoneal inflammation.

12-35   Answer B

Grey Turner's sign is a bluish discoloration over the flanks. Cullen's sign is a bluish discoloration around the umbilicus. Other findings that can result from the pancreatic inflammatory process include left-sided pleural effusion, jaundice caused by impingement on the common bile duct, and an epigastric mass secondary to pseudocyst development.

12-36   Answer C

Osteopenic bone disease may occur in celiac disease because there is decreased calcium absorption by the small intestine, decreased absorption of the fat-soluble vitamin D, and binding of calcium and magnesium in the intestinal lumen by unabsorbed dietary fatty acids. Clients should be identified as having celiac disease before menopause so that therapy to increase bone mass can be instituted before clients develop osteopenia.

12-37   Answer C

Clients with celiac disease have an allergy to gliadin, a component of gluten; therefore, they are placed on a gluten-free diet in which wheat and other grains containing analogues to wheat gluten, such as oats, barley, and rye, must be avoided.

12-38   Answer B

Self-care measures to teach a client with an ileostomy how to relieve food blockage include massaging the peristomal area, which may stimulate peristalsis and fecal elimination; assuming a knee-chest position to reduce intra-abdominal pressure; taking a warm shower or tub bath to relax the abdominal muscles; and drinking warm fluids or grape juice to produce a mild cathartic effect.

12-39   Answer A

All of the drugs listed are used in the eradication of *Helicobacter pylori*. Traditional 14-day "triple therapy" with bismuth subsalicylate (Pepto-Bismol), tetracycline (Tetracap) or amoxicillin (Amoxil), and metronidazole (Flagyl) has consistently produced eradication rates of approximately 90% and is the least expensive therapy.

12-40   Answer C

A rapid onset of severe right upper quadrant (RUQ) abdominal cramping pain with nausea and vomiting is a classic presentation of acute cholecystitis; 90%–95% of clients with acute cholecystitis also have gallstones. Other symptoms include low-grade fever, epigastric tenderness, guarding, and pain on inspiration during palpation of the RUQ (Murphy's sign). Pain associated with appendicitis would typically be near the navel progressing to the right lower quadrant. In irritable bowel syndrome (IBS) and Crohn's disease, the pain and cramping is more diffuse in the abdomen and is not usually accompanied by nausea and vomiting. The pain with IBS originates over some area of the colon, with the lower left quadrant (LLQ) being most often affected.

12-41   Answer C

No treatment is necessary for physiological jaundice unless the bilirubin level exceeds 20 mg/dL. In this case, the breastfeeding should be discontinued for 24 hours because this will result in a decreased bilirubin level.

12-42   Answer C

The most common causes of upper gastrointestinal hemorrhage, in descending order, are peptic ulcer disease, esophageal varices, esophagitis, erosive gastritis, carcinomas, and arteriovenous malformations.

12-43   Answer C

During the incubation period of viral hepatitis, there are no subjective or objective complaints. During the prodromal stage, there is anorexia, nausea, vomiting, malaise, upper respiratory infection (nasal discharge, pharyngitis), myalgia, arthralgia, easy fatigability, fever (hepatitis A virus), and abdominal pain. In the icteric stage of viral hepatitis, there is jaundice, dark urine, and light-colored stools. There are continued prodromal complaints with gradual improvement. During the convalescent stage, there is an increased sense of well-being; the appetite returns; and the jaundice, abdominal pain, and fatigability abate.

12-44   Answer C

The pain associated with pelvic inflammatory disease can be palpated in both the right and left lower quadrants. Pain in the left upper quadrant may signify a gastric ulcer, gastritis, pancreatitis, splenic abscess, or pleurisy.

12-45   Answer B

Vomiting is more common with gastric ulcers than duodenal ulcers. Stools are more often altered with duodenal ulcers. The possibility of perforation and obstruction of the gastrointestinal tract is present in both types of ulcers. Approximately half of the clients report relief of pain with food or antacids (especially with duodenal ulcers). Many clients deny the relationship of meals to the pain. Two-thirds of clients with duodenal ulcers and one-third with gastric ulcers have nocturnal pain that awakens them.

12-46   Answer C

A pyloroplasty surgically enlarges the opening between the stomach and duodenum to improve gastric emptying. A Billroth I is a gastroduodenostomy. A total gastrectomy is removal of the entire stomach and is rarely performed. It results in an anastomosis connecting the esophagus to the duodenum or jejunum. A vagotomy severs a portion or all of the vagus nerves to the stomach.

12-47   Answer C

For the client who has just had a hemorrhoidectomy, teaching would include advising the client to maintain an adequate intake of dietary fiber to maintain stool bulk; to take a sitz bath after each bowel movement for 1–2 weeks after surgery to promote relaxation and aid with discomfort; to drink at least 2,000 mL of fluids per day; to take stool softeners as prescribed (for short-term relief only); and to exercise regularly to maintain stool bulk, softness, and regularity.

12-48   Answer C

Rotavirus causes 15%–35% of all the cases of diarrhea in the United States. It is followed by enteric adenovirus and Norwalk-like viruses. *Giardia lamblia* is a parasite that causes a high incidence of diarrhea in day-care centers.

12-49   Answer B

Cushing's ulcers are stress ulcers that occur after a head injury or intracranial disease. A Cushing's ulcer may also occur after a severe burn.

12-50   Answer D

Antacids may contain magnesium, which decreases bowel transit time and may contain poorly absorbed salts that result in an osmotic draw of fluid into the bowel. Fructose, sorbitol, and caffeine are not usually contained in antacids. Fructose is present in apple juice, pear juice, grapes, honey, dates, nuts, figs, and fruit-flavored soft drinks. Sorbitol or mannitol is present in apple juice, pear juice, sugarless gums, and mints. Caffeine is present in coffee, tea, cola drinks, and over-the-counter analgesics.

12-51   Answer D

The rate of *Clostridium difficile* colitis has increased 109% in the past decade. The case fatality rate among *C. difficile* colitis patients climbed as well. Awareness of this must be heightened if we are to help control the public health ramifications of this important and morbid nosocomial infection.

12-52   Answer D

The American Cancer Society (ACS) recommends a flexible sigmoidoscopy for colon cancer screening in persons at average risk beginning at age 50 every 5 years, *or* a colonoscopy every 10 years, *or* a double-contrast barium enema every 5 years, *or* a CT colonography (virtual colonoscopy) every 5 years. If the flexible sigmoidoscopy or the barium enema are positive, a colonoscopy should be done. The multiple stool take-home test (fecal occult blood test [FOBT]) should be done every year. One test done in the office is not adequate for testing. A colonoscopy should be done if the test is positive.

12-53   Answer A

Striae are silvery-white, linear, jagged marks (stretch marks) about 1–6 cm in length that result when elastic fibers in the reticular layer of the skin are broken as a result of rapid or prolonged stretching. This stretching most commonly occurs with pregnancy but may also occur with excessive weight gain, or ascites.

12-54   Answer D

Bulking agents such as psyllium preparations may cause flatulence and bloating and requires adequate fluid intake. Saline laxatives may cause dehydration and electrolyte imbalance. Lubricants such as mineral oil may cause lipid pneumonia if aspirated. Stool softeners when combined with irritant laxatives may be hepatotoxic.

12-55   Answer A

Diarrhea is a common problem after a gastroplasty because of the induced malabsorption. Clients usually do not end up losing too much weight because sometimes the only foods they can tolerate are high-caloric foods (simple sugars) such as ice cream.

12-56   Answer B

Several studies show that intensive lifestyle changes in the form of diet and exercise can go miles in reducing death and events in high-risk patients. Studies on managing diabetes show that these modifications are more effective than drug therapy. Exercise, for example, is a strong deterrent for developing diabetes and heart disease. Some easy fixes in the diet are staying away from high-fructose corn syrup and trans fats, which are two of the biggest metabolic syndrome antagonists. Patients need to understand the association of what goes in the mouth and what goes on with their blood chemistry. Teaching must help patients understand and manage all the factors that put them in the metabolic danger zone.

12-57   Answer C

Susan has a constellation of symptoms known as metabolic syndrome. The World Health Organization (WHO), National Cholesterol Education Program Adult Treatment Panel (NCEP-ATP III), and International Diabetes Federation (IDF) have slightly different criteria for this diagnosis. They all, however, include hypertension, dyslipidemia, and central obesity.

12-58   Answer B

A middle-aged or older client with an abrupt change in defecation pattern must be evaluated for colorectal cancer.

12-59   Answer C

Once gastric cancer has been diagnosed, accurate staging can be determined by an endoscopic ultrasound. Ranson's criteria is a classification system to assess the severity of pancreatitis.

12-60   Answer D

Fecal output from an ileostomy is a malodorous, continuous, soft-to-watery effluent material that contains intestinal enzymes, which are very irritating to the skin around the stoma. Stomas farther along the large colon will have more formed stools, and a sigmoid colostomy will result in stools that are almost normal in consistency.

12-61   Answer D

Because the hepatitis C virus is transmitted in blood, including menstrual blood, clients should abstain from sex during menstruation. Clients should not donate blood, and there is a possibility of transmission through razors, toothbrushes, and tattoo instruments. No vaccine is available.

12-62   Answer B

The following drugs may cause acute hepatitis: acetaminophen, allopurinol, aspirin in high doses, captopril, carbamazepine, isoniazid, ketoconazole, methyldopa, NSAIDs, procainamide, and sulfonamides.

12-63   Answer D

An incisional or ventral hernia may develop at a previous surgical incision site. An umbilical hernia may be congenital or acquired as the tissue around the umbilical ring weakens. Conditions resulting in umbilical hernias include pregnancy, including multiple pregnancies with prolonged labor; obesity; ascites; and large intra-abdominal tumors.

12-64   Answer A

Constant periumbilical pain shifting to the right lower quadrant; vomiting following the pain; a small volume of diarrhea; no systemic symptoms such as a headache, malaise, or myalgia; a mild elevation of the white blood cell count with an early left shift; and white blood cells (WBCs) or red blood cells (RBCs) in the urine are indications of appendicitis. The WBC count becomes high only with gangrene or perforation of the appendix. The urine may have WBCs or RBCs if the bladder is irritated and ketonuria if there is prolonged vomiting.

12-65   Answer B

An infant's umbilical cord stump dries within 7 days, then hardens and falls off in 10–14 days. It then takes 3–4 weeks for skin to cover the area.

12-66   Answer D

Hernias account for more cases of mechanical bowel obstruction in all ages than do volvulus, intussusception, or cancer.

12-67   Answer B

The client with gastroesophageal reflux disease should avoid taking NSAIDs because they tend to aggravate the already-irritated gastric mucosa.

12-68   Answer B

Hyperactive bowel sounds (borborygmi) are present with laxative use, early mechanical bowel obstruction, gastroenteritis, and brisk diarrhea.

12-69   Answer A

Crohn's disease would show transmural inflammation, granulomas, focal involvement of the colon with some skipped areas, and sparing of the rectal mucosa. Ulcerative colitis would show acute inflammatory infiltrates, depleted goblet cells, negative cultures, and involvement of the rectum. Infectious colitis, because of the toxic products released, may induce periportal inflammation, mild hepatomegaly, and low-grade liver enzyme abnormalities, but usually without trophozoites in the liver. Ischemic colitis seen on colonoscopy reveals segmental inflammatory changes most often in the rectosigmoid and the splenic flexure, where there is more collateral circulation.

12-70   Answer D

There is no such thing as a "normal" pattern of defecation. Patterns of defecation vary widely and may in part be affected by dietary habits, fluid intake, bacteria in the stool, psychological stress, or voluntary postponement of defecation. Defecating every third day could be the routine pattern for Simon.

12-71   Answer C

Infants with gastrointestinal reflux should be placed on their left side to prevent aspiration. They should be fed a formula thickened with rice cereal while being held in an upright position and kept in an elevated prone position for 1 hour after feeding so that gravity helps prevent reflux.

12-72   Answer A

Pruritus indicates that biliary obstruction is present with the liver disease. Increased abdominal girth indicates ascites is present from portal hypertension or hypoalbuminemia. Right upper quadrant pain may indicate hepatitis, cholecystitis, hepatocellular carcinoma, or abscess. Easy bruising may indicate splenomegaly secondary to portal hypertension with platelet sequestration, or coagulopathy secondary to decreased synthesis of clotting factors.

12-73   Answer A

Three-dose cefmetazole administration is significantly more effective for prevention of incisional surgical site infection (SSI) than single-dose administration for clients undergoing colorectal surgery. Use of prophylactic antibiotics in elective colorectal surgery is essential. The incidence of incisional SSI among clients undergoing colorectal surgery may be as high as 30%–50% without prophylactic antibiotics.

12-74   Answer B

Enterotoxigenic *Escherichia coli* (ETEC) is the most common cause of traveler's diarrhea that occurs from contaminated food or water. It is usually self-limiting, requiring no treatment other than supportive care. It is common in developing countries. Traveler's diarrhea caused by *E. coli* used to be frequently treated with a 3- to 5-day course of a quinolone antibiotic such as ciprofloxacin (Cipro). Metronidazole may be used for *Clostridium difficile* and for *Entamoeba histolytica* (Amebiasis). Quinolone antibiotics may also be used for *Salmonella* if associated with a fever or systemic disease. Gastric lavage may be used for *Clostridium botulinum*.

12-75   Answer A

Hepatitis A (HAV) is transmitted by the fecal-oral route, sewage, contaminated water and shellfish, and possibly by blood. Hepatitis B (HBV) is transmitted by the percutaneous route (permucosal) through infected blood and body fluids and sexual contact. Hepatitis C (HCV) is transmitted by the percutaneous route, in the community, and a large percentage of those infected have no known risk factors. Hepatitis D (HDV) is transmitted by the percutaneous route, but most have coinfection with HBV. Hepatitis E (HEV) is transmitted by the fecal-oral route.

12-76   Answer A

Achalasia is an absence of peristalsis of the esophagus and a high gastroesophageal sphincter pressure. After initial noninvasive treatments, clients may require a balloon dilation of the lower esophageal sphincter. Calcium channel blockers, not beta blockers, may be used to decrease symptoms of dysphagia. A fundoplication is done for a hiatal hernia. An esophagogastrectomy is performed for esophageal cancer.

12-77   Answer C

Although some clients report a significant subjective drop in taste function following surgery, none have ongoing taste dysfunction. Sweet, sour, salty, and bitter taste abilities may be temporarily affected, but there is no lasting change in taste seen after a tonsillectomy.

12-78   Answer D

Celiac disease, also known as celiac sprue, may begin during early childhood or adulthood. Clients with sprue usually have steatorrhea, abdominal bloating and cramps, and diarrhea. Clients with celiac disease are often small in stature and have delayed maturity. The malabsorption that results may cause deficiencies such as anemia.

12-79   Answer C

Polyethylene glycol (GoLYTELY) should be taken in the early evening so as not to interfere with sleep because the first bowel movement begins within 1 hour and continues until the sigmoid colon is clear. The solution should be chilled to enhance

palatability, taken on an empty stomach, and administered in 8-oz servings every 10 minutes until 1 gallon is consumed.

12-80   Answer A

Rebound tenderness at McBurney's point, located midway between the umbilicus and the anterior iliac crest in the right lower quadrant, would alert you to appendicitis.

12-81   Answer B

Older adults have a diminished response to painful stimuli that may mask abdominal health problems. Older adults may have difficulty assuming some positions necessary for the physical examination, so positions may need to be modified to meet their needs. As people age, many of their body systems slow down and become less efficient. In the gastrointestinal tract, there is a reduction of saliva, stomach acid, gastric motility, and peristalsis that causes problems with swallowing, absorption, and digestion. These changes, along with a general reduction of muscle mass and tone, also contribute to constipation. The liver becomes smaller and liver function declines, making it harder to process medications.

12-82   Answer C

There are many systemic causes of acute abdominal pain that also result in a rash. In the infectious category, these include Rocky Mountain spotted fever, measles, mumps, anaphylaxis, acute rheumatic fever, and infectious mononucleosis. A food allergy may also present itself as abdominal pain along with dermatitis. Appendicitis does not present with a rash.

12-83   Answer B

A Schilling test is a timed urine test that evaluates the ability to absorb vitamin B_{12} from the gastrointestinal tract. It is used to diagnose pernicious anemia and malabsorption syndromes. The normal values range from 10%–40%. A value less than 7% indicates pernicious anemia and some gastric lesions.

12-84   Answer D

Women tend to develop cirrhosis more quickly with less alcohol intake than men, which suggests that a smaller, leaner body mass and enhanced absorption are both factors in the development of alcoholic cirrhosis. Alcoholic cirrhosis, also known as Laënnec's, portal, fatty, or micronodular cirrhosis, is the most common type of cirrhosis in the United States. Alcoholic cirrhosis is often associated with nutritional and vitamin deficiencies but occurs in well-nourished individuals as well as alcoholics. Cirrhosis is the irreversible end stage of liver injury and may be caused by a variety of insults.

12-85   Answer D

Antibiotic therapy is not indicated for an uncomplicated salmonellosis because it is generally a self-limiting illness.

12-86   Answer B

About 95% of gastric ulcers are benign, even though some of these seem to look malignant on x-ray.

12-87   Answer A

Cullen's sign is a bluish periumbilical color that may indicate intra-abdominal bleeding.

12-88   Answer B

Performed for clients with ulcerative colitis, a Koch pouch (continent ileostomy) is the surgical removal of the rectum and colon and construction of an internal ileal reservoir, nipple valve, and stoma, allowing for intermittent drainage of ileal contents.

12-89   Answer D

Tenesmus is the spasmodic contraction of the anal or bladder sphincters, producing pain and the persistent desire to empty the bowel or bladder via involuntary, ineffectual straining efforts. Rectal tenesmus is often experienced in ulcerative colitis.

12-90   Answer B

Food substances that reduce the lower esophageal sphincter pressure or irritate the gastric mucosa include alcohol, caffeinated beverages, chocolate, citrus fruits, decaffeinated coffee, fatty foods, onions, peppermint and spearmint, tomatoes, and tomato-based products. Nonfood substances that irritate gastroesophageal reflux disease include anticholinergic drugs, beta-adrenergic blocking agents, calcium channel blockers, diazepam, estrogens, nicotine, and theophylline.

12-91   Answer A

Weight loss is usually the presenting symptom of gastric cancer, followed by dysphagia. Hematemesis occurs in 10%–15% of all clients with gastric cancer. Gastrointestinal bleeding is uncommon with gastric cancer, although common with colorectal cancer.

12-92   Answer B

If the patient is treated empirically for an ulcer, follow up is only indicated if symptoms recur. A urea breath test is the easiest, least expensive, and most reliable test for *Helicobacter pylori*, which causes peptic ulcers. Its average sensitivity is 96% and specificity is 98%. An enzyme-linked immunosorbent assay titer, a rapid urease test (*Campylobacter*-like organism [CLO]) test, and an endoscopy may also be used. The CLO test and endoscopy require biopsy specimens and are therefore more invasive.

12-93   Answer A

Although the colon is the major site of gastrointestinal involvement in Crohn's disease (inflammatory bowel disease), the disease can affect all areas from the mouth to the anus.

12-94   Answer B

Diphenoxylate (Lomotil) and loperamide (Imodium), like all opiates and opium derivatives, help to relieve diarrhea by decreasing the motility of the ileum and colon, slowing the transit time, and promoting more water absorption. Anticholinergics such as atropine (Donnatal) and other belladonna alkaloids (Donnagel) reduce bowel spasticity and acid secretion in the stomach.

12-95   Answer C

The liver produces and secretes bile to emulsify fats. The salivary glands moisturize food and release enzymes that initiate the digestion process. The pancreas secretes cells that regulate blood sugar levels, store carbohydrates, and inhibit insulin and glucagon secretion. The gallbladder stores and concentrates bile.

12-96   Answer A

The majority of the population in the United States has antibodies against hepatitis A virus (HAV). Besides immunity, there is also a vaccine available.

12-97   Answer C

Serum chloride level is increased with significant diarrhea when the diarrhea causes sodium loss that is greater than chloride loss. However, when there is severe diarrhea and vomiting, serum chloride levels may be decreased. Serum potassium and chloride levels are decreased as a result of loss through stool, and bicarbonate level is decreased in a metabolic acidotic state.

12-98   Answer B

Escherichia coli is the pathogen most often responsible for traveler's diarrhea (infectious diarrhea). Other causes may include viruses, other bacteria, protozoa, or parasites.

12-99   Answer B

A ventral hernia, also known as an epigastric hernia, occurs along the midline between the xiphoid process and the umbilicus. The fibers along the linea alba are brought together in a patchwork-type closure; the defect exists within this decussation. As these fibers weaken, the contents can herniate through the abdomen. Epigastric hernias are three times more likely to occur in men than women. Umbilical hernias that develop in adulthood occur through a weakening in the abdominal wall around the umbilical ring. Incisional hernias can occur anywhere along a surgical incision into the abdomen. An inguinal hernia may be indirect or direct. Indirect inguinal hernias result when tissue herniates through the internal inguinal ring, which extends the length of the spermatic cord. A direct inguinal hernia occurs when the transversus abdominis and internal oblique muscles are attached, forming a high arch on the inferior border that results in a faulty shutter mechanism.

12-100   Answer B

A history of irritable bowel syndrome has no association with diverticulitis. A client with diverticulitis would have left lower quadrant abdominal pain, a tender mass in the left lower quadrant, and an elevated temperature.

12-101   Answer C

To help clients with dumping syndrome, suggest that they eat foods with a moderate fat and protein content. These foods tend to leave the stomach more slowly and do not draw fluid into the intestine. Also suggest that they reduce the amount of carbohydrates consumed, eat six small meals per day, and take fluids between meals and not at mealtime.

12-102   Answer A

Bulking agents such as psyllium preparations or methylcellulose preparations are used for irritable bowel, chronic constipation, and diverticulitis. Stool softeners such as docusate sodium are frequently used for the prevention of constipation but most likely are not effective for chronic use. Saline laxatives such as magnesium hydroxide are indicated for intermittent use in chronic constipation and as a bowel preparation; stimulant irritant laxatives such as bisacodyl, senna, and cascara are used in acute constipation and should not be used for chronic constipation. Lubricants such as mineral oil are used in intermittent chronic constipation.

12-103   Answer D

Patients with irritable bowel syndrome are 22%–26% more likely to have lactose malabsorption in addition to irritable bowel syndrome. The percentage of patients who also have thyroid dysfunction is 6%; colorectal cancer, 0%–0.51%; and celiac sprue, 4.7%.

12-104   Answer C

Clients taking phenytoin (Dilantin) should also be taking 0.4–1 mg/day of folic acid because Dilantin promotes a folate deficiency. Phenytoin may also contribute to demineralization of the bone, so the serum calcium levels should also be checked. If demineralization is detected, then vitamin D should be added.

12-105   Answer B

A strict gluten-free diet is the only treatment for celiac disease. There is no pharmaceutical cure. Patients with first- or second-degree relatives affected by celiac disease are at higher risk for developing it. The prevalence of celiac disease in the United States has increased dramatically. Approximately 1% of today's U.S. residents are affected by it.

12-106   Answer C

Metoclopramide (Reglan) is used for diabetic gastroparesis and postoperative nausea and vomiting. It works by affecting the chemoreceptor trigger zone, thereby stimulating upper gastrointestinal motility and increasing lower esophageal sphincter pressure. Anticholinergics work at the site of the labyrinth receptors and the chemoreceptor trigger zones—that is, the vomiting center. Antidopaminergic agents work at the chemoreceptor trigger zone. The site and mechanism of tetrahydrocannabinols are unknown.

12-107   Answer B

Advise clients who are lactose intolerant to avoid foods containing whey. Whey is a lactose-rich ingredient found in some foods; therefore, labels need to be read on all foods for clients who are lactose intolerant. To control symptoms, dietary lactose should be reduced or restricted by using lactose-reduced and lactose-free dairy products or by eating lactose-rich food in small amounts or in combination with low-lactose or lactose-free foods. Fermented dairy products such as aged or hard cheeses and cultured yogurt are easier to digest and contain less lactose than other dairy products. Most stores carry milk that has been pretreated with lactase, making it more than 70% lactose free. Lillian can eat oranges.

12-108   Answer B

To elicit information concerning nausea in a young child, ask the child about hunger because a young child cannot usually differentiate between hunger and mild nausea. Young children sometimes equate being "sick to their tummy" with vomiting and thus might answer no when questioned about nausea.

12-109   Answer D

A peritoneal friction rub, which sounds like a rough, grating sound, occurs over organs with a large surface area in contact with the peritoneum when there is peritoneal inflammation (peritonitis). When a peritoneal friction rub is heard over the lower right rib cage, it may be caused by an abscess or tumor of the liver. When heard over the lower left rib cage in the left anterior axillary line, it may indicate infection of the spleen or an abscess or tumor of the spleen. Irritable bowel syndrome does not produce a friction rub.

12-110   Answer C

The obturator sign is elicited when, with the patient's right hip and knee flexed, the examiner slowly rotates the right leg internally, which stretches the obturator muscle. Pain over the right lower quadrant (RLQ) is considered a positive sign. Rovsing's sign is pain elicited with deep palpation over the left lower quadrant (LLQ) with sudden

resultant pain in the RLQ. This causes tenderness over the RLQ and is considered a positive finding. Psoas sign is pain when the patient is instructed to try to lift the right leg against gentle pressure applied by the examiner or by placing the patient in the left lateral decubitus position and extending the patient's right leg at the hip. An increase in pain is considered positive and is an indication of the inflamed appendix irritating the psoas muscle. McBurney's sign is pain elicited when pressure is applied to McBurney's point, which is located halfway between the umbilicus and the anterior spine of the ilium.

12-111   Answer C

A palpable spleen 2 cm or less below the left costal margin is a normal finding in a child younger than age 3 and may be a normal finding in an older child. Other symptoms would have to be present to warrant further evaluation.

12-112   Answer C

Hepatocellular damage from chronic alcohol abuse is the most frequent cause of elevated liver function tests (LFTs) in adults. Other causes include biliary tract obstruction, hepatitis, drug-induced injuries, vascular changes caused by anoxia, and congestive heart failure; however, chronic alcohol abuse remains the number one cause of abnormal LFTs.

12-113   Answer D

In 80% of the cases, gastroenteritis is viral in nature. This viral infection causes diarrhea by stimulating the secretion of electrolytes into the intestine. This is rapidly followed by water along the osmotic gradient, resulting in watery stools.

12-114   Answer A

Ursodiol (Actigall) is an oral bile acid that dissolves gallstones. For dissolution, 8–10 mg/kg per day is given in two to three divided doses; for prevention, 300 mg twice per day is given. The safety of its use after 24 months has not been established. NSAIDs such as ibuprofen (Advil) may be very irritating to the gastrointestinal mucosa. Steroids such as prednisone (Deltasone) may mask an infection as well as be irritating to the gastric mucosa.

12-115   Answer C

Cryptosporidiosis, a common protozoal infection of the bowel, is common in immunocompromised clients. It causes villous atrophy and mild inflammatory changes and may secrete an enterotoxin. Giardiasis and amebiasis are also protozoal infections affecting the intestine, but because the question mentioned that Martina has AIDS, the answer must be cryptosporidiosis. *Escherichia coli (E. coli)* is a gram-negative bacterium.

12-116   Answer B

A false-positive result with the fecal occult blood test can result from a high dietary intake of rare-cooked beef or fruits and vegetables that contain peroxidases. Oral iron preparations have also been shown to produce a false-positive result in some, but not all, studies. False-negative results can occur in clients who ingest large amounts of vitamin C or have a colon neoplasm that is not bleeding. A false-negative result can also occur if the stool has been stored before testing.

12-117   Answer A

Although depression might be a contributing factor to Nora's wasting away, megestrol (Megace) can produce weight gain by stimulating appetite and food intake and by decreasing the nausea and vomiting that usually accompany terminal cancer.

12-118   Answer B

Clostridium botulinum is an anaerobic gram-positive bacillus that produces toxins. The primary source is canned foods. *Campylobacter jejuni* is found primarily in eggs and poultry but may be found in domestic animals. *Clostridium perfringens* is found in soil, feces, air, and water. Outbreaks are caused most often by contaminated meat. *Staphylococcus* is a common cause of food poisoning. It is caused by the ingestion of an enterotoxin found in improperly handled or stored foods.

Bibliography

Barclay, L, and Lie, D: Three-dose cefmetazole may be better than a single dose for colorectal surgery. www.medscape.com/viewarticle/560045, accessed July 20, 2007.

Dunphy, LM, et al: *The Art and Science of Advanced Practice Nursing,* ed 3. FA Davis, Philadelphia, 2011.

Landsmann, MA: Weighing in on metabolic syndrome. *Healthy Aging* 2(5):54–59, January/February 2007.

No lasting change in taste seen after tonsillectomy. www.medscape.com/viewarticle/560045, accessed July 20, 2007.

Pearson, G: Celiac disease: Furor in the small intestine. *NPs & PAs* 2(5):43–45, May 2011.

Talley, NJ: Irritable bowel syndrome: Rational therapy. *Consultant* 51(6):341–347, June 2011.

How well did you do?

85% and above, congratulations! This score shows application of test-taking principles and adequate content knowledge.

75%–85%, keep working! Review test-taking principles and try again.

65%–75%, hang in there! Spend some time reviewing concepts and test-taking principles and try the test again.

GREYSCALE

BIN TRAVELER FORM

Cut By_____EW_____ Qty__10__ Date_8/15/24_

Scanned By_____ Qty_____Date_____

Scanned Batch IDs

_____   _____   _____

Notes / Exception

_____

_____

_____

_____

_____

Chapter 13: *Renal Problems*

Jill E. Winland-Brown

Questions

13-1 The aging process begins to affect the kidneys with a progressive loss of nephron units by age

A. 40 years.

B. 50 years.

C. 60 years.

D. 70 years.

13-2 The most common cause of sepsis in older adults is

A. urinary stasis.

B. a urinary tract infection.

C. a kidney stone.

D. a common cold.

13-3 Cloudy urine is usually indicative of which of the following conditions?

A. Diabetes

B. Proteinuria

C. Malignancy

D. Urinary tract infection (UTI)

13-4 Rita, age 16, has a 3-day history of red urine. You want her to go home for a few days and then return for some lab work. In teaching her what to avoid, you know she has misunderstood the directions when she tells you she shouldn't ingest any

A. blackberries.

B. ibuprofen.

C. red food color.

D. watermelon.

13-5 Urine specific gravity is increased in clients with

A. dehydration.

B. diabetes insipidus.

C. chronic renal failure.

D. overhydration.

13-6 Cardiovascular failure is a major cause of which type of acute renal failure?

A. Prerenal

B. Intrarenal

C. Postrenal

D. Perirenal

13-7 Jessica, age 79, has been on dialysis for 6 years due to chronic kidney disease. She has been on an oral iron preparation and now asks you if she should think about switching to the intravenous (IV) iron preparation. How do you respond?

A. "If it ain't broke, don't fix it."

B. "There are more side effects with IV administration than oral administration."

C. "You have many more problems than iron deficiency anemia. Let's not worry about that."

D. "Let's try it. It corrects iron deficiency faster, more safely, and better than oral iron."

13-8 Clinical manifestations of metabolic alkalosis include

A. tetany.

B. nausea and vomiting.

C. weakness.

D. bradycardia.

13-9 Most calcium phosphate kidney stones are caused by

A. a high dietary calcium intake.

B. a high phosphorus dietary intake.

C. primary hyperparathyroidism.

D. hyperthyroidism.

13-10   You should be concerned about the use of diuretics, chronic renal failure, a high-protein diet, gout, leukemia, or lymphoma when a serum uric acid level is

A. 4.0 mg/dL.

B. 5.0 mg/dL.

C. 6.0 mg/dL.

D. greater than 7.0 mg/dL.

13-11   Leslie, age 13, says that her mother has polycystic kidney disease and asks about her chances of developing it. How do you respond?

A. "It is hereditary, but if you develop it, a cure is possible."

B. "It is hereditary and, unfortunately, incurable, but there are many measures we can use in dealing with it."

C. "It is not hereditary, but you may develop it anyway."

D. "It is hereditary, but skips generations."

13-12   Martha has been on peritoneal dialysis and is going to the operating room for placement of an arteriovenous (AV) fistula to begin hemodialysis. How do you respond when she asks you what this is?

A. "This is where an artery and a vein are sewn together internally."

B. "This is where a tubing is connecting an artery and a vein underneath the skin."

C. "This is where a catheter is tunneled underneath the skin with a little cuff on the outside."

D. "You'll have an exterior loop of tubing connecting an artery and a vein."

13-13   Which of the following groups is most prone to developing nephrolithiasis?

A. White men

B. White women

C. Black men

D. Black women

13-14   Doug, age 6, appears with abdominal distention and pain, an abdominal mass on the right side, fever, and slight hematuria. There is no precipitating event. What do you suspect?

A. A urinary tract infection

B. Appendicitis

C. Wilms' tumor

D. An intestinal obstruction

13-15   In an assessment of renal function, what is the maximum amount of urine in a 24-hour period that a client would produce for a diagnosis of anuria to be considered?

A. No urine output at all

B. Less than 100 mL

C. 100–150 mL

D. 151–200 mL

13-16   Which of the following renal hormones regulates intrarenal blood flow by vasodilation or vasoconstriction?

A. Renin

B. Prostaglandins

C. Bradykinins

D. Erythropoietin

13-17   The clinical presentation of a client with urolithiasis would include

A. a gradual onset of nagging pain.

B. marked leukocytes in the urine.

C. a fever of 101°F or above.

D. pain starting in the flank and localizing in the costovertebral angle.

13-18   A renal mass was accidentally found on George, a 70-year-old man, during his hospitalization for an episode of diverticulitis. Which of the following statements is true?

A. The malignancy risk is related to the size of the lesion.

B. The treatment of choice is a radical nephrectomy.

C. Because of an increase in the discovery of tumors (such as the incidental discovery in this case), rates of death from kidney cancer continue to decline significantly.

D. The total mortality rate at 5 years is less than 10% in patients like George.

13-19   About 80% of all cases of dysuria are caused by ascending bacterial infection of the urinary tract by which organism?

A. *Klebsiella*

B. *Proteus*

C. *Escherichia coli*

D. *Staphylococcus saprophyticus*

13-20   What is the most common cause of chronic renal failure (CRF)?

A. Glomerulonephritis

B. Hypertension

C. Diabetic nephropathy

D. A combination of urological diseases

13-21   Which nephrotoxic agent should be avoided in clients with chronic renal failure (CRF)?

A. NSAIDs

B. Kayexalate

C. Calcium carbonate

D. Erythropoietin

13-22   Which type of bloody urine is characteristic of bleeding from the upper urinary tract?

A. Grossly bloody urine

B. Urine with blood clots

C. Brown, smoky, or tea-colored urine

D. Blood noted at the beginning or end of the stream

13-23   Mary Lou, who has stress urinary incontinence, is desperate for some relief and asks for your help. She already takes several pills a day and does not really want to take any more, but she wants to do something about her problem. What do you suggest?

A. Propantheline bromide (Pro-Banthine)

B. Dicyclomine hydrochloride (Bentyl)

C. Estrogen vaginal cream

D. Imipramine hydrochloride (Tofranil)

13-24   The most frequent sign of bladder cancer is

A. hematuria.

B. flank pain.

C. nocturia.

D. dysuria.

13-25   Alice, age 29, is having an intravenous pyelogram (IVP). In teaching her about the procedure, you tell her that an IVP

A. takes about 30 minutes and uses x-rays to show the structures of the kidney, ureters, and bladder after injection of a dye that is rapidly excreted in the urine.

B. involves first filling the bladder with a dye solution, then taking x-rays of the filled bladder and of the bladder and urethra during urination.

C. involves the use of radioisotopes.

D. is the same as a renal arteriogram.

13-26   Urine tends to become colonized when indwelling urinary catheters are left in place for more than

A. 24 hours.

B. 36 hours.

C. 48 hours.

D. 72 hours.

13-27   What is the percussion tone heard over a distended bladder?

A. Dullness

B. Resonance

C. Hyperresonance

D. Tympany

13-28   Among the following genetic diseases, which is the most common cause of chronic renal disease?

A. Cystic fibrosis

B. Sickle cell disease

C. Huntington's chorea

D. Polycystic kidney disease

13-29   The best index of kidney function is

A. a midstream urinalysis.

B. serum creatinine levels.

C. urine protein level.

D. glomerular filtration rate (GFR).

13-30   The inability to empty the bladder, resulting in overdistention and frequent loss of small amounts of urine, describes which type of urinary incontinence?

A. Stress incontinence

B. Urge incontinence

C. Overflow incontinence

D. Reflex incontinence

13-31   Decreased bladder capacity; bladder irritation from a urinary tract infection, tumor, stones, or irritants such as caffeine and alcohol; and central nervous system disorders or spinal cord lesions are all contributing factors to

A. stress urinary incontinence.

B. urge urinary incontinence.

C. overflow urinary incontinence.

D. reflex urinary incontinence.

13-32   Which of the following in the urinary sediment signifies an allergic reaction in the kidney?

A. Leukocytes

B. Eosinophils

C. Crystals

D. Erythrocytes

13-33   An acidic urine pH favors precipitation of which type of kidney stone?

A. Cystine stones

B. Calcium phosphate stones

C. Struvite stones

D. Magnesium stones

13-34   The most common cause of nephrotic syndrome is

A. systemic lupus erythematosus.

B. diabetes mellitus.

C. routine use of NSAIDs.

D. glomerulosclerosis.

13-35   Which of the following renal exams identifies the size of the kidneys or obstruction in the kidneys or the lower urinary tract and may detect tumors or cysts?

A. Computed tomography (CT)

B. Voiding cystourethrography (VCUG)

C. Renal arteriogram

D. Ultrasonography (US)

13-36   Which history is commonly found in a client with glomerulonephritis?

A. Beta-hemolytic streptococcal infection

B. Frequent urinary tract infections

C. Kidney stones

D. Hypotension

13-37   Maury has renal failure and his arterial blood gas readings show a decreased pH, normal PCO_2, and decreased HCO_3. What do you suspect?

A. Respiratory acidosis

B. Respiratory alkalosis

C. Metabolic acidosis

D. Metabolic alkalosis

13-38   A urinary tract infection is best detected by performing

A. a nitrite dipstick test.

B. a urinalysis.

C. a urine culture.

D. urine sensitivity.

13-39   Which of the following radiological studies provides direct imaging in several planes conducive to detecting renal cystic disease, inflammatory processes, and renal cell carcinoma?

A. Cystoscopy

B. Ultrasonography

C. Computed tomography

D. Magnetic resonance imaging

13-40   Extracorporeal shock wave lithotripsy is not recommended for which type of kidney stones?

A. Oxalate stones

B. Uric acid stones

C. Struvite stones

D. Cystine stones

13-41   Dietary management for the client in acute renal failure includes

A. decreasing carbohydrate intake.

B. increasing dietary sodium intake.

C. limiting protein intake.

D. increasing potassium.

13-42   What is the most common cause of death in dialysis clients?

A. Infection

B. Bleeding from the access site

C. Cardiovascular failure

D. Sepsis

13-43   The most common cause of urinary tract obstruction is

A. edema resulting from trauma.

B. a tumor.

C. ureterolithiasis.

D. a vascular problem.

13-44   Who is at risk of developing a prerenal type of acute renal failure?

A. Joey, age 2, who is dehydrated from gastroenteritis

B. Tommy, age 3, who accidentally took an overdose of acetaminophen (Tylenol)

C. Justine, age 5, who nearly drowned in a swimming pool

D. Buddy, age 12, who was born with one kidney and just injured the other in a football game

13-45   Which of the following is defined as a pathophysiological process that occurs when there is a primary excess in the extracellular fluid of bicarbonate as a result of a loss of acid or the addition of excess bicarbonate?

A. Metabolic acidosis

B. Metabolic alkalosis

C. Respiratory acidosis

D. Respiratory alkalosis

13-46   Which of the following diagnostic studies for the evaluation of renal function assesses for the lack of erythropoietin?

A. Urine creatinine clearance

B. Blood urea nitrogen

C. Serum albumin

D. Serum hemoglobin and hematocrit

13-47   A factor contributing to stress incontinence is

A. a decreased estrogen level.

B. bladder irritation from a urinary tract infection.

C. prostatic hypertrophy.

D. a spinal cord lesion or trauma above S2.

13-48   Samuel wants his son circumcised, but it is noted that the baby has hypospadias. What do you tell Samuel?

A. "Your son should be circumcised as soon as possible."

B. "Wait until your son is 1 month old; then he can be circumcised."

C. "We first have to check to see where the opening is; then we can determine if your son can be circumcised or not."

D. "Your son should not be circumcised."

13-49   The most frequent complication during hemodialysis is

A. bleeding.

B. infection.

C. dialysis dementia.

D. hypotension.

13-50   Eric, age 5, has enuresis. The probable cause is

A. anatomical disease.

B. neurological disease.

C. a psychological problem.

D. maturational delay.

13-51   Sara, age 82, was unable to breathe for several minutes after choking on a piece of meat. A successful Heimlich maneuver was done and her arterial blood gases now are pH, 7.39; PaCO$_2$, 48; PaO$_2$, 92; and HCO$_3$, 24. What do you suspect?

A. Respiratory alkalosis

B. Respiratory acidosis

C. Metabolic alkalosis

D. Metabolic acidosis

13-52   Which is the least expensive method for evaluating renal mass size?

A. Palpation

B. Ultrasound imaging

C. Computed tomography (CT)

D. Magnetic resonance imaging (MRI)

13-53 *Which class of antihypertensive drugs is contraindicated in clients with renal artery stenosis?*

A. Calcium channel blockers

B. Beta blockers

C. ACE inhibitors

D. Cardiac glycosides

13-54 *Martha, age 42, states that she has intercourse only about once a month, but immediately afterward she usually gets a urinary tract infection. She is frustrated with having to come to the office frequently to have an examination with a urine test. She says that she is ready to "kick her husband out of bed." How do you respond?*

A. "By taking a low-dose antibiotic every day, you can prevent a urinary tract infection."

B. "Take 200 mg of ofloxacin with a large glass of water after intercourse."

C. "I'll write you a prescription for a 3-day pack of antibiotics with several refills to take when you need it."

D. "Yes, not having sexual intercourse will resolve the problem."

13-55 *Which of the following is associated with an elevated risk of renal cell carcinoma (RCC)?*

A. High levels of lead exposure

B. Several episodes of kidney stones

C. Frequent urinary tract infections

D. A permanent indwelling urinary catheter

13-56 *Joyce is being treated conservatively for her low back pain with NSAIDs, muscle relaxants, and physical therapy. She has recently been diagnosed with chronic kidney disease. Which of the following statements is true?*

A. She should switch to a different NSAID because some are safer than others.

B. She should not be taking anything for pain other than narcotics.

C. We should just increase her physical therapy and hope for the best.

D. She could try acetaminophen 650 mg three times daily.

13-57 *Which diagnostic finding(s) may lead to a diagnosis of nephrolithiasis?*

A. Urinary uric acid output of less than 750 mg/24 hr

B. Urinary pH greater than 5.5

C. Urinary calcium output of greater than 300 mg/24 hr

D. Serum calcium of 8 mg/dL

13-58 *After a renal biopsy, the client should be instructed*

A. that there may be some blood in the urine for the next several days.

B. to avoid strenuous activities for at least 2 weeks.

C. to drink 3–4 glasses of water per day.

D. to measure urine output for the first week.

13-59 *Which statement is true regarding acute tubular necrosis (ATN)?*

A. It is a slow, progressive disease.

B. Creatinine clearance is greatly increased.

C. Peritoneal dialysis or hemodialysis should be reserved for severe cases.

D. The removal of the offending agent may allow renal function to return gradually to normal.

13-60 *The increased presence of which of the following in a urinalysis indicates the presence of bacteria or protein, which is seen in severe renal disease and could also indicate urinary calculi?*

A. Crystals

B. Casts

C. Nitrates

D. Ketones

13-61 *The most frequent reason why a person would come to your office complaining of burning on urination is*

A. prostatitis.

B. urethritis.

C. a urinary tract infection.

D. a sexually transmitted disease.

13-62   *Transient urinary incontinence in women may be caused by*

A. hypertrophy of the vaginal or urethral walls.
B. diarrhea.
C. use of anticholinergic agents.
D. hypoglycemia.

13-63   *A 24-hour urine test for vanillylmandelic acid and catecholamines is done to diagnose*

A. a renal tumor.
B. hypertension secondary to pheochromocytoma.
C. renal artery stenosis.
D. hydronephrosis.

13-64   *Marvin, age 59, is going to have a total cystectomy to remove his bladder tumor. He states that when the surgeon was talking to him, he was not really listening, and he asks you about the incidence of impotence after such a surgery. How do you respond?*

A. "You'll have to talk to the surgeon; every case is unique."
B. "This surgery requires the removal of the prostate and seminal vessels, which does result in impotence. Let's talk about it."
C. "I'm not sure if this will be the case, but if it is, how would you feel about it?"
D. "How does your wife feel about the possibility?"

13-65   *If a client with acute renal failure (ARF) excretes 400 mL of urine on Tuesday, how much fluid intake (both oral and intravenous) should the client have on Wednesday?*

A. 400 mL
B. 600 mL
C. 900 mL
D. 1,200 mL

13-66   *What amount of urine in a 24-hour period in an adult represents oliguria?*

A. No urine output
B. Urine output less than 50 mL/day
C. Urine output less than 100 mL/day
D. Urine output less than 500 mL/day

13-67   *Which type of hematuria in an older adult is an ominous sign?*

A. Painless, gross hematuria
B. Flank pain with hematuria
C. Hematuria following trauma
D. Intermittent hematuria

13-68   *General recommendations for the prevention of kidney stones, regardless of the type of stone the client has, include*

A. drinking 3–4 L of mineral water per day.
B. reducing protein in the diet.
C. increasing vitamin C in the diet.
D. decreasing fiber in the diet.

13-69   *Why do middle-aged men not incur as many urinary tract infections as middle-aged women?*

A. Women are more prone to urinary stasis than men.
B. Men have the bacteriostatic effect of prostatic fluid and a longer urethra.
C. Women have a higher urine pH.
D. Men take more baths than women.

13-70   *Which of the following drugs is not associated with acute renal failure?*

A. Angiotensin-converting enzyme (ACE) inhibitors
B. Cimetidine (Tagamet)
C. NSAIDs
D. Erythromycin (E-Mycin)

13-71   *Sam, age 42, has had persistent proteinuria on the previous two office visits. Which action is warranted next?*

A. Schedule extensive blood work.
B. Order an intravenous pyelogram.
C. Admit Sam to the hospital.
D. Have Sam collect one urine specimen on first arising and then another 2 hours later.

13-72   *Goodpasture's syndrome is*

A. characterized by glomerulonephritis and pulmonary hemorrhage resulting from immune complex damage to the glomerular and alveolar basement membranes.

B. characterized by massive proteinuria, hypoalbuminemia, hyperlipidemia, and edema.

C. an inflammatory autoimmune disorder affecting the connective tissue of the body with inflammatory lesions involving the supportive tissues of the glomerulus.

D. typically the end stage of other glomerular disorders, such as rapidly progressive glomerulonephritis, lupus nephritis, or diabetic nephropathy.

13-73 *Urine that appears brownish in color may result from which of the following?*

A. Beets

B. Bile

C. Rifampin (Rifadin)

D. Phenazopyridine (Pyridium)

13-74 *Janet has stress urinary incontinence and has been doing Kegel exercises with some success. What other simple action might help in relieving some of the problem?*

A. Stopping smoking

B. Limiting fluids

C. Taking a daily multivitamin

D. Beginning lifting 2-lb weights

13-75 *Sally, age 24, has frequent urinary tract infections. You are teaching her about measures to prevent them. You know she has misunderstood your directions when she tells you that she'll*

A. void after intercourse.

B. avoid bubble baths.

C. wear underwear with pantyhose.

D. drink 4–6 glasses of water per day.

13-76 *Who is at a higher risk for developing nephrolithiasis?*

A. Jean, who exercises every day and drinks copious amounts of water

B. Bill, who runs every day and takes excessive amounts of vitamin C

C. Mary Ann, who watches her weight and eats a low-sodium diet

D. Harvey, a "couch potato" who drinks a lot of no-sodium soda

13-77 *Which of the following is the likeliest outcome in clients with chronic kidney disease (CKD)?*

A. End-stage renal disease (ESRD)

B. Dialysis

C. Hypertension

D. Death

13-78 *Which diuretic acts by inhibiting sodium chloride reabsorption in the thick ascending limb of the loop of Henle?*

A. Furosemide (Lasix)

B. Mannitol (Osmitrol)

C. Hydrochlorothiazide (HydroDiuril)

D. Acetazolamide (Diamox)

13-79 *What is the first step in the treatment of uric acid kidney stones?*

A. Encouraging hydration

B. Alkalinizing the urine

C. Prescribing allopurinol (Zyloprim)

D. Reducing protein intake

13-80 *In the older adult, which physiological change affects pharmacokinetics?*

A. Decreased creatine clearance

B. Increased lean muscle mass

C. Decreased total body fat

D. Increased serum albumin level

13-81 *Which of the following changes in laboratory values is associated with kidney disease?*

A. Serum creatinine greater than 4 mg/dL

B. Serum albumin 0.5–1.0 mg/dL

C. Serum sodium greater than 150 mEq/L

D. Serum calcium greater than 6.0 mEq/L

13-82 *Samuel, age 67, is a diabetic with worsening renal function. He has frequent hypoglycemic episodes, which he believes means that his diabetes is getting "better." How do you respond?*

A. "You've watched your diet for all these years and as a result, your body is using less insulin."

B. "I'll have to change your oral hyperglycemic agents as it seems your body is making more insulin."

C. "Because your kidneys are not functioning well, your insulin is not being metabolized and excreted as it should, so you need less of it."

D. "You're right; it seems like your diabetes is improving."

13-83 *Which type of kidney stone is the most common?*

A. Calcium oxalate

B. Uric acid

C. Calcium phosphate

D. Cystine

13-84 *Marie, age 16, fell off her bicycle and sustained a contusion of her left kidney. The treatment of choice is*

A. surgery.

B. urethral catheterization.

C. conservative therapy.

D. to continue normal activity because it is only a contusion.

13-85 *Which type of white blood cell may be present in the urine and activated by antigens and antigen-induced hypersensitivity reactions?*

A. Lymphocytes

B. Monocytes

C. Basophils

D. Eosinophils

13-86 *What is the most common cause of end-stage renal disease (ESRD)?*

A. Hypertensive nephropathy

B. Glomerulonephritis (GN)

C. Diabetic nephropathy

D. Acute tubular necrosis

13-87 *Your client is on a low-protein diet for end-stage renal disease (ESRD). Because of this, which of the following is essential that he include in his diet?*

A. A phosphate binder

B. Supplemental iron

C. Potassium supplements

D. Vitamin and mineral supplements

13-88 *Before using the radial artery to draw blood for arterial blood gas (ABG) testing, which test should be performed?*

A. The ABG test

B. The Thomas test

C. The Weber test

D. The Allen test

13-89 *Which of the following accounts for half of the bladder tumors among men and one-third in women?*

A. Cigarette smoke, both active and passive inhalation

B. Chemicals from plastic and rubber

C. Chronic use of phenacetin-containing analgesic agents

D. Working long hours and not voiding often

13-90 *What condition may result from clients taking NSAIDs on a long-term basis?*

A. Hemodynamically induced acute renal failure

B. Diabetes insipidus

C. Neurogenic bladder

D. Hypokalemia

13-91 *Which of the following drugs is an analgesic used to treat dysuria?*

A. Hyoscyamine (Levsin)

B. Oxybutynin (Ditropan)

C. Propantheline (Pro-Banthine)

D. Phenazopyridine (Pyridium)

13-92 *Jake is having a urinary diversion procedure performed because of a urinary tract tumor. He states that he heard about a Koch pouch and asks you what it is. You respond,*

A. "It is a cutaneous ureterostomy in which one or both of the ureters create a stoma on the skin surface."

B. "It is an ileal conduit in which the ileum is formed into a pouch with an open stoma and the ureters are inserted into the pouch."

C. "It is a continent internal ileal reservoir in which nipple valves are formed on the skin. The filling pressure closes the valves, preventing leakage and reflux."

D. "It is a ureterosigmoidostomy in which the ureters are inserted into the sigmoid colon. Urine empties into the rectum and is expelled with defecation."

13-93   Thiazide diuretics are used for the treatment of which type of renal calculi?

A. Calcium phosphate and/or oxalate stones

B. Struvite stones

C. Uric acid stones

D. Cystine stones

13-94   The kidneys excrete increased amounts of HCO_3 to lower the pH as a mode of compensation for which acid-base disturbance?

A. Respiratory acidosis

B. Respiratory alkalosis

C. Metabolic acidosis

D. Metabolic alkalosis

13-95   The most common metabolic condition that predisposes to the formation of kidney stones is

A. idiopathic hypercalciuria.

B. hyperuricosuria.

C. hyperoxaluria.

D. a low urinary citrate excretion.

13-96   Jim has had several episodes of kidney stones. The last stone he passed was examined and found to be an oxalate stone. You tell him to avoid foods high in oxalate such as

A. beans and lentils, chocolate and cocoa, dried fruits, canned or smoked fish except tuna, flour, milk, and milk products.

B. cheese, cranberries, eggs, grapes, meat and poultry, plums and prunes, tomatoes, and whole grains.

C. asparagus, beer, beets, cabbage, celery, chocolate and cocoa, fruits, green beans, nuts, tea, colas, and tomatoes.

D. goose, organ meats, sardines, herring, and venison and to have a moderate intake of beef, chicken, crab, pork, salmon, and veal.

13-97   Which group of persons experience more rapid age-related decreases in glomerular filtration rate (GFR) than do Caucasians?

A. African Americans

B. Asians

C. Europeans

D. Native Americans

13-98   You explain to Yolanda that pelvic floor (Kegel) exercises help to restore and maintain continence by improving pelvic muscle strength, increasing urethral pressure, and decreasing abnormal detrusor muscle contractions. These exercises are used for her diagnosis of

A. stool incontinence.

B. full-bladder incontinence.

C. cystitis-related incontinence.

D. stress incontinence.

13-99   Which diagnostic procedure can visualize the renal outline and identify lower rib fractures?

A. Intravenous pyelogram

B. Renal angiography

C. Computed tomography

D. A kidneys, ureters, and bladder film

13-100   Jill, who has had urinary incontinence for several months, wants to have an evaluation to determine if any therapy will be beneficial. After having an initial pelvic examination, she has a postvoid residual catheterization. A residual volume of more than how many milliliters is abnormal?

A. 10 mL

B. 30 mL

C. 50 mL

D. 100 mL

13-101   Which finding in urinary sediment is indicative of pyelonephritis and interstitial nephritis?

A. Hyaline casts

B. Granular casts

C. Red blood cell casts

D. White blood cell casts

13-102   Which of the following conditions does not cause flank pain?

A. Pyelonephritis

B. Ureterolithiasis

C. Vascular occlusion of the kidney (renal vein thrombosis)

D. Renal cysts

13-103 *Postmenopausal women tend to have more recurrent urinary tract infections because of*

A. frequent urination.

B. estrogen depletion–related changes.

C. an increase in lactobacilli.

D. a decrease in *Escherichia coli.*

13-104 *Why is the right kidney slightly lower than the left kidney?*

A. The spleen pushes the left kidney upward.

B. The liver pushes the right kidney downward.

C. The diaphragm displaces the left kidney.

D. The right kidney is structurally larger than the left kidney.

13-105 *The most common factor predisposing a woman to a urinary tract infection is*

A. the use of an oral contraceptive.

B. the use of a diaphragm.

C. urinary stasis.

D. calculi.

13-106 *Which of the following does NOT cause urine to appear reddish in color?*

A. Cascara sagrada

B. Phenazopyridine (Pyridium)

C. Phenytoin (Dilantin)

D. Multivitamins

13-107 *Excessive alcohol ingestion can cause*

A. metabolic acidosis.

B. metabolic alkalosis.

C. respiratory acidosis.

D. respiratory alkalosis.

13-108 *Clinical manifestations including microscopic or gross hematuria, a palpable abdominal mass, fever, and flank pain may indicate a*

A. pancreatic tumor.

B. liver tumor.

C. colon mass.

D. renal tumor.

13-109 *The best test to determine microalbuminuria to assist in the diagnosis of diabetic nephropathy is*

A. a dipstick strip done during a routine urinalysis in the office.

B. a 24-hour urine collection.

C. an early morning spot urine collection.

D. a serum albumin test.

13-110 *Which medication is used primarily in the treatment of acute postoperative and postpartum urinary retention and for neurogenic bladder atony with urinary retention?*

A. Bethanechol chloride (Urecholine)

B. Neostigmine (Prostigmin)

C. Propantheline bromide (Pro-Banthine)

D. Oxybutynin (Ditropan)

13-111 *Which category of diuretic has the following side effects: hyperkalemia, headache, hyponatremia, nausea, diarrhea, urticaria, and menstrual disturbances?*

A. Osmotic diuretic

B. Loop diuretic

C. Potassium-sparing diuretic

D. Thiazide diuretic

13-112 *In clients receiving dialysis, which is the most common cause of end-stage renal disease in the United States?*

A. Diabetic nephropathy

B. Chronic renal failure secondary to vascular disorders

C. Acute tubular necrosis

D. Kidney trauma

Answers

13-1   Answer A

The aging process begins to affect the kidneys with a progressive loss of nephron units by age 40. The kidneys lose about 20% of their mass between ages 40 and 80.

13-2 Answer B

The most common cause of sepsis in the older adult is a urinary tract infection (UTI). An older adult who is ill with hypothermia (below normal body temperature) or high fever, has a change in mental status and a documented UTI, or has a suspected UTI and sepsis should be treated vigorously with adequate hydration, immediate use of potent antibiotics, and support of blood pressure. Urinary stasis may precipitate a UTI, and kidney stones may accompany one, along with genitourinary problems, but a UTI alone is the most common cause of sepsis in the older adult.

13-3 Answer D

The appearance of urine may indicate ingestion of certain products and/or lead to possible common differential diagnoses. For the following urine colors, the following may apply: Cloudy urine may indicate UTI, hematuria, bilirubin, and mucus. For colorless urine, the differential diagnoses would be diabetes insipidus, diuretic agents, and fluid overload. For dark urine, they are hematuria, malignancy, stones, and acidic urine. For pink/red urine, they are hematuria, hemoglobin, myoglobin, beets, and food coloring. For orange/yellow urine, the differentials are phenazopyridine, rifampin, and bile pigments. For brown/black urine, they are myoglobin, bile pigments, melanin, cascara, and iron preparations. For green urine, they are bile pigments, methylene blue, indigo, carmine. For foamy urine, they are bile salts and proteinuria.

13-4 Answer D

Eating watermelon will not cause the urine to change color. Ingesting blackberries or beets, taking ibuprofen or phenazopyridine (Pyridium), and eating foods with red food color all may cause the urine to be pink, red, burgundy, or cola colored.

13-5 Answer A

Urine specific gravity is increased in clients who are dehydrated; in those who have a pituitary tumor that causes the release of excessive amounts of antidiuretic hormone; and in those with decreased renal blood flow, glycosuria, or proteinuria. The specific gravity of urine is decreased in clients who are overhydrated and in those who have diabetes insipidus or chronic renal failure.

13-6 Answer A

Cardiovascular failure and hypovolemia are the two major causes of prerenal acute renal failure. Vascular disease, glomerulonephritis, interstitial nephritis, and acute tubular necrosis are causes of intrarenal acute renal failure. Extrarenal obstruction, intrarenal obstruction, and bladder rupture are causes of postrenal acute renal failure. There is no such thing as perirenal failure.

13-7 Answer D

Ferumoxytol, a semisynthetic iron oxide formulated with mannitol and administered IV, corrects iron deficiency anemia in clients with CKD more quickly and more safely than do oral iron preparations. Oral iron does not raise hemoglobin that much because clients with CKD, whether or not they're on dialysis, don't absorb iron well. About 25%–50% of clients with CKD taking oral iron do not tolerate it well in the doses needed and have resulting gastrointestinal (GI) side effects. In one study, twice the number of clients taking oral iron had adverse side effects compared with those taking the IV drug.

13-8 Answer A

Clinical manifestations of metabolic alkalosis include tetany, hypotension, tachycardia, confusion, decreasing level of consciousness, hyperreflexia, dysrhythmias, seizures, and respiratory failure. Nausea and vomiting, weakness, and bradycardia are manifestations of metabolic acidosis.

13-9 Answer C

Most calcium phosphate stones are caused by primary hyperparathyroidism. Treatment involves surgical excision of the parathyroid adenoma. If the surgery is not successful or is impossible, treatment involves hydration and the administration of orthophosphate. The client is then observed for hypertension and sodium and water retention.

13-10 Answer D

When a client has an elevated serum uric acid level (greater than 7.0 mg/dL), the following should be considered as possible causes: the use of diuretics, chronic renal failure (CRF), a high-protein diet, gout, leukemia, and lymphoma. To specifically look for CRF, a serum creatinine level and a 24-hour urinary uric acid test need to be performed.

13-11   Answer B

Polycystic kidney disease is a hereditary, incurable renal disease in which multiple outpouchings (cysts) of the nephrons occur in both kidneys. The cysts may be filled with urine, serous fluid, blood, or a combination of these. As the cysts enlarge, they distort and compress surrounding renal tissue and blood vessels, causing ischemia and necrosis. Eventually, too few normal nephrons remain to support the client and end-stage renal disease slowly develops.

13-12   Answer A

An AV fistula is an internal anastomosis of an artery to a vein. An AV graft is a synthetic vessel tubing tunneled beneath the skin, connecting an artery and a vein. A dual-lumen hemodialysis catheter is an extended-use catheter, surgically tunneled under the skin with a barrier cuff. An AV shunt is an external loop of tubing connecting an artery and a vein. Each section of tubing is sutured into a vessel and brought through a skin stab wound.

A dual-lumen hemodialysis catheter is an extended-use catheter, surgically tunneled under the skin with a barrier cuff. An AV shunt is an external loop of tubing connecting an artery and a vein. Each section of tubing is sutured into a vessel and brought through a skin stab wound.

13-13   Answer A

White men are most prone to developing nephrolithiasis. The incidence of nephrolithiasis (stone in the kidney) is four times higher in men than women, with white men having three times more attacks than black men, except for struvite stones, which occur more often in black men.

13-14   Answer C

A child with Wilms' tumor commonly has abdominal distention or an abdominal mass. There may also be fever, abdominal pain, or hematuria. This kidney tumor requires surgical removal, followed by chemotherapy. Radiation therapy is not necessary.

13-15   Answer B

Anuria refers to a 24-hour urine volume of less than 100 mL. It indicates a severe reduction in urine volume commonly associated with obstruction, renal cortical necrosis, or severe acute tubular necrosis. It is important to make the distinction between oliguria (less than 500 mL in a 24-hour period) and anuria so that the appropriate treatment may be initiated early.

13-16   Answer B

All of the answer options are renal hormones. Prostaglandins regulate intrarenal blood flow by vasodilation or vasoconstriction. Renin raises blood pressure as a result of angiotensin (local vasoconstriction) and aldosterone (volume expansion) secretion. Bradykinins increase blood flow (vasodilation) and vascular permeability. Erythropoietin stimulates bone marrow to make red blood cells.

13-17   Answer D

The clinical presentation of a client with urolithiasis includes pain that typically starts in the flank and may localize at the costovertebral angle. The pain may radiate to the lower abdomen, groin, or perineum and is often associated with nausea and vomiting. Fever is unlikely unless there is a coexisting urinary tract infection. Hematuria may be present, but the urine should not have any leukocytes unless an infection is also present. Because the question is asked only about a client with urolithiasis and does not mention any infection, an assumption of an infection being present should not be made.

13-18   Answer A

The malignancy risk is related to the size of the lesion. The larger the lesion, the higher the cancer risk. Small renal masses join the growing list of "incidental" findings detected on imaging studies usually performed for other reasons. Despite improvements in radiologic and surgical techniques in recent years, renal cancer mortality rates continue to climb. Among patients older than 70 years, one-third die within 5 years of noncancer causes.

13-19   Answer C

In women, approximately 80%–90% of cases of uncomplicated UTI are the result of the gram-negative rod bacteria *Escherichia coli*. The second-most common cause (5%–20%) of uncomplicated bacterial infection is the gram-positive coccus *Staphylococcus saprophyticus*, although this agent is rare in complicated UTI. Other gram-negative rods identified as causative pathogens in a smaller number of cases, but particularly in complicated UTI, are *Proteus mirabilis*, *Klebsiella*, *Enterobacter*, *Serratia*, and *Pseudomonas*. In addition, the gram-positive coccus *Enterococcus* has been identified.

13-20   Answer C

The most common cause of chronic renal failure (CRF) is diabetic nephropathy. Diabetic nephropathy makes up about 34% of all cases of CRF, followed by hypertension (29%), glomerulonephritis (11%), and other urological diseases (6%).

13-21   Answer A

All nephrotoxic agents, such as NSAIDs and radiocontrast dye, should be avoided in clients with CRF. Low-dose Kayexalate (sodium polystyrene sulfonate) 5 mg PO one to three times a day with meals may be used as a potassium binder for hyperkalemia. Given the kidney's reduced ability to synthesize activated vitamin D in CRF and the propensity for subsequent hypocalcemia and renal osteodystrophy, oral 1.25-dihydroxyvitamin D (Calcitrol 0.25 mg every day) and calcium carbonate (600 mg twice a day) supplements should be given, along with a renal-specific multivitamin (Nephrocaps). Anemia should be treated with erythropoietin (80–120 unit/kg SC per week).

13-22   Answer C

Brown, smoky, or tea-colored urine indicates blood coming from the upper urinary tract. The color is the result of the acidic urine changing the hemoglobin to hematin, which has a brown color. Grossly bloody urine and urine with blood clots come from the lower urinary tract. Blood noted at the beginning or end of the stream also indicates lower tract bleeding, whereas blood throughout the stream may suggest upper urinary tract bleeding.

13-23   Answer C

Propantheline bromide (Pro-Banthine), dicyclomine hydrochloride (Bentyl), and imipramine hydrochloride (Tofranil) all help urinary incontinence. However, if the client does not like taking pills, the best (and least invasive) agent to suggest is estrogen vaginal cream. One type of stress urinary incontinence is anatomical incontinence, which may be caused by hormone deprivation and atrophic vaginitis. Using estrogen replacement cream to correct the vaginal dryness will also improve bladder outlet function.

13-24   Answer A

The most frequent sign of bladder cancer is hematuria. With gross hematuria, an intravenous

pyelogram should be performed to detect bladder cancer as early as possible. Flank pain is usually a sign of glomerulonephritis or kidney stones; nocturia is the number one symptom of benign prostatic hypertrophy; and dysuria is present with a urinary tract infection.

13-25   Answer A

The intravenous pyelogram is an examination that takes about 30 minutes and uses x-rays to show the structures of the kidney, ureters, and bladder after injection of a dye that is rapidly excreted in the urine. In a voiding cystourethrogram, the bladder is filled with dye solution and then x-rays of the filled bladder and of the bladder and urethra during urination are taken. Radioisotope studies provide information regarding renal anatomy; blood flow; and glomerular, tubular, and collecting system function. Renal arteriography or venography is indicated in children only when it is necessary to define vascular abnormalities such as renal artery stenosis before a surgical intervention. Usually other less invasive measures are used.

13-26   Answer D

Urine tends to become colonized with bacteria when indwelling urinary catheters are left in place for more than 72 hours. If catheters are left in place only temporarily and removed quickly when the client can void, infection will usually not result. Antibacterial coverage is warranted if catheters are left in place for 5–10 days.

13-27   Answer A

A distended bladder sounds dull when percussed. You should not be able to percuss the bladder above the level of the symphysis pubis after the client has voided. Tympany indicates the presence of gas in organs.

13-28   Answer D

Autosomal dominant polycystic kidney disease (ADPKD), is the most common genetic cause of chronic renal disease. It is 20 times more common than Huntington's chorea, 15 times more common than cystic fibrosis, and 10 times more common than sickle cell disease to cause chronic renal disease.

13-29   Answer D

The best index of kidney function is the glomerular filtration rate (GFR). Kidney function used to be assessed by serum creatinine level. Both diet and muscle mass influence generation of creatinine, however, making it an inaccurate indicator of renal function. Lower serum creatinine levels are typically observed with older age, female gender, vegetarian diet, and muscle-wasting states, while higher values are associated with muscular habitus and a high-protein diet. Serum creatinine levels can underestimate kidney disease. The National Kidney Foundation defines chronic kidney disease (CKD) as the presence of kidney damage and/or reduced GFR for 3 or more months. The most precise method to measure the GFR is to measure iothalamate or insulin clearance. This is the gold standard for investigational studies, but it is not practical in clinical practice. The 24-hour urine creatinine clearance test is an alternative in clinical practice, and that measurement is required for the calculation of the GFR. Clients often have difficulty conducting this 24-hour test. Recently, the Modification of Diet in Renal Disease (MDRD) equation has been recommended by the National Kidney Foundation to better estimate the GFR. Besides serum creatinine, the MDRD GFR requires input of client age, gender, and ethnicity.

13-30   Answer C

Overflow incontinence is the inability to empty the bladder, resulting in overdistention and frequent loss of small amounts of urine. Stress incontinence is the loss of urine associated with increased intra-abdominal pressure such as occurs with sneezing, coughing, and lifting; the quantity of urine lost is usually small. Urge incontinence is the inability to inhibit urine flow long enough to reach the toilet after the urge sensation. Reflex incontinence is the involuntary loss of a moderate volume of urine without stimulus or warning. It may occur during the day or night.

13-31   Answer B

Decreased bladder capacity; bladder irritation from a urinary tract infection, tumor, or stones; irritants such as caffeine and alcohol; central nervous system disorders; and spinal cord lesions contribute to urge urinary incontinence. Contributing factors of stress urinary incontinence include multiple pregnancies; decreased estrogen levels; a short urethra; weakness of the abdominal wall; prostate surgery; and increased intra-abdominal pressure as a result of tumor, ascites, or obesity. For overflow urinary incontinence, contributing factors include spinal cord injuries below S2; diabetic neuropathy; prostatic hypertrophy; fecal impaction; and drugs, especially those with an anticholinergic effect. For reflex urinary incontinence, contributing factors include a spinal cord lesion or trauma above S2, history of a cerebrovascular accident, neurological disorders such as Parkinson's or Alzheimer's disease, and multiple sclerosis.

13-32   Answer B

Eosinophils in the urinary sediment signify an allergic reaction in the kidney. Leukocytes are present in an infection and interstitial nephritis. Crystals are present in diseases of stone formation or following ethylene glycol intoxication. Erythrocytes are present in large amounts in active glomerulonephritis, interstitial nephritis, and infections.

13-33   Answer A

An acidic urine pH favors precipitation of organic stones: uric acid and cystine stones. An alkaline urine pH favors the precipitation of inorganic stones: calcium phosphate and magnesium ammonium phosphate (struvite) stones.

13-34   Answer B

Diabetes mellitus is the most common cause of nephrotic syndrome. Systemic lupus erythematosus, the routine use of NSAIDs, glomerulosclerosis, and diabetes mellitus are all causes of proteinuria.

13-35   Answer D

A renal ultrasound identifies the size of the kidneys or obstruction in the kidneys or the lower urinary tract and may detect tumors or cysts. A CT scan measures the size of the kidneys and may evaluate the contour to assess for masses or obstruction. A VCUG outlines the bladder's contour and evaluates abnormal bladder emptying and incontinence. A renal arteriogram identifies vascular abnormalities within each kidney and adjacent aorta.

13-36   Answer A

Clients with glomerulonephritis commonly have a history of beta-hemolytic streptococcal infections, as well as a history of systemic lupus erythematosus or other autoimmune diseases. Glomerulonephritis is usually caused by an immunological response.

13-37   Answer C

A decreased pH, normal PCO_2, and decreased HCO_3 indicated metabolic acidosis. Renal failure, diabetes, shock, and intestinal fistulas all cause metabolic acidosis because of an increased production of metabolic acids from diabetic ketoacidosis, impaired excretion of metabolic acids from renal failure, an increased bicarbonate loss from loss of intestinal secretions and increased renal losses, or an increased chloride level from abnormal renal function.

13-38   Answer C

A urine culture is still the gold standard for detecting a urinary tract infection. In the primary care setting, a urinalysis is typically done, and empiric treatment is started if a UTI is diagnosed.

13-39   Answer D

Magnetic resonance imaging provides direct imaging in several planes conducive to detecting renal cystic disease, inflammatory processes, and renal cell carcinoma. Cystoscopy detects bladder or urethral pathological processes. Ultrasonography identifies hydronephrosis and fluid collections. Computed tomography identifies tumors and other pathological conditions that create variations in body density.

13-40   Answer C

Extracorporeal shock wave lithotripsy is not recommended for struvite stones because bacteria or endotoxins inside the stone may be systemically dispersed during the procedure. Appropriate antibiotics are required.

13-41   Answer C

Dietary management for the client in acute renal failure (ARF) includes limiting protein intake to 0.7–1.0 g/kg of body weight per day to minimize the degree of azotemia. Carbohydrate intake is increased to maintain adequate calorie intake and provide a protein-sparing effect. Dietary sodium intake is decreased to assist in preventing fluid retention. Unless serum potassium levels are low, there should be no change in potassium intake.

13-42   Answer C

The most common cause of death in dialysis clients is cardiovascular failure, with hypotension and diabetes as predisposing factors. Sepsis is the next leading cause of death, followed by bleeding complications, cerebrovascular accidents, pericardial effusion with tamponade, and trauma. The mortality

in dialysis clients remains significant, about 15% in the first year.

13-43   Answer C

Ureterolithiasis—a stone in the ureter—is the most common cause of urinary tract obstruction. Pain with ureteral obstruction is compounded by the stretching of the renal capsule by edema and swelling. Edema does not usually cause complete obstruction. Although a tumor may cause an obstruction, it is not as common as an obstruction caused by ureterolithiasis. Vascular problems may aggravate or potentiate a problem leading to an obstruction but not be the actual cause.

13-44   Answer A

The prerenal classification (problems occurring prior to reaching the kidney) of acute renal failure (ARF) may be caused by dehydration secondary to gastroenteritis, malnutrition, or diarrhea, as well as by hemorrhage, hypovolemia, shock, and heart failure. Therefore, Joey, who is dehydrated, is at risk for developing a prerenal type of ARF. The renal classification (within the kidney) of ARF may be caused by nephrotoxins such as acetaminophen (Tylenol), near drowning (especially in fresh water), acute glomerulonephritis, severe infections, and diseases of the kidney and blood vessels; this applies to Tommy and Justine. Postrenal causes of ARF include obstructions caused by tumor, hematoma, stones, renal vein thrombosis, or trauma to a solitary kidney or collecting system (Buddy).

13-45   Answer B

Metabolic alkalosis is a pathophysiological process that occurs when there is a primary excess of bicarbonate in the extracellular fluid because of loss of acid (hydrogen ions) or the addition of excess bicarbonate. Metabolic acidosis results from an accumulation in the blood of keto acids (derived from fat metabolism) at the expense of bicarbonate. Respiratory acidosis occurs with a reduction of alveolar ventilation, resulting in an accumulation of carbonic acid. Respiratory alkalosis occurs with an increase of alveolar ventilation, resulting in a decrease of carbonic acid.

13-46   Answer D

Serum hemoglobin and hematocrit testing assesses bleeding or the lack of erythropoietin. A urine creatinine clearance rate measurement is a very specific indicator of renal function and is used to evaluate the glomerular filtration rate. Blood urea nitrogen level measures the nitrogen portion of urea, a product formed in the liver from protein metabolism. Serum albumin measurement is used to assist in the diagnosis of nephrotic syndrome.

13-47   Answer A

A decreased estrogen level contributes to stress incontinence. Bladder irritation from a urinary tract infection contributes to urge incontinence; prostatic hypertrophy contributes to overflow incontinence; and spinal cord lesion or trauma contributes to reflex incontinence.

13-48   Answer D

A circumcision should never be done on a baby with hypospadias because the surgeon who may ultimately correct hypospadias may need the prepuce to repair the defect. Surgical correction should be undertaken by the time the child enters the first grade.

13-49   Answer D

Hypotension is the most frequent complication seen during hemodialysis. It is related to many factors, such as changes in serum osmolality, rapid removal of fluid from the vascular compartment, and vasodilation. Bleeding is the next most common complication because of both altered platelet function associated with uremia and the use of heparin during dialysis. Infection may either occur locally, at the site of the arteriovenous fistula, or be systemic. Dialysis dementia is a progressive, potentially fatal neurological complication that affects clients on long-term hemodialysis.

13-50   Answer D

Most children with voiding disturbances do not have an anatomical or neurological disease or a psychological problem causing their enuresis. Although the cause of primary nocturnal enuresis has not been clearly established, it appears to be related to maturational delay of mechanisms involved in sleep and arousal or to a delay in the development of increased bladder capacity. Most children can be helped through parental involvement, such as restricting fluids after dinner, encouraging bladder training, awakening the child during the night to void, and using electronic devices that establish a conditioned reflex

response to waken the child the moment urination starts. (Such devices are only mildly successful.) Imipramine (Tofranil) is effective (50 mg PO at bedtime), as well as desmopressin acetate (DDAVP) nasal spray (one spray in each nostril at bedtime).

13-51   Answer B

The arterial blood gas values of pH 7.39, PaO_2 92, and HCO_3 24 are within normal range. However, the $PaCO_2$ level of 48 is elevated, which would indicate acute respiratory acidosis.

13-52   Answer B

Ultrasound imaging works as well as computed tomography (CT) and magnetic resonance imaging (MRI) for evaluating renal mass size. While the urologist may like to interpret cross-sectional images, particularly CT, comparable modalities with less morbidity for the client and reduced costs for the health-care system need to be explored, especially if they are just as effective.

13-53   Answer C

ACE inhibitors are the antihypertensive drugs contraindicated in clients with renal artery stenosis. In bilateral renal artery stenosis or stenosis to a solitary kidney, the renal perfusion pressure and the glomerular filtration rate depend on the local renin-angiotensin system. When the system is blocked by an ACE inhibitor, a marked decrease in the efferent arterial pressure with subsequent decrease in renal perfusion pressure results, causing a diminished GFR.

13-54   Answer B

Clients who recognize an association between a urinary tract infection and recent sexual intercourse can be instructed to take a single small dose of an antibiotic, such as ofloxacin (Floxin), with a large glass of water after intercourse.

13-55   Answer A

Higher blood lead levels are associated with an elevated risk of renal cell carcinoma (RCC). In this study, interestingly, higher total serum calcium was associated with a significantly reduced risk of RCC.

13-56   Answer D

Acetaminophen 650 mg taken three times daily routinely and not on a PRN basis may provide pain relief with less risk for kidney injury. Unfortunately, all NSAIDs increase the risk for acute kidney injury (AKI) and may exacerbate progression to chronic renal failure. Narcotics are often necessary when treating severe pain in patients with high risk for NSAID-associated kidney injury, but acetaminophen should be tried before narcotics.

13-57   Answer C

A urinary calcium output greater than 300 mg in 24 hours (hypercalciuria) may lead to a diagnosis of nephrolithiasis. The following disorders and diagnostic findings may also lead to a diagnosis of nephrolithiasis: hyperuricosuria (urinary uric acid output greater than 750 mg in 24 hours), hyperoxaluria (urinary oxalate output greater than 40 mg in 24 hours), hypocitraturia (urinary citrate output less than 320 mg/day), gouty diathesis (urinary pH less than 5.5 and gouty arthritis), and hypomagnesuria (urinary magnesium output less than 50 mg in 24 hours). Serum calcium of 8 mg/dL is within normal range.

13-58   Answer B

After a renal biopsy, the client should be instructed to avoid strenuous activities for at least 2 weeks. These activities include heavy lifting, contact sports, or any other activity that will cause jolting of the kidney. The client should also be warned that he or she may notice some blood in the urine for the first 24 hours following the procedure and should be instructed to drink large amounts of fluid, such as 8–10 glasses of water per day, to prevent clot formation and urine retention. Caution should be used in an oliguric client in renal failure who might develop pulmonary edema with increased fluid intake.

13-59   Answer D

In many cases of ATN, which is often caused by nephrotoxic agents, the removal of the offending agent will allow renal function to return gradually to normal. In the meantime, supportive measures should be provided, often in the form of peritoneal dialysis or hemodialysis. Because most cases of ATN are reversible, it is essential for diagnosis and aggressive management to begin early. ATN is characterized by altered renal ability to conserve sodium. Clinically, ATN is seen as a urinary sodium level greater than 20 mEq/L. Laboratory serum sodium levels vary in ATN, depending on the state of hydration. Oliguria is usually associated with postischemic ATN, whereas either oliguria or

nonoliguria may be associated with nephrotoxic ATN. Creatinine clearance is severely decreased, and plasma creatinine rises about 0.5–1 mg/dL per day in ATN. The clinical course of ATN is often divided into three phases: initial injury, maintenance, and recovery. The maintenance phase is expressed as either oliguric or nonoliguric. Nonoliguric ATN has a better outcome.

13-60   Answer B

The presence of casts in a urinalysis in increased amounts indicates the presence of bacteria or protein, which is seen in severe renal disease and could also indicate urinary calculi. The presence of ketones reflects incomplete metabolism of fatty acids, as in diabetic ketoacidosis, prolonged fasting, and anorexia nervosa. The presence of normal or abnormal crystals may indicate that the specimen has been allowed to stand. The presence of nitrates suggests bacteria, usually *Escherichia coli*.

13-61   Answer C

Urinary tract infections (UTIs) are the most common cause of burning on urination. UTIs cause approximately 7 million episodes of acute cystitis per year.

13-62   Answer C

The use of anticholinergic agents may be responsible for transient urinary incontinence in women. Etiologies for transient urinary incontinence may be stated using a DIAPERS mnemonic: *D* for drugs, such as hypnotics, sedatives, anticholinergic agents, diuretics, and adrenergic agents, and delirium or altered mental status; *I* for infection; *A* for atrophy of the vagina or urethra; *P* for psychological disorders such as functional depression; *E* for endocrine disorders, such as hyperglycemia or hypercalcemia; *R* for restricted mobility; and *S* for stool impaction.

13-63   Answer B

A 24-hour urine test for vanillylmandelic acid (VMA) and catecholamines is done to diagnose hypertension secondary to pheochromocytoma. A pheochromocytoma is an adrenal tumor that frequently secretes abnormally high levels of epinephrine and norepinephrine, resulting in episodic or persistent hypertension from arterial vasoconstriction. A renal tumor would be diagnosed by an intravenous pyelogram (IVP). To test for renal artery stenosis, duplex ultrasound, captopril renal scintigraphy, and magnetic resonance angiography (MRA) are used. Nuclear medicine and radiological tests will assess and measure kidney function and structure to determine the amount of hydronephrosis present.

13-64   Answer B

With a total cystectomy in a man, the prostate and seminal vessels are also removed, resulting in impotence. With Marvin, it is important to state the facts, then explore his feelings. Referring to the surgeon when you know the answer is an evasive tactic. Asking Marvin how his wife feels negates his own feelings.

13-65   Answer C

If a client with acute renal failure (ARF) excretes 400 mL of urine on Tuesday, the amount of fluid intake (both oral and intravenous) the client should have on Wednesday is 900 mL. A client with ARF is initially managed conservatively by fluid and dietary management. The permitted daily intake is calculated by allowing 500 mL for insensible losses (respiration, perspiration, bowel losses) and adding the amount excreted as urine in the previous 24 hours. The client excreted 400 mL as urine, so adding 500 mL for insensible loss equals 900 mL total intake for the next 24 hours.

13-66   Answer D

While many sources differ, oliguria (diminished urination) in an adult is typically defined as less than 500 mL urine output per day. Anuria, although defined as "without urine," is an output of less than 100 mL per day. The body makes 1 mL of urine per minute, or 1,440 mL per day. In the hospital, the least acceptable amount of urine is 30 mL per hour, but we actually produce 60 mL per hour.

13-67   Answer A

Painless, gross hematuria in an older adult is an ominous sign. It is usually the result of a malignancy (prostate cancer, transitional cell cancer, or renal cell carcinoma). Flank pain with hematuria is commonly caused by the presence of a kidney stone in the upper collecting system of the affected kidney. Hematuria after trauma is quite common. Isolated asymptomatic hematuria is often found on a routine screening urinalysis with no apparent source determined by history and physical examination.

The possibility of occult malignancy or other potentially serious etiology increases with age, and if the client is older than 40, he or she should be evaluated for urological tumor. Clients younger than 40 should be monitored at least monthly for 3 months and if the hematuria persists, then a more aggressive workup is indicated.

13-68   Answer B

General recommendations for the prevention of kidney stones, regardless of the type of stone the client has, include reducing protein in the diet because protein enhances calcium, urate, and oxalate excretion; drinking 3–4 L of water per day with the avoidance of nonsoftened and mineral water; avoiding vitamin C supplements because they stimulate oxalate excretion; increasing fiber to decrease calcium absorption; restricting sodium to 2.5 g/day to decrease excretion of urinary calcium; restricting the consumption of oxalate-containing foods; limiting calcium intake to 800–1,000 mg/day; and restricting alcohol to no more than one to two drinks per day.

13-69   Answer B

Middle-aged men do not incur as many urinary tract infections as middle-aged women because men have the bacteriostatic effect of prostatic fluid and a longer urethra. However, prostatic hypertrophy commonly associated with aging increases the risk of cystitis for older men. Men and women are equally prone to urinary stasis and have the same urinary pH.

13-70   Answer D

Erythromycin (E-Mycin) is not associated with acute renal failure (ARF). It is one of the safest antibiotics, even in pregnancy. NSAIDs and ACE inhibitors can cause the prerenal type of ARF by causing a decreased intrarenal arteriolar resistance. Cimetidine (Tagamet) can cause an elevation in serum creatinine levels without a change in glomerular filtration. Although this is not a problem in clients with normal renal function, there is a more profound effect on serum creatinine concentrations in clients with borderline renal dysfunction.

13-71   Answer D

Before beginning an extensive work-up for proteinuria, the syndrome of postural proteinuria should be ruled out. In this benign condition, which occurs in healthy, otherwise asymptomatic clients, urine collected first thing in the morning does not show any protein. If protein is present in the urine after the client has been ambulating for several hours, the syndrome of postural proteinuria is confirmed. The prognosis is excellent because clients with postural proteinuria do not develop renal disease with any greater frequency than that seen in the general population.

13-72   Answer A

Goodpasture's syndrome is characterized by glomerulonephritis and pulmonary hemorrhage resulting from immune complex damage to the glomerular and alveolar basement membranes. Nephrotic syndrome is characterized by massive proteinuria, hypoalbuminemia, hyperlipidemia, and edema. Lupus nephritis is an inflammatory autoimmune disorder affecting the connective tissue of the body with inflammatory lesions involving the supportive tissues of the glomerulus. Chronic glomerulonephritis is typically the end stage of other glomerular disorders such as rapidly progressive glomerulonephritis, lupus nephritis, or diabetic nephropathy.

13-73   Answer B

Bile produces urine that is brownish in color. Beets, rifampin (Rifadin), and phenazopyridine (Pyridium) can cause reddish or reddish-orange urine.

13-74   Answer A

If Janet stops smoking, her stress urinary incontinence may improve. Studies have shown that clients who smoke increase their risk of stress incontinence by 28% despite increased urethral sphincter tone. Limiting fluids, which may result in dehydration, may cause further problems. Although taking a multivitamin is good, it will not help with stress incontinence. In postmenopausal women not on hormone replacement therapy, using an estrogen vaginal cream has been shown to be effective. Lifting weights will not help with the urinary sphincter muscles. Kegel exercises have proved effective.

13-75   Answer D

Clients with frequent urinary tract infections (UTIs) and, in fact, all persons should drink 8–10 glasses of water per day to help distribute the body's own antibodies. Other measures that should be taught to women prone to developing UTIs include voiding after intercourse, avoiding bubble baths, wearing underwear with pantyhose, avoiding tight jeans, and using methods of contraception other than diaphragms with spermicidal agents. All women should avoid douching.

13-76   Answer B

Bill is at a higher risk for developing nephrolithiasis because of his intake of excessive amounts of vitamin C. Other risk factors for nephrolithiasis include use of certain medications, such as vitamin D supplements, calcium, corticosteroids, and acetazolamide (Diamox); a diet high in oxalate or sodium; a low fluid intake; and a history of chronic diarrhea, peptic ulcer disease, gout, recurrent urinary tract infection, skeletal fractures, jejunoileal bypass, or renal tubular acidosis.

13-77   Answer D

Clients with chronic kidney disease (CKD) are more likely to die from the disease than to start dialysis or progress to end-stage renal disease (ESRD), as most people would think is the likeliest outcome. It is now evident that CKD is a major risk factor for death from cardiovascular disease (CVD) and that this risk increases with worsening CKD. Clinicians need to focus their attention on preventing CKD progression, maximizing CVD risk reduction, and aggressively treating comorbidities associated with CKD. These comorbid conditions include anemia, volume overload, abnormal calcium phosphate homeostasis, hypertension, dyslipidemia, and metabolic syndrome, many of which predispose to CVD.

13-78   Answer A

Loop diuretics, such as furosemide (Lasix), bumetanide (Bumex), and ethacrynic acid (Edecrin), all act to inhibit sodium chloride reabsorption in the thick ascending limb of the loop of Henle. Mannitol (Osmitrol) is an osmotic diuretic, hydrochlorothiazide (HydroDIURIL) is a thiazide diuretic, and acetazolamide (Diamox) is a carbonic anhydrase inhibitor; these diuretics exert their effects through different mechanisms.

13-79   Answer A

Encouraging hydration is the first step in the treatment of uric acid kidney stones. Additional steps include alkalinizing the urine with potassium citrate

(Urocit-K) to keep the urine pH above 6.5. Reducing protein intake to 56 g/day will also help. As a last resort, allopurinol (Zyloprim) may be added. Usually clients with uric acid kidney stones will have a normal serum uric acid level but an elevated urine uric acid concentration. If no medical treatment is provided after removal of a uric acid kidney stone, stones will generally recur in 50% of patients within 5 years.

13-80   Answer A

Pharmacokinetics refers to the absorption, distribution, metabolism, and elimination of drugs and their metabolites. It is affected by the following physiological changes in the older adult: decreased creatine clearance, decreased lean muscle mass, increased total body fat, decreased hepatic blood flow, decreased renal blood flow, decreased serum albumin level, and decreased total body water. Serum albumin levels typically decrease, not increase, in the older adult.

13-81   Answer A

A serum creatinine level greater than 4 mg/dL is associated with kidney disease and is indicative of severe impairment of renal function. A decreased serum level of albumin occurs in nephrotic syndrome. Serum sodium is decreased in nephrotic syndrome and serum calcium is decreased in renal failure. Normal values are as follows:

- Serum creatinine: 0.5–1.0 mg/dL
- Serum albumin: 3.3–4.5 g/dL
- Serum sodium: 135–145 mEq/L
- Serum calcium: 4.5–5.5 mEq/L

13-82   Answer C

Clients with worsening kidney function may have frequent hypoglycemic episodes and have a decreased need for insulin or oral antihyperglycemic agents. The clinician must explain to the client that the kidneys metabolize and excrete insulin and when renal function declines, the insulin is available for a longer period of time and thus less of it is needed. As in this case, the end result is that many clients think that their diabetes is improving. It usually means that end-stage renal disease is approaching.

13-83   Answer A

The most common type of kidney stones are calcium oxalate stones. They make up about 75% of all kidney stones and are usually less than 2 cm in diameter. Uric acid stones, which are radiolucent, make up about 5% of all stones. Calcium phosphate stones, which occur with renal tubular acidosis, make up about 5% of all stones. Cystine stones, which are hexagonal crystals, are the result of an autosomal recessive genetic trait and make up less than 1% of all kidney stones. There are actually seven types of stones made of different types of crystals: calcium oxalate, calcium phosphate, a combination of calcium oxalate and calcium phosphate, magnesium ammonium phosphate (struvite or infection stones), uric acid, cystine, and miscellaneous types such as occur with drug metabolites.

13-84   Answer C

The treatment of choice for a contusion of the kidney after trauma is conservative therapy, including bedrest and observation. With these injuries, bleeding is typically minor and self-limiting. Treatment of major renal injuries is usually surgical to stop hemorrhaging. A urethral catheterization will be done to assess the characteristics of the urine (quantity and color), but this is a procedure to assess the condition, not to treat the kidney contusion.

13-85   Answer D

Eosinophils are present in the urine in interstitial nephritis, urinary tract infections, and acute tubular necrosis (ATN). They are not present in normal urine but are activated by antigens and antigen-induced hypersensitivity reactions. Normally only a few white blood cells are found in urine. Increased numbers of leukocytes in the urine generally indicate either renal or genitourinary tract disease.

13-86   Answer C

Diabetic nephropathy is the most common cause of ESRD. Hypertensive nephropathy is the second-most commonly occurring cause of renal failure, and glomerulonephritis is the third-most common cause.

13-87   Answer B

Anemia is a chronic problem in clients with ESRD. Because of the limited iron content of low-protein diets and decreased erythropoietin production by the kidneys, supplemental iron is needed in the diet. Most clients with renal failure also require daily vitamin and mineral supplementation, but this question specified that the client was on a low-protein diet, thus making one think of iron.

Potassium is usually restricted because hyperkalemia can cause dangerous cardiac dysrhythmias. Control of phosphate levels is begun early in chronic renal failure to avoid osteodystrophy.

13-88   Answer D

Before using the radial artery to draw blood for measurement of arterial blood gas values, the Allen test should be performed to evaluate the presence of the ulnar artery. To perform the Allen test, first cause the hand to blanch by obliterating both the radial and ulnar pulses. Then, release the pressure over the ulnar artery only. If the flow is adequate, flushing will immediately be seen. The Allen test is then considered positive and the radial artery may be used to draw the blood. ABGs are arterial blood gases. The Thomas test assesses hip motion, and the Weber test assesses hearing.

13-89   Answer A

Cigarette smoke, from both active and passive inhalation, is a significant risk factor for urinary tract neoplasms and may account for half of the incidence of bladder tumors among men and a third among women. Other factors implicated in the formation of urinary tract neoplasms include chemicals and dyes used in the plastics, rubber, and cable industries; the chronic use of phenacetin-containing analgesic agents; and substances in the environment of textile workers, leather finishers, spray painters, hairdressers, and petroleum workers. The breakdown products of these chemicals and those from cigarette smoke are stored in the bladder and excreted in the urine, which causes a local influence on abnormal cell development. Working long hours with inability to void may often result in a bladder infection, not a neoplasm.

13-90   Answer A

For clients taking NSAIDs on a long-term basis, hemodynamically induced acute renal failure; acute interstitial nephropathy, with or without nephrotic syndrome; salt and water retention; papillary necrosis and chronic renal injury; hyperkalemia; vasculitis; and glomerulitis may be found.

13-91   Answer D

Phenazopyridine (Pyridium) is the only analgesic listed. For the first few days of a urinary tract infection (UTI), all of the drugs listed may be prescribed, in addition to antibiotics, to decrease the pain and discomfort of a UTI. Use of these agents should not be prolonged, however, given their significant side-effect profile. Analgesics such as phenazopyridine (Pyridium) may be prescribed, but this alters the color of urine to orange and may cause urinary leakage secondary to anesthetization of the urethra and sphincter. Anticholinergics, including atropine (Donnatal), hyoscyamine (Levsin, Cystospaz), propantheline (Pro-Banthine), or oxybutynin (Ditropan), produce an antispasmodic effect, relieving pain. However, anticholinergics may also contribute to urinary retention (especially in the elderly), which is a clear risk factor for UTI, and should thus be used with caution.

13-92   Answer C

A Koch pouch is a continent internal ileal reservoir or continent ileal bladder conduit in which a pouch is created to be an ileal conduit. Nipple valves are formed on the skin by intussuscepting tissue backward into the reservoir to connect the pouch to the skin and the ureters to the pouch. The filling pressure closes valves, preventing leakage and reflux.

13-93   Answer A

Thiazide diuretics, along with phosphates and calcium-binding agents, are used for calcium phosphate and oxalate stones. Antibiotic therapy is used for the urinary tract infections that occur with struvite stones; allopurinol is used for uric acid stones; and penicillamine and sodium bicarbonate are used for cystine stones.

13-94   Answer B

The kidneys excrete increased amounts of HCO_3 to lower the pH as a mode of compensation for respiratory alkalosis. In respiratory acidosis, renal compensatory mechanisms elevate the bicarbonate level, and eventually the pH approaches normal. Signs of compensation in metabolic acidosis are hyperventilation (causing increased intake of oxygen and increased blowing off of carbon dioxide), decreased $PaCO_2$, and increased amounts of ammonia in the urine. The compensatory response to metabolic alkalosis is retention of carbon dioxide.

13-95   Answer A

The most common metabolic condition that predisposes clients to the formation of kidney stones is idiopathic hypercalciuria. Idiopathic hypercalciuria is present in approximately 50% of stone-forming clients, followed by a low urinary citrate excretion at a slightly lower percentage. Hyperuricosuria is present in approximately 30% of stone-forming clients and hyperoxaluria in approximately 15% of all stone-forming clients.

13-96   Answer C

Foods high in oxalate that a client with oxalate kidney stones should avoid include asparagus, beer, beets, cabbage, celery, chocolate and cocoa, fruits, green beans, nuts, tea, colas, and tomatoes. Foods high in calcium are beans and lentils, chocolate and cocoa, dried fruits, canned or smoked fish except tuna, flour, milk, and milk products. Acid ash foods to avoid with calcium phosphate or oxalate stones and struvite stones include cheese, cranberries, eggs, grapes, meat and poultry, plums and prunes, tomatoes, and whole grains. A low-purine diet is often effective in reducing stones formed from excess uric acid. This diet is achieved by limiting intake of purine-rich foods such as organ meats, red meats, seafood (especially sardines, anchovies, and scallops), poultry, legumes, whole grains, and alcohol (which decreases uric acid clearance).

13-97   Answer A

The GFR is affected more in older African Americans than in Caucasians. Sodium is not excreted as well by the kidneys in hypertensive African Americans who have high sodium intake, and the kidneys have approximately 20% less blood flow as a result of anatomical changes in small renal vessels. End-stage renal disease (ESRD) is three to four times more common in African Americans, Native Americans, and Mexican Americans than in Caucasians.

13-98   Answer D

Pelvic floor (Kegel) exercises are essential for the advanced-practice nurse (APN) to teach clients with stress incontinence to improve their quality of life. Kegel exercises help to restore and maintain continence by improving pelvic muscle strength, increasing urethral pressure, decreasing abnormal detrusor muscle contraction, and decreasing pressure within the bladder. Kegel exercises are recommended for women with urinary stress incontinence, for some men who have urinary incontinence after prostate surgery, and for people who have fecal incontinence.

13-99   Answer D

A kidneys, ureters, and bladder (KUB) film can visualize the renal outline and identify lower rib fractures. An intravenous pyelogram compares the kidneys and shows distortion of the calyces and incomplete filling. Renal angiography provides information on the integrity of the renal vasculature. Computed tomography can determine the extent of injury in three dimensions.

13-100   Answer B

A postvoid residual catheterization volume of more than 30 mL is abnormal.

13-101   Answer D

White blood cell casts are seen in pyelonephritis and interstitial nephritis. Hyaline casts may be present in normal urine; granular casts may be present in a wide variety of renal disorders; and red blood cell casts indicate glomerular bleeding that is strongly suggestive of glomerulonephritis.

13-102   Answer D

Renal cysts are usually asymptomatic and usually do not cause flank pain. Pyelonephritis, ureterolithiasis, and vascular occlusion of the kidney (renal vein thrombosis) all usually cause flank pain.

13-103   Answer B

Postmenopausal women tend to have more recurrent urinary tract infections because of postvoid residual urine secondary to anatomical changes such as a dropped bladder or uterus; estrogen depletion–related changes such as a dry, thin vaginal lining; a decrease in lactobacilli; and an increase in the colonization of the vagina by *Escherichia coli*.

13-104   Answer B

The liver on the right side displaces the right kidney slightly downward.

13-105   Answer C

Urinary stasis is the most common factor predisposing a woman to a urinary tract infection (UTI). It is followed by calculi and the presence of catheters, stents, and other foreign bodies. The use of an oral contraceptive (if the male partner is not using a condom) also predisposes a woman to a UTI because sexual intercourse increases the likelihood of developing a UTI. The use of a diaphragm also increases the risk of a UTI because of the properties of the spermicidal agents used in conjunction with the diaphragm. Women should be encouraged to empty their bladders when they get the urge to go and not to "hold" it.

13-106　Answer D

Multivitamins do not cause urine to appear reddish in color. Cascara sagrada, a stimulant laxative, may cause urine color to be red in alkaline urine and yellow-brown in acid urine; phenazopyridine (Pyridium), a urinary tract analgesic, will cause urine to appear orange to red; and phenytoin (Dilantin), an anticonvulsant, may cause urine to appear pink, red, or red-brown.

13-107　Answer A

Excessive alcohol ingestion can cause metabolic acidosis because alcohol results in excess acid levels in the blood.

13-108　Answer D

Clinical manifestations of renal tumors include microscopic or gross hematuria, a palpable abdominal mass, fever, flank pain, fatigue, weight loss, and anemia or polycythemia.

13-109　Answer C

Microalbuminuria is the earliest indicator of impaired renal function. The best way to determine microalbuminuria to assist in the diagnosis of diabetic nephropathy is a timed overnight urine collection or albumin-creatinine ratio in an early morning spot urine collected upon awakening. At least two of three timed overnight or early morning spot urine collections over a period of 3–6 months should be abnormal prior to making a diagnosis of microalbuminuria. The urine dipstick is not sensitive enough and a 24-hour urine collection, while being inconvenient, also shows a wide variety of albumin excretion due to factors such as sustained erect posture, protein intake, and exercise. These all tend to increase albumin excretion rates.

13-110　Answer A

Cholinergic drugs such as bethanechol chloride (Urecholine) are used primarily in the treatment of acute postoperative and postpartum urinary retention and for neurogenic bladder atony with urinary retention. Anticholinesterase agents such as neostigmine (Prostigmin) and pyridostigmine (Mestinon) are used primarily in the treatment of myasthenia gravis, but they are also useful in the treatment of urinary retention because they stimulate contraction of the detrusor muscle. Anticholinergic agents such as propantheline bromide (Pro-Banthine), dicyclomine (Bentyl), flavoxate hydrochloride (Urispas), and oxybutynin (Ditropan) act to relax the detrusor muscle and increase contraction of the internal sphincter. They serve to increase the bladder capacity of clients with spastic or hyperreflexive neurogenic bladder.

13-111　Answer C

Potassium-sparing diuretics, such as spironolactone (Aldactone), have the following side effects: hyperkalemia, headache, hyponatremia, nausea, diarrhea, urticaria, and menstrual disturbances. Osmotic diuretics may precipitate congestive heart failure, high doses of loop diuretics may cause hearing loss, and thiazide diuretics may cause hypokalemia and hyperglycemia.

13-112　Answer A

In clients in the United States receiving dialysis, diabetic nephropathy (Kimmelstiel-Wilson syndrome) is the most common cause of end-stage renal disease (about 25%). Both type 1 and type 2 diabetes are implicated, indicating the need for good diabetes control throughout clients' life spans. Most clients with acute tubular necrosis recover with conservative management (fluid monitoring, protein restriction, drug adjustments, and dietary and potassium control). Dialysis may become necessary; however, it is usually temporary. In clients with major renal vascular occlusive disease, vascular repair or percutaneous angioplasty has been shown to slow the progression of the disease. Kidney trauma is not an end-stage renal disease.

Bibliography

Bloom, RD, and Bress, J: Chronic kidney disease: A primary-care guide. *Clinical Advisor* 10(4):31–38, April 2007.

Charnow, JA: Increased lead exposure may raise kidney cancer risk. *Renal and Urology News.*www. renalandurologynews.com/increased-lead-exposure-may-raise-kidney-cancer-risk/article/221287/, accessed January 10, 2012.

Charnow, JA: Ultrasound not inferior for sizing renal masses. www.renalandurologynews.com/ultrasound-not-inferior-for-sizing-renal-masses/article/221975/, accessed January 10, 2012.

Dunphy, LM, et al: *Primary Care: The Art and Science of Advanced Practice Nursing*, ed 3. FA Davis, Philadelphia, 2011.

Foody, JM, Cleary, JK, Davis, LL, McGinnity, JG, and Zuber, K: Chronic kidney disease and cardiovascular risk: A perfect storm. *Clinical Advisor* (suppl.): 3–14, November 2011.

Koncicki, H, and Radbill, B: Diabetic kidney disease in the elderly: Diagnosis, treatment goals, and management. *Consultant* 51(11):797–803, 2011.

Moon, CM, Gunder, L, and Steele, AR: Adult polycystic kidney disease management. *Clinical Advisor*, 37–46, June 2011.

Rubin, RN: What's the "take home"?: An older man with a small renal mass. *Consultant* 51(11):837–839, 2011.

VanLeeuwen, AM, Kranpitz, TR, and Smith, L: *Davis's Comprehensive Handbook of Laboratory and Diagnostic Tests With Nursing Implications*, ed 2. FA Davis, Philadelphia, 2006.

Zuber, K, and Davis, JS: Renal consult: Medications and the renal patient. *Clinician Reviews* 21(6):50–53, 2011.

How well did you do?

85% and above, congratulations! This score shows application of test-taking principles and adequate content knowledge.

75%–85%, keep working! Review test-taking principles and try again.

65%–75%, hang in there! Spend some time reviewing concepts and test-taking principles and try the test again.

Chapter 14: *Male Genitourinary Problems*

Sharon K. Byrne
Lynne M. Dunphy

Questions

14-1   When teaching Tom how to do a testicular self-examination, which of the following do you tell him?

A. "Examine your testicles when you are cold because this makes them more sensitive."

B. "Make sure your hands are dry to create friction."

C. "If you feel firmness above and behind the testicle, make an appointment."

D. "Make an appointment if you note any hard lumps directly on the testicle, whether they are tender or not."

14-2   Sidney states that he was recently given a diagnosis of prostate cancer and that he has to return to the urologist for staging. He doesn't understand why because he says, "Cancer is still cancer. I just want to get rid of it." You tell him,

A. "Staging determines the type of tests required."

B. "You have time to decide on treatment until the cancer gets to the last stage."

C. "Staging will determine the extent of the spread of the cancer and treatment options."

D. "You already know you have prostate cancer; you don't need another test unless you want to know how long you've had it."

14-3   Austin has been on finasteride (Proscar) for 6 months for benign prostatic hypertrophy. A decrease in his prostate-specific antigen (PSA) from the original value of 5.4 has not occurred. Your initial expectation is

A. that his PSA would remain stable, neither increasing nor decreasing.

B. Austin's dosage should be reduced only after he has been on the medication for approximately 12 months.

C. that a significant reduction in the overall PSA would occur if the level is associated with true benign prostatic hypertrophy.

D. that an elevation of the antigen would occur because of the effect of the alpha-adrenergic antagonist.

14-4   Which technique uses a learned method to target muscle contraction and relaxation to assist with urinary continence?

A. Biofeedback

B. Kegel exercises

C. Bladder training

D. Prompted voiding

14-5   Which statement is true about the use of alpha blockers in the treatment of symptomatic benign prostatic hypertrophy?

A. They are safe and effective and should be given in the morning before breakfast.

B. They do not lower blood pressure in normotensive clients.

C. Pedal edema is the most common adverse effect.

D. Blood counts should be monitored periodically for reduction in the platelet count.

14-6   You are performing a school physical examination on Damon, age 5. You are unable to retract his foreskin over the glans penis while inspecting his penis. This is referred to as

A. phimosis.

B. paraphimosis.

C. microphallus.

D. priapism.

14-7   Which of the following statements is true about older men with HIV?

A. They have a slower disease progression when compared with their younger cohorts.

B. They have a more rapid disease progression when compared with their younger cohorts.

C. They are rarely if ever injection drug users.

D. They cannot undergo treatment with antiretrovirals.

14-8 *The bladder tumor antigen test may also be positive with*

A. testicular torsion.

B. the use of steroids for bodybuilding.

C. scrotal trauma.

D. symptomatic sexually transmitted disease.

14-9 *Milton, a 72-year-old unmarried, sexually active white man, presents to your clinic with complaints of hesitancy, urgency, and occasional uncontrolled dribbling. Although you suspect benign prostatic hypertrophy, what else should your differential diagnoses include?*

A. Antihistamine use

B. Urethral stricture

C. Detrusor hyperreflexia

D. Renal calculi

14-10 *Joe comes in for an evaluation after a testicular self-examination. He states that it is probably nothing to worry about because his testicle is not tender, but he does have a tiny, hard nodule on the testicle. You confirm that there is a hard, fixed nodule on his testicle. Your next course of action would be to*

A. order a urinalysis.

B. schedule Joe for a recheck next month.

C. refer Joe to a specialist.

D. tell Joe that it is a cyst and if it does not resolve by itself, he will have to have it excised.

14-11 *Josh has a no-scalpel vasectomy and asks if he can proceed immediately with sexual relations with his wife without worrying about getting her pregnant. You tell him,*

A. "Yes, you are now sterile."

B. "You must use protection for at least 2 weeks after the procedure."

C. "You must use protection for at least 6 weeks after the procedure."

D. "In 6 months, we'll do a sperm count to see if you can discontinue other precautions."

14-12 *Urinary tract infections in the male client are divided into upper- and lower-tract infections. A classic example of an upper-tract infection includes*

A. cystitis.

B. pyelonephritis.

C. prostatitis.

D. epididymitis.

14-13 *Bill appears with a tender, ulcerated, exudative, papular lesion on his penis. It has an erythematous halo, surrounding edema, and a friable base. What do you suspect?*

A. A chancre

B. A chancroid

C. Condylomata acuminatum

D. Genital herpes

14-14 *Which type of urinary incontinence results from Parkinson's disease and multiple sclerosis?*

A. Overflow incontinence

B. Stress incontinence

C. Urge incontinence

D. Functional incontinence

14-15 *The action of a 5-alpha-reductase inhibitor in the treatment of benign prostatic hypertrophy is to*

A. relax smooth muscle of the prostatic capsule.

B. reduce action of androgens in the prostate.

C. relieve bladder obstruction.

D. improve urinary flow rates.

14-16 *Which of the following medications causes retention of urine by inhibiting bladder contractibility and may cause overflow incontinence in certain individuals?*

A. Antispasmodics

B. Drugs that affect the sympathetic nervous system

C. Diuretics

D. Antihistamines

14-17 *The most common type of genitourinary dysfunction after a transurethral resection of the prostate is*

A. erectile dysfunction.

B. urinary incontinence.

C. retrograde ejaculation.

D. decreased libido.

14-18　*Transillumination of fluid in the scrotum may be seen with*

A. a varicocele.

B. a hydrocele.

C. testicular torsion.

D. testicular cancer.

14-19　*Harry has benign prostatic hypertrophy and complains of some incontinence. Your first step in diagnosing overflow incontinence would be to order a*

A. urinalysis.

B. cystometrogram.

C. cystoscopy.

D. postvoid residual (PVR) urine measurement.

14-20　*Precocious puberty is present if*

A. a delay in any of the Tanner stages takes longer than 2 years from one stage to the next.

B. the adolescent has had sexual relations.

C. puberty starts before age 9.5 years.

D. an adolescent rushes through all Tanner stages in less than 2 years.

14-21　*Erectile dysfunction is a complex phenomenon with a variety of causes. The predominant cause is*

A. psychological.

B. vascular.

C. neurogenic.

D. drug related.

14-22　*You are referring a 73-year-old client for management of his prostate cancer with hormonal therapy. It is understood that goserelin acetate (Zoladex) acts as a method of androgen ablation by*

A. blocking the release of follicle-stimulating hormone (FSH) and luteinizing hormone (LH).

B. blocking 5-alpha-reductase, which converts testosterone into dihydrotestosterone.

C. inhibiting the binding of testosterone to the cancer cells.

D. inhibiting the progression of cancer cells through the cell cycle.

14-23　*Principles of management of genital herpes include which of the following?*

A. Antiviral chemotherapy can control the signs and symptoms.

B. Antiviral chemotherapy, if prescribed early in a first clinical episode, is curative.

C. Antiviral chemotherapy does not control recurrent episodes.

D. Antiviral topical therapy offers minimal clinical benefit.

14-24　*Lower urinary tract symptoms (LUTS) in males can present as a constellation of storage or voiding symptoms. Storage symptoms include*

A. hesitancy and poor flow.

B. intermittency and postvoid dribble.

C. straining and dysuria.

D. urgency and nocturia.

14-25　*You are performing a rectal examination on James for follow-up of his melena. What do you expect his stool to look like if his condition has not resolved?*

A. Grayish tan

B. Bright red

C. Pale yellow, greasy, and fatty

D. Black and tarry

14-26　*A 63-year-old man presents to you with hematuria, hesitancy, and dribbling. Digital rectal examination (DRE) reveals a moderately enlarged prostate that is smooth. The client's prostate-specific antigen (PSA) is 1.2. What is the most appropriate management strategy for you to follow at this time?*

A. Prescribe an alpha adrenergic blocker.

B. Recommend saw palmetto.

C. Prescribe an antibiotic.

D. Refer the client to urology.

14-27　*Morris is in a new relationship and is not sure whether his erectile dysfunction is caused by stress about his performance or is organic. What simple test could you suggest to determine if he has the ability to have an erection?*

A. Nocturnal penile tumescence and rigidity test

B. Penile duplex ultrasonography

C. Intraspongiosum injection

D. Serum PSA

14-28   *Tommy, age 15, comes to the clinic in acute distress with "belly pain." When obtaining his history, you find that he fell off his bike this morning and has vomited. Upon closer examination, you determine the belly pain to be left-sided groin pain, or pain in his left testicle. He is afebrile and reports no dysuria. You suspect*

A. testicular torsion.

B. epididymitis.

C. a hydrocele.

D. a varicocele.

14-29   *Herb, who has diabetes, is complaining of a rash on his penis. Before examining him, you suspect that he may have*

A. tinea cruris.

B. genital herpes.

C. *Candida.*

D. intraepithelial neoplasia.

14-30   *Which sexually transmitted diseases are cofactors for HIV transmission?*

A. Syphilis and chlamydia

B. Herpes and chlamydia

C. Chancroid and genital herpes

D. Chancroid and gonorrhea

14-31   *In deciding whether to treat Morrison, who has benign prostatic hypertrophy, you use the American Urological Association (AUA) scale. No treatment is indicated if the AUA score is*

A. 36 or higher.

B. 20–35.

C. 8–19.

D. 7 or lower.

14-32   *Jack and Jane have been married for 6 months and are unable to conceive. They ask you to recommend an infertility specialist. What do you tell them?*

A. "Infertility is not an issue until you have had unprotected sex for at least 1 year."

B. "Let's run some routine tests first; then I'll recommend someone."

C. "Tell me about your sexual experiences."

D. "It's usually a problem with the woman, so let's have Jane examined first."

14-33   *Jeff, age 20, presents to the college health clinic with complaints of difficulty passing his urine and a discharge from his penis. Upon further investigation you note that the discharge is urethral in origin. The most common cause of these symptoms in the young adult male population is*

A. chronic prostatitis.

B. prostatic abscess.

C. acute prostatitis.

D. prostatic hypertrophy.

14-34   *When performing a newborn assessment of a male infant, you note that the urethral opening is on the dorsal side of the glans. This is referred to as*

A. hypospadias.

B. Peyronie's disease.

C. priapism.

D. epispadias.

14-35   *Martin is complaining of erectile dysfunction. He also has a condition that has reduced arterial blood flow to his penis. The most common cause of this condition is*

A. epilepsy.

B. multiple sclerosis.

C. diabetes mellitus.

D. Parkinson's disease.

14-36   *Cancer of the prostate often begins with subtle symptoms that develop very slowly over time and, if left untreated, will lead to metastasis. What prognostic finding is a significant indicator of probable metastatic disease?*

A. Gleason score of 2

B. Sudden onset of weakness of the legs in a man with known prostate cancer

C. TNM staging T1a, N0, M0

D. Bladder outlet obstruction

14-37   Manny has been taking finasteride (Proscar) and states that he has had dramatic relief. He previously took terazosin (Hytrin), which also helped, and he asks you about taking that again. You tell him,

A. "Yes, let's try the combination therapy because two are better than one."

B. "No, they are absolutely contraindicated together."

C. "There is no evidence to support combination therapy."

D. "When symptoms get so bad that you need two different medications, it's time for surgery."

14-38   Gerard is complaining of a scrotal mass; however, the scrotum is so edematous that it is difficult to assess. How do you determine if it is a hernia or a hydrocele?

A. You can always return a hernia's contents to the abdominal cavity.

B. Bowel sounds may be heard over a hernia.

C. You can transilluminate a hernia.

D. With a hydrocele, a bulge appears on straining.

14-39   Bloody penile discharge is most likely to be associated with which of the following?

A. Cancer of the penis

B. Herpes zoster

C. Epididymitis

D. Peyronie's disease

14-40   A history of urinary tract infections in males is often seen in men with chronic bacterial prostatitis. Other signs and symptoms of chronic bacterial prostatitis include

A. irritative voiding symptoms, low back pain, and perineal pain.

B. nausea and vomiting, as well as fever.

C. loss of appetite and weight loss.

D. irritative voiding symptoms, inability to ambulate, and fever.

14-41   Benign prostatic hypertrophy is a common finding as men age. Classically, this condition may begin with difficulty initiating the urinary stream, hesitancy, urgency, postvoid dribbling, urinary frequency, nocturia, urinary retention, sensation of a full bladder immediately after voiding, and incontinence. These preceding symptoms would also cause you to consider what other condition on your differential list?

A. Epididymitis

B. Testicular cancer

C. Cancer of the prostate

D. Balanitis

14-42   Which statement is true about prostatitis and prostatodynia?

A. The terms are interchangeable.

B. Prostatodynia may be acute, chronic, or nonbacterial.

C. The symptoms of both are extremely irritating.

D. Prostatodynia results in the same symptoms as prostatitis, but there is no evidence of infection.

14-43   When performing a prostate examination, you note a tender, warm prostate. What do you suspect?

A. Benign prostatic hypertrophy

B. Prostatic abscess

C. Prostate cancer

D. Bacterial prostatitis

14-44   John asks for a prescription for sildenafil (Viagra). He says that the only medication he takes is isosorbide mononitrate (Monoket) oral tablets and that he has diabetes, but it is controlled by diet alone. What do you tell him?

A. "Let's try a sample and see how you do."

B. "It's contraindicated with isosorbide mononitrate; let's discuss other options."

C. "Because of your history of diabetes, we can't use it."

D. "I'd better refer you to a urologist."

14-45   The initial diagnostic and/or laboratory testing that you should order to rule out organic causes of erectile dysfunction in men includes

A. color Doppler sonography.

B. CBC, blood chemistry profile, TSH, and PSA.

C. nocturnal penile tumescence and rigidity test (NPTR).

D. FBS, lipid profile, TSH, testosterone.

14-46   Erectile dysfunction (ED), which affects 18–30 million men in the United States, increases with age. In men older than the age of 50, what are the most commonly found contributors to ED?

A. Endocrine diseases

B. Vascular disorders

C. Neurogenic diseases

D. Psychiatric conditions

14-47   Samuel, who takes many different medications, is complaining of erectile dysfunction. You know that several medications could be the cause of Samuel's problem. Which of his medications is most likely the culprit?

A. Lasix

B. Reserpine

C. Prilosec

D. Isosorbide

14-48   Abnormalities of the scrotum are usually painless or nontender. Which of the following is an exception and is usually tender?

A. Hydrocele

B. Tumor of the testis

C. Spermatocele

D. Tuberculous epididymitis

14-49   At what age does the foreskin become fully retractable?

A. 3 months

B. 6 months

C. 9 months

D. 1 year

14-50   Mr. S. comes to you with scrotal pain. The examinations of his scrotum, penis, and rectum are normal. Which of the following conditions outside of the scrotum may present as scrotal pain?

A. Inguinal herniation and peritonitis

B. Renal colic and cardiac ischemia

C. Pancreatitis and Crohn's disease

D. Polyarteritis nodosa and ulcerative colitis

14-51   Common clinical symptoms of testosterone deficiency include

A. erectile dysfunction and a decrease in visceral fat.

B. an increase in lean body mass and infertility.

C. erectile dysfunction and a decrease in bone mineral density.

D. loss of libido and increased body hair.

14-52   Tim, age 12, asks you how long it will take him to make the complete change from preadolescence to adulthood once he starts puberty. You tell him it will take approximately

A. 2 years.

B. 3 years.

C. 4 years.

D. all of his teen years.

14-53   Which of the following men is more prone to prostatitis?

A. Jim, age 52, who wears tight jeans and sits at a computer all day

B. Jerry, age 30, who is a cross-country runner

C. Marvin, age 46, who is a dog trainer

D. Justin, age 39, who is a boat salesman

14-54   The aging lower urinary tract in men undergoes which changes that can result in increased urinary symptoms?

A. Bladder capacity is increased with lower postvoid residuals.

B. Bladder capacity is increased with increased detrusor (bladder muscle) contractility.

C. Bladder capacity is decreased with increased obstructive changes from the prostate.

D. Detrusor contractility is decreased, resulting in lower post-void residuals.

14-55   What is inflammation of the glans and prepuce called?

A. Balanitis.

B. Balanoposthitis.

C. Phimosis.

D. Paraphimosis.

14-56   An obstructive cause of lower urinary tract symptoms in males is

A. bladder cancer.

B. bladder stones.

C. infection.

D. prostate cancer.

14-57   If a client appears with symptoms of benign prostatic hypertrophy, a digital rectal examination is indicated in order to

A. screen for prostate or rectal malignancy.

B. evaluate for hypospadias.

C. rule out any neurological problems that may cause the symptoms.

D. detect the presence of urethritis.

14-58   The most common cause of androgen deficiency in older men is decreased testosterone production by the Leydig cells within the testes. Various systemic disorders can also affect circulating testosterone levels. These disorders include

A. diabetes and hyperthyroidism.

B. HIV and urinary tract infection.

C. hypertension and heart disease.

D. tobacco use and cholecystitis.

14-59   You have just treated Jay's condylomata acuminata with podophyllum in benzoin. What instructions do you give him?

A. "Refrain from sexual relations for 48 hours."

B. "Don't take a shower until tomorrow morning."

C. "Wash the medication off within 1–2 hours."

D. "Go into the bathroom now and wash the medication off."

14-60   The most common cause of urinary incontinence in men is

A. urethritis.

B. prostate cancer.

C. benign prostatic hypertrophy.

D. chronic bacteriuria.

14-61   Jeb, a 72-year-old male, is seen at the practice for follow-up of several episodes of orthostatic hypotension. It also appears through a review of his systems and a digital rectal examination that he has benign prostatic hypertrophy (BPH) with lower urinary tract symptoms. You review his recent ultrasonic evaluation that reports a prostate over 40 ml and the results of the American Urological Association (AUA) symptom index for BPH, and find his score to be 12. Based on the preceding information and the client's desire for noninvasive medical therapy, what management would you offer him?

A. Prazosin

B. Doxazosin

C. Finasteride

D. Phenoxybenzamine

14-62   Your client's chief complaint is blood in the urine. You know that the most common cause of gross hematuria in the male population is

A. a bladder infection.

B. benign prostatic hypertrophy.

C. bladder tumor.

D. prostatitis.

14-63   You are rolling your fingers along the inguinal ligament and you encounter small, freely mobile lymph nodes in this area. What do you suspect?

A. Nothing; this is not a cause for concern.

B. Something is abnormal and warrants further evaluation and possible referral.

C. The lymph nodes should be biopsied.

D. The lymph nodes must be congenital in origin.

14-64   Jake, age 62, has a low International Prostate Symptom Score for lower urinary tract symptoms associated with his benign prostate hypertrophy. You recommend

A. no treatment at this time.

B. immediate referral to urology.

C. balloon dilation.

D. starting him on an alpha blocker.

14-65   What is the most common site of prostate metastasis?

A. Lungs

B. Spine

C. Heart

D. Blood vessels

14-66   *Tim asks you about returning to his normal sex life after surgery for benign prostatic hypertrophy. You tell him,*

A. "You probably won't be able to have an erection after surgery; we need to discuss alternative ways of lovemaking."

B. "You need to wait several months after surgery to make sure the site has healed."

C. "You may resume sexual activity 4–6 weeks after surgery."

D. "You'll have to ask the surgeon."

14-67   *Cryptorchidism is a risk factor for*

A. cancer of the prostate.

B. testicular cancer.

C. bladder cancer.

D. a benign testicular tumor.

14-68   *Drew has an erectile dysfunction and says that a friend told him about a method that uses a constricting ring around the base of the penis. What is he referring to?*

A. Intracavernous injection therapy

B. External vacuum device

C. Urethral suppositories

D. Surgery

14-69   *Which of the following is an important question that you should ask to assess for urge urinary incontinence (UUI) in men?*

A. "Do you frequently have strong urges to urinate?"

B. "Do you urinate more than you think you should?"

C. "Do you have urges to urinate that sometimes result in wetting accidents?"

D. "Are you bothered by waking up at night to go to the bathroom?"

14-70   *Jerry, age 13, notices a sparse growth of long, slightly pigmented, downy pubic hair at the base of his penis; slightly larger testes; and a larger, red scrotum with a different texture. What Tanner stage is he in?*

A. Stage 1

B. Stage 2

C. Stage 3

D. Stage 4

14-71   *Jordan appears with a rapid onset of unilateral scrotal pain radiating up to the groin and flank. You are trying to differentiate between epididymitis and testicular torsion. Which test to determine whether swelling is in the testis or the epididymis should be your first choice?*

A. X-ray

B. Ultrasound

C. Technetium scan

D. Physical examination

14-72   *Most lesions of the penis are nontender and painless. Which of the following conditions begins with a tender, painful lesion?*

A. Syphilitic chancre

B. Genital herpes

C. Carcinoma of the penis

D. Peyronie's disease

14-73   *Balanitis may evolve into a chronic problem. If this occurs and the client experiences severe purulence and phimosis, treatment should involve*

A. a stronger topical antifungal ointment.

B. change from an antifungal ointment to a powder.

C. oral antibiotics.

D. an antiviral ointment.

14-74   *The seminal vesicles secrete*

A. a clear mucus.

B. urine.

C. fluid rich in fructose.

D. semen.

14-75   *Urinary stone disease, or urolithiasis, afflicts a large number of clients every year, exceeded in frequency as a urinary tract disorder only by infections and prostate disease. This disorder affects men more frequently than women with a ratio of 3:1. Common presenting signs and symptoms include which of the following?*

A. Guarding of the abdomen

B. Fever

C. Pain that is present during the daytime hours

D. Nausea and vomiting

14-76 *Which client will most likely never develop prostate cancer?*

A. Jacob, age 79, who had a transurethral resection of the prostate for benign prostatic hypertrophy

B. Jeffrey, age 11, who recently had an orchiectomy after a traumatic accident

C. Sid, age 70, who has a normal prostate-specific antigen level

D. Johnny, age 32, who is taking steroids for bodybuilding

14-77 *The testes in male infants descend from the retroperitoneal space through the inguinal canal and into the scrotal sacs. This most commonly occurs*

A. during the second trimester.

B. during the third trimester.

C. during the neonatal period.

D. by age 6 months.

14-78 *Bernard presents to the emergency department with a diagnosis of priapism. Despite application of cold compresses and pain medications, relief is unsuccessful. What is the treatment of choice?*

A. Terbutaline 0.25 mg subcutaneously

B. Phenylephrine injection 0.3–0.5 mL into the corpora cavernosa

C. Doxazosin 5 mg sublingually

D. Lidocaine 1% via the glans

14-79 *Barry, a 32-year-old gay man, has been diagnosed with acute bacterial prostatitis. In addition to providing education, you would encourage him to avoid*

A. rest.

B. NSAIDs.

C. hydration and stool softeners.

D. engaging in any activity that would elicit prostatic massage.

14-80 *Harris is complaining of crooked, painful erections. He has palpable, nontender, hard plaques just beneath the skin of his penis. What do you suspect?*

A. Carcinoma of the penis

B. Genital herpes

C. Syphilitic chancre

D. Peyronie's disease

14-81 *Elliot's chief complaint is heaviness in the scrotum. You assess swelling of the testicle, along with warm scrotal skin. What do you suspect?*

A. Cryptorchidism

B. Orchitis

C. Testicular torsion

D. Epididymitis

14-82 *Low-grade, localized prostate cancer can be treated successfully with*

A. radical prostatectomy or radiation.

B. chemotherapy.

C. cryosurgery (freezing) of a small part of the gland.

D. watchful waiting.

14-83 *At what point of fetal development does sexual differentiation occur?*

A. As soon as fertilization occurs

B. By 4 weeks' gestational age

C. By 8 weeks' gestational age

D. By 12 weeks' gestational age

14-84 *Which of the following scrotal disorders is most common in adolescents?*

A. Acute epididymitis

B. Testicular torsion

C. Atrophic testes

D. Scrotal edema

14-85 *According to the American Urological Association (AUA) Guideline on the Management of Benign Prostatic Hyperplasia: Diagnosis and Treatment Recommendations, when is referral for invasive surgery automatically warranted?*

A. With an AUA symptom index of 7 or lower

B. With an AUA symptom index 8 or greater

C. With irritative symptoms such as urgency, frequency, or nocturia

D. With presence of refractory retention and bladder stones

14-86   *The most common type of hernia is a(n)*

A. indirect inguinal hernia.

B. direct inguinal hernia.

C. femoral hernia.

D. umbilical hernia.

14-87   *Harvey is complaining of stress urinary incontinence. To assess the autonomic arch innervating the bladder, you test the*

A. inguinal reflex.

B. neuronal reflex.

C. bulbocavernous reflex.

D. meatal resistance.

14-88   *Roger, a healthy 68-year-old man, comes in to see you with a complaint of sudden episodes of an urgent need to void. He has had several episodes of moderate amounts of unintentional urine loss during these times. Other than these episodes, he is voiding in amounts "normal" for him, with no leakage when he coughs or sneezes. Your initial diagnosis is which type of incontinence?*

A. Stress incontinence

B. Urge incontinence

C. Overflow incontinence

D. Mixed incontinence

14-89   *Which of the following can cause phimosis?*

A. Paraphimosis

B. Smegma

C. Adhesions from infection

D. Priapism

14-90   *The most common gram-negative bacteria that causes both acute and chronic bacterial prostatitis is*

A. *Staphylococcus aureus.*

B. *Klebsiella.*

C. *Escherichia coli.*

D. *Enterobacteriaceae.*

14-91   *The single-most effective method of treating urinary calculi is*

A. prescribing an antibiotic.

B. having the client increase his fluid intake.

C. performing lithotripsy.

D. performing cystoscopy.

14-92   *Which of the following would enable you to rule out a diagnosis of testicular cancer when examining a client?*

A. Transillumination of the suspected mass

B. White race

C. Scandinavian background

D. History of cryptorchidism

14-93   *Sidney, age 72 presents to the clinic with complaints of a weak urine stream, hesitancy, and painful ejaculation. On digital rectal examination, you note that his prostate is boggy. The most common cause of his symptoms is*

A. acute bacterial prostatitis.

B. chronic bacterial prostatitis.

C. chronic nonbacterial prostatitis with chronic pelvic pain syndrome.

D. noninflammatory prostatitis.

14-94   *You percuss for pain at the costovertebral angle when examining Marlin. What condition are you assessing for?*

A. Urethritis

B. Pyelonephritis

C. Kidney stone

D. Bladder tumor

14-95   *When performing a rectal examination on the aging man, you may normally note*

A. fissures.

B. a smaller prostate.

C. a decrease in sphincter tone.

D. a longer anal canal.

14-96   *Max, age 70, is obese. He is complaining of a bulge in his groin that has been there for months. He states that it is not painful, but it is annoying. You note that the origin of swelling is above the inguinal ligament directly behind and through the external ring. You diagnose this as a(n)*

A. indirect inguinal hernia.

B. direct inguinal hernia.

C. femoral hernia.

D. strangulated hernia.

14-97   What differentiates prostate cancer symptoms from benign prostatic hypertrophy (BPH) symptoms?

A. Urinary frequency, hesitancy, and intermittency are much worse with prostate cancer.

B. Nocturia is worse with BPH.

C. Dribbling and a weak stream are more indicative of BPH.

D. Symptoms of prostate cancer in general tend to progress more rapidly than those of BPH.

14-98   The most accurate diagnostic tool for prostate cancer is

A. a digital rectal examination.

B. a prostate-specific antigen test.

C. a transrectal ultrasound examination.

D. a needle biopsy.

14-99   Mikey had an undescended testicle at birth, and at age 2 it remains in the inguinal region. His mother is afraid of surgery and asks for your advice. How do you respond?

A. "In many children, the testicle descends close to the sixth birthday."

B. "Even with only one normal testicle, he will have normal development."

C. "If it hasn't descended by now, it probably won't. He needs to have surgery by age 6."

D. "Don't worry; it can remain in that position forever with no problems."

14-100   Michael complains of a urinary tract infection (UTI). Which of the following is a risk factor for a UTI in men?

A. A history of circumcision

B. A history of testicular torsion

C. Homosexuality

D. Presence of a left inguinal hernia

14-101   What is the most common prostatitis syndrome found in males of any age?

A. Nonbacterial prostatitis

B. Prostatodynia

C. Acute bacterial prostatitis

D. Chronic bacterial prostatitis

14-102   George states that he heard that if he takes a certain pill, it is less likely he will need surgery for his benign prostatic hypertrophy, as well as less likely he will develop acute urinary retention. Which of the following medications has these positive outcomes because it is actually disease modifying?

A. Hytrin (terazosin)

B. Viagra (sildenafil citrate)

C. Proscar (finasteride)

D. Flomax (tamsulosin)

14-103   Marty, age 16, states that he feels like he has a "bag of worms" on his left scrotum. Even before examining him, what do you suspect?

A. A varicocele

B. A hydrocele

C. Cystic nodules

D. A spermatocele

14-104   Josh and Martha have five children and do not want any more. Josh said he heard about a no-scalpel vasectomy and asks how it works. What do you tell him?

A. "For the vasectomy to be permanent, you must have the vas deferens excised."

B. "It's safer for Martha to be sterilized."

C. "A loop of vas deferens is occluded through the scrotal skin."

D. "The testes are twisted, which occludes the vas deferens."

14-105   Mycoses commonly affect the skin in the groin. Which fungus commonly affects the scrotum?

A. Tinea cruris

B. *Candida albicans*

C. *Trichomonas*

D. *Trichophyton*

14-106   What is the most common cause of male infertility?

A. Azoospermia

B. A problem with sperm motility

C. A varicocele

D. Antisperm antibodies

14-107 *While cystitis is more commonly seen in women, there are specific risk factors for urinary tract infection in males, including which of the following?*

A. Hypospadias

B. Lack of circumcision

C. High sperm count

D. Varicocele

14-108 *Which drug reduces the size of the prostate, reduces the risk of urinary retention by increasing urinary flow rate, and reduces some of the symptoms of benign prostatic hypertrophy?*

A. Doxazosin (Cardura)

B. Prazosin (Minipress)

C. Finasteride (Proscar)

D. Terazosin (Hytrin)

14-109 *For inspecting the male genitalia, what is the ideal position for the client and examiner?*

A. The client should be in a modified lithotomy position with the examiner at the foot of the table.

B. The client should be in the dorsal recumbent position, and the examiner should approach from the left side.

C. The client should stand, and the examiner should assume a seated position in front of the client.

D. The client and examiner should both stand.

14-110 *Mr. S. is a frail, 87-year-old gentleman in your nursing home. He has a history of multiple strokes, diabetes type 2, heart disease managed medically, and hyperthyroidism. He has a life expectancy of less than 10 years. He has no overt urinary symptoms. His anxious daughter, Karen, is requesting prostate cancer screening. What would be your most appropriate response?*

A. Discuss how a positive test would not change Mr. S.'s treatment plan because his life expectancy is less than 10 years. Review the risk-benefit ratio of treatment should cancer be found and discuss this together with Mr. S.

B. Order a prostate-specific antigen (PSA) test and perform a direct rectal examination (DRE) on Mr. S.

C. Send Mr. S. for a CT scan.

D. Send Mr. S. for an MRI.

14-111 *Sildenafil (Viagra) 50 mg taken 1 hour before sexual activity is ordered for Mitchell for his erectile dysfunction. What medication must you make sure he is not taking before writing the prescription?*

A. An antihistamine

B. A nitrate

C. A stool softener

D. An anticoagulant

Answers

14-1 Answer D

Men should be advised to perform a monthly testicular self-examination and to call if they notice any hard lumps directly on the testicle, whether the lumps are tender or not. Testicles should be examined when taking a warm shower or bath with soapy hands to allow easy manipulation of the tissue. If parts of the testicle above and behind feel rather firm, this is the epididymis and is normal. The spermatic cord, a small, round, movable tube, extends up from the epididymis and feels firm and smooth.

14-2 Answer C

Staging will determine the extent of the spread of the cancer. The prostate cancer tissue is sometimes graded histologically, but the most widely used system is the Gleason system, which grades the architectural pattern of the cancer in the largest segment of the specimen and in the second-next largest area occupied, rather than histology. Five grades, which correlate to tumor volume, pathologic stage, and prognosis, are possible in each area. The scores are added together to produce a Gleason score on a scale of 1 to 10 with a score of 8–10 indicating a poorly differentiated cancer that is aggressive in nature. Another method is the TNM classification of the American Joint Cancer Committee. The TNM judges the size of the primary tumor (T), regional lymph nodes (N), and distant metastases (M). Staging does not determine the type of treatment required but helps the provider and the client discuss options available. Clients with localized prostate cancer should probably either have a surgical prostatectomy or radiotherapy. Watchful waiting has also been used at this stage. Advanced disease requires systemic chemotherapy or hormonal manipulation. Staging will not be able to establish how long a client has had prostate cancer.

14-3   Answer C

After 6 months of therapy with finasteride (Proscar) for benign prostatic hypertrophy, the prostate-specific antigen (PSA) level will decrease by about 50%. Testing can then be repeated annually. If the PSA level has not decreased, you should suspect prostate cancer and proceed to evaluate for such. Finasteride is a 5-alpha-reductase inhibitor and will affect PSA levels, as opposed to other agents such as alpha-adrenergic antagonists, which do not affect PSA levels.

14-4   Answer B

Kegel exercises are a learned technique of pelvic muscle exercises that help with urinary incontinence after 4–5 weeks of consistent daily exercise. When used with biofeedback, they can improve pelvic floor tone and reduce uninhibited bladder contractions. Biofeedback consists of capturing information about a normally unconscious physiological process and subsequently using it in an educational process to accomplish specific therapeutic results, in this case, continence. Bladder training is a form of behavioral modification that helps to restore a normal pattern of voiding and normal bladder function. Clients void at fixed intervals whether the urge to void is present or not. Prompted voiding is also a form of behavioral modification that uses a toileting schedule, verbal feedback, and reinforcement.

14-5   Answer B

Alpha blockers are an effective treatment of symptomatic benign prostatic hypertrophy. They reduce symptoms in 60%–70% of clients with nearly 50% improvement in urinary flow rates. They do not lower the blood pressure in normotensive clients. Dosing must begin with the lowest dose, preferably at bedtime, so the client will sleep through any mild adverse effects such as malaise, fatigue, dizziness, or orthostatic hypotension. Pedal edema is a rare adverse effect. Blood counts should be monitored occasionally for reduction in white or red blood cell counts.

14-6   Answer A

An unusually long foreskin or a foreskin that cannot be retracted over the glans penis during physical examination is referred to as phimosis. It occurs in uncircumcised males and is normal in infancy. At Damon's age, however, one should be able to retract the foreskin. He needs referral to a urologist. Paraphimosis occurs when the foreskin is retracted and is unable to be returned to the original position. The penis distal to the foreskin usually will become swollen and gangrenous. A microphallus is a normally formed penis that is smaller in size than expected. Priapism is a continuous and pathological erection of the penis that does not occur as a result of sexual desire.

14-7   Answer B

Men have been affected by HIV/AIDS at a significantly higher rate than women among both younger and older people but that is slowly changing. Physiologically, older adults experience a natural decline in their immune systems in addition to the process of HIV infection; there is a more rapid loss of naive CD4 cells and decrease in T-lymphocyte proliferation. Consequently, there is a more rapid disease progression found among older persons. HIV-transmission risk factors in the late middle-aged and older adult population continue to be injection drug use and same-sex relations. Transfusion of blood products has decreased to negligible as a risk factor in the United States. Recent research finds that older adults are prescribed antiretroviral therapy at equal proportions to their younger counterparts, and these treatments are equally as effective. However, persons with liver problems and on certain medications that affect the liver need to be monitored carefully.

14-8   Answer D

Bladder tumor antigen in urine is a qualitative agglutination test for bladder cancer that detects basement membrane proteins. It tests positive for symptomatic sexually transmitted disease and is also positive within 14 days of prostate biopsy or resection, with renal or bladder calculi, and with genitourinary tract cancers.

14-9   Answer B

Urethral strictures may develop as a result of sexually transmitted diseases and should be considered in a sexually active individual no matter what the age. Antihistamine use generally will result in hesitancy and urinary retention but not in incontinence. Detrusor hyperreflexia involves urge incontinence characterized by a strong, sudden urgency (not hesitancy), immediately followed by a bladder contraction, resulting in an involuntary loss of urine. Renal calculi commonly present as pain.

14-10   Answer C

Testicular cancer is suspected if a hard, fixed, nontender area or nodule is palpated on the testicle. The client should be referred for further evaluation and probably surgery. Testicular self-examination should be taught to all male clients beginning in adolescence. Testicular cancer is most common among men ages 16–35.

14-11   Answer C

A man is still capable of fertilizing an egg for weeks after a no-scalpel vasectomy; therefore, a sperm count should be obtained after 4 weeks. Sperm cannot survive in the ampulla of the vas for more than 3 weeks, and it takes about 15 ejaculations for most men to clear the ampulla of sperm. A repeat sperm count is done 2 weeks after the first, and if both show azoospermia, other contraceptive practices may be discontinued at that time.

14-12   Answer B

Pyelonephritis is a classic example of upper-tract urinary infections in the male. Pyelonephritis results from hematogenous or ascending infection. Bacteremia, particularly with virulent organisms such as *Staphylococcus aureus*, can result in pyelonephritis with focal renal abscesses. Prostatitis, epididymitis, cystitis, and urethritis are some of the lower-tract diseases that affect males.

14-13   Answer B

A chancroid is a tender, ulcerated, exudative, papular lesion with an erythematous halo, surrounding edema, and a friable base. It is caused by inoculation of *Haemophilus ducreyi* through tiny breaks in epidermal tissue. A chancre is a small papular lesion that enlarges and undergoes superficial necrosis to produce a sharply marginated ulcer on a clean base and is the lesion of primary syphilis. *Condylomata acuminatum* (genital warts) range from pinhead-size papules to cauliflower-like groupings of skin-colored, pink, or red lesions. They are caused by human papillomavirus infection of the epithelial cells. Genital herpes simplex virus appears as erythematous plaques, developing into vesicular lesions that may become pustular.

14-14   Answer C

There are five types of urinary incontinence: overflow, stress, urge, and functional, which are considered established causes of incontinence, and transient or potentially reversible causes of urinary incontinence. Overflow incontinence is caused by detrusor underactivity. There is frequent leakage of urine from the failure to fully empty the bladder, such as occurs with prostatic hypertrophy. Stress incontinence is a failure to store urine related to urethral incompetence. It may be caused by weak pelvic musculature or intrinsic or neurogenic sphincter deficiency and is commonly seen in men after radical prostatectomy. Urge incontinence caused by detrusor overactivity results in the failure to store urine, and can coexist with urethral obstruction from benign prostatic hypertrophy or be due to conditions such as Parkinson's disease, multiple sclerosis, urinary tract infection, bladder stones or tumors. Functional incontinence is caused by the effects of medications, fecal impaction, manual dexterity, or immobility. Transient incontinence is characterized by a sudden onset. Its causes in older males can include delirium, infection, pharmacologic agents, psychological factors, excess urinary output, restricted mobility, and stool impaction in hospitalized or immobile persons.

14-15   Answer B

5-Alpha-reductase inhibitors are prescribed for their ability to induce apoptosis and atrophy, as well as reduce the action of androgens in the prostate. Alpha-adrenergic blockers relax smooth muscle of the bladder and prostatic capsule, improve flow rates, and relieve obstruction.

14-16   Answer D

Antihistamines cause retention of urine by inhibiting bladder contractibility and may cause overflow incontinence in certain individuals. Other medications that may cause overflow incontinence include anticholinergics, antipsychotics, and antidepressants. Antispasmodics may cause excessive muscular relaxation and sphincter incompetency. Drugs that affect the sympathetic nervous system, such as alpha blockers, may relax the smooth muscle of the sphincter and decrease urethral pressure, which increases bladder emptying. Alpha stimulants may increase urethral closure pressure, which may lead to urinary retention. Diuretics may affect continence by causing frequent and large bladder volume that overwhelms the ability of the individual to reach the toilet in time.

14-17   Answer C

The most common type of genitourinary dysfunction occurring after a transurethral resection of the prostate is retrograde ejaculation (65%), followed by erectile dysfunction (15%), urinary incontinence (2.1%), and decreased libido (less than 2%).

14-18   Answer B

A hydrocele is a collection of fluid within the scrotum around the testes. It can be assessed by transillumination of the fluid, which should be performed in a darkened room using a penlight. The fluid will appear light pink, yellow, or red. The mass can be illuminated to show the full size and shape. Masses of the testicles, such as testicular cancer, do not transilluminate, nor do hematomas or testicular torsion. A varicocele is venous dilation of the pampiniform plexus above the testes; it is typically painful and may not be transilluminated. In infancy, observation is the therapy of choice for a hydrocele. For adults, no treatment is required unless complications are present. If the hydrocele is painful, large, unsightly, or uncomfortable, then several options are available: surgery, sclerotherapy, or an endoscopic procedure.

14-19   Answer D

The first step in diagnosing overflow incontinence is to perform a postvoid residual (PVR) urine measurement. Clients with overflow incontinence cannot empty their bladders completely, so after voiding, residual urine remains and this measurement is elevated. A urinalysis, cystometrogram, and cystoscopy are also commonly performed to confirm the cause and diagnosis, but a PVR measurement is the most important component of the diagnosis.

14-20   Answer C

Precocious puberty is present if puberty starts before age 9.5 years. Puberty is considered delayed if no testicular increase has occurred by age 13½ and if

pubic hair has not reached Tanner stage 2. Pubertal delay also occurs if the boy has not reached stage 3 within 4 years of reaching stage 2.

14-21   Answer B

Erectile dysfunction has an organic origin in approximately 70% of cases. Of those cases, approximately 80% are related to vascular problems. The most common problem is generalized atherosclerosis that interferes with normal arterial function. Other vascular etiologies include hypertension, peripheral vascular disease, arterial insufficiency, trauma, or congenital abnormalities. Neurogenic disorders of the somatic, parasympathetic (cholinergic), sympathetic, and central nervous systems can cause or contribute to erectile dysfunction. Other diseases associated with erectile dysfunction include Parkinson's disease, cerebrovascular accident, Alzheimer's disease, and diseases that create perfusion neuropathies such as diabetes and alcoholism. Erectile dysfunction is drug related in 25% of cases, with the common offenders being antihypertensive agents, NSAIDs, digoxin, antidepressants, sedatives, and antiandrogens.

14-22   Answer A

Goserelin acetate (Zoladex) and leuprolide (Lupron) block the release of FSH and LH. These preparations are administered intramuscularly. Oral antiandrogen agents such as bicalutamide (Casodex) and flutamide (Eulexin) inhibit the binding of testosterone to the cancer cells. Finasteride (Proscar) is used to block the enzyme 5-alpha-reductase, which converts testosterone into dihydrotesterone. Chemotherapy versus hormonal therapy exerts an affect on the cell cycle.

14-23   Answer A

Antiviral chemotherapy, by mouth, is the mainstay of management of genital herpes. These drugs are Acyclovir, Famciclovir, and Valacyclovir. They can partially control the signs and symptoms of herpes when used to treat the first clinical episode, as well as recurrent episodes. These drugs, however, neither eradicate latent virus nor affect the risk, frequency, or severity of recurrences after the drug is discontinued. Counseling about the natural history, sexual transmission, and methods to reduce transmission is also an important principle of management.

14-24   Answer D

Urgency, frequency, nocturia, stress incontinence, and urgency incontinence are all related to storage symptoms associated with overactive bladder in men. Voiding symptoms are related to issues with the urethra and sphincter control and include hesitancy, poor flow, intermittency, straining, and dysuria. Postmicturition symptoms include postvoid dribble and a sense of incomplete emptying.

14-25   Answer D

Melena is black, tarry stool caused by upper gastrointestinal bleeding. Grayish-tan stool is caused by obstructive jaundice; bright-red stool results from rectal bleeding; and pale-yellow, greasy, fatty stool (steatorrhea) is caused by malabsorption syndromes such as cystic fibrosis or celiac disease.

14-26   Answer A

The patient's symptoms appear to be related to benign prostatic hypertrophy (BPH) and not a urinary tract infection. An alpha-adrenergic blocker will relax prostate and bladder smooth muscle to improve flow and relieve symptoms. Saw palmetto extract is an alternative treatment that has not been proven to improve urinary symptoms in men with BPH, and its long-term side effects have not been studied. BPH can be successfully treated by primary health-care providers, and a referral is not appropriate until standard treatment is no longer effective.

14-27   Answer A

The NPTR (nocturnal penile tumescence and rigidity test) is a simple test the client may do at home by himself to determine if he has the ability to have a nocturnal erection, which would rule out an organic and psychogenic cause of erectile dysfunction. At night, have the client place a simple device attached to the penis before sleep. This device records the frequency, as well as the rigidity, of erections. Other tests that may be done to determine the cause of erectile dysfunction, but are not as simple, include the penile Doppler test (a noninvasive procedure comparing the penile pressure with the brachial artery pressure), a penile duplex ultrasonography (to assess the penile arteries and diagnose a vascular cause of erectile dysfunction), and an intracavernosal injection (to test for an erection, thus ruling out vascular disease). A PSA does not evaluate erectile dysfunction.

14-28   Answer A

Testicular torsion is a condition in which the testes twist on the spermatic cord, thereby compromising blood flow to the testes. This is a surgical emergency. Examination usually reveals a tender scrotal mass high in the hemiscrotum, and there is frequently a reactive hydrocele around the testes obscuring anatomical detail. The scrotum can become erythematous and edematous. The cremaster reflex is frequently blunted on the side of the torsion. Epididymitis usually is accompanied by fever, as well as urethral discharge, and usually occurs in boys older than Tommy. Although a hydrocele may develop secondary to the torsion, the intense discomfort and acute onset accompanied often by nausea distinguish the possibility of testicular torsion. A varicocele, which usually occurs in young men, may cause pain but does not usually develop acutely.

14-29   Answer C

A *Candida* infection is fairly common in clients with diabetes. *Candida* on the penis appears as multiple, discrete, flat pustules with slight scaling and surrounding edema. It is a superficial mycotic infection that occurs in moist cutaneous sites. Other predisposing factors may include moisture, antibiotic therapy, and immunosuppression. Tinea cruris is a fungal infection of the groin that appears as erythematous plaques whose scaling, papular lesions have sharp margins and occasionally clear centers. Genital herpes is caused by skin-to-skin contact with the herpes simplex virus. It causes epidermal degeneration and erythematous plaques; the plaques develop into vesicular lesions that may become pustular. Intraepithelial neoplasia is associated with chronic human papillomavirus (HPV) infection and presents as multiple red maculopapular plaque–like lesions on the glans and inner aspect of the foreskin.

14-30   Answer C

Chancroid, genital herpes, and syphilis are cofactors for HIV transmission. In the United States, about 10% of persons who have chancroid are co-infected with *Treponema pallidum* (syphilis) or HSV (herpes simplex virus). This percentage is higher in persons who have acquired chancroid outside the United States.

14-31   Answer D

If surgery for benign prostatic hypertrophy is not mandated by obstruction or severe symptoms, it is based on the results of the client's American Urological Association (AUA) scale and the client's choice. If the AUA score is 7 or lower, no treatment is indicated. If the score is 8–19 (moderate) or 20–35 (severe), then medical treatment or surgery can be presented to the client as an option.

14-32   Answer A

Infertility is defined as 1 year of unprotected intercourse in which conception has not occurred. Although routine tests, such as thyroid studies, may be performed, a specialist will usually not see a couple until they have been trying to conceive for 1 year. Although you may ask how often they have been having intercourse—because once a month is certainly different from 3 times a week—the definition of infertility remains the same. The cause of infertility is found in the man 26%–30% of the time, and most specialists perform a comprehensive diagnostic evaluation on both members of the couple.

14-33   Answer C

A client presenting with a urethral discharge or difficulty voiding can include acute and chronic prostatitis and prostatic abscess. Young adult males in their 20s usually have acute prostatitis from gonorrhea or other bacterial infections. Chronic prostatitis occurs in middle age males as a result of nonspecific prostatitis or a previous gonorrhea infection. Older males may have prostatic hypertrophy or prostatic cancer and these diagnoses are not related with urethral discharge.

14-34   Answer D

Epispadias means that the urethral meatus opens on the dorsal side of the glans. Hypospadias means that the urethral meatus opens on the ventral side of the glans. Both must be reported to the physician because a circumcision should not be performed until these conditions are corrected. Peyronie's disease is a condition of penile curvature that occurs with erection. Priapism is a continuous and pathological erection of the penis.

14-35   Answer C

About 50% of men who have had diabetes for longer than 6 years develop erectile dysfunction to some extent as a result of pathological changes in the vascular wall, which lead to a reduction of arterial blood flow to the penis. Many other conditions can cause erectile dysfunction. They include cerebrovascular accidents, spinal cord injury, temporal lobe epilepsy, multiple sclerosis, chronic obstructive pulmonary disease, angina, chronic renal failure, and Parkinson's disease.

14-36   Answer B

Sudden onset of weakness in the lower extremities can indicate metastasis to the spine with possible cord compression. Bladder outlet obstruction (BOO) can have either a bacterial or physiological etiology and does not necessarily indicate a metastatic process. Gleason scores have been used to stage cancers; a score of 4–5 (not a 2) would indicate that a metastatic process is likely. Likewise, the TNM staging system (tumor, node, and metastasis) indicates tumor size and gland involvement, node metastasis, and distant metastasis. T1a, N0, M0 indicates carcinoma in 5% or less of tissue resected with a normal DRE, no regional lymph node metastasis, and no distant metastasis.

14-37   Answer C

Combination therapy with an alpha blocker such as terazosin (Hytrin) or finasteride (Proscar) is not supported by the literature. One study showed no improvement when combination therapy was tried. Combination therapy involves extra expense and increased risk of adverse effects and has unproven effectiveness; therefore, it should not be used until successful trials have ensued.

14-38   Answer B

Bowel sounds may be heard over a hernia but not over a hydrocele. Some hernias are not able to be returned to the abdominal cavity. A hernia is incarcerated when its contents cannot be returned; it is strangulated when the blood supply to the entrapped contents is compromised. Scrotal swellings containing serous fluid such as a hydrocele transilluminate, whereas those containing blood or tissue do not. A bulge that appears on straining suggests a hernia.

14-39   Answer A

Bloody penile discharge requires close investigation, including the length of time of the discharge. Ulcerations, neoplasms, and urethritis are all common causes of bloody penile discharge. Bloody penile discharge is not usually seen in herpes zoster, epididymitis or Peyronie's disease.

14-40   Answer A

Chronic bacterial prostatitis may have a variety of clinical presentations, but nausea and vomiting, loss of appetite and weight loss, as well as an inability to ambulate are rarely among the presenting symptoms of this disorder. Even fever is typically not present in chronic cases. Typically, there are irritative voiding symptoms that have persisted over time, low back pain, and perineal pain, although any one, or all, may be present. Sometimes clients are completely asymptomatic, although bacteria might be present on urinalysis, and expressed prostatic secretions usually demonstrate increased numbers of leukocytes. Physical examination may be unremarkable as well, although in some cases the prostate will feel boggy or indurated. There is often a history of repeated urinary tract infections. Cystitis and/or chronic urethritis may be secondary or mimic prostatitis; however, cultures of the fractionated urine may localize the source of infection. Anal disease may share some of the symptoms of prostatitis, but physical examination should permit a distinction between the two.

14-41   Answer C

Other differential diagnoses for symptoms classically seen in men with benign prostatic hypertrophy, such as difficulty initiating stream, hesitancy, urgency, post void dribbling, frequency, nocturia, retention, sensation of a full bladder immediately after voiding, and incontinence, include diabetes mellitus, cancer of the prostate, and some neurological diseases that can lead to voiding disorders. Testicular cancer, balanitis, and epididymitis do not typically cause this array of symptoms.

14-42   Answer D

Prostatodynia is a condition in which the client experiences the symptoms of prostatitis but demonstrates no evidence of infection or inflammation. Prostatitis may be acute bacterial, chronic bacterial, or nonbacterial (the most common type).

14-43   Answer D

Bacterial prostatitis, in which the prostate feels very tender and warm, is usually caused by *Escherichia coli*. Clients with bacterial prostatitis usually also have a sudden onset of high fever, chills, malaise, myalgias, and arthralgias. In benign prostatic hypertrophy, the prostate gland would feel soft and nontender and would be enlarged. With prostatic abscess, the prostate feels like a firm, tender, or fluctuant mass. With prostate cancer, the prostate may have single or multiple nodules that are firm, hard, or indurated and are usually nontender.

14-44   Answer B

Because sexual stimulation leads to the release of nitric oxide in the corpus cavernosum of the penis and sildenafil (Viagra) potentiates that release, there is a double hypotensive effect between sildenafil and the presence of an existing nitric oxide such as isosorbide mononitrate (Monoket, Imdur, Ismo). Therefore, the use of sildenafil with Monoket is contraindicated. Sildenafil is not contraindicated in clients who consume nitrates in food.

14-45   Answer D

A fasting blood sugar to rule out diabetes mellitus, lipid profile to rule out dyslipidemia, and thyroid-stimulating hormone and testosterone levels are the initial laboratory test that should be done to rule out causes of erectile dysfunction (ED). If the testosterone level is below 300 ng/dl, then a serum prolactin level is warranted. In a male with established ED, a CBC, blood chemistry profile including fasting glucose or glycosylated hemoglobin level, TSH and PSA are frequently recommended. Specialized tests such as the color Doppler sonogram or NPRT can be done if the cause of ED is not apparent from the above standard tests.

14-46   Answer B

Vascular diseases account for nearly half of all cases of erectile dysfunction. These include atherosclerosis, peripheral vascular disease, myocardial infarction, and arterial hypertension. Less frequent but nonetheless important factors include systemic diseases such as diabetes, scleroderma, renal failure, and liver cirrhosis and neurogenic diseases such as epilepsy, stroke, multiple sclerosis, and Alzheimer's disease. Other contributing factors include psychiatric conditions and penile, endocrine, nutritional, hematological, and medication-associated causes.

14-47   Answer B

The following medications have been shown to cause erectile dysfunction (ED): antiandrogens; antihypertensives such as beta blockers and central sympatholytics (Reserpine); anticholinergics;

antidepressants; antipsychotics; central nervous system depressants; and drugs of abuse such as alcohol, tobacco, and heroin. Diuretics, proton pump inhibitors, and vasodilators have not been shown to cause ED.

14-48 Answer D

Tuberculous epididymitis is a chronic inflammation of tuberculosis. It produces a firm enlargement of the epididymis, which is usually tender, and thickening or beading of the vas deferens. A hydrocele is a nontender, fluid-filled mass that is in the space within the tunica vaginalis. A spermatocele is a painless, movable cystic mass just above the testis. A tumor of the testis is usually a painless nodule.

14-49 Answer D

The foreskin of the penis is not fully retractable until age 1 year. Diaper rash can cause balanitis, an acute inflammation of the glans penis. Uncircumcised clients may develop phimosis after balanitis.

14-50 Answer A

Conditions outside of the scrotum that may present with scrotal pain are abdominal aortic aneurysm, inguinal herniation, pancreatitis, renal colic, peritonitis, intraperitoneal hemorrhage, and polyarteritis nodosa. Keep in mind that any client with scrotal pain should be considered to have testicular torsion until proved otherwise, especially in the age groups of the neonate and adolescents.

14-51 Answer C

A subnormal level of testosterone causes metabolic changes that produce changes in male physiology, growth, and behavior. Common clinical symptoms of testosterone deficiency are loss of libido, erectile dysfunction, decreased lean body mass, body hair and skin alterations, decreased bone mineral density, increased visceral fat, infertility, depression, and reduced cognition.

14-52 Answer B

The complete sequence of anatomical changes that occur in the male genitalia from preadolescence to adulthood requires approximately 3 years (with a range of 1.8–5 years). There are five Tanner stages related to sex maturity in boys. The first change begins in preadolescence with fine vellus hair in the pubic area. In stage 2 there is sparse growth of pigmented hair at the base of the penis with an increase in the size of the testes. The pubic hair becomes darker and coarser as it spreads over the pubic symphysis in stage 3. The penis lengthens with the testes and scrotum becoming further enlarged. Next, pubic hair coverage continues except for the thigh area. Also in stage 4 the penis enlarges in length and breadth with development of the glans. The scrotal skin darkens. Finally, in Tanner stage 5, the pubic hair spreads to the medial surface of the thighs and the penis, testes and scrotum are adult size and shape.

14-53 Answer B

Athletes who run long distances and those who perform vigorous exercises and workout regimens have a predisposition to prostatitis. Prostatitis, both bacterial and nonbacterial, occurs predominantly between ages 30 and 50 in sexually active men.

14-54 Answer C

In the aging male, the physiological changes that occur include bladder capacity reduction, a decreased ratio of density of smooth muscle to connective tissue, decreased detrusor contractility, and increased postvoid residual volumes. With benign prostatic hypertrophy, lower urinary tract symptoms increase because of obstructive changes.

14-55 Answer B

Balanoposthitis is inflammation of the glans and prepuce. Balanitis is inflammation of the glans. Phimosis is a tight prepuce that cannot be retracted over the glans. Paraphimosis is a tight prepuce that, once retracted, gets caught behind the glans and cannot be returned, resulting in edema.

14-56 Answer D

The obstructive causes of lower urinary tract symptoms (LUTS) are bladder outlet obstruction from benign prostatic hypertrophy, a poorly contractile bladder, prostate cancer, bladder neck or urethral strictures, and neurogenic bladder. Bladder cancer, bladder stones, and infection are classified as irritative or storage causes of LUTS.

14-57 Answer A

If a client has symptoms of benign prostatic hypertrophy, a digital rectal examination (DRE) is performed to detect prostate or rectal malignancy and evaluate anal sphincter tone. Hypospadias is a disorder in which the meatus of the urethra is inferiorly located on the glans. A DRE does not rule out urethritis.

14-58   Answer A

Various disorders, including diabetes, hyperthyroidism, and HIV infection, can affect circulating testosterone levels. Neither urinary tract infections, heart disease, nor cholecystitis has been known to cause androgen deficiency. Other causes include a decrease in secretion of gonadotropin-releasing hormone from the hypothalamus; certain medications; and lifestyle factors including morbid obesity, tobacco use, alcoholism, and psychological stress.

14-59   Answer C

The treatment of choice for the client with condylomata acuminata (warts) on the external genitalia is to "paint" them with podophyllum in benzoin. The client should wash the medication off in 1–2 hours because normal tissue may be destroyed along with the warts. Sometimes a repeat treatment is necessary. Carbon dioxide laser treatment might be more effective.

14-60   Answer C

Benign prostatic hypertrophy is the most common cause of urologic incontinence in men. The enlarged prostate obstructs the bladder neck, resulting in a sensation of incomplete emptying. This results in hypertrophy of the pelvic muscle, which produces more forceful and uninhibited contractions, leading to urgency. Overflow incontinence is concomitant with this obstruction of the bladder neck. Urethritis, or inflammation of the ureter, can be a transient cause of incontinence, but it is not that frequent. Although prostate cancer does not usually cause incontinence, the surgery for it might. If the nerves that supply the bladder or urethral sphincter are damaged during surgery, incontinence may persist after surgery. Chronic bacteriuria is common in older adults, but research has not shown a link between urinary incontinence and the presence of chronic asymptomatic bacteriuria.

14-61   Answer C

Finasteride is a 5-alpha reductase inhibitor and recommended for individuals with prostate greater than 40 ml to help decrease its size.

According to the current AUA guideline for the management of benign prostatic hypertrophy (BPH), there is insufficient evidence to support the use of either phenoxybenzamine or prazosin in the management of BPH with lower urinary tract symptoms. Doxazosin is associated with a risk of orthostatic hypotension and thus would not be recommended in this client.

14-62   Answer A

The most common cause of gross hematuria is bladder infection (22%), followed by bladder tumor (14.9%), benign prostatic hyperplasia (12.5%), and prostatitis (9%).

14-63   Answer A

Lymph nodes in the inguinal area, if small and mobile, are not considered abnormal. The lymphatics from the perineum, legs, and feet drain into this area, and thus it is not surprising that small lymph nodes are frequently encountered.

14-64   Answer A

Asymptomatic clients with benign prostatic hypertrophy (BPH) rarely require treatment. Watchful waiting is an appropriate strategy for following the disease's progression and the development of any complications. Prostate surgery offers the best choice for symptom improvement. A transurethral resection of the prostate is the most commonly used surgical treatment for BPH. Balloon dilation of the prostatic urethra has fewer complications than surgery but is not as effective in relieving the symptoms. Alpha blockers relax the bladder neck and prostate smooth muscle and offer relief for many clients, particularly in regard to nocturia.

14-65   Answer B

The axial skeleton is the most common site of metastasis in prostate cancer. Be alert to signs such as back pain, pathological fractures, or radiculopathies. The lymph nodes are also sites of metastasis, causing lymphedema.

14-66   Answer C

Many clients feel more comfortable talking to their primary care provider, with whom they have an established relationship, than to their surgeon, and the question of when to resume sex after prostate surgery for benign prostatic hypertrophy is no exception. They may not feel comfortable asking their surgeon; thus, they may resume sexual activity too early or wait an exorbitant amount of time. Within 4–6 weeks after surgery, it is safe to resume a full sex life including intercourse. Before this time, the spasmodic contractions that occur in the prostatic urethra at the time of ejaculation could trigger delayed bleeding. After 6 weeks, the risk of delayed bleeding is very slight. There may be slight discomfort because of the spasm if the area has not completely healed.

14-67 Answer B

Cryptorchidism, failure of one or both of the testes to descend into the scrotum, is a risk factor for testicular cancer. Most testicular tumors are malignant. Testicular cancer is the most common solid tumor in young men ages 16–35. It begins as an irregular, nontender mass fixed on the testes that does not transilluminate.

14-68 Answer B

An external vacuum device is a viable method for alleviating erectile dysfunction regardless of the cause of the disorder. A plastic cylinder is placed around the penis, a vacuum pump causes cavernosal engorgement, and a constrictor ring is applied around the base of the penis, allowing the client to hold an erection for 30 minutes. Intracavernous injection therapy consists of injecting the vasoactive drug alprostadil (Caverject) directly into the corpus cavernosum of the penis, causing an erection that lasts 40–60 minutes. Urethral suppositories such as alprostadil are also effective in causing an erection when inserted into the urethra after voiding. Surgery involves inserting a penile prosthesis, of which there are many different types.

14-69 Answer C

Asking about leakage or wetting accidents are useful questions about urge urinary incontinence that will assist in the diagnosis of overactive bladder in men. The other questions also are used to diagnosis the condition but are specific to urgency, frequency and nocturia.

14-70 Answer B

In Tanner stage 2, there is sparse growth of long, slightly pigmented, downy hair, straight or only slightly curled, chiefly at the base of the penis. There is slight or no enlargement of the penis, the testes are larger, and the scrotum is larger, somewhat reddened, and altered in texture.

14-71 Answer B

If your client has a rapid onset of unilateral scrotal pain radiating up to the groin and flank and you are trying to differentiate between epididymitis and testicular torsion, an ultrasound test is useful to determine whether the swelling is in the testis or the epididymis and should be your first choice. Initially, before the swelling has reached its peak, a physical examination will probably differentiate, but within a few hours, when the testis also swells, it may not be possible to differentiate between epididymis and testis by palpation. A reactive hydrocele may also develop. A technetium scan will show an increased uptake in the case of epididymitis and decreased uptake in the case of torsion, but the least invasive and most inexpensive test is an ultrasound.

14-72 Answer B

Genital herpes begins with a tender, painful ulcer on the penis. Most other conditions begin with nontender, painless lesions such as those found with syphilitic chancre, carcinoma of the penis, Peyronie's disease, and venereal warts.

14-73 Answer C

Balanitis is a cutaneous inflammation of the glans penis, and *Candida* usually plays a role. Treatment usually involves a topical antifungal ointment as initial treatment if lesions show mild erythema or shallow erosions. Chronic balanitis suggests relapse, especially from a sexual partner. This suggests the partner needs to be treated. Severe purulent balanitis suggests a bacterial cause. If severe enough to cause phimosis, oral antibiotics are indicated.

14-74 Answer C

The two seminal vesicles project above the prostate and secrete a fluid rich in fructose, which nourishes the sperm. They also contain and release prostaglandins. Semen is produced by the testicles. The bulbourethral (Cowper's) glands secrete clear mucus for motility of sperm.

14-75 Answer D

Colic is the main presenting symptom of urinary stone disease and usually occurs suddenly, even awakening clients from sleep. The pain is sudden and severe and often accompanied by nausea and vomiting. These clients are constantly moving in contrast to those with acute abdominal pain who "guard" their abdomen and try not to move, each movement eliciting increased pain. Although the pain may occur episodically, it is not a chronic pain.

14-76   Answer B

In the early stages of prostate cancer, the tumor is androgen dependent. Testosterone is the major androgen, and clients who have undergone an orchiectomy before puberty never develop adenocarcinoma of the prostate.

14-77   Answer B

The testes most commonly descend from the retroperitoneal space through the inguinal canal and into the scrotal sacs during the third trimester. In some cases, one or both testes may still lie within the inguinal canal at birth, with the final descent into the scrotum occurring during the early neonatal period. Descent of the testicles may be arrested at any point or may follow an abnormal path.

14-78   Answer B

Phenylephrine (Neo-Synephrine) is the drug of choice for first-line treatment of low-flow priapism because the drug has almost pure alpha-agonist effects and minimal beta activity. In short-term priapism (less than 6 h), especially for drug-induced priapism, intracavernosal injection of phenylephrine alone may result in detumescence. Terbutaline is considered for refractory priapism of greater than 6 hours in duration. Doxazosin is used to treat benign prostatic hypertrophy. Lidocaine is not considered to be efficacious for relief of priapism.

14-79   Answer D

The prostate should not be massaged in acute bacterial prostatitis because it may cause bacteremia and sepsis. In homosexual relationships among men, this is an important educational component. Antibiotics should be ordered, as well as supportive therapy such as rest, analgesics, hydration, and stool softeners.

14-80   Answer D

In Peyronie's disease, the client has palpable, nontender, hard plaques just beneath the dorsal skin of the penis and usually complains of crooked, painful erections. With carcinoma of the penis, there is usually an indurated, nontender nodule or ulcer, and usually the man is uncircumcised. Genital herpes appears as a cluster of small vesicles, followed by shallow, painful, nonindurated ulcers on red

bases. They may appear anywhere on the penis, and the initial outbreak is usually the worst. A syphilitic chancre is an oval or round, dark red, painless erosion or ulcer with an indurated base. It feels like a button that is lying directly underneath the skin. It may also be associated with nontender, enlarged inguinal lymph nodes.

14-81   Answer B

Orchitis is an acute, painful onset of swelling of the testicle accompanied by warm scrotal skin. The client usually complains of a heavy feeling in the scrotum. It is typically unilateral but after 1 week may progress to the other testicle. In cryptorchidism, one or both testicles are undescended. Testicular torsion is a twisting or torsion of the testis. The testicle is enlarged, retracted, in a lateral position, and extremely sensitive. The result is venous obstruction, secondary edema, and eventual arterial obstruction. It is a surgical emergency. Epididymitis is caused by a retrograde spreading of pathogenic organisms from the urethra to the epididymis. It results in an indurated, swollen, and tender epididymis. The testes are also usually enlarged and tender.

14-82   Answer A

Although watchful waiting is an option for very slow-growing, localized lesions, a radical prostatectomy or radiation can be curative. The age of the client and other factors are taken into consideration and in some cases, watchful waiting is considered a better option. Chemotherapy is palliative and reserved for later stages of metastasis. Cryosurgery is most successful when the entire gland is frozen.

14-83   Answer D

The external genitalia are identical for males and females at 8 weeks' gestational age, but by 12 weeks sexual differentiation has occurred. Any fetal insult during weeks 8 and 9 of gestation may lead to major anomalies of the external genitalia.

14-84   Answer B

Testicular torsion or torsion of the testicle on its spermatic cord is the most common scrotal disorder in adolescents. It produces an acutely painful, tender, and swollen scrotum. Because of the potential of circulation being constricted, it is a surgical emergency. Acute epididymitis occurs chiefly in adults and is an acutely inflamed epididymis that is tender and swollen. Atrophic testes are small, soft testes associated with several conditions, such as cirrhosis, myotonia dystrophia, administration of estrogens, and hypopituitarism. Scrotal edema is usually associated with generalized edema in adults and is usually related to cardiac or nephrotic conditions.

14-85 Answer D

With mild symptoms of benign prostatic hyperplasia (BPH) and an AUA index of 7 or lower, watchful waiting is recommended. If a client has moderate to severe symptoms and AUA index of 8 or higher, noninvasive medical therapy is still an option as is minimally invasive therapies or surgery. The presence of refractory retention or any of the following clearly related to BPH require referral to surgery; persistent gross hematuria, bladder stones, recurrent urinary tract infections, and/or renal insufficiency. Irritative symptoms are usually what the client will present with for further assessment to diagnosis BPH or other conditions.

14-86 Answer A

An indirect inguinal hernia is the most common type of hernia affecting all ages and both genders and accounts for 50% of hernias treated. The point of origin is above the inguinal ligament and often travels into the scrotum. A direct inguinal hernia is less common (accounts for about 25% of hernias seen) and usually occurs in men older than age 40. The point of origin is above the inguinal ligament and rarely travels into the scrotum. The femoral hernia is the least common (about 10% of hernias seen) and occurs more often in women than in men. The point of origin is below the inguinal ligament and never travels into the scrotum in men. An umbilical hernia occurs more frequently in infants and is a protrusion of part of the intestine at the umbilicus.

14-87 Answer C

After palpating the prostate gland, which is the first step in evaluating a male client complaining of stress urinary incontinence, you should evaluate the autonomic arch innervating the bladder by testing the bulbocavernous reflex. By squeezing the glans penis, you should note contraction of the anal sphincter in an individual without incontinence. An absent reflex suggests that there has been an interruption of the normal neuronal arch. If the individual is able to contract the rectal sphincter voluntarily, neuronal competence is also positive.

14-88 Answer B

Urge incontinence results from overactive bladder (OAB) and has many possible etiologies, each of which causes the bladder muscle (detrusor) to contract spontaneously. Common nonneurogenic causes are bladder irritants, infection, medications, urethritis, and pelvic tumors. Neurogenic causes involve the loss of cortical inhibition of the voiding reflex; this is seen in conditions such as dementia, Parkinson's disease, multiple sclerosis, and stroke. Stress incontinence is a result of failure of the urethral sphincter, producing leakage with maneuvers that increase intra-abdominal pressure, such as coughing or sneezing. Overflow incontinence is the result of leakage when the bladder is overdistended due to states such as a spinal cord injury (causing abnormal innervation between the bladder and spinal cord) or obstruction from a large prostate or tumor. Mixed incontinence is a combination of stress and urge types.

14-89 Answer C

Phimosis, defined as inability to retract the foreskin of the penis, may be caused by a congenital malformation or, secondarily, by adhesions resulting from infections. It normally takes until age 1 year for complete retraction of the foreskin. Paraphimosis is the term used to refer to the inability to replace the foreskin, once retracted, because of edema of the glans. (If examining an unconscious client, be sure to return the foreskin to its usual state; failure to do this may result in severe edema). Smegma refers to the cheesy, white material under the foreskin, which does not in and of itself cause phimosis. Priapism is a prolonged, generally painful erection, usually unaccompanied by sexual desire.

14-90 Answer C

The most common gram-negative bacterium that causes both acute and chronic bacterial prostatitis is *Escherichia coli*. The other aerobic gram-negative bacteria include *Klebsiella*, *Pseudomonas*, *Enterobacteriaceae*, *Proteus mirabilis*, and *Neisseria gonorrhoeae*. Occasionally other bacteria (*Staphylococcus aureus* and *Streptococcus faecalis*) are causes.

14-91 Answer B

The single-most effective method of treating urinary calculi is having the client increase fluid intake to 3–4 L/day. If increased hydration is not effective, a cystoscopy, lithotripsy, or other surgery may need to be performed. Antibiotics are not indicated.

14-92   Answer A

Transillumination is not clinically significant because a cancerous tumor cannot be successfully transilluminated. The only undisputed risk factors that have been proved for testicular cancer are white race, especially Scandinavian background, and a history of undescended or partially descended testicles (cryptorchidism).

14-93   Answer B

Chronic bacterial prostatitis, a recurrent bacterial infection of the prostate and urinary tract affects men aged 50–80. It is accompanied by bladder obstruction symptoms such as weak urine stream, hesitancy or dribbling, hematuria, hematospermia, and/or painful ejaculation. The most common offending pathogen is *Escherichia coli*. Acute bacterial prostatitis primarily affects men in the fourth to sixth decade of life. It manifests with sudden onset of symptoms including fever, malaise, dysuria, low back pain and/or perineal prostatic pain. The prostate usually feels tender, warm, and edematous. Chronic nonbacterial prostatitis with chronic pelvic pain syndrome is manifested by pelvic pain and maybe accompanied by various complaints such as mild low backache, hematospermia but may or may not have obstructive voiding symptoms. This condition is subdivided into inflammatory or noninflammatory prostatitis. The prostate usually feels normal on examination with noninflammatory chronic prostatitis.

14-94   Answer B

Pyelonephritis typically begins with costovertebral angle (CVA) pain, fever, low back pain, general malaise, and often dysuria, nausea, and vomiting, or diarrhea. Physical examination may reveal flushing, tachycardia, hypotension, fever, and signs of dehydration. With urethritis, there is typically burning on urination and a urethral discharge. Kidney stones usually result in pain that "travels" as the stone moves from the kidney to the bladder to the urethra. A bladder tumor usually causes no pain and the initial sign is typically hematuria.

14-95   Answer C

An aging person may have decreased sphincter control. You may also note a relaxation of the perianal musculature during Valsalva's maneuver. Otherwise, the examination is the same as in younger men.

14-96   Answer B

A direct inguinal hernia usually occurs in middle-aged to older men and is the result of an acquired weakness caused by heavy lifting, obesity, or chronic obstructive pulmonary disease (COPD). The origin of swelling is above the inguinal ligament directly behind and through the external ring. An indirect inguinal hernia is congenital or acquired and is more common in infants younger than 1 year of age and in men ages 16–25. The origin of swelling is above the inguinal ligament. The hernia sac enters the canal at the internal ring and exits at the external ring. A femoral hernia, which occurs more frequently in women, is acquired and results from an increase in abdominal pressure, as well as muscle weakness. The origin of swelling is below the inguinal ligament. Because Max is not having any pain and the condition has been this way for months, you know that the hernia is not strangulated. A strangulated hernia, which requires immediate referral to a surgeon, results in no blood supply to the affected bowel and causes nausea, vomiting, and tenderness.

14-97   Answer D

Symptoms of prostate cancer can mimic the symptoms of benign prostatic hypertrophy (BPH); however, with prostate cancer in general, the symptoms tend to progress more rapidly as compared with those of BPH. Symptoms of both prostate cancer and BPH include urinary frequency, hesitancy, intermittency, nocturia, dribbling, and a weak urinary stream.

14-98   Answer D

A needle biopsy takes a histological sampling of the prostate gland and is diagnostic for prostate cancer. Digital rectal examination (DRE) detection rates are low and find most cancers in the later stages. Additionally, a large number of actual prostate cancers are associated with a normal DRE. An extremely elevated prostatic-specific antigen (PSA) level usually indicates prostate cancer; however, about 25% of men with prostate cancer will have a normal PSA level. Other conditions, such as benign prostatic hypertrophy, may raise the PSA level. Transrectal ultrasound is most commonly used to guide the needle biopsy; however, it is not a very accurate screening or diagnostic tool in and of itself.

14-99   Answer C

In boys with undescended testes, less than 1% have their testes descend after the first year. Orchiopexy needs to be performed before age 6 to promote normal spermatogenesis and hormone production, prevent tumor formation, and leave the testis in a location where it can be easily palpated. Testes that remain undescended by puberty should be removed.

14-100   Answer C

Young men can develop a urinary tract infection (UTI), similar to the type of uncomplicated UTI seen in women, which does not require any additional work-up. Risk factors include homosexuality, lack of circumcision, a history of prostatitis, unprotected intercourse with a woman who harbors pathogens in her vagina, and sex with men with AIDS with a CD4 count less than 200/mL. Testicular torsion, a surgical emergency, is not a risk factor. Inguinal hernias have no documented impact on the development of urinary tract infections given anatomical proximity.

14-101   Answer A

Chronic nonbacterial prostatitis is the most common of the prostatitis syndromes. It is eight times more frequent that bacterial prostatitis. The cause is not completely understood, though atypical organisms, viruses, inflammatory processes, and autoimmune disorders have been postulated. Prostatodynia presents with signs and symptoms of prostatitis but no evidence of inflammation. Acute and chronic bacterial prostatitis are both caused by an infection from either aerobic gram negative or gram positive bacteria.

14-102   Answer C

In a long-term (4-year) study in men with symptoms of urinary obstruction and prostatic enlargement, treatment with finasteride (Proscar), a 5-alpha-reductase inhibitor, reduced symptoms and prostate volume, increased urinary flow rate, and reduced the probability of surgery and acute urinary retention. No other therapies have been shown to decrease the incidence of acute urinary retention in long-term studies. Reducing the risk of acute urinary retention has implications for reducing morbidity, as well as reducing the number of men who need surgery. Previously, finasteride was used only for short intervals, but current data show that it is safe for long-term trials. Although alpha-adrenergic blockers (terazosin, tamsulosin) also provide symptomatic relief, they have not been shown to reduce the need for surgery.

14-103   Answer A

A varicocele is enlargement of the veins of the spermatic cord that commonly occurs on the left side in adolescent males. It seldom requires treatment. A hydrocele is an accumulation of fluid between the two layers of the tunica vaginalis. It may occur on its own or in response to trauma, inguinal surgery, epididymitis, or testicular tumor. Cystic nodules are round, firm sebaceous cysts that are confined within the scrotal skin. A spermatocele results from blockage of the efferent ductules of the rete testis. It causes a sperm-filled cyst to be formed at the top of the testis or in the epididymis.

14-104   Answer C

A no-scalpel vasectomy (NSV) is a method of delivering a loop of vas deferens through the scrotal skin for occlusion. The skin is stretched to create an opening, which speeds the procedure and avoids the need for cutting through tissue. Postoperative complications are minimized this way. It does result in permanent sterility. Because there is no excision, the NSV is safer than a tubal ligation would be for a woman. Minimal postoperative complications include swelling, bruising, and pain in the scrotal area.

14-105   Answer B

Tinea cruris ("jock itch") tends to affect the groin, whereas *Candida albicans* commonly affects the scrotum. *Trichomonas* infection does not evidence itself as a skin rash. *Trichophyton* causes tinea of the feet.

14-106   Answer C

The most common cause of male infertility is a varicocele. Other causes include oligospermia or azoospermia, problems with sperm function or motility, abnormalities of sperm morphology, and, rarely, an antisperm antibody.

14-107   Answer B

There is a higher incidence of urinary tract infections (UTIs) in the uncircumcised male. The mucosal surface of the foreskin has a propensity for colonization with P-fimbriated bacteria in a fashion analogous to that of the female introitus. Hypospadias does not increase the risk of UTI. There is no correlation between a high sperm count and UTI, although the prostate in normal males secretes zinc, a potent antibacterial agent. Varicocele is also not considered a risk factor for UTI.

14-108   Answer C

Finasteride (Proscar) is a 5-alpha-reductase inhibitor that blocks conversion of testosterone to dihydrotestosterone. It reduces the size of the prostate, relieves pressure on the bladder and urethra, reduces the risk of urinary retention, and results in a reduction of the symptoms of benign prostatic hypertrophy. Usually 6 months or more of treatment are required for maximal effects. Doxazosin (Cardura), prazosin (Minipress), and terazosin (Hytrin) are all alpha-adrenergic receptor blockers that relax the bladder neck and prostate smooth muscle. They also relieve some of the symptoms but do not affect the size of the prostate.

14-109   Answer C

To allow an effective visual inspection of the male genitalia, the client should stand in front of the examiner and the examiner should assume a seated position in front of the client. If the client is unable to stand or the examination continues with the client lying, a supine position is best.

14-110   Answer A

The position of the American Urological Association and the American Medical Association is an annual PSA test for all men older than 50 years of age and after age 40 for men in high-risk populations, such as African Americans and those with a positive family history. In practice, and suggested by the American College of

Physicians and other groups, testing is usually limited to those with a life expectancy of more than 10 years because of treatment risks. If this client had obstructive symptoms, a consult to urology would be appropriate. If this client were a nonfrail 87-year-old with minimal comorbidities, a PSA and DRE would be acceptable practice if agreed to by the client.

14-111   Answer B

Sildenafil (Viagra) has shown promise in clients with erectile dysfunction. It is not effective in men with psychogenic impotence or those with neurological or arterial disease. It potentiates the hypotensive effect of nitrate and is contraindicated for clients receiving nitrates, such as nitroglycerin.

Bibliography

American Urological Association: *American Urological Association Guideline: Management of Benign Prostatic Hyperplasia (BPH)*. American Urologic Association Education and Research, Linthicum, MD. www.auanet.org/content/clinical-practice-guidelines/clinical-guidelines.cfm?sub=bph.

Bickley, LS: *Bates' Guide to Physical Examination and History Taking*, ed 10. Lippincott, Williams & Wilkins, Philadelphia, 2009.

Collins-Bride, GM, and Saxe, JM: *Clinical Guidelines for Advanced Practice Nursing: An Interdisciplinary Approach*. Jones & Barlett Learning, Burlington, MA, 2012.

Dunphy, LM, et al: *Primary Care: The Art and Science of Advanced Practice Nursing*, ed 3. FA Davis, Philadelphia, 2011.

Jarvis, J: *Physical Examination and Health Assessment*, ed 6. Elsevier, St. Louis, 2011.

LeBlond, RF, et al: *DeGowin's Diagnostic Examination*, ed 9, McGraw Hill, New York, 2009.

McPhee, J, and Papadakis, MA (eds): *2011 Current Medical Diagnosis and Treatment (CMDT)*, ed 50. Lange Books/McGraw-Hill, New York, 2011.

Rakel, RE, and Rakel, DP: *Textbook of Family Practice*, ed 8. Elsevier, St. Louis, 2011.

Roehorn, CG, et al: *AUA Guideline on the Management of Benign Prostatic Hyperplasia: Diagnosis and Treatment*

Recommendations. American Urological Association Education and Research, Linthicum, MD, 2003. www.auanet.org/content/guidelines-and-quality-care/clinicalguidelines.cfm?sub=bph.

Taylor, RB, et al: *Manual of Family Practice,* ed 3. Lippincott, Williams & Wilkins, Philadelphia, 2008.

U.S. Department of Health and Human Services: *Diagnosis and Treatment of Erectile Dysfunction* (AHRQ publication No. 08(09)-E016). U.S. Department of Health and Human Services, Rockville, MD, 2009.

Wein, J, et al: *Campbell-Walsh Urology,* ed 10. Elsevier, New York, 2011.

How well did you do?

85% and above, congratulations! This score shows application of test-taking principles and adequate content knowledge.

75%–85%, keep working! Review test-taking principles and try again.

65%–75%, hang in there! Spend some time reviewing concepts and test-taking principles and then try the test again.

Chapter 15: *Female Genitourinary Problems*

Kymberlee A. Montgomery
Jill E. Winland-Brown

Questions

15-1 *A sexually active woman should be aware that genital herpes simplex virus*

A. may be transmitted to a partner or newborn even in the absence of lesions because of viral shedding.

B. is suppressed during menstruation, physical or emotional stress, immunosuppression, sexual intercourse, and pregnancy.

C. recurrences usually last the same length of time as the initial outbreak.

D. requires the use of condoms only during outbreaks.

15-2 *Susan is 9 months pregnant and asks you about using umbilical cord blood after birth for newborn DNA identification. What do you tell her?*

A. "This cord blood sample is identical to the genetic profile of the infant."

B. "Fingerprinting and footprinting that have been done in the past work perfectly."

C. "A better method of obtaining newborn DNA is with a buccal swab."

D. "The traditional method of a newborn heel stick for a DNA sample is 'tried and true.'"

15-3 *A 17-year-old female patient requests to start Depo-Provera injections as her method of birth control. She discloses that she has had four sexual partners in the past year. Her last menstrual period was 12 days ago and she had unprotected intercourse 3 days ago. The appropriate management for this patient would be to*

A. administer the injection today.

B. advise her to use another method for now and return with her next menses.

C. give the injection after a negative pregnancy test and tell her to use condoms for the next 7 days.

D. give the injection and tell her to use a barrier method for 7 days.

15-4 *The simplest and safest method of suppressing lactation after it has started is to*

A. wear a snug brassiere.

B. use ice packs.

C. gradually wean the baby to a bottle or a cup over a 3-week period.

D. begin oral hormones or long-acting hormonal injections.

15-5 *In a premenopausal woman, the biggest heart attack risk factor is*

A. cigarette smoking.

B. family history.

C. sedentary lifestyle.

D. obesity.

15-6 *First-line treatment for polycystic ovary syndrome is*

A. a bilateral oophorectomy.

B. oral testosterone therapy.

C. a combination of diet modification, weight loss, and stress management.

D. a laparoscopy with a bilateral wedge resection.

15-7 *If a woman is using the basal body temperature (BBT) method of birth control and does not want to become pregnant, when would you tell her to avoid unprotected intercourse?*

A. From the beginning of the menstrual cycle until the BBT has been elevated for 3 days

B. Whenever the BBT is elevated

C. Whenever the BBT is lowered

D. From the end of the menstrual cycle until the BBT has been low for 5 days

15-8   Which of the following is a sexually transmitted infection?

A. *Candida* vaginitis

B. Trichomonal vaginitis

C. Atrophic vaginitis

D. *Lactobacilli* vaginitis

15-9   In a patient diagnosed with cervical gonococcal infection, you would also suspect a co-infection with

A. candidiasis.

B. syphilis.

C. trichomoniasis.

D. chlamydia.

15-10   Jennifer, age 27, is complaining of lower abdominal pain. After doing some laboratory studies, you find leukocytosis, an elevated erythrocyte sedimentation rate, and an elevated C-reactive protein level. Which is the most appropriate diagnosis?

A. Ovarian cyst

B. Pelvic inflammatory disease

C. Tubal pregnancy

D. Diverticulitis

15-11   Human papillomavirus may lead to

A. pelvic inflammatory disease.

B. molluscum contagiosum.

C. cervical dysplasia.

D. genital herpes.

15-12   Gerri, a 33-year-old female patient, complains of external vaginal irritation after adding new fabric softener to her laundry. You have diagnosed her with reactive vaginitis. The treatment of choice for this condition includes

A. metronidazole (Flagyl) 500 mg twice a day for 7 days.

B. conjugated vaginal estrogen cream externally every day for 1 week.

C. rewashing undergarments without fabric softener and applying petroleum jelly to the affected area.

D. rewashing undergarments without fabric softener and applying corticosteroids to the affected area.

15-13   A dancer from an adult club down the street comes in for a renewal of her birth control pill prescription. She says that everything is fine. On examination, you find grayish-white vaginal discharge, greenish cervical discharge, and cervical motion tenderness. Which of the following differential diagnosis is most unlikely?

A. Gonorrhea

B. Interstitial cystitis

C. Bacterial vaginosis

D. Chlamydia

15-14   Leiomyomas are found

A. within the uterine wall.

B. on the vaginal wall.

C. within the cervix.

D. on the fallopian tube.

15-15   When a woman complains of dyspareunia in the lower back during orgasm, you should consider

A. endometriosis.

B. cystitis.

C. vaginitis.

D. causes related to pelvic inflammatory disease.

15-16   A 27-year-old female presents to your office for a Mirena (levonorgestrel intrauterine system) insertion. She reports that her menses started 3 days ago and is normal. How soon after insertion will she be able to safely rely on it for contraception?

A. Immediately

B. After 48 hours

C. In 1 week

D. In 1 month

15-17   Mary, age 50, desires hormone replacement therapy (HRT) for her hot flashes, which she can't stand. You've discussed the pros and cons and given her some alternative suggestions. Her mother had a history of osteoporosis. You have decided to initiate therapy for 1 year. She asks you if she also needs to take calcium or vitamin D for prevention of osteoporosis. How do you respond?

A. "Research has shown that HRT alone is sufficient to protect against osteoporosis."

B. "Yes, calcium intake should be increased to 1,200 mg/day along with 600 mg of vitamin D to decrease bone turnover and increase intestinal absorption."

C. "If you decide to take calcium and vitamin D, you can stop the HRT."

D. "If you are getting sufficient exercise, you don't need to take calcium and vitamin D."

15-18   *Julia, age 60, asks you about taking alendronate (Fosamax). What do you tell her about using this medication?*

A. "If you decide to take it, stick with a lower dose of 5 mg because the side effects are much worse with a 10 mg dose."

B. "Fosamax works better in younger women, so you should start this now rather than wait until you're 70."

C. "You should take a daily dose because the weekly dose is not as effective."

D. "In addition to its efficacy in the treatment of osteoporosis in postmenopausal women, it is also useful for the prevention of osteoporosis."

15-19   *Which type of breast cancer involves infiltration of the nipple epithelium and has an initial symptom of itching or burning of the nipple?*

A. Ductal cancer

B. Paget's disease

C. Mammary duct ectasia

D. Fibroadenoma

15-20   *Which type of incontinence has an associated symptom of recurrent cystitis?*

A. Stress incontinence

B. Urge incontinence

C. Overflow incontinence

D. Functional incontinence

15-21   *The most common type of vaginal infection is*

A. candidiasis.

B. trichomoniasis.

C. gonorrhea.

D. bacterial vaginosis.

15-22   *Which of the following is an indication for a colposcopy?*

A. A Pap smear showing dysplasia

B. Recurrent STIs

C. HIV infection

D. History of leiomyomas

15-23   *Which of the following statements do you use when instructing women about their fertile period (when they are most likely to become pregnant)?*

A. Ovulation occurs on the 14th day, plus or minus 2 days, before the next menses.

B. Sperm are viable for 24 hours.

C. The ovum is viable for 6 hours.

D. The ovaries always release one ovum per month.

15-24   *Jennifer, a 25-year-old female patient, complains of dysuria. In taking a thorough history to formulate a diagnosis, it is most important to ask,*

A. "Do you have painful intercourse?"

B. "Do you have an associated vaginal discharge or irritation?"

C. "Do you also have a problem with defecation?"

D. "Do you have stress incontinence?"

15-25   *Sydney, age 21, is taking an oral contraceptive (OC). She complains of acne. How should you adjust the estrogen in the OC?*

A. Increase the estrogen content.

B. Decrease the estrogen content.

C. Delete the estrogen content.

D. No adjustment should be made to the estrogen content.

15-26   *Marcia, age 59, presents with depression. According to the diagnostic criteria for a major depressive disorder, which of the following criterion needs to be met?*

A. The depression must have a specific cause, like alcohol, drugs, medication side effects, or physical illness.

B. The symptoms must be severe enough to upset the client's daily routine or to impact his or her work or interfere with relationships.

C. The depression may be a normal reaction to the death of a loved one.

D. There must be some type of sleep disturbance.

15-27   The best method to diagnose uterine polyps is a

A. hysteroscopy.

B. dilation and curettage.

C. colposcopy.

D. laparoscopy.

15-28   Darcy is to undergo a cone-needle biopsy for a suspicious breast mass. This procedure includes

A. a 21- or 22-gauge needle that is used to aspirate cells from the lesion for analysis.

B. removal of a large core of tissue from the lesion for histological evaluation utilizing a large-gauge cutting needle.

C. removal of a wedge of tissue for examination.

D. removal of the entire lesion.

15-29   Which of the following lifestyle factors is associated with an increased risk for breast cancer?

A. Being underweight

B. Having one to two drinks of alcohol per day

C. Smoking

D. Eating a low-fat diet

15-30   Sandra says that her previous doctor never discussed why he took her off hormone replacement therapy (HRT). You share with her some of the results of the Women's Health Initiative (WHI). Which statement is true regarding the study?

A. Estrogen plus progestin increased the risk of a cardiac event in apparently healthy women.

B. Persons on HRT are at a higher risk of colorectal cancer.

C. Postmenopausal hormones do not actually prevent fractures of the hip.

D. Estrogen alone is associated with a greater risk of breast cancer than a combination of estrogen plus progestin.

15-31   Mrs. Williams would like to schedule an appointment to bring her 18-year-old daughter in to see you for her first gynecological exam and Pap smear. The most appropriate reply would include

A. "I would be happy to see your daughter and complete her gynecological exam and Pap smear."

B. "Your daughter does not need a gynecological exam and Pap at this time."

C. "Your daughter only needs a gynecological exam and Pap smear when she becomes sexually active."

D. "I would be happy to see your daughter and complete her gynecological exam; however, she does not need a Pap smear until the age of 21."

15-32   Women who take oral contraceptives are less likely to experience

A. human papillomavirus infection.

B. migraine headache.

C. iron-deficiency anemia.

D. herpes simplex virus.

15-33   The average age of menopause in the United States is

A. 45 years.

B. 48 years.

C. 50 years.

D. 53 years.

15-34   A 26-year-old female comes to your office to discuss birth control options. Her history includes migraine headaches with aura while on combination oral contraceptives in the past. She does not want to become pregnant. Which of the following birth control options would be the best choice for her?

A. Combined hormonal contraceptive pills

B. Ortho Evra Patch

C. Mirena IUD

D. Vaginal NuvaRing

15-35   Unilateral galactorrhea may be present with

A. an intraductal papilloma.

B. a woman who is lactating.

C. a ruptured breast implant.

D. pregnancy.

15-36   Which of the following drugs may have their effects enhanced when used in combination with an oral contraceptive?

A. Beta blockers

B. Oral anticoagulants

C. Antacids

D. Anti-convulsants

15-37   Which of the following drugs may diminish the effectiveness of oral contraceptives?

A. Beta blockers

B. Oral anticoagulants

C. Antibiotics

D. Oral hypoglycemics

15-38   During a pelvic examination, you ask Mrs. Krane to Valsalva (strain). While doing this, a pouching is seen on the anterior wall of the vagina. This is indicative of

A. a cystocele.

B. a rectocele.

C. an enterocele.

D. a uterine prolapse.

15-39   Samantha has a diagnosis of a chlamydia vaginal infection. You believe that it is questionable whether she will fill the prescription that you write or take it for 7 days as ordered. What would you do?

A. Give azithromycin (Zithromax) 1 g PO now.

B. Emphasize the importance of the drug and tell her the consequences of not taking it.

C. Send out the public health nurse to follow up on whether she takes the drug for 7 days.

D. Assume that Samantha is an adult and will follow your instructions.

15-40   Infertility is best defined as the

A. inability to conceive with multiple sex partners.

B. inability to conceive for 9 months of unprotected intercourse when both partners are younger than 30 years of age.

C. state of voluntary childlessness.

D. inability to conceive after 1 full year of unprotected intercourse.

15-41   Reiter's syndrome is a complication of

A. bacterial vaginosis.

B. syphilis.

C. chlamydia.

D. gonorrhea.

15-42   Mrs. Henderson inquires about why she needs progesterone in addition to her estrogen for hormone replacement. Women who have an intact uterus need to add progesterone to their prescribed estrogen because progestin

A. assists in relieving the typical hot flashes of menopause.

B. reduces the incidence of endometrial hyperplasia and cancer.

C. decreases the risk of osteoporosis.

D. controls mood swings.

15-43   A 21-year-old woman comes to your office and reports a history of genital warts. In reference to the HPV vaccination (Gardasil or Cervarix), she should be educated that

A. she is not in the correct age group and is not a candidate for the vaccination.

B. she should receive the HPV vaccination.

C. she already has been exposed to HPV; therefore, she is not a candidate for the vaccine.

D. there is a vaccine coming out shortly specifically for those who have been exposed. She should wait.

15-44   Joanne wants to use some form of birth control, but because she is getting married next year, she wants to be able to stop the birth control method after the wedding and have her fertility restored almost immediately. Which method do you recommend for her?

A. Birth control pills

B. Vaginal ring

C. Depot-medroxyprogesterone acetate (DMPA) injections

D. Lea's Shield

15-45   Beth is breastfeeding her 3-month-old infant with no supplementation. She says she has heard that she cannot get pregnant during this time. What do you tell her?

A. "It's highly likely that you may become pregnant, so you should use another method of birth control."

B. "Yes, you're safe for as long as you breastfeed."

C. "For the first 6 months, if you breastfeed and have very little supplementation, your chances are less than 2% that you'll get pregnant."

D. "You're more at risk for getting pregnant now because of your fluctuating hormone levels."

15-46   Which of the following drugs may have their effects diminished when used in combination with an oral contraceptive?

A. Corticosteroids

B. Oral anticoagulants

C. Antibiotics

D. Anticonvulsants

15-47   The most common reason for surgery for macromastia is

A. back and shoulder pain.

B. breast cancer.

C. fibrocystic breast disease.

D. inability to breastfeed.

15-48   You've just finished a Pap smear on Sadie, age 39. During the wet mount, you see cells with bacteria adherent to the cell wall giving it a stippled, granular appearance. What do you suspect?

A. Candidiasis

B. Bacterial vaginosis

C. Trichomoniasis

D. Cervicitis

15-49   The majority of breast carcinomas are found in which anatomical site in the breast?

A. Around the areola

B. In the upper outer quadrant

C. In the lower half of the breast

D. Toward the sternum

15-50   Ursula, age 19, is going to begin taking birth control pills. She asks you if she is "safe" immediately. How do you respond?

A. "Yes, you should not get pregnant once you start taking the pill. However, it doesn't protect you from STIs."

B. "For the first month, you need to be on a backup birth-control method. However, the pill doesn't protect you from STIs."

C. "A second birth control method needs to be used during intercourse for the first 7 days while taking the pill. However, the pill doesn't protect you from STIs."

D. "Until you have your second period (cycle) with the pill, you are not considered safe."

15-51   The most common type of invasive breast carcinoma is

A. infiltrating ductal carcinoma.

B. medullary carcinoma.

C. lobular carcinoma.

D. infiltrating papillary carcinoma.

15-52   Jennifer, age 42, presents for her well-woman examination and you notice "dimpling" on her left breast. Your initial reaction is that it may possibly be

A. breast cancer.

B. fibrocystic breast disease.

C. Paget's disease.

D. striae from recent dieting.

15-53   What is the most common cause of mastitis in breastfeeding women?

A. Escherichia coli

B. Streptococcus

C. Mycobacterium tuberculosis

D. Staphylococcus aureus

15-54   Which of the following drugs given to nursing mothers may cause a reduction in the milk supply?

A. Antihistamines

B. Antithyroid medication

C. Oral contraceptives

D. Laxatives

15-55 *Jenna has been diagnosed with a generalized anxiety disorder (GAD). You know that she may experience which of the following?*

A. She may be worried or anxious about having a panic attack.

B. She may be worried about being separated or about being away from home or close relatives.

C. She may have been excessively anxious and worried on most days for more than 6 months.

D. She may have multiple physical complaints or believe she has a physical illness.

15-56 *Judy has severe pain monthly with her fibrocystic breast disease. Which medication do you suggest she try?*

A. Micronized estradiol (Estrace)

B. Danazol (Danocrine)

C. Paroxetine (Paxil)

D. Venlafaxine (Effexor)

15-57 *Emotional support is best given to the client with a sexually transmitted infection by*

A. offering many alternatives.

B. authentic active listening.

C. assuring the client that everything will be okay.

D. emphasizing the duration of the disease.

15-58 *Marsha, age 40, has been given a diagnosis of rheumatoid arthritis. She asks you whether she should continue taking her birth control pills. You tell her*

A. to check with her rheumatologist.

B. to stop.

C. to continue.

D. the dose will have to be altered.

15-59 *Mrs. Peterson would like to be fitted for a diaphragm. She has been on numerous hormones in the past and does not like the side effects. It is important to remember that when properly fitting a patient for a diaphragm, it should*

A. allow a fingertip between it and the pubic arch.

B. be small enough to allow for vaginal expansion.

C. lie snugly over the pubic arch and under the cervix.

D. provide firm tension against the vaginal walls.

15-60 *Herpes simplex virus can be potentially acquired through maternal transmission. This is least likely to occur*

A. before labor.

B. during delivery.

C. postnatally.

D. during the neonatal period.

15-61 *A treatment used to improve the chance of pregnancy in an infertile woman who has minimal or mild endometriosis is*

A. laparoscopic resection or ablation of the lesions.

B. dilation and curettage.

C. the use of gonadotropin-releasing hormone analogues.

D. the use of birth control pills for 3 months and then abruptly stopping.

15-62 *Sarah, age 29, complains of premenstrual syndrome. She states she was told that changing her diet might help in managing some of the symptoms. What changes in her diet do you recommend?*

A. Increase her intake of protein.

B. Increase her intake of complex carbohydrates.

C. Increase her intake of salt and salty foods.

D. Decrease her intake of fatty foods.

15-63 *Joy has been breastfeeding and has developed puerperal mastitis. You tell her,*

A. "Using cool compresses to the affected breast before pumping will increase milk expression."

B. "Continue breastfeeding the baby to avoid milk stasis."

C. "Continue doing your normal activities during the acute phase to keep things flowing."

D. "Do not massage the breasts."

15-64 *Minnie, age 52, states that she is going to have a TRAM procedure after her breast surgery. However, she was in shock from the diagnosis when the surgeon explained the procedure. She asks you to explain it. How do you respond?*

A. "It's when a breast implant is inserted under the pectoris muscle."

B. "It's an autogenous procedure that uses skin from the latissimus dorsi muscle to fashion a breast."

C. "It's an autogenous procedure that uses skin from the rectus abdominis muscle to fashion a breast."

D. "It's a breast implant that is done after the mastectomy scar heals."

15-65   *Which form of estrogen is secreted in the greatest amount by the ovaries during the reproductive years and considered most potent?*

A.   Estrone (E1)

B.   Estradiol (E2)

C.   Estriol (E3)

D.   The potency and secretion of all of the above are in equal amounts.

15-66   *Janice, age 26, who has genital herpes, asks if her partner has to use a condom during sexual intercourse even if she does not have a visible lesion. How do you respond?*

A.   "Yes, we're not sure if it's still transmitted when the lesions are not visible, so it's better to be on the safe side."

B.   "No, you're not 'contagious' when the lesions are not visible."

C.   "No, use of a spermicidal agent is all that is required."

D.   "Yes, shedding of the herpes simplex virus from mucocutaneous surfaces in the absence of visible lesions is a primary mode of transmission."

15-67   *When a woman has extreme spasticity, which position should she assume for a Pap smear?*

A.   "OB" stirrups position

B.   Knee-chest position while prone

C.   V-shaped position without stirrups

D.   Side-lying position

15-68   *On physical exam, Judy has pubic hair that spreads over her mons pubis with a slight lateral spread. In addition, her breast development shows breast enlargement with secondary mound formation by the developing areola. Which Tanner best describes Judy's development?*

A.   Stage II

B.   Stage III

C.   Stage IV

D.   Stage V

15-69   *Of the symptoms listed below, the most commonly expressed symptom of women with premenstrual syndrome is*

A.   fatigue.

B.   depression.

C.   breast tenderness.

D.   swelling of the extremities.

15-70   *The Mobiluncus species is responsible for which sexually transmitted infection?*

A.   Condylomata acuminata

B.   Bacterial vaginosis

C.   Human papillomavirus

D.   Lymphogranuloma venereum

15-71   *An occurrence of genital herpes is*

A.   cured with acyclovir (Zovirax).

B.   best managed with trichloroacetic acid 80%–90% applied directly to the lesion.

C.   expected to be completely resolved within 21 days (for the primary lesion).

D.   not a factor in continuing with intercourse.

15-72   *Lynne, age 43, comes to your office in tears, stating that last night she had unprotected sex and forgot to take her birth control pill. She wants to know about the "morning-after pill." You tell her,*

A.   "If your period does not start at the scheduled time, come back to see me."

B.   "I'll go ahead and order the estrogen-only postcoital contraception pill."

C.   "I'll go ahead and order the Yuzpe regimen."

D.   "I'll refer you to a gynecologist."

15-73   *Lori, age 38, states that she has not had a pelvic examination in 5 years because she does not like having the digital rectal examination. How do you respond?*

A.   "Let's schedule an examination now because women no longer need a rectal exam with routine pelvic examinations."

B.   "OK, we'll do a pelvic, and I'll just put 'refused' on the chart to cover my liability."

C. "We really need to do one because the rectal examination has been shown to pick up many abnormalities such as rectal polyps."

D. "I'll try to be quick with the rectal examination and get it over with."

15-74   Lactobacilli *in the vagina*

A. decreases glycogen metabolism.

B. maintains an acid pH range.

C. increases the development of white blood cells.

D. maintains an alkaline pH range.

15-75   *Dana is a 23-year-old patient diagnosed with dyspareunia. Which of the following is NOT a cause for this condition?*

A. Vulvovaginitis

B. An incompletely stretched hymen

C. Vaginismus

D. Multiple pregnancies

15-76   *There are many causes of amenorrhea. In ballet dancers or marathon runners, which anatomical structure is the probable cause?*

A. Outflow tract

B. Ovary

C. Anterior pituitary

D. Hypothalamus

15-77   *What is the most common virus to be transmitted in utero?*

A. Cytomegalovirus

B. Rubella

C. Varicella

D. Toxoplasmosis

15-78   *Susan has been diagnosed with fibrocystic breast disease. Which of the following may exacerbate the condition?*

A. Daily dose of aspirin

B. Spicy foods

C. Chocolate

D. Wearing tight bras

15-79   *How long can the vaginal contraceptive ring (Nuvaring) be out of the vagina before an additional form of contraception is necessary?*

A. 30 minutes

B. 1 hour

C. 2 hours

D. 3 hours

15-80   *Which of the following ovarian tumors or cysts has the potential for malignancy?*

A. Follicle cysts

B. Brenner's tumor

C. Fibroma

D. Secondary ovarian tumors

15-81   *The Joneses are thinking about going for infertility counseling because they have been married for 5 years and have been unable to conceive. They ask you whether the man or the woman is usually the cause of the infertility. What do you tell them about the etiology of infertility?*

A. "In most cases, infertility is related to a female factor."

B. "In most cases, infertility is related to a male factor."

C. "In the majority of cases, the etiology cannot be identified."

D. "Male and female infertility rates are almost the same in the majority of cases."

15-82   *Brianne, age 24, complains of urgency, frequency, and dysuria. Your dipstick test shows no hematuria, and her urine culture shows no growth. What is your next action?*

A. You suspect a sexually transmitted infection, so you obtain a culture of the urethra, do a potassium hydroxide wet prep, and obtain another urine culture.

B. You suspect urethra irritation, so you tell her to take showers, not bubble baths, and wear white, dry underwear and loose-fitting clothing.

C. You suspect a urinary tract infection not visible yet on culture, so you start her on Bactrim DS.

D. You suspect that the vulva is irritated. You tell her to take a relaxing shower and dry the area well and come back in 1 week if there is no improvement.

15-83   *Judi has a seizure disorder and wants to get pregnant. What is the drug of choice for her during pregnancy?*

A. Valproate (Depakene)

B. Trimethadione (Tridione)

C. Phenobarbital (Luminal)

D. Phenytoin (Dilantin)

15-84   *When premenstrual syndrome symptoms do not respond to dietary and nonmedical therapies, which of the following drugs might you try?*

A. Antidepressants

B. Antihistamines

C. Corticosteroids

D. Anticholinergics

15-85   *A vaginal ph of 4.2 is an expected finding in*

A. a healthy prepubertal age girl.

B. a woman with trichomoniasis vaginalis.

C. a postmenopausal woman with atrophic vaginitis.

D. a healthy woman of reproductive age.

15-86   *Julia is nursing her 8-week-old baby and states that he is very irritable and sleeps poorly. What medication or substance do you ask her if she is taking or using?*

A. Cimetidine (Tagamet)

B. Ergotamine (Ergostat)

C. Nicotine

D. Caffeine

15-87   *Which of the following conditions is a contraindication to using the copper intrauterine device (IUD)?*

A. History of ectopic pregnancy

B. Nulliparity

C. Treated cervical dysplasia

D. Heart disease

15-88   *Jane is 7 weeks pregnant and experiencing morning sickness. The most common cause for this condition is*

A. production of human chorionic gonadotropin.

B. suppression of estrogen.

C. suppression of linea alba.

D. suppression of progesterone.

15-89   *Candidiasis is more common in*

A. teenage girls.

B. women on low-fat diets.

C. women with diabetes.

D. women with frequent urinary tract infections.

15-90   *Which blood tumor marker is highly specific to epithelial ovarian cancer?*

A. PSA

B. CA 125

C. CA 15-3

D. CA 19-9

15-91   *Emergency contraception refers to*

A. an induced abortion in an emergency room (ER).

B. quickly starting on birth control pills in anticipation of sexual intercourse.

C. having a medroxyprogesterone (Depo-Provera) injection in the ER every 12 weeks.

D. taking emergency contraceptive pills (ECPs).

15-92   *Stein-Leventhal syndrome, one of the leading causes of female infertility, is more commonly known as*

A. pelvic inflammatory disease.

B. polycystic ovary disease.

C. multiple sex partners.

D. ectopic pregnancy syndrome.

15-93   *Toxic shock syndrome (TSS) may be caused by which of the following?*

A. Tampon contamination with *Staphylococcus aureus*

B. A short vaginal canal

C. The use of superabsorbent tampons

D. A urinary tract infection involving the bladder and kidneys

15-94   *Mrs. Green called the office to make an appointment for her annual Pap smear. She needs to be given the following instructions prior to her appointment:*

A. "Insert nothing in the vagina for 24 hours before the examination."

B. "Douching enhances visualization of the cervix and should be done before the appointment."

C. "An infection or menstrual period is no reason to cancel the appointment."

D. "The procedure is completely painless."

15-95   *Procidentia is a*

A. cystocele.

B. rectocele.

C. vaginal fistula.

D. third-degree uterine prolapse.

15-96   *Endometrial cancer, hirsutism, acne, breast cancer, increased risk of diabetes, infertility, menstrual bleeding problems, and an increased risk of cardiovascular disease are clinical consequences of*

A. mastalgia.

B. menorrhagia.

C. endometriosis.

D. persistent anovulation.

15-97   *Menses at irregular intervals with excessive flow and duration is defined as*

A. oligomenorrhea.

B. polymenorrhea.

C. menorrhagia.

D. metrorrhagia.

15-98   *The most likely cause of amenorrhea is*

A. an anatomical deviation.

B. a genetic factor.

C. an endocrine abnormality.

D. pregnancy.

15-99   *Marsha, age 42, is having dysfunctional uterine bleeding (DUB) and cannot take oral contraceptives due to a history of a blood clot (emboli). Management includes which medication?*

A. Medroxyprogesterone

B. Ethinyl estradiol

C. Conjugated estrogen

D. Piroxicam

15-100   *Characteristics of polycystic ovary syndrome include*

A. hirsutism, thinness, hypoinsulinemia.

B. menopausal onset, vitiligo, hyperinsulemia.

C. alopecia, thinness, abdominal cramping.

D. premenarchial onset, obesity, hyperinsulinemia.

15-101   *Dysfunctional uterine bleeding is usually associated with*

A. pregnancy.

B. anovulation.

C. genital tumor.

D. inflammation.

15-102   *Sharon states that she has heard that douching effectively washes out the sperm after intercourse and that she has been using this as a method of birth control. Which of the following statements about douching is true?*

A. Douching prevents sperm from entering the uterus.

B. Douching should be used at least once a month after menses if not used after intercourse.

C. Douching is a reliable contraceptive.

D. Douching may increase the risk of ectopic pregnancy.

15-103   *Cynthia says that her health-care provider wants to do a colposcopy. She asks you what this is. You tell her that a colposcopy*

A. visualizes the cervical, vaginal, or vulvar epithelium under magnification to identify abnormal areas that may require a biopsy.

B. involves removal of one or more areas of the endometrium by means of a curette or small aspiration device without cervical dilation.

C. allows visual examination of the uterine cavity with a small fiber-optic endoscope passed through the cervix.

D. allows visualization of the abdominal and pelvic cavity through a small fiber-optic endoscope passed through a subumbilical incision.

15-104 Which type of cyst of the female reproductive system usually results in pain, redness, a perineal mass, and dyspareunia?

A. Ovarian cyst
B. Bartholin's cyst
C. Gardner's cyst
D. Nabothian cyst

15-105 What is the position of the uterus when the cervix is on the anterior vaginal wall?

A. Midposition
B. Retroverted
C. Retroflexed
D. Anteverted

15-106 Small-quantity incontinence with nearly continuous dribbling is symptomatic of which kind of incontinence?

A. Stress incontinence
B. Urge incontinence
C. Overflow incontinence
D. Functional incontinence

15-107 Which of the following terms describes the bluish or purplish discoloration of the vulva, vagina, and a portion of the cervix that occurs in pregnancy?

A. Goodell's sign
B. Hegar's sign
C. Piskacek's sign
D. Chadwick's sign

15-108 Which glands are posterior on each side of the vaginal orifice and open onto the sides of the vestibule in the groove between the labia minora and hymen?

A. Bartholin's glands
B. Skene's glands
C. Paraurethral glands
D. Cystocele

15-109 Thelarche is the first sign of puberty in most girls. It usually occurs at about what age?

A. 8 years
B. 10 years
C. 11 years
D. 13 years

15-110 Which of the following signs and/or symptoms of a genital herpes infection usually occurs first?

A. Painful or pruritic vesicles
B. Dysuria
C. Prodromal tingling or pruritus of the genital region
D. White, curdlike plaques on a red base in the vagina

15-111 A 17-year-old female presents to your office with the complaint of lower abdominal pain since her period ended 2 days ago. She has a new sexual partner in the past 3 months and does not use condoms. On physical examination, you find that she has cervical motion tenderness. You are concerned that she may have pelvic inflammatory disease (PID). To meet the Centers for Disease Control and Prevention's minimum criteria for empiric treatment of PID, she must also have

A. an oral temperature greater than 101°F and mucopurulent cervicitis.
B. a positive test for cervical infection and an adnexal mass.
C. lower abdominal tenderness and adnexal tenderness.
D. mucopurulent cervicitis and an elevated white blood cell count.

Answers

15-1   Answer A

A sexually active woman should be aware that genital herpes simplex virus may be transmitted to a partner or newborn even in the absence of lesions because of viral shedding. Genital herpes may be transmitted to a partner at any time; therefore, condoms should always be used. Menstruation, physical or emotional stress, immunosuppression, sexual intercourse, and pregnancy may actually trigger herpes recurrences. Herpes recurrences usually do not last as long as the initial occurrence.

15-2 Answer A

DNA is the only reliable source of newborn identification and is easily obtained from an umbilical cord blood sample at birth. The American Academy of Pediatrics (AAP) and the American College of Obstetricians and Gynecologists (ACOG) stopped recommending the use of fingerprinting or footprinting for newborn identification purposes because babies don't produce well-defined fingerprints until 4–6 years of age and newborn footprinting has been shown to be inaccurate. A buccal swab is another possible method of obtaining newborn DNA but, if not processed or frozen soon after collection, degradation may occur. Many additional factors can influence buccal cell DNA as well. A newborn heel stick is commonly used to obtain the blood specimen for a newborn DNA sample. The procedure is painful, some parents are hesitant to agree to this, and there are many potential complications that may result, with some being permanent.

15-3 Answer B

Depo-Provera is the most commonly used injectable contraceptive that contains depot medroxyprogesterone acetate (DMPA). Given by intramuscular injection, DMPA 150 mgs is given every 12 weeks and provides highly effective contraception when used properly. The DMPA injection can be given anytime during the menstrual cycle *as long as the woman can be reasonably certain that she is not pregnant* (World Health Organization). If DMPA is given within 5–7 days of a normal last menstrual period, no backup is needed. If it is given after the 7th day in the menstrual cycle, back up contraception is needed. In this scenario, this patient had unprotected intercourse 3 days ago, so a pregnancy test would not provide accurate results at this time.

15-4 Answer C

The simplest and safest method of suppressing lactation after it has started is to gradually wean the baby to a bottle or a cup over a 3-week period. If nursing must be stopped abruptly, avoiding nipple stimulation, refraining from expressing milk, and wearing a snug brassiere will help. Ice packs and analgesics are also helpful. The practice of using oral and long-acting injections of hormonal preparations has been abandoned because of their questionable efficacy and their associated adverse effects, such as thromboembolic episodes and hair growth.

15-5 Answer A

In a premenopausal woman, the biggest heart attack risk factor is cigarette smoking. If a woman is premenopausal, her own estrogen is most likely to protect her from heart disease, but there are still risk factors associated with heart disease. The more risk factors that apply, the greater the danger. Smoking is the biggest risk factor. Others include a family history of premature heart disease (paternal side before age 55, maternal side before age 65), being older than age 54, going through premature menopause, sedentary lifestyle, and a history of diabetes or high blood pressure.

15-6 Answer C

First-line treatment for polycystic ovary syndrome (PCOS) is a combination of diet modification, weight loss, and stress management because obesity and stress alone can contribute to androgen excess. Oral estrogens are considered the first-line treatment for hyperandrogenism, with combination (estrogen and progesterone) oral contraceptives being the medication of choice. Treatment of uncomplicated amenorrhea in PCOS requires, at a minimum, monthly or bimonthly administration of medroxyprogesterone acetate (Depo-Provera). A laparotomy with a bilateral wedge resection is a treatment for anovulation. Because of the possibility of adhesions and ovarian atrophy, surgical interventions are used only in women who have tried and failed clomiphene citrate ovulation induction and when all other noninvasive options have been considered.

15-7 Answer A

If a woman is using the basal body temperature (BBT) method of birth control and does not want to become pregnant, tell her to avoid unprotected intercourse from the beginning of the menstrual cycle or at least from day 4 (the day a period starts is considered day 1 until the BBT has been elevated for 3 days). When using the BBT method, the temperature is taken daily after a minimum of 3 hours of sleep, before rising, eating, or drinking, and is recorded. The preovulatory temperatures are suppressed by estrogen, whereas postovulatory temperatures are increased under the influence of heat-inducing progesterone. Temperatures typically rise within a day or two after ovulation has occurred and remain elevated for 2 weeks until menstruation begins.

15-8 Answer B

Trichomonal vaginitis is a sexually transmitted infection. Monilial vaginitis, atrophic vaginitis, and bacterial vaginosis (BV) are all nonsexually transmitted types of vaginitis. Vulvovaginal candidiasis (formerly *Monilia* species), although not an STI, may be transmitted between partners and between mother and newborn. Atrophic vaginitis is present in postmenopausal women who are not on hormone replacement therapy. BV is the most common vaginitis in women of reproductive age, of which almost 50% are asymptomatic. It results in changes in the vaginal bacterial flora with a loss of lactobacilli, an increase in vaginal pH (pH 4.5), and an increase in multiple anaerobic and aerobic bacteria. BV may be caused by multiple bacteria and some cases may be transmitted sexually.

15-9 Answer D

Simultaneous chlamydial infections are present in 30%–50% of clients who have cervical gonococcal infections. Treatment should automatically be done for both when one has been diagnosed. The most common therapies are azithromycin (Zithromax) 1 g PO for one dose for *Chlamydia* infection and ceftriaxone (Rocephin) 125 mg IM for one dose for gonorrhea.

15-10 Answer B

In clients with pelvic inflammatory disease, leukocytosis is present in about 50% of the cases, the erythrocyte sedimentation rate is classically elevated, and the C-reactive protein level is usually elevated (exceeding 20 mg/L) in about 74% of the cases.

15-11 Answer C

When human papillomavirus (*Condylomata acuminata*) causes genital warts, it may lead to cervical dysplasia and cervical cancer. Pelvic inflammatory disease is usually secondary to gonorrhea or *Chlamydia* infection. Molluscum contagiosum is a sexually transmitted disease that causes a benign viral skin infection. Genital herpes is caused by herpes simplex virus.

15-12 Answer D

Elimination of the offensive agent and use of corticosteroids is the treatment of choice for reactive vaginitis. An antifungal agent needs to be administered for candidiasis, and topical estrogen is used for atrophic vaginitis. No treatment or povidone-iodine is used for normal cervical or vaginal-discharge vaginitis.

15-13 Answer B

Interstitial cystitis is a chronic disease with none of the symptoms given in the stem of the question. A client who presents with grayish-white vaginal discharge, greenish cervical discharge, and cervical motion tenderness may have gonorrhea, bacterial vaginosis, or *Chlamydia* infection. Gonorrhea may be asymptomatic or the client may present with yellowish urethral or vaginal discharge. The discharge of bacterial vaginosis is typically gray-white, malodorous or fishy smelling, and pruritic. *Chlamydia* infection may present with or without a vaginal or urethral discharge.

15-14 Answer A

Leiomyomas are commonly called uterine fibroids; they are the most common benign tumor of the uterus. Most are small and asymptomatic. Leiomyomas are classified by location within the uterine wall and can be subserous, submucous, and/or intramural. Rarely, a leiomyoma can be intraligamentous, cervical, or parasitic (deriving its blood supply from an organ to which it becomes attached). Most uterine fibroids are surrounded by compressed (otherwise normal) myometrium. When leiomyomas outgrow their blood supply, they can become necrotic and ulcerate.

15-15 Answer A

When a client complains of dyspareunia in the lower back during orgasm, you should consider a diagnosis of endometriosis. Cystitis and vaginitis should be considered when pain occurs at the vaginal canal and adjacent structures with the penis in midvagina. Pelvic inflammatory disease should be considered if pain occurs in the deep pelvis when there is deep penile penetration with thrusting. Causes of dyspareunia are many and diverse and depend on when and where the pain occurs.

15-16   Answer A

The levonorgestrel intrauterine system (Mirena IUD) is a small T-shaped contraceptive device that was approved for use in the United States in 2000. This system releases levonorgestrel (progestin) directly into the endometrial cavity at an initial rate of 20 mcg per day and is utilized as a safe and effective contraceptive method that can provide continuous pregnancy prevention for up to 5 years and can be removed any time within that 5-year period. Although this IUD can be inserted at any time during the menstrual cycle, Mirena is effective immediately if inserted within 7 days after the start of menses. If Mirena is inserted at any other time during the menstrual cycle, another method of birth control during the first week after insertion should be used. Pregnancy protection will begin after 7 days.

15-17   Answer B

Hormone replacement therapy (HRT) may be used for short-term effectiveness in treating hot flashes in the absence of a personal or family history of breast cancer or a previous problem with venous thrombosis. It is no longer considered cardioprotective. It is effective in preventing bone loss. Prevention of osteoporosis includes HRT, exercise to help decrease bone turnover, and 1,200 mg of calcium and 600 mg of vitamin D per day. For women not on HRT, calcium should be increased to 1,500 mg/day.

15-18   Answer D

In addition to its efficacy in the treatment of osteoporosis in postmenopausal women, alendronate (Fosamax) is useful for the prevention of osteoporosis. Weekly administration of Fosamax is as effective as daily dosing. The risk of side effects is similar for doses of 5 mg, 10 mg, or greater. Fosamax appears to be equally effective in older and younger postmenopausal women with osteoporosis.

15-19   Answer B

Paget's disease (Paget's carcinoma) is a rare type of breast cancer involving infiltration of the nipple epithelium. It begins with itching or burning of the nipple combined with superficial erosion, crusting, or ulceration. It is usually misdiagnosed as an infection. It has an excellent prognosis if the cancerous changes are confined to the nipple. Mammary duct ectasia, also known as plasma cell mastitis, is a palpable lumpiness found beneath the areola. Duct ectasia involves periductal inflammation, dilation of the ductal system, and an accumulation of fluid and dead cells that block the involved ducts. It is sometimes difficult to differentiate from cancer because it also occurs in perimenopausal or late premenopausal women. Fibroadenomas are overgrowths of periductal stromal connective tissue that compress ducts into well-defined lumps with circumscribed edges and smooth boundaries. They are mobile, firm, and nontender lumps and usually occur in women younger than age 25.

15-20   Answer A

Recurrent cystitis is an associated symptom of stress incontinence. Recurrent cystitis occurs more frequently in clients who have persistent residual urine resulting from an atonic bladder, cystocele, or diabetes mellitus. An associated symptom of urge incontinence (unstable detrusor contractions) is the inability to delay voiding long enough to reach the toilet. Neurogenic disorders are frequently associated with urge incontinence. Overflow incontinence is usually associated with benign prostatic hyperplasia and neurogenic conditions. Functional incontinence is incontinence caused by functional disabilities such as those associated with Alzheimer's disease or a cerebrovascular accident rather than any problem with structure.

15-21   Answer D

Bacterial vaginosis (BV) is the most common vaginal infection (about 40% of all cases). The infecting organisms are identified as *Gardnerella vaginalis*, *Mobiluncus* species, and other anaerobes. Bacterial vaginosis results in an overgrowth condition within the vagina for as-yet-unknown reasons. The incubation period is 5–10 days. About half of all clients with BV are asymptomatic. Those with symptoms typically describe a gray-white, malodorous or fishy-smelling, pruritic discharge that is accompanied by burning. It may be scant to profuse and adheres to the vaginal walls. The differential diagnoses include any other known cause for vaginitis (such as trichomoniasis or candidiasis) and cervicitis (such as gonorrhea or *Chlamydia* infection). Diagnosis is made through microscopic examination of the specimen by wet mount. The practitioner should look for clue cells; the presence of these cells, which look like pepper on the surface of cells, is diagnostic of BV.

15-22   Answer A

Indications for a colposcopy include a Pap smear showing dysplasia or cancer; history of diethylstilbestrol exposure; persistent unexplained atypia of a Pap with evidence of human papillomavirus; suspicious visible lesion of the cervix, vagina, or vulva; and as a follow-up for previously treated clients. It is also highly recommended for clients with visible condylomata, unexplained vaginal discharge, or a sexual partner with condylomata.

15-23   Answer A

When instructing women about their fertile period (when they are most likely to become pregnant), tell them that ovulation occurs on the 14th day, plus or minus 2 days, before the next menses. Sperm are viable for 3 days, and the ovum is viable for 24 hours. It is essential for women to know these facts if they are using the calendar or rhythm method for preventing a pregnancy. The ovaries may release more than one ovum per month or none at all, depending on the fertility status of the woman.

15-24   Answer B

Women with dysuria should be questioned about an associated vaginal discharge or irritation. Dysuria often represents a vaginal infection rather than a urinary tract infection. Women with dysuria from cystitis usually describe an internal discomfort, whereas women with dysuria from vaginitis usually describe a more external discomfort with the burning sensation in the vagina or labia, a result of urine flow over an inflamed vaginal mucosa.

15-25   Answer A

If a client taking an oral contraceptive (OC) complains of acne, the estrogen in the OC should be increased or the progestin decreased. In addition, you should also discuss hygiene, diet, and topical antibiotic drug therapy.

15-26   Answer B

For a diagnosis of major depressive disorder (MDD) to be made, the symptoms must be severe enough to upset the client's daily routine or to impact his or her work or interfere with relationships. The depression should not have a specific cause, like alcohol, drugs, medication side effects, or physical illness, and the depression is not just a normal reaction to the death of a loved one.

15-27   Answer A

The best method to diagnose uterine polyps is a hysteroscopy. A hysteroscopy is visualization of the endometrium through a scope to assess for some types of uterine fibroids, polyps, or structural abnormalities. Tissue sampling and removal of the polyps can be done through the hysteroscope. A dilation and curettage consists of scraping the walls of the uterus. A colposcopy is used to examine the vulva, vagina, and cervix. A laparoscopy examines the peritoneal cavity.

15-28   Answer B

In a cone-needle biopsy, a large-gauge cutting needle is used to provide a large core of tissue from the lesion for histological examination. The results of a core-needle biopsy are as accurate as a surgical biopsy, but the procedure is less invasive with better cosmetic results. A stereotactic or ultrasound-guided biopsy can be performed on nonpalpable lesions. A 21- or 22-gauge needle is used to aspirate a cyst or extract cells from a palpable solid lesion for analysis in a fine-needle aspiration (FNA). An incisional biopsy in which a large wedge of tissue is removed for histological examination may be done when a mass is very large and cannot be removed without major surgery. An open surgical excisional biopsy (lumpectomy) involves the entire removal of a palpable mass or a nonpalpable lesion (after stereotactic or ultrasound-guided biopsy or mammographic needle localization).

15-29   Answer C

Smoking is one of the lifestyle factors associated with an increased risk for breast cancer. Others include a high-fat diet, two or more drinks of alcohol per day, obesity, a high socioeconomic status, and breast trauma.

15-30   Answer A

The Women's Health Initiative (WHI) found that estrogen plus progestin increased the risk of a cardiac event in apparently healthy women. Users of postmenopausal hormones are actually at a lower risk of colorectal cancer; the mechanisms by which hormone use might reduce risk are unclear. The WHI was the first trial with definitive data supporting the ability of postmenopausal hormones to prevent fractures of the hip, vertebrae, and other sites. Estrogen plus progestin appears to be associated with greater risk of breast cancer than estrogen alone.

15-31   Answer D

In the past, the American Cancer Society, the American College of Obstetricians and Gynecologists (ACOG), and the American Society of Colposcopy and Cervical Pathology (ASCCP) recommended the initiation of cervical cytology screening in an adolescent based on time since onset of vaginal intercourse. However, there was much confusion and nonadherence to the guidelines. Many adolescents were being screened inappropriately. A study by Barnholtz-Sloan and colleagues shows that screening in adolescents does not appear to change the rate of cervical cancer in these groups, and the ACOG and ASCCP now recommend that cervical cytology screening begin at age 21 years, regardless of the age of onset of sexual activity. The few rare cases of cervical cancer in this population do not appear to have been preventable by screening.

15-32   Answer C

Iron-deficiency anemia is usually helped when women take an oral contraceptive (OC) because women on an OC tend to lose less blood each month. Other noncontraceptive benefits or conditions for which OC use offers protection include ovarian and endometrial carcinoma, ectopic pregnancy, pelvic inflammatory disease, functional ovarian cysts, menstrual irregularities, dysmenorrhea, benign breast disease, and premenstrual syndrome.

15-33   Answer C

The average age of menopause in the United States is 50 years. Menopause is defined by the World Health Organization as the permanent cessation of menstruation resulting from loss of ovarian follicular activity and 12 months of amenorrhea at the time of midlife.

15-34   Answer C

Women who have a history of migraine headaches with aura on combination oral contraceptives should not take estrogen containing contraception. Combined oral contraceptive pills, the Ortho Evra patch, and the vaginal NuvaRing all contain an estrogen hormone. The Mirena IUD contains levonorgestrel, which is a progestin.

15-35   Answer A

Galactorrhea (lactation not associated with pregnancy or nursing) is sometimes associated with a pituitary tumor. However, when the discharge is unilateral, from one or two ducts, a differential diagnosis of fibrocystic breast disease, intraductal papilloma, or carcinoma must be considered.

15-36   Answer A

The effects of beta blockers, as well as the effects of alcohol, corticosteroids, theophylline, and diazepam (Valium), may be enhanced when they are used in combination with oral contraceptives. Other drugs whose effects may be enhanced when used in combination with an oral contraceptive include tricyclic antidepressants and some benzodiazepines.

15-37   Answer C

Antibiotics, antacids, anticonvulsants, and barbiturates may diminish the effectiveness of oral contraceptives. Clients should be urged to use other methods of birth control when taking antibiotics.

15-38   Answer A

A cystocele is the prolapse into the vagina of the anterior vaginal wall and the bladder. Clinically, a pouching is seen on the anterior wall as the client strains. A rectocele is a prolapse into the vagina of the posterior vaginal wall and the rectum and is seen on the posterior wall as the client strains. An enterocele is a hernia of Douglas' pouch into the vagina and would be seen as a bulge emerging from the posterior fornix. In first-degree uterine prolapse, the cervix appears at the introitus when the client strains.

15-39   Answer A

An appropriate first-line drug for a *Chlamydia* vaginal infection is azithromycin (Zithromax) 1 g PO. Although doxycycline (Vibramycin) 100 mg PO twice daily for 7 days is the most tried-and-true and least expensive treatment, azithromycin is the most convenient option for single-dose administration. Azithromycin is contraindicated in pregnant women. For this population, erythromycin 500 mg PO four times a day for 7 days should be ordered.

15-40   Answer D

Infertility is a disease that affects approximately 15% of reproductive age couples (ages 15–44) in the United States. Although pregnancies do occur outside this age range, they are less frequent. Infertility is defined as the failure of a couple to conceive after 12 months of frequent, unprotected intercourse.

15-41   Answer D

Gonorrhea may precipitate Reiter's syndrome (reactive arthritis). Bacterial vaginosis seldom results in complications. Syphilis may result in disseminated disease, but not Reiter's syndrome. Left untreated in women, *Chlamydia* infections may cause scarring in the uterine tubes, leading to infertility and ectopic (tubal) pregnancies.

15-42   Answer B

A woman with an intact uterus needs to add progestin to her estrogen replacement therapy—estrogen plus progestin therapy (EPT)—because it reduces the incidence of endometrial hyperplasia and cancer, both of which are associated with long-term estrogen use. Decreased estrogen levels account for hot flashes. Discussion about discontinuing hormone replacement therapy should begin.

15-43   Answer B

The human papillomavirus is the most common sexually transmitted infection (STI). There are more than 40 HPV types that can infect the genital areas, mouth, and throat of males and females. According to the Centers for Disease Control and Prevention (CDC), females should get the vaccine before they become sexually active and prior to becoming exposed to HPV. Females who are sexually active may also benefit from the vaccine, but they may get less benefit from it. Women who have an existing history of genital warts have generally been exposed to HPV types 6 and 11, which are not oncogenic. However, few sexually active young women are infected with all HPV types prevented by the vaccines, so most young women could still get protection by getting vaccinated.

15-44   Answer D

Lea's Shield is the only product listed that does not contain hormones that may delay pregnancy after discontinuing use. Lea's Shield is similar to the diaphragm and cervical cap but is more user friendly. The dome-shaped silicone device covers the cervix, allowing for secretions to exit without sperm entering in. The shield is used with spermicide. There may be a temporary delay in conception after discontinuing oral contraceptives, although the exact time is unclear. Return to fertility with depot-medroxyprogesterone acetate (DMPA) may be delayed regardless of the duration of its use. DMPA injections are given every 3 months. A vaginal ring (NuvaRing) releases synthetic hormones and is worn for 21 days and then removed for 7 days to allow for a menstrual period. The vaginal ring has similar side effects to that of oral contraception.

15-45   Answer C

Women have less than a 2% chance of getting pregnant as long as they are amenorrheic for 2 months postpartum; are fully breastfeeding, with a supplementation not exceeding 15%; and are less than 6 months postpartum. If any of these conditions is not present, the woman needs to begin to use another form of contraception.

15-46   Answer B

The effects of oral anticoagulants, acetaminophen, some benzodiazepines, oral hypoglycemic agents, and methyldopa may be diminished when used in combination with oral contraceptives.

15-47   Answer A

Breast surgery reduction for macromastia is performed to reduce breast size and relieve back and shoulder pain caused by heavy, pendulous breasts. Many women with large breasts or macromastia complain of neck strain, occipital headache, shoulder pain, disfigurement caused by brassiere straps that burrow into the skin, low back pain, anterior chest discomfort, and paresthesia of the little fingers.

15-48   Answer B

With the wet mount for bacterial vaginosis (BV), you will see clue cells—characteristic epithelial cells with bacteria adherent to the cell wall giving a stippled, granular appearance. BV is the most prevalent form of vaginitis among childbearing women. With candidiasis, the microscopic examination of the vaginal solution diluted with saline or 10% KOH (potassium hydroxide) preparations will demonstrate hyphal forms or budding yeast cells in 50%–70% of infected women. With trichomoniasis, you will visualize motile flagellated trichomonads.

15-49   Answer B

Of all breast carcinomas, 60% are found in the upper outer quadrant of the breast, 5% around the areola and nipple, 15% in the upper inner quadrant (toward the sternum), 15% in the lower outer quadrant, and 5% in the lower inner quadrant.

15-50   Answer C

When a client is first starting to take birth control pills, she should be instructed to use a second birth control method during intercourse, such as condoms or a diaphragm used with spermicide, for the first 7 days. Another contraceptive method should always be kept on hand to use in case of missed pills; when taking another medication that might interfere with pill effectiveness, such as an antibiotic; or when vomiting or diarrhea occurs.

15-51   Answer A

The most common type of invasive breast carcinoma is infiltrating ductal carcinoma (70%–80%). This is followed by lobular (5%–10%); medullary (5%–7%); and Paget's, inflammatory, infiltrating papillary, tubular, and mucinous breast carcinomas (less than 5%).

15-52   Answer A

Dimpling on the breast is known as *peau d'orange* because it looks like an orange peel and may indicate a breast tumor due to pulling and retraction of the underlying tissue by the tumor. A nodule in fibrocystic breast disease is benign, tender, movable, and may be soft to firm. Mammary Paget's disease is cancer of the mammary ducts. Striae are streaks of light-colored skin that occur after rapid skin stretching.

15-53   Answer D

Although all the organisms listed may cause mastitis, the causative organism of sporadic puerperal mastitis is *Staphylococcus aureus* in at least 50% of reported cases. It is frequently found on skin and cultured from the neonate's mouth. The incidence of mastitis in breastfeeding women has been reported from 1%–9%. One study found an incidence of 26% in a population of long-term breastfeeding mothers.

15-54   Answer C

Oral contraceptives, even in low doses, may cause a reduction in the milk supply to an infant. The progestin-only minipill can be used. Antihistamines are contraindicated because of the increased sensitivity of newborns and infants to antihistamines. Antithyroid medications such as methimazole (Tapazole) are contraindicated because they may cause goiter or agranulocytosis. However, the antithyroid drug propylthiouracil is considered safe. Laxatives may cause diarrhea in an infant.

15-55   Answer C

According to *DSM-IV*, the diagnostic manual from the American Psychiatric Association (APA), generalized anxiety disorder (GAD) is present if excessive anxiety and worry (apprehensive expectation) occurs more days than not for 6 months about a number of events or activities such as work or school performance, if the client finds it difficult to control the worry, and if three or more of the following six symptoms are present: restlessness, fatigability, difficulty in concentration, irritability, muscle tension, and sleep disturbances.

15-56   Answer B

For clients with severe pain with their fibrocystic breast disease, danazol (Danocrine) 100–200 mg twice per day has been found helpful. Danazol is an androgen derivative that suppresses pituitary gonadotropins. With its androgenic effects, such as acne, edema, and hirsutism, most women find that the treatment is worse than the condition and prefer to try milder forms of pain relief. A daily dose of 400 IU of vitamin E may also help. Paroxetine (Paxil) and venlafaxine (Effexor) are both selective serotonin reuptake inhibitors (SSRIs) that have been shown in some studies to relieve hot flashes as well as hormone therapy can.

15-57   Answer B

Emotional support is best given to the client with a sexually transmitted infection (STI) by authentic active listening. During times of increased psychological stress, minimizing choices is better than offering too many choices. The client with an STI needs support from others, and emphasis should focus on the prevention of recurrences rather than the specifics of the duration of the disease.

15-58   Answer C

If your client with rheumatoid arthritis (RA) is taking birth control pills, she should continue taking them, as well as any medications for her RA.

15-59   Answer A

The diaphragm is a barrier method of contraception that may provide up to 6 hours or more of birth control. It is a dome-shaped rubber cup that has a flexible rim and is inserted into the vagina before intercourse so the posterior rim rests in the posterior portion of the vagina and the anterior rim fits snugly behind the pubic bone. The diaphragm covers the cervix and is used in conjunction with spermicide. When fit correctly, there should be just enough space to insert one fingertip comfortably between the inside of the pubic arch and the anterior edge of the diaphragm rim.

15-60   Answer D

Herpes simplex virus may be acquired before labor, during delivery, or postnatally. About 5% of infants with neonatal herpes acquire the virus before labor (intrauterine infection) and 85% by direct contact with the maternal genitalia or secretions during delivery. Postnatal acquisition occurs by direct contact with an infected caretaker and accounts for the other 10% of neonatal herpes infections.

15-61   Answer A

A treatment used to improve the chance of pregnancy in an infertile woman who has minimal or mild endometriosis is laparoscopic resection or ablation of the lesions. Although dilation and curettage remove tissue, it may not be the specific endometrial tissue involved. Gonadotropin-releasing hormone analogues suppress endometriosis by creating a pseudomenopause, which is not desired in a woman who wants to become pregnant.

15-62   Answer B

In the client complaining of premenstrual syndrome, advise her to increase her intake of complex carbohydrates. A diet high in complex carbohydrates, such as whole grains and cereals, fruits, and vegetables, helps prevent low blood sugar levels and reduces fatigue, jitteriness, and irritability. It may also raise serotonin levels, thus improving mood. Eating several small meals at frequent intervals rather than three large ones also keeps blood sugar on an even level and reduces the feeling of bloating. Women should also restrict their intake of salt, caffeine, and alcohol during the week before their period.

15-63   Answer B

Puerperal mastitis is a cellulitis that develops in the lactating or nonlactating breast after parturition. It is vital that the infant continue to breastfeed during puerperal mastitis to avoid milk stasis. Because the infection is extraductal, there is no risk to the infant on continuing breastfeeding. Massage of the breasts during feeding helps to better drain the breast, and additional pumping may be needed. Bedrest is imperative during the acute phase of the illness. The mother should be assisted with her household duties and rest in bed with her infant. Moist heat to the affected breast can be useful before feeding and pumping to increase mild expression. Cold application may be comfortable between feedings. Antibiotic therapy is traditionally recommended to treat the infection.

15-64   Answer C

A transverse rectus abdominis musculocutaneous (TRAM) flap procedure is a type of breast reconstruction surgery. It is an autogenous procedure in which skin is transferred from the rectus abdominis muscle to fashion a breast. It is performed immediately after the removal of the breast cancer. The abdominal muscle is fashioned into a new breast and a new nipple is created or the client's own one is used. Women seem to prefer this type of breast reconstructive surgery because a "tummy tuck" is done at the same time.

15-65   Answer B

Estradiol (E2) is the most potent form of estrogen and is secreted in the greatest amount by the ovaries during the reproductive years. Estrogens are secreted throughout the menstrual cycle, although at varying levels. They are essential for the development and maintenance of secondary sex characteristics and, along with progesterone and androgen, stimulate the female reproductive organs to prepare for the growth of a fetus. As ovarian function decreases, the production of estradiol decreases and is ultimately replaced by estrone (E1) as the major ovarian estrogen. Estrone has only a fraction of the potency of estradiol. During this time, the second ovarian hormone, progesterone, also is markedly reduced. Estrone is metabolized to estriol, which is the least potent of the three estrogens.

15-66   Answer D

A condom should be worn during sexual intercourse when one partner has genital herpes, even though there may not be a visible lesion. Shedding of the herpes simplex virus from mucocutaneous surfaces in the absence of visible lesions is a primary mode of transmission both horizontally (to sexual partners) and vertically (to the fetus).

15-67   Answer B

The woman who has extreme spasticity should assume a knee-chest position while prone for a Pap smear. Assistance may be required to keep the legs away from the perineal area. The OB stirrups position allows a woman who has difficulty using foot stirrups to assume the standard pelvic examination position. The client may need assistance in putting her legs into the stirrups up to the knees, which can be padded for comfort. The V-shaped position may be used without stirrups or with one foot in a stirrup. One or two assistants may be required to help the woman maintain this position by supporting each straightened leg at the knee and ankle. The client's comfort may be increased by elevating her legs slightly or by using a pillow under the small of her back or coccyx. The speculum must be inserted with the handle up. The side-lying position does not require stirrups and is most appropriate for the client who feels most comfortable and balanced lying on her side. This position is also good for the extremely obese woman. An assistant may help elevate one leg if the client cannot spread her legs. The speculum can be inserted with the handle pointing either toward the woman's back or front, but the clinician should be sure to angle the speculum toward the small of the client's back and not straight up toward her head.

15-68   Answer C

When a girl has pubic hair of adult type but over a smaller area with none on the medial thigh, she is in Tanner's sexual maturity rating stage IV. In girls, stage I is preadolescent with no pubic hair. In stage II, pubic hair growth is sparse and mostly on the labia. The hair is long and downy, slightly pigmented, and straight or only slightly curly. In stage III, the pubic hair is sparse and spreads over the mons pubis. The hair is darker, coarser, and curlier. In stage V, pubic hair is adult in type and patterned as an inverse triangle. Hair also appears on the medial thigh surface.

15-69   Answer A

Of the symptoms listed in the question, the most commonly expressed symptom of women with premenstrual syndrome is fatigue (90%). Depression occurs about 80% of the time; breast tenderness, about 85%; and swelling of the extremities, about 67%. Other common symptoms include irritability (91%) and abdominal bloating (90%).

15-70   Answer B

The *Mobiluncus* species causes bacterial vaginosis. The human papillomavirus is responsible for condylomata acuminata (genital warts). Lymphogranuloma venereum is a sexually transmitted infection characterized by localized lymphatic infection with a *Chlamydia* origin.

15-71   Answer C

Although the primary lesion of genital herpes normally resolves within 21 days, the client usually has recurrent episodes. Acyclovir (Zovirax) is a palliative management option, but the drug does not cure herpes simplex. Topical trichloroacetic acid is the treatment for genital warts, not herpes. Intercourse should be avoided when a lesion is present.

15-72   Answer C

Emergency contraception, referred to as postcoital contraception, prevents pregnancy after unprotected sexual intercourse. It should ideally be taken within 72 hours after unprotected intercourse. Waiting for menses to start or referring the client to a gynecologist is too late. In the United States, three methods are available. The Yuzpe regimen consists of taking two birth control pills within 72 hours and two more 12 hours later. This is 75% effective. A medication for nausea should be taken before the birth control pills. An alternative plan is to take progestin-only postcoital contraceptives, which reduce the risk of pregnancy by 89%. One pill (levonorgestrel 75 mg) is taken within 72 hours of unprotected sex and another 12 hours later. The third method of postcoital contraception involves inserting a copper IUD up to 7 days after unprotected sex. This method reduces the risk of pregnancy by 99%. Another choice would be a single dose of 200 mg of mifepristone, a synthetic antiprogestational-antiglucocorticoid pill to be used as an oral abortifacient. It induces abortion during the first 9 weeks of pregnancy. If it is followed in 36–48 hours with a prostaglandin vaginal suppository, the success rate in terminating the pregnancy is increased.

15-73   Answer A

The American College of Obstetricians and Gynecologists (ACOG) recommends that women age 50 and older should be screened for colorectal cancer using one of five recommended screening strategies. If fecal occult blood testing (FOBT) is used, patients should collect two or three samples at home and return them for laboratory analysis. Single samples obtained by digital rectal examination in the OB-GYN's office are not adequate for colorectal cancer screening.

15-74   Answer B

Vaginal flora of a normal reproductive aged female includes multiple anaerobic and aerobic species (10 to 1). The typical vagina pH ranges between 4 and 4.5. Lactobacilli in the vagina helps to maintain an acidic pH range to help protect against reproductive pathogens.

15-75   Answer D

Multiple pregnancies are not associated with dyspareunia. Dyspareunia (painful intercourse) may be caused by vulvovaginitis, an incompletely (or inadequately) stretched hymen during the initial intercourse, vaginismus, endometriosis, tumors or other pathological conditions, or psychosexual conflicts.

15-76   Answer D

In exercise-induced amenorrhea, such as occurs in dancers and marathon runners, the location of the problem is the hypothalamus. The outflow tract is the location of the problem with developmental absence of the vagina or uterus, obstruction of the outflow tract, scarred uterine lining, and cervical obstruction. The ovary is the location of the problem in primary amenorrhea if the etiology is a congenital chromosomal abnormality, such as Turner's syndrome. The anterior pituitary is the location of the problem with amenorrhea resulting from prolactin-secreting tumors or nonfunctioning adenomas.

15-77   Answer A

The most common virus known to be transmitted in utero is cytomegalovirus (CMV). Transmission of CMV can take place as a consequence of either primary or reactivated infection in the mother. Children in day-care settings can also transmit the virus to their mothers or day-care workers.

If the woman is infected in pregnancy, there is a 40% chance of transmission to the fetus, and 15% of infants born with CMV have symptoms such as hepatosplenomegaly, petechiae, small size for gestational age, direct hyperbilirubinemia, or thrombocytopenia. The risk is even higher for the infant if the mother acquires the disease early in the pregnancy. If a mother is infected with rubella in the first trimester, the rate of infection in utero is as high as 80%, but after the first trimester, the rate drops drastically. Congenital varicella is very rare. Toxoplasmosis is caused by a parasite, not a virus. When mothers are infected with toxoplasmosis during pregnancy, almost 40% of their infants become infected in utero, and about 15% of those children have severe clinical damage.

15-78   Answer C

There are many interventions that will alleviate the pain of fibrocystic breast disease, as well as help decrease the proliferation of breast tissue. Caffeine, chocolate, tea, colas, and drugs containing caffeine should be reduced to help alleviate breast tenderness and reduce nodularity. Vitamin E has been shown to decrease the pain and tenderness associated with fibrocystic change, as well as the proliferation of breast tissue. Daily aspirin therapy and spicy foods have not been associated with fibrocystic breast disease. Wearing a tight-fitting bra does not exacerbate the condition but may increase tenderness.

15-79   Answer D

A vaginal contraceptive ring (NuvaRing) is a soft, transparent, flexible ring of ethylene vinyl acetate copolymer. The ring releases 120 mcg of etonogestrel and 15 mcg of ethinyl estradiol daily. The ring is placed in the vagina once every 28 days and kept in place for 21 days. The ring is then removed for a 7-day period to allow for a withdrawal bleed. If the ring is accidentally expelled from the vagina for less than 3 hours, instruct the woman to rinse it with lukewarm water and reinsert it into her vagina. No backup method is needed. If the ring is expelled from the vagina for 3 hours or more, instruct the woman to discard the ring and (a) insert a new ring immediately and use backup method for an additional 7 days, or (b) have a withdrawal bleed and insert a ring no later than 7 days from when the last ring was removed and use backup methods for 7 days.

15-80   Answer D

Secondary ovarian tumors account for about 10% of the fatal malignant diseases in women. They are usually the result of bowel or breast metastases to the ovary, and all of the tumors are malignant. Follicle cysts are frequent in the menstrual years, never occur in the postmenopausal years, and do not have a potential for malignancy. Follicle cysts often disappear after a 2-month regimen of oral contraceptives. Fibromas account for less than 5% of the ovarian tumors and very rarely have the potential for malignancy. Brenner's tumor accounts for about 1% of ovarian tumors, occurs more than 50% of the time in postmenopausal women, and very rarely has the potential for malignancy.

15-81   Answer D

The etiology of infertility can be identified in 90% of couples. Male and female factor infertility are almost the same (males 30%, females 35%), and in 20% of cases there is a combination of male and female factors. It should also be stressed that infertility is no one's "fault" and that many things may be tried to assist the couple to conceive.

15-82   Answer A

You suspect an sexually transmitted infection (STI) because although the symptoms are suspicious for a urinary tract infection (UTI), the diagnosis is not supported by the dipstick and urine culture results. Your next action for Brianne is to obtain a culture of the urethra, do a potassium hydroxide wet prep to test for bacterial vaginosis, and obtain another urine culture. Doing so is the most efficient way of treating Brianne now. Discussing her social history might help you determine which course of action is most appropriate. However, if you do only one test now and it is negative, you might have to perform another diagnostic test, thereby delaying treatment again. A diagnosis of *Chlamydia* infection is accomplished by culture or smears for Gram staining, but this is expensive and takes 2–6 days to obtain results. Other techniques include direct immunofluorescence assay and enzyme immunoassay. Diagnosis of gonorrhea is accomplished through cultures of the discharge (urethral, endocervical, rectal, pharyngeal, or conjunctive) using a modified Thayer-Martin medium or by Gram staining to look for typical gram-negative intracellular diplococci. Diagnosis

of herpes simplex viruses is accomplished by the enzyme-linked immunosorbent assay technique or viral cultures. Another, less reliable method of diagnosis consists of serological antibody testing. The diagnosis of human papillomavirus infection is made by colposcopy. Trichomoniasis is diagnosed by pH that, as in bacterial vaginosis, is greater than 4.5 and by a microscopic finding of flagellated motile organisms resembling whips that are larger than white blood cells. By just treating the symptoms as a UTI or irritation, you could be ignoring the true problem, giving an STI time to spread. Medicating with antibiotics without identifying a definitive organism leads to antibiotic resistance.

15-83   Answer C

Phenobarbital (Luminal) is the drug of choice in a pregnant woman with a seizure disorder. Ideally, if the woman has not had a seizure for 5 years before the pregnancy, a prepregnancy trial of withdrawal from seizure medication should be tried. Valproate (Depakene) and trimethadione (Tridione) are contraindicated during pregnancy, and phenytoin (Dilantin) is teratogenic during the first trimester. If phenobarbital is used, serum levels should be measured in each trimester, and the dosage should be such that it maintains the serum levels in the low-normal therapeutic range.

15-84   Answer A

When premenstrual syndrome symptoms do not respond to other treatments, you may prescribe any of the following drugs to aid in alleviating the symptoms: antidepressants, such as paroxetine (Paxil), fluoxetine (Prozac), or sertraline (Zoloft) to raise the levels of serotonin; diuretics to help relieve bloating; gonadotropin-releasing hormone agonists to suppress the menstrual cycle; antianxiety agents such as alprazolam (Xanax); and an oral progesterone to help relieve bloating and moodiness.

15-85   Answer D

The normal vaginal discharge has a pH of 3.8–4.2. The vaginal pH in prepubescent girl is usually above 7 due to lack of estrogen. The vagina of a postmenopausal woman with atrophic vaginitis lacks estrogen and is usually greater than 6. Women infected with trichomoniasis vaginalis have a vaginal pH of greater than 4.5.

15-86 Answer D

Caffeine in large amounts will make the infant who is being nursed irritable and give him or her a poor sleep pattern. Cimetidine (Tagamet) and ranitidine (Zantac) are concentrated in breast milk and may suppress the infant's gastric acidity and cause central nervous system stimulation. Ergotamine (Ergostat) in doses sufficient to treat a migraine may cause vomiting, diarrhea, and convulsions, as well as suppress lactation. Nicotine increases the incidence of respiratory disease in infants exposed to smoke.

15-87 Answer D

Heart disease is considered a contraindication to the use of a copper intrauterine device (IUD) because the client may be susceptible to bacterial endocarditis. The following conditions were previously believed to preclude the use of IUDs, including the copper IUD, but they are no longer contraindications: history of ectopic pregnancy (remains a contraindication to use with the progesterone-containing IUDs), nulliparity, treated cervical dysplasia, diabetes mellitus, valvular heart disease, irregular menses as a result of anovulation, breastfeeding, corticosteroid use, and age under 25 years. The conditions that preclude systemic hormonal methods (breast cancer, venous thromboembolism or phlebitis, arterial vascular disease, active liver disease, and age older than 35 combined with smoking) do not preclude intrauterine contraception.

15-88 Answer A

Nausea and vomiting occurring during the first trimester are probably a result of hormonal changes such as the production of human chorionic gonadotropin. Women also experience pyrosis because of esophageal reflux caused by a decrease in gastrointestinal motility, leading to prolonged gastric emptying time.

15-89 Answer C

Candida albicans infection is more common in women with diabetes, as well as those who are pregnant, immunosuppressed, or using antibiotics or oral contraceptives.

15-90 Answer B

CA 125 is a tumor marker that is highly specific to epithelial ovarian cancer. Increased levels (greater than 35 U/mL) may indicate peritoneal diseases such as endometriosis, although significant elevations are usually found with ovarian cancer. The prostrate-specific antigen (PSA) is the tumor marker for prostate cancer, although high levels have also been shown with benign prostatic hypertrophy, prostate massage, prostate surgery, and prostatitis. CA 15-3 level is elevated in metastatic breast disease and may be elevated in benign breast or ovarian disease. CA 19-9 level is elevated in pancreatic and hepatobiliary cancer.

15-91 Answer D

Emergency contraception or emergency birth control refers to keeping a woman from getting pregnant when she has had unprotected sex. Depending on when they are taken, the pills work by keeping the egg from leaving the ovary, by keeping the sperm from meeting the egg, or by keeping a fertilized egg from attaching to the uterus. They must be taken within 5 days of unprotected sex in order to work. There are two types of emergency contraception pills. Plan B is a progestin-only pill taken for the purpose of emergency contraception. One pill is taken immediately; the next is taken 12 hours later. In the second type, a higher dose of regular birth control pills is taken. The number of pills is different for each brand and, again, one dose is taken immediately and the second dose is taken 12 hours later. Plan B is sold over the counter to women older than the age of 18 without a prescription.

The abortion pill—Mifeprex, also called RU 486—is for use after a woman becomes pregnant (after a fertilized egg has already attached to the uterus). Mifeprex is used with misoprostol and can end an early pregnancy within 49 days of the start of a woman's last menstrual period. The regimen for a medical abortion through day 49 of a pregnancy is on day 1 to take Mifeprex three tabs of 200 mg together, and then on day 3 to take misoprostol two tabs of 200 mcg together. On day 14 the client should see her health-care provider to confirm that a complete termination of the pregnancy has occurred.

15-92 Answer B

One of the leading causes of female infertility, Stein-Leventhal syndrome is polycystic ovary syndrome (PCOS). It is a condition that afflicts many women during their childbearing years. Symptoms of PCOS, which are related to androgen excess and not associated with estrogen deficiency, include amenorrhea, hirsutism, acne, and obesity.

15-93   Answer A

Toxic shock syndrome (TSS) is a potentially lethal disorder that is caused in almost all cases by absorption of one or more toxins produced by colonized *Staphylococcus aureus*. Several mechanisms are implicated as causative, although not proven. They include tampon contamination with *S. aureus*, damaged cervical and vaginal mucosa, the use of superabsorbent tampons (or the synthetic materials they are made of) for an extended period of time, absorption of bacteriostatic cervical secretions, alterations in the normal vaginal flora, mechanical blockage of menstrual fluids, and the enhanced multiplication of the organism in the menstrual efflux. The incidence of TSS has decreased steadily as a result of education, altered patterns of tampon use, and the removal of extremely high-absorbency tampons from the market. A urinary tract infection involving the bladder and kidneys does not cause TSS.

15-94   Answer A

Nothing should be inserted in the vagina for 24 hours before performing a Pap smear. Douching should be discouraged in all women because it changes the normal flora, increasing the likelihood of an infection. An acute infection or heavy menses precludes Pap testing because it alters the ability of the practitioner to obtain an adequate sample. Some women find the Pap test physically or emotionally very uncomfortable; therefore, reassurance about its necessity should be provided.

15-95   Answer D

Procidentia is a third-degree uterine prolapse. Prolapse of the uterus can vary from mild to complete. In procidentia, also called hysteroptosia, the uterus prolapses completely outside the body, with inversion of the vagina. It is generally attributable to the relation of the tissues that provide support for the pelvic organs. A cystocele is a herniation of the urinary bladder into the vagina. A rectocele is a hernial protrusion of part of the rectum into the vagina. A vesicovaginal fistula is an abnormal opening between the urinary bladder and the vagina, leading to incontinent leakage of urine through the vagina. A rectovaginal fistula is an abnormal opening between the rectum and vagina, causing incontinent leakage of stool or flatus

through the vagina. This type is less common than the vesicovaginal fistula.

15-96   Answer D

The clinical consequences of persistent anovulation include infertility; menstrual bleeding problems, ranging from amenorrhea to dysfunctional uterine bleeding; an increased risk of cardiovascular disease; hirsutism and acne; an increased risk of endometrial cancer and breast cancer; and an increased risk of diabetes mellitus in clients with hyperinsulinemia. Therapy depends on the client. If the client wants to get pregnant, she is a candidate for the medical induction of ovulation. For the client who does not wish to become pregnant and does not complain of hirsutism but is anovulatory and has irregular bleeding, therapy is directed toward interruption of the steady-state effect on the endometrium and breast. Mastalgia is breast pain. The breast is a complex organ that is sensitive to hormones. Estradiol and progesterone stimulate breast tissue. Breast pain that positively correlates with menses is cyclic mastalgia. Cyclic mastalgia is the most common breast-related complaint seen in women's health practice. Menorrhagia is excessive bleeding but at the normal time during the month. Endometriosis is extrauterine growth of the endometrial glands or stroma. It is believed to occur through retrograde menstruation, or differentiation of totipotential cells, or both.

15-97   Answer D

Metrorrhagia is menses with irregular intervals and excessive flow and duration. Oligomenorrhea is menses with an interval of more than 35 days. Polymenorrhea is menses with intervals of less than 21 days. Menorrhagia is menses of regular normal intervals, but with extensive flow and duration.

15-98   Answer D

Although pregnancy seems like an obvious choice as the most likely cause of amenorrhea, it is sometimes overlooked, especially if the client denies the possibility of pregnancy and is seeking a pathological reason for the amenorrhea. The most likely physiological causes of amenorrhea that should be considered are pregnancy, lactation, and menopause, if appropriate. Among women who are in the childbearing years, amenorrhea unrelated to pregnancy may signal stress or a life-threatening disease. These conditions may include anatomical deviations, genetic factors, endocrine abnormalities or imbalances, defective enzyme systems, autoimmune diseases, tumors, eating disorders, excessive exercise, and medications. With amenorrhea, a pregnancy test should always be done first to rule out pregnancy or its related complications: ectopic pregnancies, complete or incomplete abortions, and trophoblastic neoplasms. The most accurate test for pregnancy is the serum beta human chorionic gonadotropin test.

15-99   Answer A

Management of DUB is directed toward controlling bleeding and preventing a recurrence. For women who cannot take oral contraceptives (OCs), medroxyprogesterone is offered. For teenagers, management includes observation for those with mild cases and no anemia, medroxyprogesterone for clients not sexually active, or OCs for sexually active teenagers. For women of reproductive age, treatment is based on the woman's desire for fertility or contraception. OCs containing ethinyl estradiol (EE) are used in acute bleeding episodes. For women with severe acute bleeding but who remain hemodynamically stable, conjugated estrogen is used until bleeding stops. Piroxicam is used for dysmenorrhea.

15-100   Answer D

Characteristics of polycystic ovary syndrome (PCOS) include premenarchal onset, obesity, hyperinsulinemia, hyperandrogenism (hirsutism, seborrhea, acne, alopecia), menstrual disturbances, and infertility. Visible signs of the syndrome are obesity, acne, and hirsutism. Clients with PCOS typically present with complaints of amenorrhea or irregular menstrual cycles, but some have the initial complaint of infertility. About 10%–20% of clients with PCOS are symptomatic. PCOS should be considered in all clients presenting with amenorrhea, infertility, or hirsutism.

15-101   Answer B

Dysfunctional uterine bleeding (DUB) is excessive, prolonged, and unpatterned bleeding from the endometrium in the absence of any structural pelvic pathology. It is usually associated with anovulation. DUB is not related to pregnancy, inflammation, genital tumor, or other anatomical uterine lesion. Although no organic problems are associated with DUB, a history and physical examination and

pelvic and rectal examinations are done to rule out neoplasia. These are followed by diagnostic tests and blood work.

15-102   Answer D

Douching will not prevent sperm from entering the uterus because sperm may enter the cervical canal as soon as 15 seconds after ejaculation. Douching may even enhance the movement of sperm up the canal because it washes fluids deeper into the vagina and washes away the protective mucus. Douching has been associated with an increased risk of pelvic infection and ectopic pregnancy and most gynecologists do not recommend it at any time.

15-103   Answer A

A colposcopy visualizes the cervical, vaginal, or vulvar epithelium under magnification to identify abnormal areas that may require a biopsy. It is performed in the office. An endometrial biopsy removes one or more areas of the endometrium by means of a curette or small aspiration device without cervical dilation. A hysteroscopy allows visual examination of the uterine cavity with a small fiber-optic endoscope passed through the cervix. A laparoscopy allows visualization of the abdominal and pelvic cavity through a small fiber-optic endoscope passed through a subumbilical incision.

15-104   Answer B

Bartholin's cyst is an obstruction or infection of the Bartholin's gland. It results in pain, redness, a perineal mass, and dyspareunia. An ovarian cyst may be functional or inflammatory. A functional ovarian cyst occurs during ovulation and may be asymptomatic and resolve spontaneously, or it can cause pain, menstrual irregularity, or amenorrhea. An inflammatory cyst is an infection of the ovary or uterine tube and results in an elevated white blood cell count, a low-grade fever, pain, and excessive menstrual flow. A Gardner's duct cyst is present in the vagina during fetal development and usually goes away before birth. However, it can be persistent after birth on the sidewalls of the vagina and does not cause any symptoms. A nabothian cyst is a mucus-filled lump on the surface of the cervix and is asymptomatic.

15-105   Answer D

When the uterus is anteverted, the position of the cervix is on the anterior vaginal wall. When the position of the uterus is midposition, the cervix is at the apex of the vagina. When it is retroverted, the cervix is on the posterior vaginal wall. When the uterus is retroflexed, the position of the cervix may be on the anterior or posterior vaginal wall or the apex.

15-106   Answer C

Small-quantity incontinence, which produces nearly continuous dribbling, is symptomatic of overflow incontinence. Stress incontinence is symptomized by small-quantity incontinence on coughing, sneezing, laughing, and running. Urge incontinence involves an uncontrolled urge to void and is symptomized by large-quantity incontinence. Functional incontinence involves voiding normally with assistance.

15-107   Answer D

In early pregnancy, increased vascularity, blood supply, and congestion to the cervix causes a bluish discoloration which is termed Chadwick's sign. The cervix is normally firm; however, at 6 weeks of pregnancy, there is marked softening of the cervix. This is called Goodell's sign. Hegar's sign is the softening of the lower uterine segment between the body of the uterus and the cervix and can be felt on bimanual exam. Piskacek's asymmetric enlargement of the body of the pregnant uterus due to implantation.

15-108   Answer A

Bartholin's (greater vestibular) glands are posterior on each side of the vaginal orifice and open onto the sides of the vestibule in the groove between the labia minor and hymen. Skene's (lesser vestibular, paraurethral) glands open onto the vestibule on each side of the urethra. Cystocele is a herniation of posterior bladder into the anterior vagina with a primary symptom of incontinence.

15-109   Answer C

Thelarche (breast bud development) is the first sign of puberty in most girls. It occurs at an average age of 11 years. It is considered premature if it occurs before age 8. Premature thelarche without other signs of pubertal development or accelerated growth is usually benign and requires no treatment. It should be diagnosed after a medical evaluation is performed to exclude true precocious puberty,

estrogen-producing tumors, ovarian cysts, and exogenous estrogen exposure.

15-110   Answer C

Signs and symptoms of a genital herpes infection include tender inguinal lymph nodes, as well as painful or pruritic vesicles, dysuria, prodromal tingling or pruritus of the genital region (which usually occurs first), and cervical ulcerations. White, curdlike plaques on a red base in the vagina are seen with monilial vaginitis.

15-111   Answer C

Pelvic inflammatory disease (PID) comprises a spectrum of inflammatory disorders of the upper female genital tract. Sexually transmitted organisms, especially *Neisseria gonorrhoeae* and *Chlamydia trachomatis*, are implicated in many cases. Empiric treatment for PID should be initiated in sexually active young women and other women at risk for sexually transmitted infections if they are experiencing pelvic or lower abdominal pain, if no cause for the illness other than PID can be identified, and if one or more of the following minimum criteria are present on pelvic examination: cervical motion tenderness, uterine tenderness, adnexal tenderness.

Bibliography

American College of Obstetricians and Gynecologists (ACOG): Cervical cancer in adolescents: Screening, evaluation, and management. Committee Opinion #463. August 2010.

American College of Obstetricians and Gynecologists (ACOG): Primary and preventative care. Committee Opinion #483. April, 2011.

Beckmann, C, Ling, F, Barzansky, B, Herbert, W, Laube, D, and Smith, R: *Obstetrics and Gynecology*, ed 6. Lippincott Williams & Wilkins, Philadelphia, 2010.

Centers for Disease Control and Prevention (CDC): Genital HPV fact sheet. Updated August 11, 2011. www.cdc.gov/std/HPV/STDFact-HPV.htm, accessed October 26, 2011.

Centers for Disease Control and Prevention (CDC): Sexually transmitted diseases (STDs). Updated October 11, 2011. www.cdc.gov/std/, accessed October 18, 2011.

Centers for Disease Control and Prevention (CDC): Sexually transmitted diseases 2010 treatment guidelines. Updated January 28, 2011. www.cdc.gov/std/treatment/2010/pid.htm, accessed October 26, 2011.

Crouch, SJ, Rowell, KR, and Beiser, SO: Umbilical cord blood for newborn DNA identification. *Journal of Obstetric, Gynecologic, and Neonatal Nursing* 36(4):308–312, July/August 2007.

Dunphy, LM, et al: *Primary Care: The Art and Science of Advanced Practice Nursing*, ed 2. FA Davis, Philadelphia, 2011.

Hackley, B, Kriebs, JM, and Rousseau, ME: *Primary Care of Women: A Guide for Midwives and Women's Health Care Providers*. Jones and Bartlett, Boston, 2007.

Hatcher, R, Trussell, J, Nelson, A, Cates, W, Stewart, F, and Kowal, D: *Contraceptive Technology*, ed 19. Ardent Media, New York, 2009.

March of Dimes: Pregnancy, baby, prematurity, and birth defects. Updated 2011. www.marchofdimes.com, accessed October 22, 2011.

Rosen, HN: Bisphosphonates in the management of osteoporosis in postmenopausal women. Pamphlet by American Academy of Nurse Practitioners in the series *Up-To-Date in Adult Primary Care and Internal Medicine*, January 12, 2007.

Schorge, J, Schaffer, J, Halvoron, L, Hoffman, B, Bradshaw, K, and Cunningham, FG: *Williams Gynecology*. McGraw Hill, New York, 2008.

Women's Health Initiative: Findings from the WHI postmenopausal hormonal therapy trials. Updated September 21, 2010. www.nhlbi.nih.gov/whi/, accessed October 18, 2011.

World Health Organization (WHO): Hormone contraception and bone health (2007). Updated 2011. www.who.int/reproductivehealth/publications/family_planning/pbrief1/en/index.html, accessed October 26, 2011.

How well did you do?

85% and above, congratulations! This score shows application of test-taking principles and adequate content knowledge.

75%–85%, keep working! Review test-taking principles and try again.

65%–75%, hang in there! Spend some time reviewing concepts and test-taking principles and then try the test again.

Chapter 16: *Musculoskeletal Problems*

Sharon K. Byrne
Lynne M. Dunphy
Jill E. Winland-Brown

Questions

16-1 *If any limitation or any increase in range of motion occurs when assessing the musculoskeletal system, the angles of the bones should be measured by using*

A. Phalen's test.

B. skeletometry.

C. the Thomas test.

D. a goniometer.

16-2 *Jake, age 16, comes into the office with a human bite on his fist. What is the first course of action?*

A. De-bride and irrigate the wound thoroughly.

B. Initiate broad-spectrum antibiotics.

C. Leave the wound open for drainage.

D. Administer a tetanus injection.

16-3 *Sandy, age 49, presents with loss of anal sphincter tone, impaired micturition, incontinence, and progressive loss of strength in the legs. You suspect cauda equina syndrome. What is your next action?*

A. Order physical therapy.

B. Order a lumbar/sacral x-ray.

C. Order extensive lab work.

D. Refer to a neurosurgeon.

16-4 *In assessing the skeletal muscles, you turn the forearm so that the palm is up. This is called*

A. supination.

B. pronation.

C. abduction.

D. eversion.

16-5 *Ethan, a 10-year-old boy, jumps off a 2-foot wall, twisting his foot and ankle upon landing. His ankle x-ray demonstrates a fracture of the distal tibia over the articular surface into the epiphysis and physis. Based on the Salter-Harris classification for growth plate injuries, you know this is a*

A. Salter-Harris II.

B. Salter-Harris III.

C. Salter-Harris IV.

D. Salter-Harris V.

16-6 *Karen, who is postmenopausal, is taking 1,500 mg of calcium but does not understand why she also needs to take vitamin D. You tell her that*

A. a deficiency of vitamin D results in an inadequate mineralization of bone matrix.

B. all vitamins need to be supplemented.

C. vitamin D increases intestinal absorption of dietary calcium and mobilizes calcium from the bone.

D. vitamin D binds with calcium to allow active transport into the cells.

16-7 *The American College of Obstetricians and Gynecologists' guidelines for exercise during pregnancy and after delivery include which of the following?*

A. Women should try to exercise moderately for at least 30 minutes on most, if not all, days of the week.

B. Exercise in the supine position is the position of choice.

C. Anaerobic exercise during pregnancy is preferred over aerobic exercise.

D. Exercise should be discontinued upon discovery of pregnancy and be resumed after delivery.

16-8 *Colchicine may be used to terminate an acute attack of gouty arthritis, as well as to prevent recurrent episodes. The mechanism of action is to*

A. interrupt the cycle of urate crystal deposition and inflammatory response.

B. increase serum uric acid levels.

C. potentiate the excretion of uric acid.

D. inhibit the tubular reabsorption of urate, promoting the excretion of uric acid.

16-9   Lois, age 52, who has just been given a diagnosis of sarcoidosis, has joint symptoms including arthralgias and arthritis. Your next plan of action would be to

A. order a bone scan.

B. obtain a tissue biopsy.

C. begin a course of glucocorticoids.

D. obtain an electrocardiogram.

16-10   Greg, age 26, runs marathons and frequently complains of painful contractions of his calf muscles after running. You attribute this to

A. hypercalcemia.

B. hyponatremia.

C. heat exhaustion.

D. dehydration.

16-11   Steve, age 15, has only one testicle. When he asks you if he can play on the soccer team at school, how do you respond?

A. "No, you'd be taking too much of a chance of injuring your remaining testicle."

B. "You can play any noncontact sport; however, soccer is too strenuous."

C. "As long as you can protect the remaining testicle, go for it."

D. "It should have no bearing on any activity."

16-12   There are many precursors of deep venous thrombosis (DVT), such as decreased blood flow, injury to the blood vessel wall, and altered blood coagulation. Which clinical risk factor for DVT is the result of hypercoagulability?

A. High estrogen states, such as with oral contraceptives

B. Trauma that results in orthopedic surgery

C. An indwelling intravenous catheter of a lower extremity

D. Prolonged sedentary position related to immobility

16-13   Heidi, age 29, is a nurse who has an acute episode of back pain. You have determined that it is a simple "mechanical" backache and order

A. bedrest for 2 days.

B. muscle relaxants.

C. "let pain be your guide" and continue activities.

D. back-strengthening exercises.

16-14   Daniel, who is 45 and of northern European ancestry, has a dysfunctional and disfiguring condition affecting the palmar tissue between the skin and the distal palm and fourth and fifth fingers. What do you suspect?

A. Hallux valgus

B. De Quervain's tenosynovitis

C. Dupuytren's contracture

D. Hallux rigidus

16-15   For your client with a knee injury, you order an NSAID to be taken on a routine basis for the next 2 weeks. Your teaching should include which of the following?

A. "You may take this medication on an empty stomach as long as you eat within 2–3 hours of taking it."

B. "If one pill does not seem to help, you can double the dose for subsequent doses."

C. "If you notice nausea/vomiting or black or bloody stools, take the next dose with a glass of milk or a full meal."

D. "If you have additional pain, an occasional acetaminophen (Tylenol) is permitted in between the usual doses of the NSAID."

16-16   Joyce, age 87, broke her wrist after falling off a curb. She just had a plaster cast applied to her wrist. In instructing her family on allowing the cast to dry properly, tell them to

A. continuously elevate Joyce's arm on a pillow.

B. change the position of Joyce's arm every hour.

C. position a fan near Joyce during the night to ensure even drying of the cast.

D. put a blanket over the cast to absorb the dampness.

16-17 *James, age 17, has been complaining of a painful knob below his right knee that has prevented him from actively participating in sports. He has recently been given a diagnosis of Osgood-Schlatter disease and asks you about his treatment options. You tell him that the initial treatment is*

A. relative rest; he could benefit from hamstring stretching, heel cord stretching, and quadriceps stretching exercises.

B. immobilization; a long-leg knee immobilizer is recommended.

C. surgical intervention; removal of the bony fragments is necessary.

D. bedrest for 1 week.

16-18 *Which of the following tests assesses the patency of the radial and ulnar arteries?*

A. Allen test

B. Finkelstein's test

C. Phalen's test

D. Tinel's sign

16-19 *Mrs. Matthews has rheumatoid arthritis. On reviewing an x-ray of her hip, you notice that there is a marked absence of articular cartilage. What mechanism is responsible for this?*

A. Antigen-antibody formation

B. Lymphocyte response

C. Immune complex formation

D. Lysosomal degradation

16-20 *Beth, age 49, comes in with low back pain. An x-ray of the lumbar/sacral spine is within normal limits. Which of the following diagnoses do you explore further?*

A. Scoliosis

B. Osteoarthritis

C. Spinal stenosis

D. Herniated nucleus pulposus

16-21 *In assessing an infant for developmental dysplasia of the hip (DDH), the practitioner places the infant supine, flexes the knees by holding the thumbs on the inner midthighs, with fingers outside on the hips touching the greater trochanters, stabilizes one hip, and abducts and gently pulls*

anteriorly on the other thigh. If this external rotation feels smooth with no sound present, there is no hip dislocation. This is

A. the Allis test.

B. Lasègue's sign.

C. the McMurray test.

D. Ortolani maneuver.

16-22 *A common cause of in-toeing in childhood is*

A. internal tibial torsion.

B. femoral retroversion.

C. external tibial torsion.

D. flat feet.

16-23 *A clinical manifestation of symmetric neurogenic pain may indicate*

A. radiculopathy.

B. reflex sympathetic dystrophy.

C. entrapment neuropathy.

D. peripheral neuropathy.

16-24 *Mr. Miller is a 72-year-old African American with type 1 diabetes mellitus. He has been a chronic smoker for 50 years. He has been told recently that he must have an above-the-knee amputation because of a gangrenous foot. He has lost the will to live and states, "They shoot horses, don't they?" How do you respond?*

A. "You should be thankful they can save your life, if not your leg."

B. "Your wife needs you; you must think of her at this time."

C. "How do you feel this surgery will affect you?"

D. "I will stay with you before, during, and after the surgery because I know that this is a difficult time for you."

16-25 *Mr. McKinsey was recently given a diagnosis of degenerative joint disease. Which assessment test would you use to check for effusion on his knee?*

A. Thomas test

B. Tinel's sign

C. Bulge test

D. Phalen's test

16-26   You correctly perform the obturator test when you raise the client's leg with knee flexed and internally rotate the leg. A positive obturator test is indicative of

A. avascular necrosis (AVN) of the femoral head.

B. cholecystitis.

C. hip bursitis.

D. appendicitis.

16-27   You suspect a herniated disk on Sarah, age 72. You elevate her affected leg when she is in the supine position and it elicits back pain and sciatic nerve pain, which indicates a positive test. This is known as which test or sign?

A. Femoral stretch test

B. Cross straight-leg-raising test

C. Doorbell sign

D. Straight-leg-raising test

16-28   June, a 59-year-old cashier, presents with back pain with no precipitating event. The pain is located over her lower back and muscles without sciatica, and it is aggravated by sitting, standing, and certain movements. It is alleviated with rest. Palpation localizes the pain, and muscle spasms are felt. There was an insidious onset with progressive improvement. What is your initial diagnosis?

A. Ankylosing spondylitis

B. Musculoskeletal strain

C. Spondylolisthesis

D. Herniated disk

16-29   Which of the following would be considered a common cause of sudden death in athletes younger than age 30?

A. Bronchospasm from exercise-induced asthma

B. Hypertrophic cardiomyopathy

C. Compartment syndrome

D. Meningitis

16-30   Cass, age 67, tells you that she has been diagnosed with a condition that causes sudden flares of pain, swelling, and redness of the joints in her toes. She cannot remember the name of the diagnosis but she knows that it is caused by urate crystals that "get stuck in the joint and cause

pain." Joan is on hydrochlorothiazide (HCTZ) for management of her hypertension. You suspect a diagnosis of

A. septic arthritis.

B. gout.

C. rheumatoid arthritis.

D. Charcot neuro-osteoarthropathy.

16-31   During a sports preparticipation physical examination, when you ask the client to rise up on his toes and raise his heels, you are observing for

A. calf symmetry and leg strength.

B. hip, knee, and ankle symmetry.

C. hip, knee, and ankle motion.

D. scoliosis, hip motion, and hamstring tightness.

16-32   What part of the body is affected by Dupuytren's contracture?

A. The fourth and fifth fingers

B. The great toe

C. The tibia

D. The penis

16-33   Christian, a 22-year-old carpenter who is right-hand dominant, comes to you for follow-up from the emergency department where he was seen for right forearm pain. He states he was diagnosed with right forearm tendinitis and wants you to explain this diagnosis to him. You explain that he has inflammation of one or more tendons, which are

A. the ropelike bundles of collagen fibrils that connect bone to bone.

B. the collagen fibers that connect muscle to bone.

C. the pouches of synovial fluid that cushion bone and other joint structures.

D. the fibrocartilaginous disks that separate bony surfaces.

16-34   What is the type of joint that is freely movable, such as the shoulder joint, called?

A. Synarthrosis joint

B. Amphiarthrosis joint

C. Diarthrosis joint

D. Juxtarthrosis joint

16-35   Mickey is on a chemotherapeutic antibiotic for a musculoskeletal neoplasm. Which drug do you think he is taking?

A. Cyclophosphamide (Cytoxan)

B. Doxorubicin (Adriamycin)

C. Methotrexate (Rheumatrex)

D. Cisplatin (Platinol)

16-36   Jim, age 64, has rheumatoid arthritis (RA). Which of the following drugs would be of the least benefit?

A. Disease-modifying antirheumatic drugs (DMARDs)

B. Acetaminophen (Tylenol)

C. NSAIDs

D. Glucocorticoids

16-37   First-line drug therapy for acute low back pain includes the use of

A. NSAIDs.

B. muscle relaxants.

C. opioids.

D. antidepressants.

16-38   Janine, age 69, has a class III case of rheumatoid arthritis. According to the American Rheumatism Association, her function would be

A. adequate for normal activities despite a handicap of discomfort or limited motion of one or more joints.

B. largely or wholly incapacitated, bedridden, or confined to a wheelchair permitting little or no self-care.

C. completely able to carry on all usual duties without handicaps.

D. adequate to perform only few or none of the duties of usual occupation or self-care.

16-39   A coccygeal fracture is treated with

A. traction.

B. surgical repair.

C. analgesia and by use of a "donut" cushion when sitting.

D. prolonged bedrest for 6 weeks.

16-40   Marsha, age 34, presents with symptoms resembling both fibromyalgia and chronic fatigue syndrome, which have many similarities. Which of the following is more characteristic of fibromyalgia than of chronic fatigue syndrome?

A. Musculoskeletal pain

B. Difficulty sleeping

C. Depression

D. Fatigue

16-41   You have just completed a work-up on Michael, age 13, and confirmed Osgood-Schlatter disease. You should

A. refer to orthopedics for early surgical correction.

B. recommend physical therapy for quadriceps-strengthening exercises.

C. advise him to temporarily discontinue all sports activities until his growth plates have completely fused.

D. tell Michael that he can resume his usual activities immediately without concern and should begin aggressive exercises to increase muscle bulk and strength.

16-42   John, age 17, works as a stock boy at the local supermarket. He is in the office for a routine visit. You notice that he had an episode of low back pain 6 months ago from improperly lifting heavy boxes. In discussing proper body mechanics with him to prevent future injuries, you tell him,

A. "Bend your knees and face the object straight on."

B. "Hold boxes away from your body at arm's length."

C. "Bend and twist simultaneously as you lift."

D. "Keep your feet firmly together."

16-43   Ginny, age 48, has rheumatoid arthritis and gets achy and stiff after sitting through a long movie. This is referred to as

A. longevity stiffness.

B. gelling.

C. intermittent arthritis.

D. molding.

16-44 *Which of the following statements is true regarding vertebrae?*

A. All people have only 24 vertebrae (cervical, thoracic, lumbar).

B. Due to differences in race or gender, select groups may have 23 or 25 vertebrae (cervical, thoracic, lumbar).

C. It is common to have fewer than 23 vertebrae (cervical, thoracic, lumbar).

D. It is common to have more than 25 vertebrae (cervical, thoracic, lumbar).

16-45 *Which muscle enzyme is elevated in polymyositis?*

A. Aldolase A

B. Aspartate aminotransferase

C. Creatine kinase

D. Lactate dehydrogenase

16-46 *Alexander, age 18, sprained his ankle playing ice hockey. He is confused as to whether to apply heat or cold. What do you tell him?*

A. "Use continuous heat for the first 12 hours, then use heat or cold to your own preference."

B. "Use continuous cold for the first 12 hours, then use heat or cold to your own preference."

C. "Apply cold for 20 minutes, then take it off for 30–45 minutes; repeat for the first 24–48 hours while awake."

D. "Alternate between cold and heat for 20 minutes each for the first 24–48 hours."

16-47 *Which test assesses for thoracic outlet syndrome by having the client abduct his or her arms 90 degrees externally rotated with the elbows flexed 90 degrees, and then having the client open and close his or her hands for 3 minutes?*

A. Neer test

B. Speeds test

C. Hawkins test

D. Roos test

16-48 *When wrist and finger extension causes pain over the extensor carpi radialis brevis tendon, the extensor carpi radialis longus tendon, and the extensor digitorum communis, you would suspect*

A. tennis elbow.

B. golfer's elbow.

C. de Quervain's disease.

D. intersection syndrome.

16-49 *Anne, a 67-year-old female who sustained a fall on an outstretched hand, presents holding her arm against her chest with her elbow flexed. Based on the specific location of her pain, you suspect a radial head fracture. Your best initial assessment strategy to assess for radial head fracture would be*

A. to palpate for tenderness, swelling, and crepitus just distal to the lateral epicondyle.

B. to palpate for tenderness, swelling, and crepitus along the radial wrist.

C. to palpate for tenderness in the "anatomical snuffbox."

D. to order an x-ray of the wrist.

16-50 *A 13-year-old obese (BMI greater than 95%) boy reports low-grade left knee pain for the past 2 months. He denies antecedent trauma but admits to frequent "horseplay" with his friends. The pain has progressively worsened, and he is now unable to bear weight at all on his left leg. His current complaints include left groin, thigh, and medial knee pain and tenderness. His examination demonstrates negative drawer, Lachman, and McMurray tests; left hip with decreased internal rotation and abduction; and knee flexion causing external hip rotation. Based on the above scenario, you suspect*

A. left meniscal tear.

B. left anterior cruciate ligament (ACL) tear.

C. slipped capital femoral epiphysis (SCFE).

D. Osgood-Schlatter disease.

16-51 *Steve, age 32, fell off a roof while shingling it. He is complaining of pain in his left hip and leg area. Other than an x-ray, what would make you suspect a fractured pelvis?*

A. A clicking sensation when moving the hips

B. A positive pelvic tilt test

C. Hematuria

D. Absence of distal reflexes

16-52   *You are assessing Mike, age 16, after a football injury to his right knee. You elicit a positive anterior/posterior drawer sign. This test indicates an injury to the*

A. lateral meniscus.

B. cruciate ligament.

C. medial meniscus.

D. collateral ligament.

16-53   *Margaret, a 55-year-old female, presents to you for evaluation of left hand and wrist pain and swelling after a slip and fall on the ice yesterday. On examination, you note tenderness at her "anatomical snuffbox." You know this probably indicates*

A. ulnar styloid fracture.

B. scaphoid fracture.

C. hamate fracture.

D. radial head fracture.

16-54   *Mike, a golf pro, has had chronic back pain for many years. His work-up reveals that it is not the result of a degenerative disk problem. His back "goes out" about twice per year, and he is out of work for about a week each time. Which of the following should you advise him to do?*

A. Consider changing careers to a less physical job.

B. Begin a planned exercise program to strengthen back muscles.

C. Make an appointment with a neurosurgeon for a surgical consultation.

D. Start on a daily low-dose narcotic to take away the pain.

16-55   *In analyzing synovial fluid, a yellow-green color may indicate which of the following?*

A. Trauma

B. Gout

C. A bacterial infection

D. Rheumatoid arthritis

16-56   *Jane, age 64, comes in for a visit. She has a cast on her right arm and tells you that she has a comminuted fracture of her radius. When she asks*

what that means, you tell her that in a comminuted fracture the

A. bony fragments are in many pieces.

B. broken ends of the bone protrude through the soft tissues and skin.

C. bone breaks cleanly but does not penetrate the skin.

D. bone is crushed.

16-57   *Jeffrey, age 16, was involved in a motor vehicle accident. He walks into the office with an obvious facial fracture, then collapses. What should your first action be?*

A. Call his parents for permission to treat.

B. Assess for an adequate airway.

C. Obtain head and maxillofacial CT.

D. Assess for a septal hematoma.

16-58   *When you elicit a painful Finkelstein's sign, you are testing for*

A. carpal tunnel syndrome.

B. bursitis of the shoulder.

C. de Quervain's tenosynovitis.

D. tennis elbow.

16-59   *In a client with osteomalacia, you would expect levels of*

A. serum calcium to be elevated.

B. alkaline phosphatase to be elevated.

C. creatinine excretion to be elevated.

D. serum phosphorus to be elevated.

16-60   *The straight-leg-raising maneuver can be used to diagnose*

A. nerve root compression.

B. a fractured hip.

C. an anterior cruciate ligament tear.

D. tendinitis.

16-61   *To diagnose fibromyalgia, there must be tenderness on digital palpation in at least 11 of 18 (nine pairs) tender-point sites, which would include*

A. the occiput, low cervical, trapezius, and supraspinatus.

B. the proximal interphalangeal (PIP), metacarpophalangeal (MCP) joints of the hands, and the metatarsophalangeal (MTP) and PIP joints of the foot.

C. the facet joints of the cervical, thoracic, and lumbar spine.

D. the radial and ulnar styloids and the medial and lateral malleoli.

16-62   Sandra, a computer programmer, has just been given a new diagnosis of carpal tunnel syndrome. Your next step is to

A. refer her to a hand surgeon.

B. take a more complete history.

C. try neutral position wrist splinting and order an oral NSAID.

D. order a nerve conduction study such as an electromyography (EMG).

16-63   To plan for a community education program, the nurse practitioner needs to know that persons at highest risk for developing thoracic outlet syndrome (TOS) are

A. bicycle riders.

B. dancers.

C. computer programmers.

D. swimming instructors.

16-64   Carol, age 62, has swollen, bony proximal interphalangeal joints. You describe these as

A. Heberden's nodes.

B. Bouchard's nodes.

C. Osler's nodes.

D. Murphy's nodes.

16-65   Which of the following statements is true regarding range of motion (ROM) of a joint?

A. The normal active ROM of a joint is greater than the passive ROM of the same joint.

B. If there is a limitation of active ROM, you should not attempt passive ROM to avoid further injury to the joint.

C. Active and passive ROM of a joint should be equal, full, and cause only mild discomfort.

D. Active and passive ROM of a joint should be equal, full, and pain free.

16-66   Trevor, age 4, has an apparent hypertrophy of the calf muscles, which seem doughy on palpation. His mother is concerned because Trevor is unable to raise himself from the floor without bracing his knees with his hands. What do you suspect?

A. Duchenne muscular dystrophy

B. Cerebral palsy

C. Legg-Calvé-Perthes disease

D. Multiple sclerosis

16-67   In assessing your client, you place the tips of your first two fingers in front of each ear and ask him to open and close his mouth. Then you drop your fingers into the depressed area over the joint and note for smooth motion of the mandible. With this action, you are assessing for

A. maxillomandibular integrity.

B. well-positioned permanent teeth or well-fitting dentures.

C. temporomandibular joint syndrome.

D. mastoid inflammation.

16-68   Your client has just been told that he has a primary bone tumor. He was so upset when he heard this that he focused only on the word "tumor" and not on the prognosis or type of tumor. Which of the following tumors is malignant?

A. Osteochondroma

B. Chondroma

C. Osteosarcoma

D. Giant-cell tumor

16-69   Jennifer says that she has heard that caffeine can cause osteoporosis and asks you why. How do you respond?

A. "Caffeine has no effect on osteoporosis."

B. "A high caffeine intake has a diuretic effect that may cause calcium to be excreted more rapidly."

C. "Caffeine affects bone metabolism by altering intestinal absorption of calcium and assimilation of calcium into the bone matrix."

D. "Caffeine increases bone resorption."

16-70   Matthew, age 52, is a chef who just severed two of his fingers with a meat cutter. You would recommend that he

A. wrap the severed fingers tightly in a dry towel for transport to the emergency department with him.

B. leave the severed fingers at the scene because fingers cannot be reattached.

C. immediately freeze the severed fingers for reattachment in the near future.

D. pack the fingers in a saline-soaked dressing and seal in a plastic bag.

16-71   You suspect adolescent idiopathic scoliosis in Victoria, age 15, who is in her growth spurt. You perform the Adams forward-bending test and note a right-sided rib hump. What is this indicative of?

A. Right lumbar shifting

B. Right thoracic curvature

C. Right truncal shift

D. Spondylolysis

16-72   You are assessing Maya, a 69-year-old Asian woman, for the first time. You are trying to differentiate between scoliosis and kyphosis. Kyphosis involves

A. asymmetry of the shoulders, scapulae, and waist creases.

B. a lateral curvature and vertebral rotation on posteroanterior x-rays.

C. one leg appearing shorter than the other.

D. a posterior rounding at the thoracic level.

16-73   Lillian, age 70, was told that she has osteoporosis. When she asks you what this is, you respond that osteoporosis

A. develops when loss of bone matrix (resorption) occurs more rapidly than new bone growth (deposition).

B. is a degenerative joint disease characterized by degeneration and loss of articular cartilage in synovial joints.

C. is a chronic, systemic inflammatory disorder characterized by persistent synovitis of multiple joints.

D. is a metabolic bone disorder characterized by inadequate mineralization of bone matrix.

16-74   Joan, age 76, has been give a diagnoses of osteoporosis confirmed with a dual-energy x-ray absorptiometry (DEXA) scan. You have educated her about the importance of increasing calcium and vitamin D in her diet and starting a low impact weight bearing exercise program. You are also going to start her on medial management. Joan asks you about a drug called a "SERM" that she has heard has been shown in studies to prevent vertebral factures. Which of the following pharmacological therapies for osteoporosis is classified as a selective estrogen receptor modulator (SERM)?

A. Alendronate

B. Risedronate

C. Salmon calcitonin

D. Raloxifene

16-75   You are driving home from work and stop at the scene of a motorcycle accident that must have just occurred because there are no rescue vehicles at the scene. The driver is lying at the side of the road unconscious with an obvious open fracture of his femur. Which of the following actions should take priority?

A. Stop the bleeding from the wound.

B. Determine if there has been a cervical fracture.

C. Establish an airway.

D. Palpate the peripheral pulses.

16-76   What is the largest joint in the body?

A. The hip

B. The shoulder

C. The knee

D. The elbow

16-77   Which test is routinely recommended for a preparticipation sport physical?

A. A complete blood count

B. A chest x-ray

C. An electrocardiogram

D. A Snellen test

16-78   The C5 myotome innervates

A. wrist extension.

B. elbow extension.

C. shoulder abduction and elbow flexion.

D. ulnar deviation at the wrist along with finger flexion and abduction.

16-79   A Baker's cyst is

A. an inflammation of the bursa.

B. a form of tendinitis.

C. the buildup of synovial fluid behind the knee.

D. the result of a "swollen" ligament.

16-80   When teaching Alice, age 67, to use a cane because of osteoarthritis of her left knee, an important point to stress is to tell her to

A. carry the cane in the ipsilateral hand.

B. advance the cane with the ipsilateral leg.

C. make sure that the cane length equals the height of the iliac crest.

D. use the cane to aid in joint protection and safety.

16-81   Paul has a malignant fibrosarcoma of the femur. He recently had surgery and is now on radiation therapy. You want to order a test to determine the extent of the tumor invasion of the surrounding tissues and the response of the bone tumor to the radiation. Which of the following tests should you order?

A. An x-ray

B. A magnetic resonance imaging (MRI) scan

C. A computed tomography (CT) scan

D. A needle biopsy

16-82   Tara, the mother of a 2-year-old, is concerned because her daughter walks on her toes all the time. What do you tell her?

A. "Toe walking is considered normal until age 3."

B. "Don't worry, she'll outgrow it."

C. "Toe walking is normal until she starts kindergarten."

D. "We should do further testing now."

16-83   Shane, age 26, has a cast on his right arm because of an in-line skating accident. Twelve hours after the cast was applied, he complains of severe pain even though he recently took his pain medication. His fingers are pink, yet he states that

they are tingling and feel slightly numb. What do you suspect?

A. Compartment syndrome

B. Phlebitis

C. Osteomyelitis

D. Muscle contraction

16-84   Which of the following is true regarding scoliosis?

A. Functional scoliosis is flexible; it is apparent with standing and disappears with forward bending.

B. Functional scoliosis is fixed; the curvature shows both on standing and bending forward.

C. Structural scoliosis is fixed; the curvature shows both on standing and bending forward.

D. Functional scoliosis is permanent, whereas structural scoliosis can result from outside influences such as leg length discrepancy or muscle spasms.

16-85   The knee is an example of a

A. spheroidal joint.

B. hinge joint.

C. condylar joint.

D. fibrous joint.

16-86   Jessie, age 49, states that she thinks she has rheumatoid arthritis. Before any diagnostic tests are ordered, you complete a physical examination and make a tentative diagnosis of osteoarthritis rather than rheumatoid arthritis. Which clinical manifestation ruled out rheumatoid arthritis?

A. Fatigue

B. Affected joints are swollen, cool, and bony hard on palpation

C. Decreased range of motion

D. Stiffness

16-87   Dan, age 49, developed osteomyelitis of the femur after a motorcycle accident. Which of the following statements about the clinical manifestations of osteomyelitis is correct?

A. Integumentary effects include swelling, erythema, and warmth at the involved site.

B. There is a low-grade fever with intermittent chills.

C. Musculoskeletal effects include tenderness of the entire leg.

D. Cardiovascular effects include bradycardia.

16-88 *Rose Marie has a 15-year-old son who wants to play sports; however, she is very leery because she has heard of so many accidents. Which one of the following sports does the American Academy of Pediatrics list as a limited contact/impact sport?*

A. Field hockey

B. Soccer

C. Basketball

D. Lacrosse

16-89 *Sean, age 48, has asymptomatic hyperuricemia. What is your initial therapy?*

A. NSAIDs

B. Dietary counseling

C. Colchicine

D. Allopurinol (Zyloprim)

16-90 *The most common cause of cauda equina syndrome is*

A. fracture.

B. hematoma.

C. lumbar intervertebral disk herniation.

D. space-occupying lesion.

16-91 *You are caring for a patient that has a history of psoriasis and now is showing signs of musculoskeletal signs and symptoms with joint involvement. Seropositivity provides a definitive diagnosis of psoriatic arthritis (PsA). Your initial treatment choice for management of the patient is*

A. disease-modifying antirheumatic drugs (DMARDs).

B. NSAIDs.

C. tumor necrosis factor–alpha inhibitors (TNF-α inhibitors).

D. uricosuric.

16-92 *What disorder affects older individuals, particularly women, and is characterized by pain and stiffness in the cervical spine and shoulder and hip girdles, along with signs of systemic infection such as malaise, weight loss, sweats, and low-grade fever?*

A. Fibromyalgia syndrome

B. Myofascial somatic dysfunction

C. Polymyalgia rheumatica

D. Reiter's syndrome

16-93 *Manny, age 52, is a postal worker who drives a truck every day. He presents with lower back pain and has decreased sensation to a pinprick in the lateral leg and web of the great toe. This indicates discogenic disease in the dermatomal pattern of which area?*

A. L3/L4 (L4 root involvement)

B. L4/L5 (L5 root involvement)

C. L5/S1 (S1 root involvement)

D. None of the above

16-94 *Sam, age 50, presents with Paget's disease that has been stable for several years. Recently, his serum alkaline phosphatase level has been steadily rising. You determine that it is time to start him on*

A. NSAIDs.

B. corticosteroids.

C. bisphosphonates.

D. calcitonin.

16-95 *Jim, age 22, a stock boy, has an acute episode of low back pain. You order an NSAID and tell him which of the following?*

A. Maintain moderate bedrest for 3–4 days.

B. Call the office for narcotic medication if there is no relief with the NSAID after 24–48 hours.

C. Begin lower back strengthening exercises depending on pain tolerance.

D. Wear a Boston brace at night.

16-96 *During your assessment of your client's foot, you note that the foot is in alignment with the long axis of the lower leg and that weight-bearing falls on the middle of the foot, from the heel, along the midfoot, to between the second and third toes. What do you diagnose?*

A. A normal foot

B. Hallux valgus

C. Talipes equinovarus

D. Hammertoes

16-97   *Which test is used to diagnose an Achilles tendon rupture?*

A. Boutonniere test

B. Lachman test

C. Thompson test

D. Drawer test

16-98   *You are considering a diagnosis of calcium pyrophosphate dihydrate (CPPD) crystal deposition disease or pseudogout in a 72-year-old man who presents with complaints of pain and stiffness in his wrists and knees. The most useful diagnostic test to assist you in making this diagnosis would be*

A. synovial-fluid analysis and x-ray.

B. bacterial culture.

C. bone scan and MRI.

D. anticitrullinated protein antibody (ACPA) test and RA factor.

16-99   *What pathophysiology associated with transient pain after exercising usually begins a few hours after exercise with soreness and may last up to a week?*

A. Increased lactic acid production, muscle breakdown, and minor inflammation

B. Mild musculotendinous inflammation

C. Major musculotendinous inflammation, periostitis, and bone microtrauma

D. Breakdown in soft tissue and stress fracture

16-100   *Which of the following is a modifiable risk factor for osteoporosis?*

A. Low alcohol intake

B. Low caffeine intake

C. Smoking

D. Excessive exercise

16-101   *Treatment of choice for polymyalgia rheumatica (PMR) is*

A. acetaminophen or NSAIDs.

B. low-dose steroids.

C. tricyclic antidepressants.

D. antibiotics.

16-102   *To aid in the diagnosis of meniscus damage, which test should you perform?*

A. Bulge test

B. Lachman test

C. Drawer sign

D. Apley's compression test

16-103   *Bone mineral density (BMD) testing is recommended by the National Osteoporosis Foundation for which of the following client populations to assess whether they are at high risk for osteoporosis?*

A. All women age 65 and older regardless of risk factors

B. All men age 65 and older regardless of risk factors

C. All women in their 30s for baseline

D. All women of menopausal age

16-104   *The most widely accepted screening tool for psoriatic arthritis (PsA) is the*

A. ACR (American College of Rheumatology) Criteria

B. CASPAR (Classification of Psoriatic Arthritis) Criteria

C. Psoriasis Area and Severity Index

D. Rome Criteria

16-105   *Jill, age 49, has recently begun a rigorous weight-lifting regimen. She presents in your office with a shoulder dislocation. Which of the following clinical manifestations make you suspect an anterior shoulder dislocation over a posterior dislocation?*

A. Inability to shrug the shoulder

B. Absence of pain

C. Inability to rotate the shoulder externally

D. Shortening of the arm

16-106   *Management of fibromyalgia would include*

A. giving psychotropic drugs, such as amitriptyline (Elavil), in a low dose at bedtime.

B. instructing clients to keep as busy as possible to keep their minds off the symptoms.

C. using high doses of NSAIDs.

D. avoiding exercise.

16-107   *Stan, age 34, fractured his femur when his horse tripped over a jump. With this type of injury, you know that Stan is at risk for fat emboli. Early assessment findings for this complication include*

A. fever, tachycardia, rapid respirations, and neurological manifestations.

B. neurological manifestations, temperature elevation, bradycardia, and pallor.

C. hostility; combativeness; substernal pain; and weak, thready pulse.

D. lethargy, hypothermia, paresthesia, and absent peripheral pulses.

16-108   *When Maxwell, age 12, slid into home plate while playing baseball, he injured his ankle. You are trying to differentiate between a sprain and a strain. You know that a sprain*

A. is an injury to the ligaments that attach to bones in a joint.

B. is an injury to the tendons that attach to the muscles in a joint.

C. is an injury resulting in extensive tears of the muscles.

D. does not result in joint instability.

16-109   *Harry, age 59, has Paget's disease of the bone. It was diagnosed as a result of routine blood work during his annual physical, which showed an increased serum alkaline phosphate level. You know that the most serious complication of Paget's disease is*

A. osteosarcoma.

B. nerve compression.

C. fractures.

D. bone pain.

16-110   *Martin, age 58, presents with urethritis, conjunctivitis, and asymmetric joint stiffness, primarily in the knees, ankles, and feet. Which condition do you suspect?*

A. Syphilis

B. Gonorrhea

C. HIV

D. Reactive arthritis

16-111   *When grading muscle strength on a scale of 1–5, a grade of 4 indicates*

A. full range of motion (ROM) against gravity with full resistance.

B. full ROM against gravity with some resistance.

C. full ROM with gravity.

D. full ROM with gravity eliminated (passive motion).

16-112   *Which of the following can assist in the diagnosis of myasthenia gravis?*

A. Repetitive nerve stimulation

B. The presence of cogwheel rigidity

C. Chvostek's sign

D. Trousseau's sign

16-113   *Anne Marie states that she has a maternal history of rheumatoid disease but that she has never been affected. Today she presents with complaints of dryness of the eyes and mouth. What do you suspect?*

A. Rheumatoid arthritis

B. Systemic lupus erythematosus

C. Sjögren's syndrome

D. Rosacea

16-114   *Alan, age 46, presents with a tender, red, swollen knee. You rule out septic arthritis and diagnose gout by confirming*

A. an elevated WBC.

B. hyperuricemia.

C. a significant response to a dose of ceftriaxone (Rocephin).

D. a positive antinuclear antibody test.

16-115   *Hilda, age 73, presents with a complaint of low back pain. Red flags in her history of a minor fall, having osteopenia, and prolonged steroid use for systemic lupus erythematosus suggest the possibility of which of the following serious underlying conditions as the cause of her low back pain?*

A. Cancer

B. Cauda equina syndrome

C. Neurological compromise

D. Spinal fracture

16-116   *Mrs. Kelly, age 80, has a curvature of the spine. This is likely to indicate which age-related change?*

A.   Lordosis

B.   Dorsal kyphosis

C.   Scoliosis

D.   Kyphoscoliosis

16-117   *Mary, age 72, has severe osteoarthritis of her right knee. She obtains much relief from corticosteroid injections. When she asks you how often she can have them, how do you respond?*

A.   Only once a year in the same joint

B.   No more than twice a year in the same joint

C.   No more than three to four times a year in the same joint

D.   No more than five to six times a year in the same joint

16-118   *Which of the following statements concerning developmental dysplasia of the hip (DDH) is correct?*

A.   It is often associated with being the firstborn female child.

B.   It results from an orthopedic malformation in utero.

C.   It has no genetic predisposition.

D.   It is more common in males.

16-119   *How can you differentiate between a ganglion cyst and a neoplasm?*

A.   A neoplasm is more painful.

B.   Ganglia transilluminate.

C.   Ganglia cause more swelling.

D.   A neoplasm may fluctuate in size.

16-120   *Black men have a relatively low incidence of osteoporosis because they have*

A.   increased bone resorption.

B.   a higher bone mass.

C.   wide and thick long bones.

D.   decreased bone deposition.

16-121   *What is stiffness or fixation of a joint called?*

A.   Contracture

B.   Ankylosis

C.   Dislocation

D.   Subluxation

16-122   *Anna, age 42, is pregnant and was just given a diagnosis of carpal tunnel syndrome. She is worried that this will affect her in caring for the baby. What do you tell her?*

A.   "Don't worry, we'll find a brace that is very malleable."

B.   "After childbirth, your carpal tunnel syndrome may resolve."

C.   "If we do surgery now, you'll be recovered by the time the baby arrives."

D.   "You should prepare yourself for the probability of being unable to care for your baby."

16-123   *Grating of the bones or entrance of air into an open fracture is manifested as*

A.   swelling.

B.   ecchymosis.

C.   crepitus.

D.   pain and tenderness.

16-124   *Emily, age 21, presents today with another muscle strain from one of her many sports activities. You think that she was probably never taught about health promotion and maintenance regarding physical activity. What information do you include in your teaching?*

A.   "After an activity, if any part hurts, apply ice for 20 minutes."

B.   "You must first get in shape with a rigorous schedule of weight training and then you can participate in any activity once you are physically fit."

C.   "After any strenuous activity, you must completely rest your muscles before beginning your next activity."

D.   "Stretching and warm-up exercises are an important part of any exercise routine."

Answers

16-1   Answer D

If any limitation or increase in range of motion (ROM) occurs when assessing the musculoskeletal system, the angles of the bones should be measured by using a goniometer, which gives precise measurements of joint ROM. Phalen's test is used to diagnose carpal tunnel syndrome; it is not a tool. Skeletometry does not exist. The Thomas test is for evaluation of hip ROM.

16-2   Answer A

When a client has a human bite, the first immediate course of action must be to debride and irrigate the wound. Then, an x-ray should be taken to rule out osteomyelitis, fractures, and retained teeth from the offender. A wound culture would be required only for an older injury or a wound with evidence of infection. Broad-spectrum antibiotics such as IV ampicillin/sulbactam (Unasyn) and/or PO Amoxicillin with clavulanic acid (Augmentin) should be started and the wound left open for drainage. Rabies is not a concern with human bites. Clients should then be evaluated for the need for a tetanus injection.

16-3   Answer D

A prompt referral to a neurosurgeon is required when a diagnosis of cauda equina syndrome is suspected. Cauda equina syndrome is a widespread neurological disorder in which there is loss of anal sphincter tone; impaired micturition and incontinence; saddle anesthesia at the anus, perineum, or genitals; and motor weakness or sensory loss in both legs. An x-ray is not helpful in the diagnosis of cauda equina, and precious time should not be wasted in a client with suspected cauda equina. An MRI can be a useful diagnostic tool, but prompt evaluation by a neurosurgeon is an essential first step to prevent permanent neurological damage.

16-4   Answer A

Turning the forearm so that the palm is up is supination. Turning the forearm so that the palm is down is pronation. Abduction is moving a limb away from the midline of the body. Eversion is moving the sole of the foot outward at the ankle.

16-5   Answer B

The Salter-Harris classification system of growth plate injuries divides most growth plate injuries into five categories based on the damage: Salter-Harris I is through the physis; Salter-Harris II is through the metaphysis and the physis; Salter-Harris III is through the epiphysis and the physis; Salter-Harris IV is through the metaphysis, epiphysis, and the physis; and a Salter-Harris V is a compression injury of the physis.

16-6   Answer C

Advise clients taking calcium supplements that they also need to take vitamin D because vitamin D raises serum calcium levels by increasing the intestinal absorption of dietary calcium and mobilizing calcium from the bone. Vitamin D deficiency results in an inadequate mineralization of bone matrix (rickets), more commonly seen in children.

16-7   Answer A

The guidelines from the American College of Obstetricians and Gynecologists for exercise during pregnancy and after delivery include the following: Women can and should try to exercise moderately for at least 30 minutes on most, if not all, days. Exercise in the supine position should be avoided after the first trimester because this position is associated with a decreased cardiac output. Because of decreased oxygen available for aerobic exercise during pregnancy, the intensity of the workout should be based on maternal symptoms.

16-8   Answer A

The mechanism of action of colchicine is to interrupt the cycle of urate crystal deposition and inflammatory response. Used to treat an acute attack of gout, colchicine does not alter serum uric acid levels. Colchicine is generally used as a second-line therapy in gout when NSAIDs or corticosteroids are contraindicated or ineffective. Allopurinol (Zyloprim) acts on purine metabolism to reduce the production of uric acid and decrease serum and urinary concentrations of uric acid. It is useful for prevention of gout but not in the treatment of acute gout.

16-9   Answer C

Sarcoidosis is the result of an exaggerated immune system response to a class of antigens or self-antigens. Fifty percent of clients experience joint symptoms, including myopathy and polyarthritis, and glucocorticoids are prescribed to suppress the immune process, thus relieving symptoms. About 25% show some form of cardiac dysfunction, although it is often not recognized clinically.

16-10   Answer B

Painful contractions of muscles after exertion, such as heat cramps, may be related to hyponatremia or other electrolyte imbalances. Usually the gastrocnemius and hamstring muscles are involved. Treatment of heat cramps includes passive muscle stretching, cessation of activities, transfer to a cooler environment, and drinking cool liquids. Sports drinks such as Gatorade that contain electrolytes may be beneficial. Heat exhaustion is a more serious condition, with symptoms ranging from nausea, vomiting, headache, loss of appetite, and dizziness to irritability, tachycardia, and hyperventilation. Hyperkalemia may cause muscular weakness, fatigue, and muscle cramps. Greg's dehydration is attributed to his hyponatremia and would be a good second-choice answer. Hypercalcemia may affect gastrointestinal, renal, and neurological function. Symptoms may include constipation, polyuria, and at times, nausea, vomiting, and anorexia.

16-11   Answer C

For the client with only one testicle, as long as the remaining testicle can be protected, the client can participate in any sport.

16-12   Answer A

One of the precursors of deep vein thrombosis is altered blood coagulation or hypercoagulability, which may result from the clinical risk factor of high estrogen states. Oral contraceptives or hormone replacement therapy are two causes of high estrogen states in women. Decreased blood flow or venous status can be related to prolonged sedentary positions and is common in clients who are immobilized. Venous flow can be decreased by 50% in bedridden persons. Injury to the blood vessel wall may occur as a direct result of force, such as from trauma that may occur during orthopedic surgery or with lower extremity indwelling intravenous catheter placement.

16-13   Answer C

Faster symptomatic recovery has been seen in clients with a simple "mechanical" backache who continue normal activities as much as they can with "pain being their guide" than in clients who use traditional medical treatments, such as bedrest and use of NSAIDs. Muscle relaxants should be ordered only if muscle spasms are actually present, although acetaminophen (Tylenol) and NSAIDs have also been shown to help the muscle spasms adequately. Back-strengthening exercises should be started within 6 weeks of the onset of pain.

16-14   Answer C

Dupuytren's contracture affects the palmar tissue between the skin and the distal palm and fingers, most often in the fourth and fifth fingers but also in the thumb-index finger web space. It is progressive and results in flexor contracture while not affecting the flexor tendons. Most frequently occurring in males between the ages of 40 and 60, it is common among persons of Northern European ancestry. It is dysfunctional and disfiguring. Although not actually painful, it may be tender. Surgery is recommended when the inability to straighten the fingers limits the client's hand function. Hallux valgus, commonly referred to as a bunion, is an osseous deformity at the MTP joint of the great toe with medial deviation of the toe. Hallux rigidus is a common condition of arthritis at the base of the great toe at the MTP joint, causing stiffness and decreased movement of the great toe.

16-15   Answer D

When teaching clients about NSAIDs, tell them not to take these drugs on an empty stomach but to take them with food or milk and to stop the medication and call immediately if they notice any nausea/vomiting, coffee-ground emesis, black stools, or blood in the stool. If the client is having additional pain, acetaminophen (Tylenol) may be taken in conjunction with an NSAID because it is not an NSAID and will not potentiate gastric bleeding. Clients should be taught to never take more than the prescribed dose of an NSAID due to the likelihood of increasing the chances of gastrointestinal (GI) damage and kidney damage.

16-16   Answer B

Instructions to the client and family on how to allow a cast to dry properly should include advising them to change the position of the extremity with the cast every hour. In this case, Joyce's arm should be repositioned frequently to prevent indentations in the cast itself (caused by continuous placement on a pillow) and to ensure drying on all the surfaces of the cast. Elevating her arm will prevent edema, but elevation is not needed continuously. A fan will dry only the outside of the cast. A blanket will prevent drying of the cast.

16-17   Answer A

Osgood-Schlatter disease is an overuse injury that results from excessive tension and pull of the patellar tendon on the tibial tuberosity. Treating the client conservatively while an adolescent will avoid potential problems as an active adult.

Initially, relative rest should be used with hamstring stretching, heel cord stretching, and quadriceps stretching exercises. If the problem persists, a long-leg knee immobilizer may be used. Surgical intervention is rarely required, but if so, only in an adult after bone growth is complete.

16-18   Answer A

The Allen test assesses the patency of the radial and ulnar arteries in the arterial arch. Have the client make a fist, and use your fingers to occlude both radial and ulnar arteries. Then, have the client open the hand, and you release the radial pressure. Observe for rapid refill of color to the palm indicating patency of the radial artery. Repeat the same maneuver, releasing ulnar pressure to assess ulnar artery competency. Finkelstein's test assesses for de Quervain's tenosynovitis. Phalen's test and Tinel's sign assess for carpal tunnel syndrome.

16-19   Answer D

Lysosomal degradation results when leukocytes produce lysosomal enzymes that destroy articular cartilage in rheumatoid arthritis. The collagen fibers and the protein polysaccharides of articular cartilage are broken down by the enzymes. Immune complexes initiate the inflammatory process that brings leukocytes to the cartilage. Immune complexes are formed by the combination of immunoglobulin G with rheumatoid factors that are the result of antigen-antibody formation.

16-20   Answer D

A plain x-ray film will not show a herniated nucleus pulposus or a muscle strain. It will show spondylolisthesis, scoliosis, osteoarthritis, and spinal stenosis. Note that x-rays of the spine are not indicated in low back pain unless the cause of the pain is thought to have a bony origin or to be traumatic in nature or to rule out systemic disease.

16-21   Answer D

In performing Ortolani's maneuver to assess for developmental dysplasia of the hip (formerly referred to as congenital hip dislocation), the practitioner places the infant supine, flexes the knees, places thumbs on the medial proximal thighs and fingers on the greater trochanters, and stabilizes one thigh while the other thigh is gently abducted. If this movement results in a palpable "clunk" (the hip moving back into the socket), there is dislocation of that hip. If the movement is smooth and silent, there is no hip dislocation. The Allis test is also used to check for hip dislocation or dysplasia by comparing leg lengths by checking knee heights while both knees are flexed and feet are flat on the table. Lasègue's sign is straight leg raising, which helps to confirm the presence of a herniated nucleus pulposus. The McMurray test is performed to evaluate for a torn meniscus.

16-22   Answer A

Internal tibial torsion is the most common overall cause of in-toeing. External tibial torsion is the most common overall cause of out-toeing. Femoral retroversion is a common cause of out-toeing, whereas femoral anteversion is a cause of in-toeing. Flat feet often cause out-toeing.

16-23   Answer D

Symmetric neurogenic pain (burning, numbness, tingling) will include peripheral neuropathy and myelopathy. Asymmetric neurogenic pain will include radiculopathy, reflex sympathetic dystrophy, and entrapment neuropathy. A claudication pain pattern will be present in peripheral vascular disease, giant-cell arteritis (with jaw pain), and lumbar spinal stenosis. These conditions all include the clinical manifestations of neurogenic pain.

16-24   Answer C

Exploring Mr. Miller's feelings and getting more clarification of how the surgery will affect him will allow you to know him better and be better able to assist him in dealing with the situation.

16-25   Answer C

The bulge test assesses for an effusion of the knee. If effusion is present, a bulge will appear to the sides of or below the patella when the practitioner compresses the area above the patella. The Thomas test is used to assess for hip problems. Both Tinel's sign and Phalen's test assess for carpal tunnel syndrome.

16-26   Answer D

A positive obturator test, especially with a positive McBurney's point and a positive psoas sign, is indicative of appendicitis. Although internal rotation of the hip may cause hip discomfort in a client with hip bursitis and AVN of the femoral head, the obturator test elicits right lower quadrant (RLQ) abdominal pain, which is indicative of appendicitis.

16-27   Answer D

All of the tests listed as possible options are tests done to assess for a herniated disk. In the straight-leg-raising test, you elevate the affected leg when the client is in the supine position; back pain and sciatic nerve pain (radiating leg pain) indicate a herniated disk. In the cross straight-leg-raising test, elevation of the uninvolved leg produces sciatic pain down the contralateral leg. The doorbell sign is the development of sciatica when the spinous process over the protruded disk is deeply palpated. The femoral stretch test is done with the client prone and the leg extended and the knee flexed. Pain radiating to the anterior thigh indicates an L4 radiculopathy. Suspect a herniated disk.

16-28   Answer B

Pain over the lower back and spine, as well as the muscles, without sciatica is musculoskeletal strain. Often there is no precipitating event, and there is an insidious onset. It is aggravated by sitting, standing, and certain movements. Palpation localizes the pain, and muscle spasms may be felt. It is alleviated by rest, and there is progressive improvement. Ankylosing spondylitis is back pain and stiffness over several months where there is a systemic inflammatory condition of the vertebral column and sacroiliac joints. Painful ankylosed sacroiliac joints, reduced chest wall expansion, and excessive thoracic kyphosis are also present. It most frequently affects males between the ages of 20 and 30, causing chronic low back pain that is worse in the morning. There is relief with exercise and reduced mobility of the spine. A herniated disk is often preceded by years of recurrent episodes of localized back pain and there is usually leg pain that overshadows the back pain. With spondylolisthesis, there is a defect or fracture of the pars interarticularis with forward shifting of one vertebra on top of another. This can cause nerve irritation and damage if the vertebrae are pressing on a spinal nerve root.

16-29   Answer B

Although exercise-induced asthma is common among athletes, it is not a common cause of sudden death. Cardiac conditions are responsible for the three most common causes of sudden death in athletes younger than age 30 and include hypertrophic cardiomyopathy, idiopathic left ventricular hypertrophy, and coronary artery anomalies. Many sports teams require echocardiograms to pick up potential problems.

Compartment syndrome and meningitis can occur in both athletes and nonathletes, but, by definition, they are not causative of sudden death.

16-30   Answer B

Gout is a disorder that involves abnormal metabolism of uric acid and results in hyperuricemia. High concentrations of urate precipitate into crystals that collect in tissue and joint spaces and can cause pain and inflammation. It is likely that the patient's symptoms may be aggravated by the use of HTCZ. Like gout, septic arthritis presents with an acute onset of swelling, pain, and heat in a joint. However, unlike gout, it occurs most frequently in the knee followed by the hip, shoulder, wrist, and ankle. Rheumatoid arthritis typically affects multiple joints simultaneously and is a slow and progressive disease. Charcot neuro-osteoarthropathy occurs in diabetic patients presenting as hot, swollen, and red joints. These patients usually report a history of trauma, surgery, or prior infection.

16-31   Answer A

To observe for calf symmetry and leg strength, the practitioner asks the client to rise up on the toes and raise the heels. Simple inspection and observation while the client is standing with feet together is required to assess for hip, knee, and ankle symmetry. The "duck walk" of four steps away from the examiner with buttocks on heels would be used to observe for hip, knee, and ankle motion. Standing with the knees straight and then touching the toes is to check for scoliosis, hip motion, and hamstring tightness.

16-32   Answer A

Dupuytren's contracture manifests itself by nodular thickening of the connective tissue of one or both hands, usually affecting the fourth and fifth fingers. There is tenderness with the inability to extend the fingers. Pain, tenderness, erythema, and swelling of the first metatarsal joint are the typical presentation for gout. Peyronie's disease is a connective tissue disorder that results in painful curvature of the erect penis.

16-33   Answer B

Tendons are the collagen fibers that connect muscle to bone. Ligaments connect bone to bone in the joints. Bursae are the pouches of synovial fluid that reduce friction between bones, muscles, or tendons. Fibrocartilaginous disks separate bony surfaces such as those between the vertebrae in the spine.

16-34   Answer C

The type of joint that is freely movable, such as the shoulder joint, is called a diarthrosis joint. Diarthrosis or synovial joints include the joints of the limbs, shoulders, and hips. They can be further divided onto what is noted as ball and socket, hinge, gliding, pivot, and compound joints. Synarthrosis or fibrous joints are immovable and include skull sutures, epiphyseal plates, ribs, and the manubrium of the sternum. Amphiarthrosis or cartilaginous joints are slightly movable joints, such as the vertebral bodies of the spine. There is no such thing as a juxtarthrosis joint.

16-35   Answer B

The only antineoplastic antibiotic listed is doxorubicin (Adriamycin). All of the other medications are chemotherapeutic agents of other classifications that may be used for musculoskeletal neoplasms. Cyclophosphamide (Cytoxan) is an alkylating agent, methotrexate (Rheumatrex) is an antimetabolite, and cisplatin (Platinol) is an inorganic platinum agent.

16-36   Answer B

The client with rheumatoid arthritis (RA) benefits from DMARDs, NSAIDs, and steroids because they all treat the disease of RA as well as the pain. Acetaminophen (Tylenol) is a pain reliever but does not have anti-inflammatory effects. Acetaminophen is not considered a treatment option for the disease of RA and is likely even ineffective as a pain reliever for the pain associated with RA.

16-37   Answer A

First-line drug therapy for acute low back pain includes the use of NSAIDs. NSAIDs, as well as aspirin and acetaminophen (Tylenol), have been shown to be as effective as muscle relaxants and opioids for the control of acute low back pain but without the potential for dependence and abuse. Evidence has shown that muscle relaxants are no more effective than NSAIDs in the relief of acute low back pain. Antidepressant drug therapy, particularly tricyclic antidepressants, have been trialed in patients with chronic low back pain even without clinical depression.

16-38   Answer D

The American Rheumatism Association has identified functional classes I–IV depending on the client's ability to accomplish activities of daily living. Because Janine is a class III, her function would be adequate to perform only few or none of the duties of usual occupation or self-care. Class I refers to the client who can carry on all usual duties without handicaps. Class II refers to the client whose function is adequate for normal activities despite a handicap of discomfort or limited motion at one or more joints. Class IV refers to the client who is largely or wholly incapacitated, bedridden, or confined to a wheelchair, permitting little or no self-care.

16-39   Answer C

A coccygeal fracture, usually incurred by a fall onto the sacrococcygeal area, is treated conservatively with analgesia and by using a "donut" cushion when sitting.

16-40   Answer A

Musculoskeletal pain is not characteristic of chronic fatigue syndrome; rather, it is characteristic of fibromyalgia. The musculoskeletal pain, usually an achy muscle pain that may be localized or involve the entire body, is usually gradual in onset, although the onset may be sudden, occasionally after a viral illness. Fatigue is a more significant feature of chronic fatigue syndrome. With both disorders, difficulty sleeping and depression occur.

16-41   Answer B

Osgood-Schlatter is usually a benign, self-limited knee condition in adolescent boys and girls. Treatment consists of ice, analgesics, NSAIDs, and temporary avoidance of pain-producing activities. Conservative treatment includes quadriceps-stretching exercises to decrease tension on the tibial tubercle. Surgical correction for Osgood-Schlatter disease is not recommended until all other options have been tried and have failed.

16-42   Answer A

In discussing proper body mechanics with John to prevent future injuries, you tell him to bend his knees and face the object straight on, to hold boxes close to his body and not at arm's length, and to spread his feet about shoulder-width apart. Using legs and arms, facing objects straight on, and keeping a wide stance provides a broad base of support and allows for use of supporting muscles, relieving stress on the back muscles. Never bend and twist simultaneously, but rather keep the spine straight to minimize injury.

16-43 Answer B

Gelling refers to the achiness and stiffness that occur in clients with rheumatoid arthritis after a period of inactivity.

16-44 Answer B

Although 24 vertebrae (cervical, thoracic, lumbar) are found in 85%–93% of all people, racial and gender differences reveal 23 or 25 vertebrae in select groups. There are usually 7 cervical, 12 thoracic, and 5 lumbar vertebrae. There are also 5 sacral and 3–4 coccygeal vertebrae.

16-45 Answer C

Increased levels of creatine kinase are found in polymyositis, traumatic injuries, and progressive muscular dystrophy. Aldolase A level is elevated in muscular dystrophy and dermatomyositis. Aspartate aminotransferase is found in skeletal muscle but mainly in heart and renal cells. Lactate dehydrogenase level is elevated in skeletal muscle necrosis, extensive cancer, and progressive muscular dystrophy.

16-46 Answer C

Tell a client who has sprained his ankle to apply cold for 20 minutes, then take it off for 30–45 minutes, and repeat that procedure for the first 24–48 hours while awake. Cold will cause vasoconstriction and decrease edema, preventing any further bleeding into the tissues. Ice has been proven to speed recovery in ankle sprains; however, ice should never be applied continuously because it could hinder proper circulation and cause frostbite. Therefore, always recommend a protective padding between the ice and the skin. Applying heat may increase swelling and subsequently slow recovery. After any sprain, use the principles of RICE: *R* for rest, *I* for ice, *C* for compression, and *E* for elevation.

16-47 Answer D

The Roos test suggests thoracic outlet syndrome if pain or paresthesias are present when the client positions his or her shoulders in abduction and external rotation of 90° with the elbows flexed to 90°. The client then opens and closes his or her hands for 3 minutes. The Neer test suggests inflammation or injury to the structures in the subacromial space when pain is experienced when the client is seated and maximal forced flexion of the shoulder is imposed with the forearm pronated.

The Speeds test suggests tendinitis of the long head of the biceps when there is pain at the bicipital groove with forward elevation of the shoulders plus resistance. The Hawkins test assesses for inflammation or injury to the structures in the subacromial space when pain is elicited with forced internal rotation of the shoulder.

16-48 Answer A

With tennis elbow, wrist and finger extension causes pain over the extensor carpi radialis brevis tendon, the extensor carpi radialis longus tendon, and the extensor digitorum communis. With golfer's elbow, pain is experienced on wrist flexion over the flexor carpi radialis, the flexor carpi ulnaris, and the pronator teres tendons. With de Quervain's disease, pain is experienced on thumb extension over the abductor pollicis longus and the extensor pollicis brevis tendons. With intersection syndrome, pain is experienced with a grip and wrist extension over the extensor carpi radialis brevis and the extensor carpi radialis longus tendons.

16-49 Answer A

The radial head is the proximal aspect of the radius, located in the elbow joint. Falling on an outstretched hand transfers a significant amount of force to the radial head. Often a fracture line cannot be seen on an x-ray, but presence of an anterior or posterior fat pad sign (or sail sign) indicates an occult radial head fracture. Tenderness, swelling, and crepitus at the radial wrist could indicate a distal radius fracture or fracture of the carpal bones. Tenderness in the "anatomical snuffbox" is used to assess for possible fracture of the scaphoid bone in the wrist. A wrist x-ray will demonstrate abnormalities of only the distal radius, ulna, or carpal bones. An elbow x-ray would assist in the diagnosis of a radial head fracture.

16-50 Answer C

Slipped capital femoral epiphysis (SCFE) is a displacement of the femoral head relative to the femoral neck that occurs through the physis (growth plate) of the femur. The vast majority of the clients are obese, as the added weight increases shear stress across the physis. The mean age at diagnosis is 12 years for females and 13.5 years for males. Surgery is often required via in situ pin fixation (single screw) to stabilize the growth plate to prevent further slippage and to avoid complications. There would be a positive McMurray sign and a positive Lachman and/or drawer test in meniscal or cruciate ligament tears, respectively. Osgood-Schlatter disease would result in swelling, pain, and tenderness at the tibial tubercle.

16-51   Answer C

To determine if a client has a fractured pelvis, a test for hematuria will usually prove positive. A fracture of the pelvis usually results in hypovolemia caused by a generally significant associated blood loss. Surrounding blood vessels rupture and result in a large retroperitoneal hematoma with shock. Pelvic fractures also commonly injure the urinary bladder or urethra. A client with a fracture in several locations of the pelvis may need a pneumatic antishock garment to control the blood loss and stabilize the pelvis. Only x-ray studies will confirm the diagnosis.

16-52   Answer B

A positive anterior or posterior drawer sign indicates an injury to the anterior or posterior cruciate ligaments, respectively. The drawer test, or Lachman test, are both utilized to assess for cruciate ligament injury. Meniscus tears are also a common cause of knee joint pain or injury with the medial meniscus being injured more frequently than the lateral meniscus. The most consistent physical finding of a meniscal tear is tenderness to palpation along the joint line. To examine for a meniscal tear, perform the McMurray test by fully flexing the knee with leg externally rotated for medial meniscus and internally rotated for lateral meniscus. Then firmly extend the leg. A painful cartilage click is considered a positive McMurray test for meniscal injury. The abduction or valgus stress test and adduction or varus stress test are used respectively to test the medial collateral ligament (MCL) and lateral collateral ligament (LCL).

16-53   Answer B

There is tenderness over the "anatomical snuffbox" in a scaphoid (aka navicular) fracture, the most common injury of the carpal bones. Poor blood supply puts the scaphoid bone at risk for avascular necrosis; therefore, wrist pain and tenderness in the anatomical snuffbox, even without history of antecedent trauma, warrants a wrist x-ray. A fracture of the hook of the hamate is an uncommon fracture seen in golfers and in players of other racket sports and involves pain and tenderness on the ulnar side of the palm. An ulnar styloid fracture would produce tenderness at the distal ulna. A radial head fracture would result in pain at the elbow joint where the radial head lies proximal to the distal humerus. Be sure not to confuse the radial head (proximal end of the radius) with the radial styloid (distal end of the radius at the wrist).

16-54   Answer B

In this case, Mike may benefit from a regular planned exercise program to strengthen back muscles and attempt to reduce the probability of future episodes of back pain. Surgery is recommended only for clients with low back pain caused by degenerative disk disorders, and then only when severe neurological involvement has occurred. Surgery benefits only approximately 1% of persons with low back problems. Suggesting a career change should be considered only in cases of disability or inability to safely continue one's current employment. Narcotic pain medications are not considered first-line treatment for mechanical back pain.

16-55   Answer D

Synovial fluid that is turbid and yellow-green on analysis indicates an inflammation, such as one that occurs in rheumatoid arthritis. Normal synovial fluid is clear and light yellow or straw colored. With trauma, the color would be turbid and red or xanthochromic. With osteoarthritis, it is clear and yellow or straw colored. With gout, synovial fluid is turbid and yellow/milky white in color. With a septic infection such as a bacterial infection or tuberculosis, the fluid is turbid and gray-green or greenish-yellow.

16-56   Answer A

A comminuted fracture occurs when the bony fragments are in many pieces. An open fracture occurs when the broken ends of the bone protrude through soft tissues and skin. A closed fracture occurs when the bone breaks cleanly but does not penetrate the skin. A compression fracture occurs when the bone is crushed.

16-57   Answer B

The primary concern in the management of facial fractures is to ensure an adequate and stable airway. Displaced soft tissues, blood, secretions, or other foreign material may obstruct the airway and cause asphyxia. Septal hematomas are more commonly seen in children than in adults, but the first priority is to maintain an adequate airway. Once his airway is established and he is stabilized, permission to treat Jeffrey can be obtained from his parents. Head and maxillofacial CT would then be obtained.

16-58   Answer C

Pain elicited when the Finkelstein's test is performed indicates de Quervain's tenosynovitis at the base of the thumb. The test is performed by flexion of the thumb across the palm, with ulnar deviation of the wrist. Gliding the inflamed tendons will produce pain, which is considered a positive Finkelstein's test. Tinel's sign and Phalen's test are used to diagnose carpal tunnel syndrome. The tennis elbow test evaluates for lateral epicondylitis. The client's elbow is stabilized in the examiner's hand and the thumb of that hand positioned on the client's lateral epicondyle. The client makes a fist, pronates the forearm, and radially deviates and extends the wrist while the examiner applies a resisting force at the wrist. This test is positive if pain is elicited in the area of the lateral epicondyle. There is no specific test for shoulder bursitis.

16-59   Answer B

The alkaline phosphatase level is moderately elevated in osteomalacia. Serum calcium and phosphorus, urinary calcium, and creatinine excretion levels are all low in osteomalacia.

16-60   Answer A

The straight-leg-raising maneuver can be used to diagnose nerve root compression by eliciting radiating pain down the leg in the affected dermatomal distribution. The leg is straight and lifted by the heel. The leg may also be brought across the body to increase the sensitivity of this maneuver. Leg shortening and external rotation may be present with a fractured hip. Extending the knee would elicit pain if an anterior cruciate ligament tear were present. Pressure over an affected tendon would elicit pain if tendinitis were present.

16-61   Answer A

To diagnose fibromyalgia, there must be tenderness on digital palpation in at least 11 of 18 (nine pairs) tender-point sites, including the occiput, low cervical, trapezius, supraspinatus, second rib, lateral epicondyle, gluteal, greater trochanter, and knee. PIP, MCP, and MTP joint tenderness occurs primarily in rheumatoid arthritis. Facet joints of the spine are often tender in facet arthritis. Tenderness over the bony prominences of the wrist and ankle would be specific to injury at those areas.

16-62   Answer C

For the client who has just been given a diagnosis of carpal tunnel syndrome, your next step is to try neutral position wrist splinting and order an oral NSAID. For symptoms of less than 10 months' duration, conservative treatment should be tried first. Taking a more complete history is not essential at this point because a diagnosis has already been made. Nerve conduction studies (i.e., electromyography [EMG]) confirm focal median nerve conduction delay within the carpal canal and also provide information about disease severity. For refractory cases, median nerve decompression may be accomplished by surgery, but complete recovery is not possible if atrophy is pronounced.

16-63   Answer C

Thoracic outlet syndrome (TOS) results from a compression of nerves, blood vessels, or both, into the upper extremity arising from the head, neck, shoulders, upper extremities, and chest. Predisposing factors for thoracic outlet syndrome include a history of head and neck trauma, poor posture, chronic illness, and occupations that result in compression of the neurovascular structures supplying the upper extremity such as computer programming and piano playing.

16-64   Answer B

Swollen, bony proximal interphalangeal joints are Bouchard's nodes. Bony enlargements of the distal interphalangeal joints are Heberden's nodes. Both suggest osteoarthritis. Osler's nodes are painful, raised lesions of the fingers, toes, or feet that occur with bacterial endocarditis. There are no Murphy's nodes.

16-65   Answer D

Both active range of motion (AROM) and passive range of motion (PROM) of a joint should normally be equal, full, and pain free. AROM requires strength against gravity, and PROM is performed by the examiner without the effects of muscle contraction or gravity. Any pain or limitation with range of motion should be further investigated to determine the cause. If you note a limitation of AROM, you should gently attempt passive motion to further assess the joint.

16-66   Answer A

Duchenne muscular dystrophy, inherited in a sex-linked recessive pattern, afflicts boys, with the onset usually occurring around ages 3–5. The inability of the child to raise himself without supporting his knees because of weakness beginning primarily in the calf muscles, quadriceps, and hip extensor muscles is characteristic. Cerebral palsy affects motor function along with occasionally affecting intellect, emotional behavior, speech, sight, hearing, and touch. Damage occurs to the upper motor neurons during the prenatal or neonatal period. Legg-Calvé-Perthes disease is avascular necrosis of the capital femoral epiphysis. A limp would be present. Multiple sclerosis usually appears in the client around ages 20–40. The most common symptoms involve visual, sensory, and gait disturbances.

16-67   Answer C

In assessing your client, place the tips of your first two fingers in front of each ear and ask him to open and close his mouth. Then drop your fingers into the depressed area over the temporomandibular joint (TMJ) and note for smooth motion of the mandible. With this action, you are assessing for TMJ syndrome. Clicking or popping noises, decreased range of motion, pain, or swelling may indicate TMJ syndrome. However, an audible and palpable snap or click does occur in many normal people as they open their mouths. In rare cases, this may indicate osteoarthritis.

16-68   Answer C

An osteosarcoma is the most common malignant tumor that occurs in the long bones and the knee. An osteochondroma is the most common benign tumor and usually occurs in the pelvis, scapula, and ribs. A chondroma occurs in the hands, feet, ribs, spine, sternum, or long bones. A giant-cell tumor is a tumor of the bone marrow cells in the shaft of the long bones, such as the femur, tibia, radius, and humerus.

16-69   Answer B

The effect of caffeine in causing osteoporosis is controversial, but it is postulated to result from caffeine's diuretic effect that causes calcium to be excreted more rapidly.

16-70   Answer D

If a client has severed his fingers, the fingers should be wrapped in a saline-soaked dressing, placed in a plastic bag, and transported to the emergency room along with the client. The fingers should be cooled on ice, not frozen or kept at body temperature. Severed fingers can be reattached after 1–2 days or more, if properly stored.

16-71   Answer B

When you have a client bend forward to assess the spine (the Adams forward-bending test) and you note a right-sided rib hump, this is indicative of a right thoracic curve. Adolescent idiopathic scoliosis is a lateral spinal curvature of greater than 10° when no pathological cause has been determined. Management consists of the three O's: observation, orthosis, and operation. Spondylolysis is a bony defect of the pars interarticularis.

16-72   Answer D

Kyphosis involves a posterior rounding at the thoracic level and a kyphotic curve of more than 45° on x-ray. There may be moderate pain with kyphosis. Scoliosis involves asymmetry of the shoulders, scapulae, and waist creases; a lateral curvature and vertebral rotation on the posteroanterior x-rays; and one leg may appear shorter than the other.

16-73   Answer A

Osteoporosis develops when bone resorption occurs more rapidly than bone deposition. Osteoarthritis is a degenerative joint disease characterized by degeneration and loss of articular cartilage in synovial joints. Rheumatoid arthritis is a chronic, systemic inflammatory disorder characterized by persistent synovitis of multiple joints. Osteomalacia is a metabolic bone disorder characterized by inadequate mineralization of bone matrix, often caused by vitamin D deficiency.

16-74   Answer D

Raloxifene is a selective estrogen receptor modulator. Intranasal salmon calcitonin has been shown effective for pain management of osteoporotic fracture, but data on fracture incidence with this treatment is not available. Alendronate and risedronate are classified as bisphosphonates and can be used for prevention and treatment of osteoporosis.

16-75   Answer C

Follow the ABCs of first aid: airway, breathing, circulation. Establishing the airway is the first priority, followed by breathing, then circulation. Stopping the bleeding from the wound, assessing if there has been a cervical fracture, and palpating the peripheral pulses are all important actions, but if the client is not breathing, the other actions will not be necessary.

16-76   Answer C

The knee is the largest joint in the body, with the articulation of four bones, the femur, tibia, fibula, and patella, in one common articular cavity. It is a joint that not only permits flexion and extension but also some degree of rotation. The knee also has the body's largest synovial membrane.

16-77   Answer D

Other than a gross eye examination (most commonly performed using a Snellen eye chart) and vital signs, no specific tests are routinely recommended for a preparticipation sport physical.

16-78   Answer C

In reviewing myotomes, the C5 myotome innervates shoulder abduction (deltoid) and elbow flexion (biceps). Wrist extension results from the muscles and their corresponding nerves at C6, elbow extension from C7, and ulnar deviation at the wrist along with finger flexion and abduction from C8.

16-79   Answer C

A Baker's cyst, also called popliteal cyst, is the buildup of synovial fluid behind the knee. It usually results from inflammation resulting from knee arthritis or a cartilage (especially meniscal) tear and consists of local pain, inability to extend the knee, and symptoms related to compression of surrounding structures. The latter symptoms may mimic venous thrombophlebitis.

16-80   Answer B

When teaching clients about using a cane, tell them to advance the cane with the ipsilateral (affected) leg. The cane should be carried in the contralateral hand and the cane length should equal the height of the greater trochanter. The use of assistive devices is an important strategy to protect the joints, as well as provide safety, but clients must be taught the proper use of all devices.

16-81   Answer B

For Paul, who has a malignant fibrosarcoma of the femur, a magnetic resonance imaging scan will determine the extent of the tumor invasion on the surrounding tissues and the response of the bone tumor to the radiation. It will also determine response to chemotherapy and will detect recurrent disease. A conventional x-ray will show the location of the tumor and the extent of bone involvement. Metastatic bone destruction has a characteristic "moth-eaten" pattern in which the growth has a poorly defined margin that cannot be separated from normal bone. A computed tomography scan will evaluate the extent of the tumor invasion into bone, soft tissues, and neurovascular structures. A needle biopsy, usually performed at the time of surgery, will determine the type of tumor.

16-82   Answer A

Toe walking is considered normal until age 3 years. Constant toe walking after that age is considered abnormal and requires further investigation for neuromuscular disorders.

16-83   Answer A

Compartment syndrome occurs when external pressure constricts the structures within a compartment, compromising tissue perfusion. The pressure causes compressed nerves, muscles, and blood vessels. Cellular acidosis results, followed by edema, further increasing compartment pressures. This usually develops within the first 48 hours of injury. When assessing for compartment syndrome, remembering the five P's—pain, pulselessness, pallor, paresthesias, and paralysis—can be helpful, but they are not true diagnostic criteria. Phlebitis usually involves the lower extremities. Osteomyelitis might be considered if the fracture were an open one and bacteria entered through the open wound, but it would not develop this soon after the injury. Osteomyelitis can occur at any age, but children younger than age 12 and adults older than age 50 are the usual victims. A muscle contraction is a normal physiological function and would not result in these symptoms.

16-84   Answer A

Scoliosis is a curve in the spine. It is prominent beginning between ages 8 and 10 years through adolescence and is more common in females than in males. Functional scoliosis is flexible; it is apparent with standing and disappears with forward bending.

It is due to a problem that does not involve the spine such as leg length discrepancy or muscle spasm. Structural scoliosis is fixed; the curvature shows both on standing and bending forward. When the person is standing, note unequal shoulder elevation, unequal scapulae, obvious curvature, unequal elbow length, and unequal hip level.

16-85   Answer C

In a condylar joint, such as the knee and temporomandibular joint, the articulating surfaces are convex or concave and are termed condyles. Spheroidal joints have a ball-and-socket configuration—a rounded convex surface articulating with a cuplike cavity, allowing a wide range of rotary movement, as in the shoulder and hip. Often the knee is mistakenly referred to as a hinge joint, but hinge joints are flat and uniplanar, allowing only a gliding motion in a single plane, as in flexion and extension of the interphalangeal joints. In fibrous joints, such as the sutures of the skull, intervening layers of fibrous tissue or cartilage hold the bones together. The bones are almost in direct contact, which allows no appreciable movement.

16-86   Answer B

In osteoarthritis, the affected joints are swollen, cool, and bony hard on palpation. With rheumatoid arthritis, the affected joints appear red, hot, and swollen and are boggy and tender on palpation. Fatigue, decreased range of motion, and joint stiffness are common to both diseases.

16-87   Answer A

The clinical manifestations of osteomyelitis include the integumentary effects of swelling, erythema, and warmth at the involved site, as well as drainage and ulceration through the skin and lymph node involvement, especially in the involved extremity. The client with osteomyelitis may also have tachycardia, localized tenderness, and a high fever with chills.

16-88   Answer C

Basketball is listed as a limited contact/impact sport by the American Academy of Pediatrics Committee on Sports Medicine. Field hockey, soccer, and lacrosse all involve high-speed running and have the potential for collision and serious injury and therefore are classified as contact/collision sports.

16-89   Answer B

Asymptomatic hyperuricemia does not require any therapy because most people never develop symptoms. Although diet plays a minor role, dietary counseling to avoid foods high in purine and alcoholic beverages may be helpful to prevent future gout attacks. An acute attack of gout may be treated with colchicine or an NSAID. Allopurinol (Zyloprim) decreases uric acid production and might be prescribed to clients after multiple gouty attacks but should not be given as treatment for an acute gouty attack.

16-90   Answer C

A herniated lumbar intervertebral disc is the most common cause of cauda equine syndrome (CES). Other causes of CES include trauma, fracture, hematoma, abscesses, lymphoma, tumor and other space occupying lesions that compress the spinal nerve roots.

16-91   Answer B

NSAIDs are the first-line treatment for musculoskeletal signs and symptoms with joint involvement. DMARDs such as methotrexate are used for early-stage treatment of active disease with structural damage and inflammation. Biological agents or TNF-α inhibitors are considered for patients with active disease and inadequate response to one or more systemic DMARDs or very active psoriatic arthritis (PsA). A uricosuric such as Probenecid, with the addition of the anti-inflammatory Colchicine, is indicated for chronic gouty arthritis.

16-92   Answer C

Myalgias in the cervical spine and shoulder and hip girdle with polymyalgia rheumatica (PMR) can be profound and are commonly accompanied by systemic symptoms. Arthralgias may also occur which are similar to those found in patients with rheumatoid arthritis. Fibromyalgia also occurs more commonly in women but is associated with a more chronic widespread musculoskeletal pain and trigger points. Myofascial somatic dysfunction is described as impairments of the body framework. The impairments can affect joints, skeletal, and myofascial structures along with their related vascular, lymphatic and neural function. Reiter's syndrome or reactive arthritis is a classic triad of non-gonococcal urethritis, conjunctivitis, and arthritis that follows certain infections of the gastrointestinal or genitourinary tract.

16-93   Answer B

If a client presents with lower back pain and has decreased sensation to a pinprick in the lateral leg and web of the great toe, this indicates a dermatomal pattern of discogenic disease in the L4/L5 area (L5 root involvement). L3/L4 (L4 nerve root) innervates the sensory function of the distal thigh to medial calf to the arch of the foot. L5/S1 (S1 nerve root) innervates the sensory function of the lateral lower leg/calf to the fifth toe.

16-94   Answer C

NSAIDs are helpful for clients with Paget's disease who have mild symptoms and pain. However, once the serum alkaline phosphatase level rises, which indicates that the disease has progressed, bisphosphonates, which decrease bone resorption by inhibiting osteoclast activity, are the treatment of choice. Calcitonin (Calcimar) also inhibits osteoclastic bone resorption but is not as powerful as the bisphosphonates and does not suppress the disease activity for as long after cessation. Corticosteroids do inhibit bone metabolism but are limited by the side effects of long-term therapy with high doses.

16-95   Answer C

Years ago, muscle relaxants and bedrest were the treatments of choice for low back pain. Studies have now shown that resuming normal activity within the limits imposed by the pain has an effect as good as, if not better than, 2 days of bedrest. The expression is "let pain be your guide." Exercise should begin as soon as possible after the acute injury and is directed at building endurance and stamina with consideration given to one's pain tolerance. NSAIDs, not narcotics, are generally the first-line medication treatment of low back pain without the risk of opioid dependency. A Boston brace may be used in the treatment of scoliosis.

16-96   Answer A

If you note during your assessment of your client's foot that the foot is in alignment with the long axis of the lower leg and that weight-bearing falls on the middle of the foot, from the heel, along the midfoot, to between the second and third toes, you would diagnose a normal foot. Hallux valgus is a common deformity in which a lateral or outward deviation of the toe with medial prominence of the head of the first metatarsal is present. A hammertoe deformity is common in hallux valgus and is a deformity in the second, third,

fourth, or fifth toes that includes hyperextension of the metatarsophalangeal joint and flexion of the proximal interphalangeal joint. Talipes equinovarus (clubfoot) is a congenital defect; it presents as a rigid and fixed malposition of the foot, including inversion, forefoot adduction, and the foot pointing downward.

16-97   Answer C

The Thompson test is used to diagnose an Achilles tendon rupture. With an Achilles tendon rupture, there is local swelling and bruising and a weak push-off. The Thompson test is positive when the gastrocnemius muscle belly is firmly squeezed and the foot does not plantarflex. Boutonniere deformity, not test, usually results from an injury at the proximal interphalangeal joint, involving the extensor slip that attaches to the middle phalanx. It can also develop in inflammatory disorders such as rheumatoid arthritis. The Lachman test assesses for an anterior cruciate ligament (ACL) tear. The knee is flexed 30°, the examiner places one hand on the distal femur and the other on the proximal tibia, and an anterior force is applied to the proximal tibia. An intact ACL should prevent forward movement of the tibia. Any perceived contralateral difference is usually significant. The anterior drawer test is also used to assess for an ACL tear, but it is much less reliable than the Lachman test.

16-98   Answer A

CPPD disease (pseudogout) may appear clinically similar to gouty arthritis however, in CPPD crystals form in the cartilage and lead to inflammation. The typical age of onset is later in life than for gout and initially presents in the sixth decade of life or later. Diagnosis is made through synovial-fluid analysis will reveal positive calcium pyrophosphate dihydrate crystals. An x-ray will show radiographic evidence of chondrocalcinosis or calcification in hyaline and/or fibrocartilage in the affected joint. Bacterial cultures would be warranted to aid in diagnosis of cellulitis. Bone scan and MRI are used to differentiate gouty arthritis from Charcot neuro-osteoarthropathy. ACPA and an RA factor assist in the diagnosis of rheumatoid arthritis.

16-99   Answer A

The pathophysiology associated with transient pain after exercising that usually lasts a few hours with postexercise soreness and may last up to a week is increased lactic acid production, muscle breakdown, and minor inflammation. Longer-lasting pain late in an activity or immediately after is often caused by mild musculotendinous inflammation. When there is pain in the beginning or middle of the activity, there might be major musculotendinous inflammation, periostitis, and bone microtrauma. When the pain begins before or early in the exercise, preventing or affecting the performance, it is often the result of breakdown in soft tissue or stress fracture.

16-100   Answer C

Modifiable risk factors for osteoporosis include smoking, high caffeine intake, high alcohol intake, sedentary lifestyle, calcium deficiency, and estrogen deficiency. Over the course of their lives, women tend to lose up to one-third of their original bone mass, ultimately affecting 80% of their skeletal system. It is essential that modifiable risk factors be modified because there are many that cannot, including increasing age, race (incidence is greater in white women), gender, pale complexion, and long-term glucocorticoid therapy.

16-101   Answer B

Treatment for PMR consists of low-dose steroids, starting with 10–15 mg and tapering to 5–7.5 mg daily for several weeks or months.

16-102   Answer D

To aid in the diagnosis of meniscus damage such as a torn meniscus, you should perform Apley's compression test. With the client in the prone position, the suspected knee is flexed to 90 degrees and then downward pressure is exerted on the foot so that the tibia is firmly opposed to the femur. The leg is then rotated externally and internally. If the knee locks and there is pain or clicking with this maneuver, it is a positive Apley's sign, indicating the presence of a loose body, such as a torn cartilage, trapped in the joint articulation. The bulge test assesses for effusions in the knee joint. The Lachman test is an indicator of injury to the anterior cruciate ligament. The drawer test assesses for stability of the anterior and posterior cruciate ligaments.

16-103   Answer A

The National Osteoporosis Foundation recommendations indicate that bone mineral density (BMD) testing should be performed on all women age 65 and older regardless of risk factors, on postmenopausal women under age 65 with risk factors, on women of menopausal age with risk factors, and on individuals who present with fractures after age 50 to confirm underlying disease and severity. Men age 70 or older, as well as between the ages of 50 and 69 with risk factors, should also be screened with the BMD test.

16-104   Answer B

The CASPAR Criteria is the most widely accepted tool and has a 91.4% sensitivity and 98.7% specificity rate. It assigns points from five categories: current psoriasis, personal history of psoriasis, family history of psoriasis; typical psoriatic nail dystrophy; negative rheumatoid factor; current dactylitis or history of dactylitis; and radiographic evidence of juxta-articular new bone formation. The Psoriasis Area and Severity Index (PASI) is a quantitative rating scale for measuring the severity of psoriatic lesions based on area coverage and severity. The criteria, known as ACR Criteria (American College of Rheumatology Criteria), compares the effectiveness of various arthritis medications or arthritis treatments as to improvement in tender or swollen joint counts and improvement in three of the following five parameters: acute phase reactant (such as sedimentation rate), patient assessment, physician assessment, pain scale, and disability/ functional questionnaire. The Rome Criteria is used to help diagnose irritable bowel syndrome (IBS).

16-105   Answer A

Clinical manifestations of an anterior shoulder dislocation, which is far more common than a posterior dislocation, include the inability to shrug the shoulder, pain, and lengthening of the arm. The inability to rotate the shoulder externally is a clinical manifestation of a posterior shoulder dislocation, along with the inability to elevate the arm.

16-106   Answer A

Management of fibromyalgia includes giving tricyclic antidepressants such as amitriptyline (Elavil) in a low dose at bedtime. Although clients with fibromyalgia are fatigued and have stiff joints and muscle pain, physical therapy, including exercise, is an important aspect of care. Injecting trigger points with local anesthetics and steroids can also be helpful. NSAIDs have not proven beneficial in the treatment of fibromyalgia, and NSAIDs are always associated with the risk of gastrointestinal bleeding, especially in high doses.

16-107   Answer A

Fat emboli are a serious and potentially fatal complication after a long-bone fracture. They usually occur within 72 hours after the injury. Fat emboli commonly lodge in the lung and produce sudden-onset respiratory problems resulting in hypoxemia. Symptoms include fever, tachycardia, rapid respirations, and neurological manifestations.

16-108   Answer A

A sprain is defined as an injury to the ligaments that connect bone to bone in a joint that results from a twisting motion and may cause joint instability. A strain is defined as an injury to the muscles and/or the tendons that attach muscles to bones.

16-109   Answer A

The development of osteosarcoma in pagetic lesions is the most serious complication of Paget's disease. This development is rare (less than 1%), but the incidence of osteosarcoma in patients with Paget's disease is approximately 1,000-fold greater than in age-matched persons without Paget's disease. A more significant number of patients with the disease have bone pain, skeletal deformities, fractures, high-output cardiac failure, or nerve compression syndromes.

16-110   Answer D

Reactive arthritis (formerly Reiter's syndrome) is arthritis of the lower extremities and is more common in white men. Associated symptoms include the classic triad of conjunctivitis, nongonococcal urethritis, and arthritis. A common mnemonic is the client who "can't see, can't pee, and can't climb a tree."

16-111   Answer B

In grading muscle strength on a scale of 1–5, a grade of 4 indicates full range of motion (ROM) against gravity with some resistance. A grade of 5 is full ROM against gravity with full resistance. A grade of 3 is full ROM with gravity. A grade of 2 is full ROM with gravity eliminated (passive motion). A grade of 1 indicates slight muscle contraction. A grade of 0 indicates no muscle contraction.

16-112   Answer A

Repetitive nerve stimulation (RNS) is the most frequently used electrodiagnostic test for myasthenia gravis. The nerve to be studied is electrically stimulated and the compound muscle action potential (CMAP) is recorded with surface electrodes over the muscle. Serological tests such as serum anti-AChR antibodies are also usually included along with electrodiagnostic testing. Cogwheel rigidity is present in Parkinson's disease. Chvostek's and Trousseau's signs are indications of tetany.

16-113   Answer C

Sjögren's syndrome, which affects the salivary and lacrimal glands, causes clients to have dry eyes and mouths. It is an inflammatory disease of the exocrine glands and may be an isolated entity or may be associated with other rheumatic disease, such as rheumatoid arthritis (RA) or systemic lupus erythematosus (SLE). Because Anne Marie has no other symptoms of RA or SLE, Sjögren's syndrome should be considered first. Rosacea is a chronic facial skin disorder with a vascular component.

16-114   Answer B

To diagnose gout, there should be a negative joint culture and hyperuricemia. A septic joint would likely cause an elevated white blood count (WBC) and a positive bacterial joint culture. Rocephin (Ceftriaxone) is an antibiotic used in the treatment of bacterial infections such as a septic arthritis. A positive antinuclear antibody test may indicate systemic lupus erythematosus or scleroderma.

16-115   Answer D

The red flags for spinal fracture include major trauma or a direct blow the back in adults, a minor fall or heavy lifting in a potentially osteoporotic or elderly person, prolonged steroid use, and age over 70. Low back pain accompanied by acute onset of urinary retention or overflow incontinence, loss of anal sphincter tone or fecal incontinence, loss of sensation in the buttocks and perineum, and motor weakness in the lower extremities are red flags for cauda equina syndrome or severe neurologic compromise. Cancer may be suspected if the low back pain is accompanied by unexplained weight loss and immunosuppression in a person over the age of 50.

16-116   Answer B

Dorsal kyphosis, an exaggerated convexity of the thoracic curvature, typically accompanies the aging process. Lordosis occurs when the normal lumbar concavity is further accentuated, such as with pregnancy or obesity. Scoliosis, which is more prevalent in adolescent girls, is a lateral S-shaped or C-shaped curvature of the thoracic and/or lumbar spine and can also involve vertebral rotation.

16-117   Answer C

Intra-articular corticosteroid injections provide much needed pain relief in weight-bearing joints of clients with osteoarthritis; however, they should be limited to no more than three to four in the same joint per year because of potential damage to the cartilage if given more frequently.

16-118   Answer A

Developmental dysplasia of the hip (DDH), previously referred to as congenital hip dislocation, occurs in approximately 1% of live births and is more common in females than males. Factors related to development of DDH include being the firstborn female child, a family history of congenital dislocation of the hip, and breech presentation. Orthopedic malformation in utero is not considered a developmental cause.

16-119   Answer B

Ganglia can be distinguished from neoplasms by their ability to transilluminate. Large ganglia and neoplasms may both restrict joint motion. Painless swelling is usually the main feature of ganglia. Ganglia may fluctuate in size depending on the individual's activity level and often will spontaneously resolve.

16-120   Answer B

Black men have a relatively low incidence of osteoporosis because they have higher levels of bone mass and are protected by the bone-resorptive effects of parathyroid hormone. Osteoporosis has the highest incidence in white women.

16-121   Answer B

Ankylosis is stiffness or fixation of a joint. It often involves inflammation of the connective tissue, muscles, and the joint itself. A contracture is a shortening of a muscle leading to limited range of motion of a joint. This is often the result of scar formation from trauma, genetics, or chronic disease. Dislocation is one or more bones in a joint being out of position. Subluxation is a partial dislocation of a joint.

16-122   Answer B

Pregnant women have an increased incidence of carpal tunnel syndrome (CTS) but often have their carpal tunnel syndrome resolve after delivery. Although repetitive use of the hand can lead to carpal tunnel syndrome, certain medical conditions such as diabetes, obesity, and thyroid disease also increase the likelihood of CTS. Often, the cause of CTS is unknown.

16-123   Answer C

Grating of the bones or entrance of air into an open fracture is manifested as crepitus. The extremity should not be manipulated to elicit crepitus because it may cause additional damage. Swelling is manifested by edema from localization of serous fluid and bleeding. Ecchymosis results from extravasation of blood into the subcutaneous tissue. Pain and tenderness result from muscle spasm, direct tissue trauma, nerve pressure, or movement of the fractured bone.

16-124   Answer D

Health promotion and maintenance information regarding physical activity that should be included in client teaching includes reminding the client that stretching and warm-up exercises are an important part of any exercise routine. After proper stretching and warm-up exercises, muscles should not hurt after most sports activities if engaged in on a regular basis. If the activity is new, a muscle group may be slightly sore, in which case ice applied to the area may help relieve the discomfort. Any rigorous exercise should be avoided until one is in proper physical condition. This is usually obtained after a conservative, lengthy program of physical fitness activities. After any strenuous activity, a cool-down period should be employed.

Bibliography

American Academy of Pediatrics and Council on Sports Medicine and Fitness: Medical conditions affecting sports participation. *Pediatrics* 121(4): 841–848, 2008.

Andreoli, TE, et al: *Andreoli and Carpenter's Cecil Essentials of Medicine*, ed 8. Saunders Elsevier, Philadelphia, 2010.

Bickley, L: *Bates' Guide to Physical Examination and History Taking*, ed 10. Lippincott, Williams & Wilkins, Philadelphia, 2009.

Crosby, J, and Haddow, S: Gouty arthritis: How to make the diagnosis. *Clinical Advisor* 4, 9–45, 2011.

Gossec L, et al: European League Against Rheumatism recommendations for the management of psoriatic arthritis with pharmacological therapies. *Annals of Rheumatic Diseases* (e-pub), 2011.

Grottkau, B: Top 5 orthopedic referrals from the PCP: An orthopedist's perspective. PRIMED East 2007. *Current Clinical Issues in Primary Care*, October 13, 2007.

Jarvis, C: *Physical Examination and Health Assessment*, ed 6. WB Saunders, Philadelphia, 2011.

Kinkade, S: Low back pain. In Sloane, PD, et al: *Essentials of Family Medicine*, ed 6. Lippincott, Williams & Wilkins, Philadelphia, 2012.

Martin-Plank, L. Musculoskeletal problems (chap. 15). In Dunphy, LM, et al: *Primary Care: The Art and Science of Advanced Practice Nursing*, ed 3. FA Davis, Philadelphia, 2011.

National Osteoporosis Foundation: NOF learn about osteoporosis, 2012. www.NOF.org, accessed Nov. 3, 2012.

Sass, P, and Hassan, G: Lower extremity abnormalities in children. *American Family Physician* 68(3): 461–468, 2007.

Schlesinger, N, et al: Colchicine for acute gout. *Cochrane Database of Systematic Reviews* 4: CD006190.

Sloane PD et al: *Essentials of Family Medicine*, Lippincott, Williams & Wilkins, Philadelphia, 2012.

Smith, D, and Kaul, T: Diagnostic triage and differentiation of low back pain: Cauda equina syndrome case study. *American Journal for Nurse Practitioners* 15:12, 2011.

Taylor, W, et al: Classification criteria for psoriatic arthritis: development of new criteria from a large international study. *Arthritis & Rheumatism* 54(8):2665–2673, 2006.

Wheeless, CR, Nunley, JA, and Urbaniak, JR (eds): *Wheeless' Textbook of Orthopaedics*. Data Trace Publishing, Brooklandville, MD, 2011. www.wheelessonline.com ortho/2130, accessed November 25, 2011.

How well did you do?

85% and above, congratulations! This score shows application of test-taking principles and adequate content knowledge.

75%–85%, keep working! Review test-taking principles and try again.

65%–75%, hang in there! Spend some time reviewing concepts and test-taking principles and try the test again.

This is very difficult content and some questions will probably be known only by nurses working in this specialty.

Chapter 17: *Endocrine and Metabolic Problems*

Jill E. Winland-Brown
Lynne Palma

Questions

17-1 *After a subtotal thyroidectomy, it is crucial to assess*

A. heart tones.
B. for peripheral edema.
C. speaking ability.
D. skin turgor.

17-2 *Diane has had Cushing's disease for 20 years and has been taking hydrocortisone since then. Today, she appears with a thick trunk and thin extremities. She has a "moon face," a "buffalo hump," thin skin with visible capillaries, and a number of bruises that appear to be slow in healing. To what do you attribute these symptoms?*

A. Decreased adrenal androgen levels
B. Malfunctioning of the adrenal cortex
C. Excessive levels of circulating cortisol
D. Ectopic secretion of adrenocorticotropic hormone

17-3 *You suspect myxedema in your client because she exhibits*

A. smooth, moist skin.
B. pitting edema.
C. abnormal deposits of mucin in the skin.
D. abdominal bloating.

17-4 *What is the most common cause of chronic hypocalcemia?*

A. Alkalosis
B. Burn trauma
C. Hypoalbuminemia
D. Renal failure

17-5 *Which of the following statements is true about insulin lispro?*

A. It works faster than regular insulin because its amino acid composition has been slightly modified.
B. When taken 30 minutes before a meal, it reduces after-meal hyperglycemia.
C. Its duration of action is about 4–5 hours.
D. It is taken with the first bite of food.

17-6 *Sara has diabetes and is now experiencing anhidrosis on the hands and feet, increased sweating on the face and trunk, dysphagia, anorexia, and heartburn. Which complication of diabetes do you suspect?*

A. Macrocirculation changes
B. Microcirculation changes
C. Somatic neuropathies
D. Visceral neuropathies

17-7 *A client with diabetes complains of paresthesias. Which of the following medications can cause sensory changes?*

A. Glipizide
B. Sitagliptin (Januvia)
C. Metformin
D. Exenatide (Byetta)

17-8 *Morton has type 2 diabetes. His treatment, which includes diet, exercise, and oral antidiabetic agents, is insufficient to achieve acceptable glycemic control. Your next course of action is to*

A. increase the dosage of the oral antidiabetic agents.
B. add a dosage of long-acting insulin at bedtime to the regimen.

C. discontinue the oral antidiabetic agents and start insulin therapy.

D. suggest treatment using an insulin pump.

17-9   *Alice, age 48, has a benign thyroid nodule. The most common treatment involves*

A. surgery.

B. administration of levothyroxine therapy.

C. watchful waiting with an annual follow-up.

D. radioactive iodine therapy.

17-10   *Sadie, age 40, has just been given a diagnosis of Graves' disease. She has recently lost 25 lb, has palpitations, is very irritable, feels very warm, and has a noticeable bulge on her neck. The most likely cause of her increased thyroid function is*

A. hyperplasia of the thyroid.

B. an anterior pituitary tumor.

C. a thyroid carcinoma.

D. an autoimmune response.

17-11   *Why is parathyroid hormone secretion increased during pregnancy?*

A. To meet the increased stress demands on the mother

B. To meet the increased requirements for calcium and vitamin D for fetal skeletal growth

C. To help prevent neural tube defects in the fetus

D. To help promote neurological growth of the developing brain in the fetus

17-12   *The major risk factor for development of thyroid cancer is*

A. inadequate iodine intake.

B. presence of a goiter.

C. exposure to radiation.

D. smoking.

17-13   *The following is a self-monitoring blood glucose (SMBG) log on a client receiving 20 units Novolin 70/30 in the morning (a.m.) and 20 units Novolin 70/30 in the evening (p.m.): Fasting a.m. pre-dinner: 90, 150, 105, 144, 101, 172, 98, 201. What changes would you make?*

A. Increase the p.m. insulin.

B. Increase the a.m. insulin.

C. Add NovoLog at bedtime (hs).

D. Increase the a.m. and p.m. insulin.

17-14   *Trousseau's sign assesses for*

A. hypocalcemia.

B. hyponatremia.

C. hypercalcemia.

D. hypermagnesemia.

17-15   *An elderly client presents with atrial fibrillation. Which of the following lab tests is important in forming the diagnosis?*

A. CBC

B. CRP

C. CMP

D. TSH

17-16   *Which is the only treatment option that is curative for primary hyperparathyroidism (PHPT)?*

A. Type II calcimimetic cinacalcet

B. Hormone therapy

C. Parathyroidectomy

D. Bisphosphonates

17-17   *Which of the following hormones is secreted by the posterior pituitary gland?*

A. Antidiuretic hormone (ADH)

B. Thyroid-stimulating hormone (TSH)

C. Adrenocorticotropic hormone (ACTH)

D. Growth hormone (GH)

17-18   *Which of the following statements is true about the ophthalmopathy in Graves' disease?*

A. Propranolol (Inderal) initially helps to control symptoms related to ophthalmopathy.

B. Treatment often includes prednisone.

C. Radiation or surgical decompression should never be done until the eyes are no longer bulging.

D. Radioactive iodine may be effective.

17-19   Eunice, age 32, has type 2 diabetes. She said that she heard that she should take an aspirin a day after she reaches menopause for its cardioprotective action. She does not have coronary artery disease, but her father does. How do you respond?

A. "You're right. Your hormones protect you against coronary artery diseases until menopause; then you should start on aspirin therapy."

B. "The American Diabetes Association recommends that you start on aspirin therapy now."

C. "Aspirin therapy is recommended only if you have a family history of coronary artery disease."

D. "If you maintain good glycemic control, you don't need aspirin therapy."

17-20   Pancreatitis has been associated with which of the following antidiabetic drugs?

A. Glipizide

B. Metformin

C. Glargine (Lantus)

D. Exenatide (Byetta)

17-21   Marty has pheochromocytoma. You instruct him to

A. void in small amounts.

B. not exercise for more than 30 minutes at a time.

C. avoid sleeping in the prone position.

D. take steroids.

17-22   Which of the following is a sign of hypothyroidism?

A. A thyroid bruit

B. Brittle hair

C. Gynecomastia

D. Warm, smooth, moist skin

17-23   Mary, age 72, has been taking insulin for several years. She just called you because she realized that yesterday she put her short-acting insulin in the long-acting insulin box and vice versa. She just took 22 units of regular insulin when she was supposed to take only 5 units.

She says that she tried to do a fingerstick to test her glucose level but was unable to obtain any blood. She states that she feels fine. What do you tell her to do first?

A. "Keep trying to get a fingerstick and call me back with the results."

B. "Call 911 before you collapse."

C. "Drive immediately to the ER."

D. "Drink 4 oz of fruit juice."

17-24   Jane has insulin-dependent diabetes mellitus and has been experiencing hyperglycemia before dinner. A possible solution to this problem is to

A. adjust her morning dose of rapid-acting insulin.

B. increase her midafternoon snack.

C. add physical activity between lunch and dinner.

D. reduce the amount of carbohydrates at dinner.

17-25   When you inspect the integumentary system of clients with endocrine disorders, coarse hair may be an indicator of

A. Addison's disease.

B. diabetes mellitus.

C. Cushing's syndrome.

D. hypothyroidism.

17-26   To lower the serum concentration of thyroid hormones and reestablish a eumetabolic state in the client with Graves' disease, which of the following therapies may be used?

A. Radiation

B. Antithyroid drugs

C. Chemotherapy

D. Parathyroid surgery

17-27   Margie has hypoparathyroidism. Which of the following would you assess during your examination?

A. Skin turgor

B. Heart tones

C. Chvostek's sign

D. Homans' sign

17-28 *Sandra has secondary obesity. Which of the following may have caused this?*

A. An intake of more calories than are expended

B. Polycystic ovary disease

C. Her antihypertensive medications

D. Her sedentary lifestyle

17-29 *Early-morning increases in blood glucose concentration that occur with no corresponding hypoglycemia during the night are referred to as*

A. the Somogyi phenomenon.

B. insulin shock.

C. diabetic ketoacidosis.

D. the dawn phenomenon.

17-30 *Which blood test should be obtained before initiating antithyroid drugs for Graves' disease?*

A. Serum electrolytes

B. Lipid profile

C. White blood cell count

D. Complete chemistry profile

17-31 *A client with Graves' disease is prescribed a beta-adrenergic antagonist. Which of the following comorbid conditions will be exacerbated with the initiation of the propranolol?*

A. Tachycardia

B. Hypertension

C. Hyperlipidemia

D. Asthma

17-32 *ACE inhibitors are given to clients with diabetes who have*

A. an elevated glycohemoglobin level.

B. insulin sensitivity.

C. persistent proteinuria.

D. an elevated serum creatinine level.

17-33 *Joan has severe asthma and has been on high doses of oral corticosteroids for 2 years. She has been reading some home remedy books and stops all of her medications. What condition may she develop?*

A. Myxedema crisis

B. Diabetes insipidus

C. Hypoparathyroidism

D. Addisonian crisis

17-34 *June stopped breastfeeding 2 years ago. Yesterday, when doing a breast self-examination, she noticed a small amount of yellowish liquid when she squeezed her nipples. She is concerned that this is one of the signs of breast cancer. You tell her,*

A. "Let's get a mammogram to be on the safe side."

B. "Let's wait for a month and reassess."

C. "A small amount of breast milk can be expressed from the nipple in many parous women and is not a cause for concern."

D. "We should do an ultrasound."

17-35 *The most common worldwide cause of hypothyroidism is*

A. an autoimmune process.

B. Hashimoto's thyroiditis.

C. iodine deficiency.

D. iatrogenic hypothyroidism.

17-36 *When teaching Marcy how to use her new insulin pump, you tell her that she needs to monitor her blood glucose level*

A. at least once a day.

B. only occasionally because glycemic levels are maintained very steadily.

C. at least four times a day.

D. on an as-needed basis when she feels she needs to give herself an extra dose of insulin.

17-37 *You are counseling your client with diabetes about diet. You know she misunderstands when she tells you that*

A. "I can substitute two Oreo cookies for a fresh pear."

B. "I can have an occasional glass of chardonnay."

C. "I should monitor the amount of carbohydrates I eat at each meal."

D. "As long as I monitor my blood sugar and it's normal, I can eat anything."

17-38   Jay has had diabetes for 10 years. He recently had a physical and was told he has some evidence of renal nephropathy. What is the first manifestation of this renal dysfunction?

A. Proteinuria

B. Development of Kimmelstiel-Wilson nodules

C. Decreased blood urea nitrogen levels

D. Increased serum creatine levels

17-39   A diabetic client on a sulfonylurea and metformin with an HbA1c of 6.5% is complaining of episodes of low blood sugar. Which of the following changes would be the most appropriate?

A. Decrease the dosage of the metformin.

B. Discontinue the metformin.

C. Increase carbohydrate intake.

D. Decrease the sulfonylurea.

17-40   Which of the following steps will not prevent or slow the progression of diabetic nephropathy?

A. Control of blood pressure

B. Use of ACE inhibitors

C. Restriction of protein intake

D. Use of calcium channel blockers

17-41   Ben, a client with type 1 diabetes, is hospitalized with an admitting diagnosis of diabetic ketoacidosis. Which of the following signs and symptoms would be consistent with this condition?

A. Hypoglycemia and glycosuria

B. Decreased respiratory rate with shallow respirations

C. Polydipsia and an increased blood pH

D. Ketonuria and polyuria

17-42   Joy has gout. In teaching her about her disease, which food do you tell her is allowed on the diet?

A. Asparagus

B. Beans

C. Broccoli

D. Mushrooms

17-43   Peter, age 62, has diabetes and wants to start an exercise program. Which type of exercise might be detrimental?

A. Swimming

B. Jogging

C. Tennis

D. Dancing

17-44   Marisa, age 16, is an active cheerleader who just developed type 1 diabetes. She is worried that she will not fit in with her friends anymore because she does not think she can have all the same snacks they have. How do you respond?

A. "As long as your snacks are low in fats and carbohydrates, you'll be fine."

B. "Any snacks that are sufficient in calories to maintain your normal weight are OK."

C. "Just be sure that your snacks are high in fats and proteins."

D. "Be sure to stick to snacks that are high in simple carbohydrates."

17-45   Scott has type 2 diabetes and asks if he needs to do self-monitoring of his blood glucose (SMBG) level. You tell him,

A. "No, it is indicated only in type 1 diabetes."

B. "Yes, definitely; you should be performing SMBG at least on a daily basis."

C. "You should be doing SMBG at least three times a week."

D. "We'll just test your serum glucose each month and you'll be OK."

17-46   Harriet, age 62, has type 1 diabetes that is well controlled by insulin. Recently, she has been having marital difficulties that have left her emotionally upset. As a result of this stress, it is possible that she will

A. have an insulin reaction more readily than usual.

B. have an increased blood sugar level.

C. need less daily insulin.

D. need more carbohydrates.

17-47   *Susie has insulin-dependent diabetes mellitus. To forestall hypoglycemia, how much carbohydrate must she eat if she misses a regular meal?*

A. 5–15 g

B. 15–30 g

C. 30–35 g

D. More than 35 g

17-48   *Presence of Trousseau's sign is often preceded by*

A. a spasm of the facial muscle.

B. muscle cramps in the legs and feet.

C. abdominal pain.

D. headache.

17-49   *Diabetes and coronary artery disease (CAD) have a close interrelationship. Which of the following statements about the relationship between diabetes and CAD is true?*

A. Hyperinsulinemia decreases sympathetic tone and cardiac contractility by increasing plasma catecholamines, epinephrine, and norepinephrine.

B. An increase of glucose causes the distal nephrons of the kidneys to absorb less sodium, resulting in more fluid, expanding the intravascular volume and increasing the blood pressure.

C. Hyperinsulinemia causes a large number of vascular smooth muscle cells to be formed and deposited on the walls of vessels, eventually decreasing space for blood flow.

D. An increase in glucose stimulates more secretion of epinephrine, thus raising the blood pressure (BP).

17-50   *Judy has the visiting nurse prefill her insulin syringes because of her visual and dexterity difficulties. On Judy's routine visit for her blood work, she asks you about storing these prefilled syringes. How do you respond?*

A. "Keep them at room temperature with the needle angled down, just like you do with a bottle of wine."

B. "They can be kept in the refrigerator for 1 week when the visiting nurse should fill new ones."

C. "They can be stored in a vertical position in the refrigerator for 30 days with the needle pointing upward."

D. "They should be placed in the refrigerator without the needles on—those should be added just prior to administration."

17-51   *Mindy is scheduled to have an oral glucose tolerance test. For 3 days before the test, she is instructed to discontinue many of her medications. Which one is it safe to continue taking?*

A. Vitamin C

B. Aspirin

C. Calcium

D. Her oral contraceptive

17-52   *Marsha, age 24, is preparing for radioactive iodine therapy for her Graves' disease. Which test must she undergo first?*

A. Beta human chorionic gonadotropin

B. Basal metabolism rate

C. Lithium level

D. Serum calcium

17-53   *Minnie is pregnant. She has hypothyroidism and has been on the same levothyroxine medication for years. What might you expect to do with her levothyroxine medication?*

A. Increase the dosage.

B. Maintain her established dose.

C. Decrease her dosage.

D. Increase the dose during the first trimester, then decrease it during the second and third trimesters.

17-54   *Which of the following is a characteristic of virilization in a woman?*

A. Squeaky voice

B. Decreased muscle mass

C. Clitoral enlargement

D. Excessive hair distribution

17-55   *Steve, age 42, has never been hypertensive but appears today in the office with a blood pressure of 162/100 mm Hg. He also complains of "attacks" of headache, perspiration, and palpitations with frequent attacks of nausea, pain, weakness, dyspnea, and visual disturbances. He has lost 10 lb over the past 2 months and seems very anxious today. Your next action would be to*

A. start him on an antianxiety agent.

B. obtain a 24-hour urine test for catecholamines.

C. start him on a diuretic or beta blocker.

D. recheck his blood pressure in 1 week.

17-56   Which hormone is secreted by the adrenal cortex?

A. Thyroid-stimulating hormone

B. Growth hormone

C. Follicle-stimulating hormone

D. Aldosterone

17-57   Martin, age 62, has acute nontransient abdominal pain that grows steadily worse in the epigastric area and radiates straight through to the back. The pain has lasted for days. He is also complaining of nausea, vomiting, sweating, weakness, and pallor. Physical examination reveals abdominal tenderness and distention and a low-grade fever. What do you suspect?

A. Cholecystitis

B. Acute pancreatitis

C. Cirrhosis

D. Cushing's syndrome

17-58   Older clients with diabetes are predisposed to which of the following types of ear infections?

A. Simple otitis externa

B. Malignant otitis externa

C. Otitis media

D. Serous otitis media

17-59   An elderly client with hyperthyroidism may present with atypical symptoms. Which of the following manifestations are commonly seen in the elderly with hyperthyroidism?

A. Adrenergic findings such as tachycardia

B. Weight gain, depression, heat intolerance

C. Atrial fibrillation, depression, and weight loss

D. Heat intolerance, hyperreflexia, and anorexia

17-60   You suspect that Sharon has hypoparathyroidism because, in addition to her other signs and symptoms, she has

A. elevated serum phosphate levels.

B. elevated serum calcium levels.

C. decreased neuromuscular irritability.

D. increased bone resorption, as implied by her bone density test.

17-61   Jason, age 14, appears with tender discoid breast tissue enlargement (2–3 cm in diameter) beneath the areola. Your next action would be to

A. perform watchful waiting for 1 year.

B. order an ultrasound.

C. obtain laboratory tests.

D. refer Jason to an endocrinologist.

17-62   The Diabetes Control and Complications Trial recommends intensive management of diabetes for

A. children younger than age 13.

B. older adults.

C. persons who already have a diagnosis of beginning nephropathy, neuropathy, or retinopathy.

D. individuals with a history of frequent severe hypoglycemia.

17-63   Jeremiah, age 72, has gout and is obese. When teaching him about diet, which of the following do you tell him?

A. "Beer and wine are OK because they have no effect on uric acid."

B. "Keeping your weight stable, even if you are a little overweight, is better than fluctuating."

C. "You must go on a very low caloric-restricted diet to effect immediate change."

D. "Fluid intake should exceed 3,000 mL daily to prevent formation of uric acid kidney stones."

17-64   A newly diagnosed client with diabetes who has an HbA1c of 7.5 is started on therapeutic lifestyle changes (TLC) and medical nutritional therapy (MNT). Which oral antidiabetic agent is recommended as monotherapy?

A. Glipizide

B. Sitagliptin (Januvia)

C. Exenatide (Byetta)

D. Metformin (Glucophage)

17-65   Jenny, age 46, has hypertension that has been controlled with hydrochlorothiazide 50 mg every day for the past 3 years. She is 5 ft 8 in. tall and weighs 220 lb. Her fasting blood sugar (FBS) level is 300 mg/dL, serum cholesterol level is 250 mg/dL, serum potassium level is 3.4 mEq, and she has 4+glucosuria. Your next course of action would be to

A. discontinue her hydrochlorothiazide.

B. order a glucose tolerance test (GTT).

C. repeat her FBS test and do an HbA1c.

D. start insulin therapy.

17-66   How long after the acute illness of hepatitis A do immunoglobulin M anti–hepatitis A virus titers disappear?

A. 1 week

B. 3–6 months

C. 1 year

D. 2 years

17-67   Dan, age 45, is obese and has type 2 diabetes and has been having trouble getting his glycohemoglobin under control. He's heard that exenatide (Byetta) causes weight loss and wants to try it. What do you tell him?

A. "Let's adjust your oral antidiabetic agents instead."

B. "That's a myth. People usually change their eating habits when taking this, and that's what causes the weight loss."

C. "With type 2 diabetes, you never want to be on injectable insulin."

D. "Let's try it. You're glycohemoglobin will be lowered and you may lose weight."

17-68   A client with type 2 diabetes is on the maximum dosage of three oral antidiabetic agents, and the HbA1c remains at 8.5%. The practitioner initiates basal insulin. Which of the following would be an appropriate order?

A. Insulin glargine (Lantus) 10 units nightly

B. Insulin detemir (Levemir) 10 units before each meal

C. Insulin aspart (NovoLog) 10 units before each meal

D. Regular insulin before each meal

17-69   Which of the following statements about primary hyperparathyroidism (PHPT) is true?

A. PHPT is the most common cause of hypercalcemia.

B. Hypotension is one of the first clinical manifestations.

C. On a DEXA scan, a client with PHPT will have bone cysts as a common finding.

D. The history and physical examination are crucial elements in diagnosing PHPT.

17-70   Which of the following medications can produce gynecomastia?

A. Cimetidine (Tagamet)

B. Cholesterol-lowering medications

C. Beta blockers

D. Aspirin

17-71   Mason, age 52, has diabetes and is overweight. You now find that he is hypertensive. How should you treat his hypertension?

A. You should treat it the same as in a client without diabetes.

B. Because insulin affects most of the antihypertensive drugs, you should try diet and exercise first before any antihypertensives are ordered.

C. You should treat it very aggressively.

D. Initiate therapy when the blood pressure is 5–10 mm Hg more than the conventional therapeutic guidelines.

17-72   The thyroid-stimulating hormone (TSH) test measures the

A. total serum level of thyroxine.

B. serum level of T_3 and T_4.

C. pituitary's response to peripheral levels of thyroid hormone.

D. combined serum levels of T_3 and T_4.

17-73   How do you explain the fact that someone with Cushing's disease bruises easily?

A. Decreased skin turgor

B. A loss of neurological sensation

C. Decreased prothrombin levels

D. Protein wasting and collagen loss

17-74 *Sandra has diabetes and frequently develops vaginitis. You instruct her to*

A. wipe from back to front after voiding.

B. wear white nylon underwear.

C. wear pantyhose if wearing tight jeans.

D. avoid douching.

17-75 *Sandra, who has diabetes, states that she heard that fiber is especially good to include in her diet. How do you respond?*

A. "Fiber is important in all diets."

B. "Too much fiber interferes with insulin, so include only a moderate amount in your diet."

C. "Fiber, especially soluble fiber, helps improve carbohydrate metabolism, so it is more important in the diet of persons with diabetes."

D. "You get just the amount of fiber you need with a normal diet."

17-76 *The most common cause of hyperthyroidism is*

A. Graves' disease.

B. a toxic uninodular goiter.

C. subacute thyroiditis.

D. a pituitary tumor.

17-77 *What is the medication of choice for an initial acute attack of gout?*

A. An NSAID

B. Colchicine

C. A corticosteroid

D. Allopurinol (Zyloprim)

17-78 *Sandy is being treated for chronic hypocalcemia. When her serum calcium level returns to normal, you assess her urinary calcium level and note that it is greater than 250 mg in a 24-hour sample. This indicates that*

A. her vitamin D dosage should be increased.

B. her vitamin D dosage should be decreased.

C. she needs to restrict foods high in calcium.

D. she needs to eat more foods high in calcium.

17-79 *Pancreatic juice carries all of the following digestive enzymes except*

A. pancreatic amylase.

B. pancreatic lipase.

C. pancreatic protease.

D. pancreatic trypsin.

17-80 *Which of the following statements regarding osteoporosis and gender is true?*

A. Men and women are equally prone to osteoporosis.

B. Because of menopause, women are more prone to osteoporosis.

C. Men who develop osteoporosis usually have fractures of the wrist and ankle.

D. Women who have had hysterectomies are more prone to developing osteoporosis.

17-81 *Sidney has been taking a sulfonylurea for 5 years for his type 2 diabetes. He asks how long he needs to be taking the medication before he tries another medication. You tell him,*

A. "Sulfonylureas are usually effective for 7–10 years in most clients."

B. "You'll probably be on this medication for the rest of your life."

C. "After about 5 years, you will need to start on insulin therapy."

D. "After a few years, you can stop altogether and just regulate your diabetes with your diet."

17-82 *Leah has had diabetes for many years. When teaching her about foot care, you want to stress*

A. that her calluses will protect her from infection.

B. the need to assess the bottom of her feet carefully after walking barefoot.

C. that painless ulceration might occur and feet should be examined with a mirror.

D. that mild pain is to be expected because of neuropathies.

17-83 *Which of the following statements is true regarding the epidemiology of Graves' disease?*

A. It is more common in males.

B. The diagnosis is most commonly made during the early teenage years.

C. It is the most common autoimmune disease in the United States.

D. It is more common in African Americans.

17-84   *Which type of insulin would be expected to have the earliest onset of action?*

A. NPH

B. Glargine (Lantus)

C. Aspart (NovoLog)

D. Novolin-R

17-85   *Diabetic clients with neuropathy require special foot care because most ulcers begin at the site of*

A. an ingrown toenail.

B. a previous sore.

C. a mole.

D. a callus.

17-86   *Which of the following serum laboratory findings are found in the client with Cushing's syndrome?*

A. Increased cortisol, decreased sodium, and decreased potassium levels

B. Decreased cortisol, decreased potassium, and decreased glucose levels

C. Increased cortisol, increased sodium, and decreased potassium levels

D. Normal blood urea nitrogen, increased sodium, and decreased potassium levels

17-87   *What percentage of cases of type 2 diabetes is associated with excess body weight?*

A. 20%

B. 40%

C. 60%

D. 80%

17-88   *The process of aging results in*

A. an increase in liver weight and mass.

B. a decreased absorption of fat-soluble vitamins.

C. an increase in enzyme activity.

D. constricted pancreatic ducts.

17-89   *Pathological changes that occur with diabetic neuropathies include*

A. a thinning of the walls of the blood vessels that supply nerves.

B. the formation and accumulation of amino glycosyl within the Schwann cells, which impairs nerve conduction.

C. demyelinization of the Schwann cells, which results in slowed nerve conduction.

D. increase of nutrients clogging the vessels that supply nerve endings.

17-90   *A client with hyperthyroidism presents with a complaint of a "gritty" feeling in her eyes. Over the past week, her visual acuity has diminished, and her ability to see colors has changed. She also has a feeling of pressure behind her eyes. The next step for the nurse practitioner is to*

A. order a thyroid ultrasound.

B. refer the client for immediate evaluation by an ophthalmologist.

C. order a total T4.

D. prescribe a beta-adrenergic blocker.

17-91   *Mandy has type 2 diabetes. She says she heard that if she becomes pregnant, she must go on insulin therapy. How do you respond?*

A. "You're under good glycemic control now with your oral agents. As long as you stay in good control, you'll stay on the medication you are on now."

B. "Don't worry about it now; wait until you get pregnant."

C. "Insulin is commonly used during pregnancy. Some oral agents are now being used."

D. "You need to start on insulin therapy now before you get pregnant. You'll also need it throughout your pregnancy."

17-92   *Marie, age 50, has type 1 diabetes and checks her blood glucose level several times every day. Her blood glucose level ranges from 250–280 mg/dL in the morning and is usually about 140 at lunch, about 120 at dinner, and about 100 at bedtime. In the morning she takes 30 units of neutral protamine Hagedorn (NPH) insulin and 4 units of regular insulin, and before dinner she takes 18 units of NPH insulin and 4 units of regular insulin. Although she has had her insulin dosage* adjusted several times in the past month, it has had no effect on her high morning blood glucose level. What is your next course of action?

A. Increase the evening NPH insulin dosage by 2 more units.

B. Have her check her blood glucose level between 2 a.m. and 4 a.m. for the next several days.

C. Increase the morning regular insulin dosage by 2 units.

D. Order a fasting blood sugar test.

17-93 *Your diabetic client asks you about Lantus. You tell her that*

A. it may be administered subcutaneously at home or intravenously in the hospital if need be.

B. the onset of action is 15 minutes.

C. Lantus stays in your system for 24 hours.

D. it can be mixed with any other insulin.

17-94 *Polydipsia occurs in diabetes as a result of a high serum glucose level, which*

A. interferes with the release of antidiuretic hormones.

B. has an osmotic effect on fluids and eventually triggers the thirst mechanism for compensation.

C. causes a dry mouth, increasing the client's thirst to the point of drinking compulsively.

D. disrupts fluid and electrolyte imbalance, increasing the thirst mechanism to compensate for fluid loss or gain.

17-95 *Mark has type 1 diabetes and has mild hyperglycemia. What effect does physical activity (exercise) have on his blood glucose level?*

A. It may cause it to vary a little.

B. It may decrease it.

C. It may elevate it.

D. It may fluctuate greatly either way.

17-96 *Jane, who has type 1 diabetes mellitus, has been hypoglycemic at bedtime. You know she misunderstands your teaching when she tells you,*

A. "I could adjust my insulin dose before dinner."

B. "I could try adding a carbohydrate at dinner."

C. "I could add an afternoon snack."

D. "I could change the time of dinner."

17-97 *After an oral cholecystogram, Sam complains of burning on urination. This is because of*

A. a mild reaction to the contrast medium.

B. biliary obstruction.

C. contraction of the gallbladder.

D. the presence of dye in the urine.

17-98 *One of the three P's of diabetes is*

A. paresthesias.

B. polydipsia.

C. polycythemia.

D. proteinuria.

17-99 *Kelley has a score of 8 on the Ferriman-Gallwey scale. This is diagnostic for*

A. gynecomastia.

B. hirsutism.

C. adrenal hyperplasia.

D. an ovarian cyst.

17-100 *Sigrid, age 48, appears with a 3-month history of heat intolerance, increased sweating, palpitations, tachycardia, nervousness, irritability, fatigue, and muscle weakness. Which test would you order first?*

A. A blood chemistry panel

B. Thyroid-stimulating hormone level

C. Liver function studies

D. Electrocardiogram

17-101 *After establishing clinical and biochemical euthyroidism after a thyroidectomy, you should perform a measurement of the serum thyroid-stimulating hormone (TSH) level every*

A. 3 months.

B. 6 months.

C. 1 year.

D. 2 years.

17-102 *Which class of antihypertensive agents may be problematic for clients with diabetes?*

A. ACE inhibitors

B. Calcium channel blockers

C. Beta blockers

D. Alpha blockers

17-103 *If a thyroid gland is palpable and you listen over the thyroid gland with the bell of the stethoscope while the client is holding his or her breath, what are you are listening for?*

A. A bruit, which may indicate increased vascularity of hyperthyroidism

B. Absence of sound, which may indicate a thyroid nodule

C. An echo from surrounding vessels indicating high blood pressure

D. A "thrill" indicating increased vascularity

17-104 *A fetus with intrauterine growth retardation is prone to hypoglycemia at birth because of*

A. an imbalance in insulin-glucagon secretion resulting from hyperinsulinemia from islet cell hyperplasia.

B. few carbon stores in the form of glycogen and body fat.

C. an inborn error of metabolism: glycogen storage disease.

D. a complication of birth asphyxia.

17-105 *What does a low level of thyroid-stimulating hormone indicate?*

A. Hypothyroidism

B. Myxedema

C. Hyperthyroidism

D. Thyroid nodule

17-106 *If a client has hepatitis, abdominal pain in the right upper quadrant is a result of what pathophysiological basis?*

A. Reduced prothrombin synthesis by injured hepatic cells

B. Bile salt accumulation

C. Release of pyrogens

D. Stretching of Glisson's capsule

17-107 *Betty, age 40, has had type 1 diabetes for 20 years and takes a combination of neutral protamine Hagedorn (NPH) and regular insulin every day. She comes to the office because she has developed a severe upper respiratory infection with chills, fever, and production of yellow sputum.*

Because of her acute infection, you know that Betty is likely to require

A. a decrease in her daily insulin dosage.

B. an increase in her daily insulin dosage.

C. a high-caloric dietary intake and no insulin change.

D. a change in her insulin from NPH to insulin aspart (NovoLog).

17-108 *Morris has had type 1 diabetes for 10 years. Several recent urinalysis reports have shown microalbuminuria. Your next step would be to*

A. order a 24-hour urinalysis.

B. start him on an angiotensin-converting enzyme (ACE) inhibitor.

C. stress the importance of strict blood sugar control.

D. send him to a dietitian because he obviously has not been following his diet.

17-109 *Clients with diabetes are more prone to cardiovascular disease than those without diabetes. This is probably because*

A. of their difficulty in metabolizing fats and proteins, the end products of which accumulate in the blood vessels.

B. they are usually overweight, which increases the workload on the heart and blood vessels.

C. most are older adults, who are more likely to have degenerative cardiovascular disease.

D. the high levels of glucose and fat that occur with poor control result in atherosclerotic changes in the blood vessels.

17-110 *Which of the following can increase the ocular manifestations of Graves' disease?*

A. Pregnancy

B. Hypertension

C. Smoking

D. Hyperlipidemia

17-111 *Jeffrey, age 17, has gynecomastia. You should also assess him for*

A. obesity.

B. endocrine abnormalities.

C. testicular cancer.

D. tuberculosis.

17-112 *Dena said that she read on her husband's hospital chart that he has podagra. She asks what this is. You tell her it is*

A. rheumatoid arthritis.

B. a fungal nail infection.

C. an ingrown toenail.

D. gout.

17-113 *Lynne has Cushing's syndrome. You would expect her to have or develop*

A. onychomycosis.

B. generalized increased pigmentation of the skin.

C. hair loss.

D. excitability and nervousness.

17-114 *The American Diabetes Association (ADA) recommends which of the following quarterly blood tests to be performed on all clients with diabetes?*

A. Urine

B. Liver function

C. Glycohemoglobin

D. Serum glucose

17-115 *Which of the following antithyroid drugs blocks thyroid hormone production and release?*

A. Propylthiouracil

B. Methimazole (Tapazole)

C. Saturated solution of potassium iodide

D. Radioactive iodine (^{131}I)

Answers

17-1   Answer C

Laryngeal nerve damage is a potential danger after a subtotal thyroidectomy. You should assess the client's speaking ability, including the ability to speak aloud, along with the quality and tone of the voice. The location of the laryngeal nerve increases the risk of damage during thyroid surgery. Hoarseness may be present because of edema or the endotracheal tube during surgery and will subside, but permanent hoarseness or loss of vocal volume is a sign of laryngeal nerve damage.

17-2   Answer C

Diane's symptoms today are the result of excessive levels of circulating cortisol. Ordinarily, there is a feedback loop that controls the circulating adrenocorticotropic hormone (ACTH) and cortisol levels. In Cushing's disease, the anterior pituitary is constantly producing excessive ACTH, which increases the levels of both cortisol and adrenal androgens. Her symptoms were precipitated by the administration of pharmaceutical cortisone preparations given in large doses over a long period of time.

17-3   Answer C

Myxedema is characterized by abnormal deposits of mucin in the skin and other tissues; a dry, waxy type of swelling in the skin; and nonpitting edema in the pretibial and facial areas. Myxedema is most common in hypothyroid women in their 60s. Untreated myxedema has been associated with severe atherosclerosis and has been attributed to the increase in serum cholesterol concentrations, particularly of low-density lipoprotein. Thyroid hormone replacement counters these changes.

17-4   Answer C

The most common cause of chronic hypocalcemia is hypoalbuminemia. Other causes of hypocalcemia include vitamin D deficiency, alkalosis, hypoparathyroidism, malabsorption syndromes, pancreatitis, laxative abuse, peritonitis, pregnancy, renal failure, phosphate excess, burn trauma, osteomalacia, and overwhelming infections.

17-5   Answer A

Insulin lispro is a rapid-acting human insulin whose amino acid composition has been slightly modified to make it work faster. It is administered 5–10 minutes before meals and reduces after-meal hyperglycemia to a greater extent than does regular insulin. Its duration of action is about 3 hours, rather than the 5–6 hours of regular insulin. Because of this, lispro reduces the risk of hypoglycemia between meals and during the night.

17-6   Answer D

Visceral neuropathies, also known as autonomic neuropathies, include anhidrosis (absence of sweating) on the hands and feet, increased sweating on the face or trunk, dysphagia, anorexia, heartburn, constricted pupils, nausea and vomiting, constipation, and diabetic diarrhea. Macrocirculation changes include an early onset of atherosclerosis and peripheral vascular insufficiency with claudication, ulcerations, and gangrene of the legs. Microcirculation changes include diabetic retinopathy with retinal ischemia and loss of vision and diabetic nephropathy with hypertension, albuminuria, edema, and progressive renal failure. Somatic neuropathies include changes in sensation in the feet and hands; palsy of cranial nerve III with headache, eye pain, and inability to move the eye up, down, or to the middle; pain or loss of cutaneous sensation over the chest; and motor and sensory deficits in the anterior thigh and medial calf.

17-7   Answer C

A rare adverse effect of metformin is megaloblastic anemia due to impaired absorption of vitamin B_{12}. This can be prevented by administration of vitamin B_{12} along with folic acid. Nerve degeneration often begins early in the course of diabetes and can also cause paresthesias. Nerve damage is directly related to sustained hyperglycemia, which may cause metabolic disturbances in nerves or may injure the capillaries that supply nerves. Diabetic neuropathy necessitates vigilance in the care of the extremities to prevent damage.

17-8   Answer B

If treatment with diet, exercise, and oral antidiabetic agents is insufficient to achieve acceptable glycemic control in clients with type 2 diabetes, adding a dose of insulin at bedtime to the regimen may be necessary. As a first step, the addition of a bedtime injection of long-acting insulin such as insulin glargine (Lantus) or insulin detemir (Levemir) is recommended. Intermediate-acting insulin such as neutral protamine Hagedorn (NPH) is no longer recommended because of the peaks in drug levels that can cause hypoglycemia. Initially, the dosage is 10 units at bedtime; then the dose is adjusted to reduce overnight hepatic glucose production and achieve a normal or near-normal fasting blood glucose concentration. If this regimen does not achieve the desired effect, the oral antidiabetic agents should be discontinued and mealtime analogue rapid-acting insulin can be added to the largest meal. Most clients will eventually require four injections with the basal-bolus regime.

17-9   Answer C

Thyroid specialists agree that most benign thyroid nodules require no management beyond watchful waiting and an annual follow-up to evaluate their size. In rare cases, surgery may be indicated if a nodule enlarges to the point of interfering with breathing. Surgery may also be a cosmetic choice. There are conflicting studies regarding the use of levothyroxine to shrink thyroid nodules; because of this, the practice remains unclear. The choice of treatment for malignant thyroid nodules usually calls for subtotal or total thyroidectomy followed by radioactive iodine therapy to destroy residual thyroid tissue.

17-10   Answer D

The cause of Graves' disease is an autoimmune response wherein the body produces antibodies that act against its own organs and tissues. Thyroid-stimulating immunoglobulins are found in 95% of persons with Graves' disease and are evidence of this autoimmune process. Although thyroid carcinoma and pituitary tumors can cause hyperthyroidism, they do not cause Graves' disease. Hyperplasia of the thyroid results from hyperthyroidism; it does not cause it.

17-11   Answer B

Increased parathyroid hormone peaks between 15 and 35 weeks' gestation to meet increased requirements for calcium and vitamin D for fetal skeletal growth. Folic acid is a member of the vitamin B complex and is necessary to reduce the risk of neural tube defects.

17-12   Answer C

The major risk factor for development of thyroid cancer is exposure to radiation, usually from treatment to the head and neck. Until 1950, radiation treatments were given to children for an enlarged thymus, enlarged tonsils, and acne. Several million children were exposed in this manner. It may also occur in individuals who have had radiation therapy to the face or upper chest. There is also an increased incidence of thyroid cancer in areas where iodine deficiency and goiter are more common. Cigarette smoking is a risk factor for bladder and lung cancer but not thyroid cancer.

17-13   Answer B

Insulin mixes such as NovoLog 70/30 and Novolin 70/30 were developed to deliver a more convenient medication regime. Seventy percent of the mix is NPH, and 30% is either regular or a rapid-acting insulin analogue. It is given twice a day before breakfast and dinner. If the rapid-acting portion is regular insulin, it should be injected 30 minutes before the meal. If the rapid-acting portion is aspart (NovoLog), it can be injected 5–15 minutes before the meal. It is a less flexible dosing pattern than basal-bolus because the client is required to eat midday or suffer hypoglycemia. In this case, the pre-dinner glucose levels are elevated. Increasing the morning dose by 2 units will lower the pre-dinner glucose levels. The regular insulin will also be increased and can lead to low blood sugar at lunchtime. Many providers are getting away from the insulin mixes because of the problems with hypoglycemia and are substituting the more flexible basal-bolus insulin regimes.

17-14   Answer A

Trousseau's sign assesses for hypocalcemia. It is assessed by inflating a blood pressure cuff above the client's antecubital space to occlude the blood supply to the arm, then deflating it. Decreased calcium levels (hypocalcemia/tetany) cause the client's hand and fingers to contract in a carpal spasm. Hypocalcemia may also be assessed by checking for Chvostek's sign, which is performed by tapping fingers in front of the client's ear at the angle of the jaw. If hypocalcemia is present, the client's lateral facial muscle will contract.

17-15   Answer D

Atrial fibrillation is a common presentation in elderly clients with hyperthyroidism. If the thyroid-stimulating hormone (TSH) is suppressed, a free T4 and T3 should be drawn.

17-16   Answer C

The only treatment option that is curative for PHPT is a parathyroidectomy. It is successful in 90%–98% of the cases. The type II calcimimetic cinacalcet treats the underlying cause of PHPT by binding to the calcium-sensing receptor on the surface of the parathyroid glands, which increases the sensitivity to extracellular calcium, which then reduces the excess secretion of PTH. It is used for the treatment of secondary hyperparathyroidism

but not for PHPT. Although the first generation of bisphosphonates was found to be ineffective for the treatment of the skeletal manifestations of PHPT, the newer bisphosphonates such as alendronate (Fosamax) increase the bone density a little, but they do not affect PTH secretion and thus will not reduce serum calcium. Hormone therapy is not used by itself. Low doses of estrogen have been shown to reduce calcium, prevent bone loss, and improve bone density.

17-17   Answer A

Posterior pituitary hormones include antidiuretic hormone (ADH) with the kidney as the target organ and oxytocin with the uterus and breasts as the target organs. Anterior pituitary hormones include growth hormone (GH) with bones and organs as the target organ, adrenocorticotropic hormone (ACTH) affecting the adrenal cortex, thyroid-stimulating hormone (TSH) affecting the thyroid, follicle-stimulating hormone (FSH) affecting the testes and ovaries, luteinizing hormone (LH) affecting the ovaries, and prolactin affecting the breasts.

17-18   Answer B

Treatment for ophthalmopathy in Graves' disease often includes oral and ophthalmic prednisone; severe cases may require radiation or surgical decompression. Propranolol (Inderal) is usually given initially to control symptoms of tachycardia, palpitations, or tremors during the initiation of radioactive iodine therapy. It is not used to help control symptoms related to ophthalmopathy in Graves' disease. Radioactive iodine may worsen the ophthalmopathy in Graves' disease. Clients with ophthalmopathy require a referral to an ophthalmologist.

17-19   Answer B

The American Diabetes Association's position statement on aspirin therapy in diabetes recommends aspirin use as a secondary prevention strategy in men and women with diabetes who have evidence of large-vessel disease, such as a history of myocardial infarction, vascular bypass procedures, and stroke. They also recommend aspirin therapy as a primary prevention strategy in high-risk men and women with type 1 or type 2 diabetes who have a family history of coronary heart disease and for individuals who smoke, are hypertensive or obese, or who have albuminuria, cholesterol levels greater than 200 mg/dL, low-density lipoprotein cholesterol levels greater than 130 mg/dL, high-density lipoprotein cholesterol levels less than 40 mg/dL, and triglyceride levels greater than 250 mg/dL.

17-20   Answer D

The incretin-like drugs are oral agents, such as the dipeptidyl-peptidase-4 (DPP-4) inhibitors (e.g., sitagliptin [Januvia] and saxagliptin [Onglyza]), and injectable incretin mimetics or analogues, such as exenatide (Byetta) and liraglutide(Victoza). All of these agents have been associated with increased risk of pancreatitis and should not be used in clients with a history of pancreatitis. Clients and providers should be aware of the signs and symptoms of pancreatitis. Victoza has been associated with and increased risk of medullary thyroid cancer.

17-21   Answer A

Clients with pheochromocytoma should be told to void in small amounts and to avoid a full bladder. In addition, to prevent stimulating a paroxysm in pheochromocytoma, also advise the client to avoid smoking; drugs that may influence catecholamine release, such as some anesthetics, atropine, opiates, steroids, and glucagon; and activities that might displace abdominal organs, such as bending, exercising, straining, and vigorous palpation of the abdomen. For women, pregnancy should be discouraged.

17-22   Answer B

Brittle hair is a sign of hypothyroidism. A thyroid bruit; gynecomastia; and warm, smooth, moist skin are all signs of hyperthyroidism.

17-23   Answer D

The first action a client should take for treating hypoglycemia (which is assumed because Mary took more than four times the usual dose of her short-acting insulin) is to ingest 10–15 g of a rapidly absorbable carbohydrate, such as three to five pieces of hard candy, two to three packets of sugar, or 4 oz of fruit juice, to abort the episode. This should be repeated in 15 minutes, as needed. Mary should continue to try to obtain her blood glucose level and should certainly not drive. You should ask Mary to call you back in about 30 minutes to 1 hour after ingesting the carbohydrate and after checking her glucose level (or sooner if she feels any different).

17-24   Answer C

If Jane has insulin-dependent diabetes mellitus and has been experiencing hyperglycemia before dinner, a possible solution to this problem is to add physical activity between lunch and dinner. In addition, she may try the following strategies: adjust her afternoon dose of rapid-acting insulin, reduce her carbohydrate consumption at lunch, reduce or omit her midafternoon snack, or change the time of her lunch or midafternoon snack. Adjusting her morning dose of rapid-acting insulin may be necessary if she is hyperglycemic before lunch. Reducing the amount of carbohydrate at dinner may be necessary if she is hyperglycemic at bedtime.

17-25   Answer D

During inspection of the integumentary system of clients with endocrine disorders, coarse hair may be an indicator of hypothyroidism. Fine hair is seen in clients with hyperthyroidism; hirsutism with Cushing's syndrome; hyperpigmentation with Addison's disease or Cushing's syndrome; hypopigmentation with diabetes mellitus, hyperthyroidism, or hypothyroidism; and purple striae over the abdomen and bruising with Cushing's syndrome.

17-26   Answer B

The treatment of Graves' disease (hyperthyroidism) is directed toward lowering the serum concentrations of thyroid hormones to reestablish a euthyroid state. Therapies that may be used include antithyroid drugs (ATDs), radioactive iodine (^{131}I), and thyroid surgery. Chemotherapy is not used. For clients with hyperthyroidism and a low radioactive iodine uptake, none of these therapies is indicated because low-uptake hyperthyroidism usually implies thyroiditis, which generally resolves spontaneously. Therapy with beta-blocking agents is usually sufficient to control the symptoms of hyperthyroidism in these individuals. In addition, lithium carbonate and stable iodine have been used to block release of thyroid hormone from the thyroid gland in clients who are intolerant to ATDs.

17-27   Answer C

Chvostek's sign is seen in tetany and is a spasm of the facial muscles after a tap on one side of the face over the facial nerve. To diagnose hypoparathyroidism, the following are usually present: a positive Chvostek's sign and positive

Trousseau's sign, tetany, carpopedal spasms, tingling of the lips and hands, muscular and abdominal cramps, low serum calcium level, high serum phosphate level, and reduced urine calcium excretion.

17-28   Answer B

Secondary obesity is rare; possible causes include Cushing's disease, polycystic ovary disease, hypothalamic disease, hypothyroidism, and insulinoma. Some medications associated with weight gain include glucocorticoids, tricyclic antidepressants, and phenothiazines. Essential obesity is the most prevalent type and is the result of the intake of more calories than are expended. This type of obesity results from the multiple interactions of genetic and environmental factors (cultural, metabolic, social, and psychological factors).

17-29   Answer D

The dawn phenomenon is an early-morning increase in blood glucose concentration occurring with no corresponding hypoglycemia during the night. It is secondary to the nocturnal elevations of growth hormone. The Somogyi phenomenon is a rebound effect caused by too much insulin at night, resulting in hypoglycemia during the night. This results in the secretion of certain anti-insulin hormones, including epinephrine, glucagon, glucocorticoids, and growth hormones, which results in hyperglycemia. Insulin shock is a hypoglycemic reaction. Diabetic ketoacidosis implies that there is hyperglycemia at all times during the day, not only in the early morning.

17-30   Answer C

Clients should be cautioned about the adverse effects of antithyroid drugs (ATDs) before the initiation of therapy. A white blood cell (WBC) count and liver function tests are needed before initiating ATDs because of the risk of liver failure and agranulocytosis.

17-31   Answer D

Asthma may be exacerbated with the initiation of propranolol. Beta adrenergic antagonists, especially the noncardioselective type are commonly prescribed to clients with hyperthyroidism to decrease palpitations. It is recommended that beta-adrenergic blockade be initiated when the resting heart rate is in excess of 90 bpm or there

is coexistent cardiovascular disease. Worsening of asthma is a possibility because the beta receptors in the lungs are also blocked with the use of nonselective beta-adrenergic drugs leading to bronchoconstriction. In clients who cannot tolerate a noncardioselective beta blocker, a cardioselective beta blocker or a nondihydropyridine calcium channel blocker can be used. Clients with diabetes who are treated with beta blockers may not sense the tachycardia that goes along with hypoglycemia. Other symptoms such as sweating can be more reliable in clients receiving beta-blocking drugs. In general, beta blockers should be used with caution in clients with asthma, COPD, diabetes, and heart failure.

17-32   Answer C

ACE inhibitors are given to clients with diabetes who have persistent proteinuria. When diabetes is diagnosed, it may have been present for 10 years. Most clinicians will order an ACE inhibitor for clients with diabetes even without hypertension due to the renoprotective mechanism. Microalbumin measurements of greater than 30 mg/day justifies the addition of an ACE inhibitor in normotensive clients. Proteinuria is one of the early signs of diabetic nephropathy, with or without the presence of hypertension. Urine protein must be measured to monitor the effectiveness of the ACE inhibitor. ACE inhibitors may be effective in decreasing urinary excretion of albumin even in clients without hypertension; therefore, a urinalysis should be performed and a serum creatinine level determined at least yearly. Detection of microalbuminuria alerts one that nephropathy is developing. When the serum creatinine level reaches about 3 mg/dL, a referral to a diabetologist and nephrologist should be done. Intensive treatment can delay or improve diabetic nephropathy in its early stages. There is evidence that, with good control of hypertension, proteinuria can be reduced and the expected decline in the glomerular filtration rate can be slowed.

17-33   Answer D

Addisonian crisis is a serious, life-threatening response to acute adrenal insufficiency and may be precipitated by abruptly stopping glucocorticoid medications. Other causes include major stressors, especially if the person has poorly controlled Addison's disease, and hemorrhage into the adrenal glands from either septicemia or anticoagulant therapy. The primary problems in addisonian crisis are severe hypotension, circulatory collapse, shock, and coma. Treatment involves rapid intravenous replacement of fluids and glucocorticoids.

17-34   Answer C

Galactorrhea is lactation that occurs in the absence of nursing. A small amount of breast milk can be expressed from the nipple in many parous women and is not of concern. Normal breast milk may vary in color and not always be white. If there are significant amounts, or if galactorrhea occurs in nulliparous women or in conjunction with amenorrhea, headache, or visual field abnormalities, it might imply a systemic illness.

17-35   Answer C

Iodine deficiency is the most common worldwide cause of hypothyroidism. In the United States, where iodine ingestion is adequate, autoimmune processes are the primary cause of hypothyroidism. Hashimoto's thyroiditis, a type of primary hypothyroidism, is the most common form of autoimmune thyroid disease. Iatrogenic hypothyroidism, which occurs after treatment with radioactive iodine for hyperthyroidism or surgery for hyperthyroidism, thyroid nodules, or carcinoma, is the next most common cause of hypothyroidism.

17-36   Answer C

Clients using an insulin pump need to monitor their blood glucose levels at least four times a day. The client can develop diabetic ketoacidosis in as little as 4 hours if there is mechanical failure of the pump because the only insulin used in the pump is rapid acting.

17-37   Answer D

Although the diabetic diet has "relaxed" over the years, it is still not possible to eat everything. It is acceptable to substitute two Oreo cookies for a fresh pear. In the past, sugar was forbidden to clients with diabetes. The belief was that simple carbohydrates, like candy, were quickly digested, allowing blood sugar to soar, whereas the body took more time to process complex carbohydrates such as bread. Research now shows that both types of carbohydrates—simple and complex—affect glucose levels at comparable speeds. That being said, it is likely that two Oreo cookies will lead to another and then another. A pear has the additional

benefit of high soluble fiber, vitamins, and no fat. It is still important to monitor the amount of total carbohydrates per meal because they have the greatest impact on blood sugar. Drinking alcohol may increase the risk of low blood sugar, so if your client has an occasional glass of wine, stress the fact that alcohol should not be consumed on an empty stomach.

17-38   Answer A

Proteinuria is the first symptom indicative of renal nephropathy in clients who have had diabetes for about 10 years (although some studies suggest 5 years). There is increased permeability of the capillaries, with resultant leakage of albumin into the glomerular filtrate, causing albuminuria. The development of Kimmelstiel-Wilson nodules occurs in persons with type 1 diabetes but does not necessarily precede the proteinuria. As renal function deteriorates, both the serum creatine and the blood urea nitrogen levels increase.

17-39   Answer D

Metformin, DPP-4 inhibitors such as sitagliptin (Januvia) and incretin mimetics such as exenatide (Byetta) are gaining favor over sulfonylureas because the risk of hypoglycemia is less than with sulfonylureas.

17-40   Answer D

Calcium channel blockers do not slow the progression of diabetic nephropathy in clients with diabetes. The steps that can be taken to avoid or slow the progression of diabetic nephropathy include maintaining excellent blood pressure control, using ACE inhibitors, restricting protein, and maintaining excellent glucose control.

17-41   Answer D

Signs and symptoms of diabetic ketoacidosis include Kussmaul's breathing (very deep respiratory movements), hyperglycemia, glycosuria, polyuria, polydipsia, anorexia, and headache, as well as ketonuria and a decreased blood pH.

17-42   Answer C

Foods high in purine should be avoided by clients with gout. Broccoli is not high in purine. Foods high in purine include all meats and seafood, meat extracts and gravies, yeast and yeast extracts, beans, peas, lentils, oatmeal, spinach, asparagus, cauliflower, and mushrooms. Wine and alcohol in excessive amounts impair the kidney's ability to excrete uric acid and should be used in moderation.

17-43   Answer B

Jogging is not a wise choice for clients with diabetes because of the potential underlying nerve damage to their feet or eyes. Although tennis is physically taxing, it does not require a constant bouncing up and down on the feet, and even if played at night, courts are well lit. Swimming and dancing are excellent forms of exercise.

17-44   Answer B

Marisa can have snacks that are sufficient in calories to maintain her normal weight. She should consume adequate amounts of carbohydrates, fats, and proteins in a well-balanced diet. The majority of the fats should be unsaturated to decrease the incidence of vascular changes. The carbohydrates should be complex rather than simple to provide a more constant blood glucose level. She can still go out with her friends and consume most of the same snacks. Pizza, hamburgers, and many other "fast foods" are on the American Diabetes Association diet.

17-45   Answer C

Although it is generally accepted that self-monitoring of blood glucose (SMBG) is a necessary component of the management of type 1 diabetes, its use in type 2 diabetes is controversial. Although individuals with type 2 diabetes may be treated with diet, oral agents, insulin, or combination therapy, the frequency of SMBG depends on the particular therapeutic interventions. The minimum recommended frequency is three times a week at selected intervals. The frequency obviously depends on the client's success in achieving treatment goals.

17-46   Answer B

Stress causes the adrenal glands to secrete more cortisol, which leads to gluconeogenesis and insulin antagonism, raising the blood sugar. It is possible, then, that Harriet will have an increased blood sugar level. She will not need less daily insulin or more carbohydrates and will not have an insulin reaction, such as hypoglycemia, more readily than usual. Harriet may, in fact, need to increase her insulin use.

17-47   Answer B

A client with insulin-dependent diabetes mellitus who misses a meal needs to eat about 15–30 g of complex carbohydrates to forestall hypoglycemia. If the client's appetite is poor, this may be accomplished through juice, flavored gelatin, soft drinks, or frozen juice bars.

17-48   Answer B

Trousseau's sign (carpal spasm) is one of two neuromuscular signs indicative of hypocalcemia. It is often preceded by muscle cramps in the legs and feet. Carpal spasm consists of a flexed elbow and wrist, adducted thumb over the palm, flexed metacarpophalangeal joints, adduction of hyperextended fingers, and extended interphalangeal joints. The response is elicited by inflation of a blood pressure cuff to 20 mm Hg above the level of the systolic blood pressure. Inflation is maintained for 3 minutes to elicit the response, which is secondary to ulnar and median nerve ischemia. In severe hypocalcemia, spontaneous spasms may occur in the lower extremities. Chvostek's sign is the second neuromuscular sign associated with hypocalcemia. It is an abnormal unilateral spasm of the facial muscle when the facial nerve is tapped below the zygomatic arch anterior to the earlobe.

17-49   Answer C

There is a major link between diabetes mellitus and coronary artery disease (CAD). There are many theories about the pathophysiology of diabetes mellitus and how it leads to CAD. Some of these mechanisms include the following: Hyperinsulinemia causes a large number of vascular smooth muscle cells to be formed and deposited on the walls of vessels, causing buildup and eventual blockage, reducing blood flow; hyperinsulinemia increases (not decreases) sympathetic tone and cardiac contractility by increasing plasma catecholamine, epinephrine, and norepinephrine levels; and an increase in the glucose level causes the distal nephrons of the kidneys to absorb more (not less) sodium, resulting in more fluid, expanding the intravascular volume and increasing blood pressure.

17-50   Answer C

Clients with visual or dexterity difficulties may benefit from prefilling syringes. Prefilled insulin syringes may be stored in a vertical position in the refrigerator for up to 30 days with the needle pointing upward. Alternatives to syringes include jet injectors and penlike devices. Jet injectors are useful for clients who have needle phobias, but they are expensive. Penlike devices hold insulin cartridges and are useful if the client is visually or neurologically impaired, and they help to increase the accuracy of insulin administration. Another alternative is the insulin pump.

17-51   Answer C

Calcium does not affect an oral glucose tolerance test (OGTT). The following medications may interfere with the results of an OGTT and should be discontinued for 3 days before the test: vitamin C, aspirin, oral contraceptives, corticosteroids, synthetic estrogens, phenytoin (Dilantin), thiazide diuretics, and nicotinic acid.

17-52   Answer A

Radioactive iodine therapy is the most commonly used treatment in the United States for Graves' disease (hyperthyroidism); however, it is contraindicated during pregnancy. Therefore, for women, a pregnancy test (beta human chorionic gonadotropin) needs to be performed before initiating therapy. Women of childbearing age should also be told to delay conception for a few months after radioactive iodine therapy. It is also contraindicated in women who are breastfeeding. Older adults or clients at risk for developing cardiac complications may be pretreated with antithyroid drugs (ATDs) before therapy to deplete the thyroid gland of stored hormone, thereby minimizing the risk of exacerbation of hyperthyroidism because of radioactive iodine (^{131}I)–induced thyroiditis. Marsha's basal metabolism rate will be affected by her Graves' disease but has no bearing on her preparation for radioactive iodine therapy. Lithium levels are usually not performed before radioactive iodine therapy. They may be done if lithium is being used to block the release of thyroid hormone from the thyroid gland in clients who are intolerant of ATDs. Although parathyroid hormone secretion is dependent on the serum calcium level, it is usually not necessary to obtain a serum calcium level measurement before radioactive iodine therapy.

17-53   Answer A

During pregnancy, many clients with hypothyroidism require an increase in levothyroxine, which would require an increase in the dosage of levothyroxine medication by typically 30%. This need would be detected by performing a thyroid-stimulating hormone (TSH) level test. The woman's TSH level should be checked every trimester to make sure the TSH level is normal. Adjustments to the medication dosage should be made as indicated. Usually, the levothyroxine medication dosage is returned to the prepregnancy dosage immediately after delivery. A serum TSH level reading should be obtained at the 6-week postpartum visit.

17-54   Answer C

Virilization involves an increased androgen response, including increased muscle mass, clitoral enlargement, lowered voice, and behavioral changes. Hirsutism is excessive hair distribution.

17-55   Answer B

Starting Steve on an antianxiety agent, starting him on a diuretic and/or beta blocker, or rechecking his blood pressure in 1 week will only delay the correct diagnosis. Steve's signs and symptoms are diagnostic of a pheochromocytoma, which can be detected with an assay of urinary catecholamine levels (total and fractionated), metanephrine, vanillylmandelic acid, and creatinine levels. A 24-hour urine specimen is usually obtained, but an overnight or shorter collection may also be obtained. Pheochromocytoma typically causes attacks of severe headache (85%), palpitations (65%), and profuse sweating (65%). The absence of all three of these symptoms can exclude the diagnosis of pheochromocytoma to a 99% certainty.

17-56   Answer D

Aldosterone is a mineralocorticoid hormone secreted by the adrenal cortex. Follicle-stimulating hormone, thyroid-stimulating hormone, and growth hormones are all secreted by the anterior pituitary gland.

17-57   Answer B

Acute pancreatitis is an inflammation of the pancreas caused by the release of activated pancreatic enzymes into the surrounding parenchyma with the subsequent destruction of tissue, blood vessels, and supporting structures. Although pancreatitis may be acute or chronic, acute symptoms include continuous abdominal pain for several days' duration that increases in the epigastric area and radiates to the back, nausea, vomiting, sweating, weakness, pallor, abdominal tenderness, distention, and a low-grade fever. Pancreatitis occurs primarily in middle-aged adults and slightly more often in women than in men. The pain is in the upper right quadrant with cholecystitis and is intermittent, usually after a fatty meal. The gastrointestinal (GI) manifestations of cirrhosis include parotid enlargement, esophageal or rectal varices, peptic ulcers, and gastritis. The clinical manifestation of Cushing's syndrome related to the GI system is a peptic ulcer, which would result in intermittent pain related to meals.

17-58   Answer B

Older clients with diabetes are predisposed to malignant otitis externa, caused by *Pseudomonas aeruginosa*. It is an invasive and necrotizing infection with a high mortality, mainly because of meningitis. The client complains of pain in the ear with or without a purulent drainage, swelling of the parotid gland, trismus (tonic contraction of the muscles of mastication), and paralysis of the 6th through 12th cranial nerves.

17-59   Answer C

Hyperthyroidism often presents atypically in elderly clients. Expected adrenergic findings are often absent. It is more common in the elderly to see atrial fibrillation, depression, anorexia, and weight loss which is referred to as *apathetic hyperthyroidism of the elderly*.

17-60   Answer A

Signs of hypoparathyroidism include elevated serum phosphate levels; decreased serum calcium levels; increased neuromuscular activity, which may progress to tetany; decreased bone resorption; hypocalciuria; and hypophosphaturia.

17-61   Answer A

Pubertal gynecomastia is common and is characterized by tender discoid breast tissue enlargement of about 2–3 cm in diameter beneath the areola. The swelling usually subsides spontaneously within a year, and watchful waiting along with reassurance is recommended for that time period.

17-62   Answer C

The Diabetes Control and Complications Trial recommends intensive management of diabetes for persons who already have a diagnosis of beginning nephropathy, neuropathy, or retinopathy. Intensive management of diabetes is recommended for clients with diabetes to prevent or reduce the risk for developing retinopathy, nephropathy, or neuropathy. Having one of these conditions does not preclude therapy. Intensive therapy may slow the progression of the disease if already present. However, because the most significant adverse effect of intensive treatment is an increase in the risk of severe hypoglycemic episodes, intensive therapy is not recommended for children younger than age 13; older adults; or people with heart disease, advanced complications, or a history of frequent severe hypoglycemia.

17-63   Answer D

Fluid intake should exceed 3,000 mL daily to prevent formation of uric acid kidney stones. Clients should avoid dehydration because it may precipitate an acute attack. Because both wine and alcohol in excessive amounts impair the kidney's ability to excrete uric acid, they should be used in moderation. Clients must be aware that binge drinking may provoke an acute attack. If the client is obese, weight loss should be encouraged because loss of excess body fat may normalize serum uric acid without pharmacological intervention. Weight loss will also decrease stress on weight-bearing joints. Caution as to severe, rapid weight loss should be given because secondary hyperuricemia may result. A very low caloric-restricted diet may precipitate an acute attack.

17-64   Answer D

Because of its safety, efficacy, and cost, metformin is the cornerstone of monotherapy unless there is a contraindication, such as renal disease, hepatic disease, gastrointestinal intolerance, or risk of lactic acidosis. Metformin often has beneficial effects on components of the metabolic syndrome, including mild to moderate weight loss, improvement of the lipid profile, and improved fibrinolysis. It improves the effectiveness of insulin in suppressing excess hepatic glucose production and increases insulin sensitivity in peripheral tissues. Hypoglycemia with the use of metformin is low. Gastrointestinal side effects can be diminished by starting at the lowest dose of 500 mg daily and gradually increasing the dosage as needed to a maximum dose of 2,000 mg/day. Use of metformin and alcohol can increase the risk of lactic acidosis.

Insulin secretagogues such as sulfonylureas can cause hypoglycemia and are often added as a second, cost-effective choice. The dipeptidyl-peptidase-4 (DPP-4) inhibitors such as sitagliptin (Januvia) increase insulin secretion, suppress glucagon secretion, and suppress hepatic glucose production and peripheral glucose uptake and metabolism. An injectable agent, exenatide (Byetta), is an incretin mimetic that often induces weight loss. Both sitagliptin and exenatide have a lower risk of hypoglycemia, making them a good choice over a sulfonylurea as dual therapy. The cost of both of these newer agents may be prohibitive for many clients, and evidence for long-term reduction of morbidity and mortality is lacking. There is also a risk of pancreatitis with the oral and injectable incretin-like drugs.

17-65   Answer C

Jenny's fasting blood sugar (FBS) test should be repeated along with an HbA1c. An HbA1c of greater than 6.5 can now be used to diagnosis diabetes. A glucose tolerance test (GTT) to confirm a diagnosis of diabetes is usually not needed. Diabetes is not usually diagnosed with a single high glucose reading. Hyperglycemia can be an adverse reaction to high doses of hydrochlorothiazide, but the first action would be to repeat the FBS. If it is high for a second reading, the diuretic should be reduced. Insulin therapy would not be started until Jenny was given a positive diagnosis, and even then, oral antidiabetic agents would be considered first.

17-66   Answer B

Immunoglobulin M (IgM) anti–hepatitis A virus (HAV) titers peak during the first week of the infection with acute hepatitis A and usually disappear within 3–6 months. Detection of IgM anti-HAV is a valid test for demonstrating acute hepatitis A. Immunoglobulin G anti-HAV titers peak after 1 month of the disease but may stay elevated for years; therefore, they are an indicator of past infection.

17-67   Answer D

Unlike many oral antidiabetic agents, exenatide (Byetta) can cause weight loss in some individuals. The active ingredient is a protein that encourages digestion and the production of insulin.

17-68   Answer A

The preference for basal insulins, such as glargine (Lantus) and detemir (Levemir) combined with mealtime or prandial rapid-acting insulin analogues such as aspart (NovoLog), lispro (Humalog), and glulisine (Apidra), injected once a day, is based on the ability of this regime to closely mimic the normal kinetics and dynamics of endogenous insulin. This method, called *basal-bolus*, is easy to initiate, allows for flexible mealtimes, has less incidence of hypoglycemia, and helps clients reach the HbgA1c goal safely. The disadvantages of the insulin analogues are their increased price and the increased frequency of up to four injections a day. Neither detemir nor glargine can be mixed with other types of insulin. Many providers, especially endocrinologists, have abandoned the use of regular, neutral protamine Hagedorn, and combinations such as Novolin 70/30. Basal insulin is usually 50% of the calculated insulin requirement in a day. Insulin requirements range from 0.4 units/kg/day to 0.7 units/kg/day. The basal dose is half of the total daily dose. The remaining amount can be divided and given as rapid acting mealtime injections prior to breakfast, lunch, and dinner if needed. It is common to initiate basal insulin using glargine or detemir at 10 units at night (or 0.2 units/kg/day), letting the client know that additional injections will be required. The basal insulin can be adjusted by 2 units every 4–5 days until the fasting blood sugar is normalized. If the HbA1c remains elevated, the initiation of mealtime insulin with a rapid-acting analogue can be started with one injection with the largest meal. Many providers start with 4 units of a rapid-acting analogue such as aspart and have the client check blood sugar levels 2 hours after the start of the meal. If the postprandial glucose is elevated 2 hours after the start of the meal, the mealtime dosage can be increased by 1–2 units.

17-69   Answer A

In an outpatient setting, primary hyperparathyroidism (PHPT) is the most common cause of hypercalcemia. Some of the clinical manifestations include hypertension, left ventricular hypertrophy, peptic ulcer disease, pancreatitis, fatigue, and anxiety. A dual-energy x-ray absorptiometry (DEXA) scan is required to detect skeletal involvement in mild PHPT. Bone cysts and subperiosteal resorption are no longer common findings, but bone loss is usually found in varying degrees. The client's history and physical examination are not usually helpful in diagnosing this condition. Persistent hypercalcemia and an elevated parathyroid hormone (PTH) level are necessary for a diagnosis of PHPT.

17-70   Answer A

Medications such as cimetidine (Tagamet), digoxin (Lanoxin), spironolactone (Aldactone), phenothiazines, antituberculosis agents, as well as marijuana, heroin, and alcohol, can produce gynecomastia. In addition, men receiving estrogen therapy for the treatment of prostate cancer are likely to experience gynecomastia.

17-71   Answer C

Because hypertension is implicated in accelerating the microangiopathy of diabetes (especially retinopathy and nephropathy), therapy for hypertension in a client with diabetes should be more aggressive and initiated at a blood pressure 5–10 mm Hg less than the conventional therapeutic guidelines indicate (either systolic or diastolic pressure consistently over 140/90 mm Hg).

17-72   Answer C

The thyroid-stimulating hormone (TSH) test measures the pituitary's response to peripheral levels of thyroid hormone. If the circulating level of T_4 is low, the pituitary will increase the production of TSH to try to stimulate the thyroid gland to produce more thyroid hormone.

17-73   Answer D

When clients have been on long-term cortisol therapy, increased protein breakdown or catabolism leads to loss of adipose and lymphatic tissue. The collagen loss is a result of protein wasting, which causes individuals to bruise easily. The skin is susceptible to rupture because the loss of collagenous support around the vessels makes them vulnerable. The skin becomes thin and atrophic.

17-74   Answer D

Women who have diabetes and frequently develop vaginitis should avoid douching. They should also maintain good personal hygiene, wipe from front to back after voiding, wear cotton underwear, avoid wearing tight jeans with nylon pantyhose, and void after intercourse.

17-75   Answer C

Fiber is important in the dietary management of diabetes. A diet high in fiber, especially soluble fiber, helps improve carbohydrate metabolism, lowers total cholesterol level, and lowers low-density lipoprotein cholesterol. Soluble fiber is found in dried beans, oats, barley, and in some vegetables and fruits (peas, corn, zucchini, cauliflower, broccoli, prunes, pears, apples, bananas, and oranges). It should not be assumed that individuals will get enough fiber in their diet because most dietary habits are not perfect. An intake of 20–30 g of fiber per day is recommended.

17-76   Answer A

The most common cause of hyperthyroidism is an autoimmune condition known as Graves' disease. It accounts for 90% of hyperthyroid conditions in young adults. A toxic uninodular goiter is the second most common cause of hyperthyroidism. Other causes include toxic hyperfunctioning multinodular goiter, subacute thyroiditis, metastatic follicular thyroid carcinoma, ingestion of iodide-containing drugs and contrast media, a pituitary tumor, a human chorionic gonadotropin–secreting tumor, and a testicular embryonal carcinoma.

17-77   Answer A

The medication of choice for an initial acute attack of gout is an NSAID. Indomethacin (Indocin) is the most commonly prescribed NSAID for this use. An initial dose of 50–75 mg is given, followed by 25–50 mg every 8 hours for 5–10 days. An alternative to indomethacin is naproxen (Naprosyn). The first dose of naproxen is 750 mg, followed by 250 mg every 8 hours for 5–10 days. Colchicine is an effective medication to terminate an acute attack only if administered within 48 hours of the initial onset of symptoms. Unfortunately, the attack is usually not diagnosed within this time frame. Corticosteroids can provide dramatic systematic relief but are contraindicated in septic conditions; therefore, they should not be administered before analysis of the synovial aspirate. Allopurinol (Zyloprim) is used to decrease uric acid production. Although it is effective, it may take weeks to decrease the uric acid level and therefore is not the initial choice in an acute attack.

17-78   Answer B

When serum calcium levels return to normal, urinary calcium should be assessed. Hypercalciuria (greater than 250 mg in a 24-hour urine sample) indicates that the client's vitamin D dosage should be decreased. Once the dosages of calcium and vitamin D are regulated to achieve normal serum calcium levels, urinary calcium levels should be assessed every 3 months.

17-79   Answer C

Pancreatic protease is not carried in pancreatic juice. Pancreatic juice carries pancreatic amylase, pancreatic lipase, and pancreatic trypsin. Proteolytic enzymes are activated by trypsin, which is activated in the intestine. Pancreatic amylase splits carbohydrates into dextrins and maltose. Pancreatic lipase hydrolyzes fat to yield glycerol and fatty acids. Pancreatic trypsin is one of a group of enzymes, including chymotrypsin and carboxypolypeptidase, that split proteins.

17-80   Answer A

Men and women are equally prone to osteoporosis, but it usually occurs later in life in men. Men develop the classic fractures of osteoporosis: Colles', vertebral, and hip. In women, the loss of sex steroids at menopause or after a hysterectomy leads to an increase in bone turnover through activation of bone remodeling. This results in an overall bone loss and loss of cancellous (trabecular) bone. In addition, with loss of estrogen, the amount of bone resorbed is greater than that replaced, leading to a continuing decline in overall bone mass and worsening microarchitecture. Hormone replacement for older men is not an option as it is in women because of the detrimental effects of testosterone on blood pressure and serum lipids. Prevention of osteoporosis in men is limited to maintenance of exercise, calcium supplementation, and cessation of smoking.

17-81   Answer A

For sulfonylurea and other oral antidiabetic medications to be effective, reasonable pancreatic insulin reserve is necessary. This reserve tends to dwindle over time; therefore, sulfonylureas and other agents tend to be effective for only 7–10 years in most clients. The recommendations are to start metformin in most cases and then add another agent such as a sulfonylurea. It is unlikely that after being on an oral antidiabetic agent for 7–10 years, the client will no longer require it and that diet alone would be effective.

17-82   Answer C

Painless ulcerations are very common in clients with diabetes, and the only way to assess for them in the feet is for clients to use a mirror to examine the bottoms of their feet. Leah should not be walking barefoot because her sensations are probably decreased as a result of neuropathy, and she should try to avoid the development of calluses because preparations used to remove them are very caustic.

17-83   Answer C

Graves' disease is the most common autoimmune disease in the United States. It is more common than other autoimmune diseases such as rheumatoid arthritis, Hashimoto's thyroiditis, vitiligo, type 1 diabetes, pernicious anemia, muscular sclerosis, systemic lupus erythematosus, and Sjögren's syndrome. It is more common in females, and most commonly diagnosed in the third to fifth decade of life. A genetic predisposition is suspected because of familial clustering of the disease, a high sibling recurrence risk, and a 30% concordance between identical twins.

17-84   Answer C

The rapid acting insulin analogues (such as lispro, aspart, and glulisine) are preferred because they mimic endogenous secretion of insulin. When an individual with a normal functioning pancreas eats a meal, the insulin secretion is immediate. The newer analogue insulins have a very rapid onset of action of 5–15 minutes, which can match the increase in blood sugar associated with a meal. These "physiologic" insulins are more efficacious and provide greater flexibility for those clients with variable mealtimes and carbohydrate content of meals. The duration of action of the rapid-acting insulin analogues is shorter than regular insulin, and the chances of hypoglycemia is less.

17-85   Answer D

Clients with neuropathy require professional nail and callus care because most ulcers begin at the site of a callus.

17-86   Answer C

Serum laboratory findings in the client with Cushing's syndrome usually include increased cortisol, increased sodium, decreased potassium, decreased glucose, and normal blood urea nitrogen levels.

17-87   Answer D

Eighty percent of cases of type 2 diabetes are associated with excess body weight. Although heredity is an important consideration, a normal-weight client with two parents who have diabetes has a better chance of avoiding the disease than an overweight client with healthy parents.

17-88   Answer B

The process of aging results in a decreased absorption of fat-soluble vitamins. There is a decrease in the number and size of hepatic cells, leading to a decrease in liver weight and mass. There is also a decrease in enzyme activity, which diminishes the liver's ability to detoxify drugs, which increases the risk of toxic levels of many medications in older adults. There is calcification of the pancreatic vessels and the ducts distend and dilate. These changes lead to a decrease in the production of lipase.

17-89   Answer C

Diabetic neuropathies involve three pathological changes: a thickening of the walls of the blood vessels that supply nerves, which causes a decrease in nutrients; the formation and accumulation of sorbitol within the Schwann cells, which impairs nerve conduction; and demyelinization of the Schwann cells that surround and insulate nerves, which results in slowed nerve conduction. The locations of the lesions determine where the neuropathies occur.

17-90   Answer B

The practitioner should refer the client for an immediate evaluation by an ophthalmologist. Clinically recognized Graves' ophthalmopathy occurs in about 50% of cases of Graves' disease. A client with Graves' orbitopathy with these complaints is at risk of blindness if there is compression of the optic nerve. Additional symptoms include photophobia and diplopia. Autoantibodies present in Graves' disease can cause increased muscle thickness in the eye muscle, leading to edema and compression of the optic nerve. Fundal exam may reveal disk swelling. This is an emergency situation that may require hospitalization and treatment with prednisone to diminish the inflammation. Artificial tears are also helpful. The onset of Graves' orbitopathy occurs within the year before or after the diagnosis of thyrotoxicosis in 75% of clients but can sometimes precede or follow thyrotoxicosis by several years.

17-91   Answer C

Women with type 2 diabetes often need to use insulin during their pregnancy to maintain good glycemic control. There is a risk of having a malformed infant if conception occurs when the blood sugar is not well controlled. Insulin, rather than oral antidiabetic medications, is often usedto achieve good glycemic control because the effects of most of the oral antidiabetic preparations on the human embryo and fetus are not well known. Metformin appears to be safe in pregnancy and is now being used by some providers. Many clients do not require antidiabetic therapy for the first several weeks after delivery, and most women can return to their preconception regimen within 6–12 weeks. Sulfonylureas and ACE inhibitors may be transferred to the fetus via breast milk, so they should not be resumed until breastfeeding is discontinued.

17-92   Answer B

Marie is experiencing the Somogyi phenomenon (nocturnal rebound hyperglycemia). If her blood glucose level at 2 a.m. to 4 a.m. is greater than 70 mg/dL, the evening dosage of neutral protamine Hagedorn (NPH) insulin should be increased and changed from before dinner to before bedtime. These actions should prevent most cases of nocturnal rebound hypoglycemia, which results in morning hyperglycemia. A fasting blood sugar test will not confirm the Somogyi phenomenon. The blood sugar level needs to be checked during the night to "catch" the Somogyi phenomenon. Many providers prefer the longer acting insulins such as insulin glargine (Lantus) and insulin detemir (Levemir) because they are mostly "peakless" and have less risk of hypoglycemia than NPH.

17-93   Answer C

Lantus (insulin glargine) has an onset of action in just over 1 hour and stays in the system for 24 hours. Regular insulin may be administered by the intravenous route. The newer insulin analogues such as aspart (Novolog) are also approved for intravenous use. Because of the cost, there is little reason to use the more expensive agents. Lantus and Levemir may not be mixed with any other insulin.

17-94   Answer B

Polydipsia occurs in diabetes as a result of high serum glucose levels that have an osmotic effect on fluids, drawing fluid from the cells into the intravascular space and creating a dehydrated state that, in turn, triggers the thirst mechanism for compensation. With a deficiency of antidiuretic hormone, as in diabetes insipidus, copious amounts of urine are excreted by the client, stimulating the thirst mechanism to replace fluid losses. Certain drugs such as phenothiazines and anticholinergics can cause dry mouth, increasing the client's thirst to the point of drinking compulsively. Excessive ingestion of salt, glucose, and other hyperosmolar substances can disrupt fluid and electrolyte imbalance, increasing the thirst mechanism to compensate for fluid loss or gain.

17-95   Answer B

Clients with insulin-dependent diabetes mellitus (IDDM) type 1 who have mild hyperglycemia may experience a drop in their blood glucose level during physical activity, whereas those with marked hyperglycemia may experience a rise in their blood glucose level. Clients with IDDM should check their blood glucose level before exercising and refrain from exercising if their blood glucose levels are too high (greater than 300 mg). For individuals without diabetes, the blood glucose level generally varies little during physical activity unless the activity is intense and of very long duration, such as marathon running.

17-96   Answer C

Jane, who has type 1 diabetes mellitus, has been hypoglycemic at bedtime. To correct this, she could try all of the strategies listed as options except adding an afternoon snack. This would be a strategy to try if the client were hypoglycemic before dinner. Strategies to try to correct hypoglycemia at bedtime include adjusting her insulin dose before dinner, adding carbohydrates at dinner, changing the time of dinner or evening snack, or adding an evening snack.

17-97   Answer D

After an oral cholecystogram, some persons experience burning on urination because of the presence of dye in the urine. This is helped by forcing fluids. An oral cholecystogram is done to assess for biliary obstruction. Contraction of the gallbladder may be desirable during a cholecystogram to obtain a better reading and may be accomplished by having the client consume a high-fat meal during the procedure. A reaction to the contrast medium would produce symptoms such as urticaria, nausea, vomiting, or dyspnea.

17-98   Answer B

Although paresthesias (tingling or numbness in the hands or feet) may be one of the warning signs of diabetes, the classic symptoms remain the three polys—polyuria, polydipsia, and polyphagia. Proteinuria can also occur, although it is not one of the classic warning symptoms.

17-99   Answer B

The Ferriman-Gallwey scale has been used to define and grade hirsutism. The clinician evaluates hair growth in nine androgen-sensitive hair-growth areas. No hair growth is indicated by 0, and 4 is designated for frank virile hair growth. A score of 8 is diagnostic for hirsutism.

17-100   Answer B

For a client with the symptoms experienced by Sigrid, a thyroid-stimulating hormone (TSH) level measurement should be ordered first because the symptoms suggest hyperthyroidism. The TSH level is the best screening test for hyperthyroidism. Other laboratory and isotope tests for hyperthyroidism include a free T_3 or T_4 level, T_3 resin uptake, and thyroid autoantibodies including TSH receptor antibody (TSH or TRab). Tests not routinely performed but that may be helpful include radioactive iodine uptake and a thyroid scan (with iodine-123 [^{123}I] or technetium-99m), which help to determine the etiology of the hyperthyroidism and assess the functional status of any palpable thyroid irregularities or nodules associated with the toxic goiter. If antithyroid drugs are used, CBC and liver functions tests will need to be preformed. An electrocardiogram may be ordered because of the palpitations, but once the thyroid is stabilized, the cardiac rhythm usually returns to normal.

17-101   Answer C

After establishing clinical and biochemical euthyroidism after a thyroidectomy, you should perform a serum thyroid-stimulating hormone (TSH) level every year. If it is necessary to adjust a client's dosage of levothyroxine, a repeat TSH level measurement should be done in 2–3 months to assess the therapeutic response. Once clinical and biochemical euthyroidism is reestablished, you may return to obtaining an annual serum TSH level.

17-102 Answer C

Beta blockers may be problematic in clients with diabetes because they block the first sign of hypoglycemia, which is often tachycardia. Many clients with diabetes have compelling indications for the use of beta blockers, such as coronary artery disease. In these clients the need for a beta blocker outweighs any risk that occurs. Decreasing the possibility of low blood sugar by selecting appropriate agents and adjusting dosages may be necessary. If the client with diabetes is on a beta blocker, it is important to explain that instead of the tachycardia, he or she will notice other signs of hypoglycemia, such as sweating, that will still occur if the client is taking a beta blocker. ACE inhibitors are the first choice for clients with diabetes who have hypertension because they slow the progression of diabetic nephropathy. Calcium channel blockers provide pressure reduction without adverse effects on lipids and glucose control. Alpha-blocking agents provide a smooth control and an improved lipid profile.

17-103 Answer A

If the thyroid gland is palpable, the next step is to have the client hold his or her breath and listen over the gland with the bell of the stethoscope for bruits. A bruit may indicate an increased vascularity of hyperthyroidism. Although there may not be any sound, that doesn't mean that there is not a thyroid nodule. A thrill is feeling turbulent blood flow, whereas a bruit is listening to it.

17-104 Answer B

The fetus with intrauterine growth retardation has very scant carbon stores in the form of glycogen and body fat and is prone to hypoglycemia even with appropriate endocrine adjustments at birth. In addition, an infant whose mother has diabetes (and had no problem with intrauterine growth retardation) has abundant glucose stores in the form of glycogen and fat and also develops hypoglycemia because of an imbalance in insulin-glucagon secretion resulting from hyperinsulinemia caused by islet cell hyperplasia. Other causes of hypoglycemia are associated with islet cell hyperplasia, inborn errors of metabolism such as glycogen storage disease and galactosemia, and as a complication of birth, asphyxia, hypoxia secondary to cardiorespiratory disease, or other stresses such as bacterial and viral sepsis.

17-105 Answer C

A low level of thyroid-stimulating hormone (TSH) indicates hyperthyroidism. Hyperthyroidism is an excess of circulating thyroid hormones, which will suppress the level of TSH produced by the pituitary. The TSH would be increased in primary hypothyroidism. In myxedema, there would be a deficiency of thyroxine. Most thyroid nodules secrete thyroid hormone, so levels of thyroid hormones would be elevated.

17-106 Answer D

For the client with hepatitis, abdominal pain in the right upper quadrant is caused by stretching of Glisson's capsule surrounding the liver, which occurs because of inflammation; bleeding tendencies are a result of reduced prothrombin synthesis by injured hepatic cells; pruritus is caused by bile salt accumulation in the skin; and fever is the result of the release of pyrogens in the inflammatory process.

17-107 Answer B

For clients with diabetes requiring insulin, an increase in their daily insulin dosage is usually required in the presence of an acute infection. Betty should begin by increasing her regular insulin dosage by just 2 units and then monitor her blood sugar level. At some point, a more physiologic insulin regime such as basal-bolus might be considered.

17-108 Answer B

Morris should be started on an ACE inhibitor such as enalapril (Vasotec). ACE inhibitors have renoprotective effects by reducing the intraglomerular pressure. They do this by inhibiting the renin-angiotensin system, which causes efferent dilation, and by improving glomerular permeability, which causes a reduction of glomerulosclerosis. ACE inhibitors have this beneficial effect on clients with diabetes who are normotensive and hypotensive. Diabetic nephropathy is the leading cause of end-stage renal disease in the United States. Monitoring for microalbuminuria is a method for identifying early nephropathy. Ordering a 24-hour urinalysis will not give you any additional information. You do want to stress tight glycemic control and possibly send Morris to a dietitian, but he needs to be started on an ACE inhibitor now because he is already exhibiting microalbuminuria.

17-109   Answer D

Clients with diabetes are more prone to cardiovascular disease than those without diabetes. The most likely reason for this is that the high levels of glucose and fat that occur with poor control result in atherosclerotic changes in the blood vessels. The client with diabetes may also be overweight, but that is not the primary contributing factor to the development of cardiovascular disease. Diabetes is associated with a greater incidence of high blood lipid levels, high blood pressure, and obesity, all of which are risk factors for cardiovascular disease. Diabetes affects both small and large blood vessels, which contributes to the process of atherosclerosis. In women, diabetes negates the protective effects of estrogen. The amount of protein in the diet of a client with diabetes is restricted to help prevent or delay renal complications, not cardiovascular ones. The reason clients with diabetes, especially older adults, are more prone to cardiovascular disease than those without diabetes is the high levels of glucose and fat, which result in atherosclerotic changes in the blood vessels.

17-110   Answer C

Clients with Graves' disease should not smoke. The use of tobacco increases the inflammatory cytokines within the orbit and can worsen the ocular manifestations of Graves' disease. Smoking is the most important known risk factor for the development or worsening of Graves' ophthalmopathy.

17-111   Answer C

Gynecomastia may be the first sign of testicular cancer. It is also associated with breast, adrenal, pituitary, lung, and hepatic malignancies. Hypogonadism produces low testosterone levels in men with normal estrogen levels. Alteration in breast tissue responsiveness to hormonal activity can result in gynecomastia. Gynecomastia can occur secondary to cirrhosis, chronic obstructive lung disease, malnutrition, hyperthyroidism and other endocrine imbalances, tuberculosis, and chronic renal disease.

17-112   Answer D

Podagra is gout of the first metatarsophalangeal joint, the joint most frequently affected in the initial attack. Podagra is experienced by 90% of clients with gout. An acute attack of gout is usually monoarticular (affecting only one joint). Subsequent attacks may progress to include several joints (polyarticular).

17-113   Answer A

Cushing's syndrome results in an excessive amount of adrenocorticotropic hormone, which stimulates the secretion of glucocorticoids, mineralocorticoids, and androgenic steroids from the adrenal cortex. In the presence of excessive cortisol, fungal infections of the skin, nails, and oral mucosa, such as onychomycosis and tinea versicolor, are common, and skin wounds heal very slowly. Other symptoms include fatigue and weakness and excessive hair growth. Addison's disease, which is a deficiency in the secretion of adrenocortical hormones, usually results in an increased pigmentation of the entire skin.

17-114   Answer C

Although a serum glucose test is an excellent test for clients with diabetes, it reports only the serum glucose of that day. The American Diabetes Association (ADA) therefore recommends that the glycohemoglobin (hemoglobin A_{1C}) test be performed quarterly because it reports the serum glucose concentration of the previous 3 months. HbA1c can now be used for diagnosis of diabetes (greater than 6.5%). The ADA also recommends an annual urine test to assess for urine protein that might indicate an early sign of kidney damage. Liver function studies should be done on an annual basis as part of a routine examination.

17-115   Answer C

Saturated solution of potassium iodide is an antithyroid drug that blocks the production and release of thyroid hormone. It is used to treat hyperthyroidism before thyroidectomy. Propylthiouracil and methimazole (Tapazole) treat hyperthyroidism by inhibiting thyroid hormone synthesis. Radioactive iodine (^{131}I) treats hyperthyroidism and may be used to treat thyroid cancer by destroying thyroid tissue.

Bibliography

American Thyroid Association, et al: Hyperthyroidism and other causes of thyrotoxicosis: Management guidelines of the American Thyroid Association and American Association of Clinical Endocrinologists. *Endocrine Practice* 17(3):593–646, 2011.

DeNoia, V: Bisphosphonates for osteoporosis: A closer look at efficacy and safety. *Arthritis Practitioner* 3(4):20–23, 2007.

Dunphy, LM, et al: *Primary Care: The Art and Science of Advanced Practice Nursing,* ed 3. FA Davis, Philadelphia, 2011.

Fitzgerald, MA: *Nurse Practitioner Certification Examination and Practice Preparation.* FA Davis, Philadelphia, 2010.

Gharib, H, et al: American Association of Clinical Endocrinologists, Associazione Medici Endocrinologi, and European Thyroid Association Medical guidelines for clinical practice for the diagnosis and management of thyroid nodules. *Endocrine Practice* 16(suppl 1): 1–50, 2010.

Handelsman, Y, et al: American Association of Clinical Endocrinologists medical guidelines for clinical practice for developing a diabetes mellitus comprehensive care plan. *Endocrine Practice* 17(suppl 2): 1–53, 2011.

Jones, R: Primary hyperparathyroidism. *Clinician Reviews* 17(7):27–33, 2007.

Mensing, C, McLaughlin, S, Halstenson, C, and American Association of Diabetes Educators: *The Art and Science of Diabetes Self-Management Education Desk Reference* ed 2. American Association of Diabetes Educators, Chicago, 2011.

Rodbard, HW, et al: Statement by an American Association of Clinical Endocrinologists/American College of Endocrinology consensus panel on type 2 diabetes mellitus: An algorithm for glycemic control. *Endocrine Practice* 15(6):540–559, 2009.

Stern, SD, Cifu, AS, Altkorn, D: *Symptom to Diagnosis: An Evidence-Based Guide,* ed 2. McGraw-Hill, New York, 2010.

Wynne, AL, Woo, TM, and Olyaei, AJ: *Pharmacotherapeutics for Nurse Practitioner Prescribers,* ed 2. FA Davis, Philadelphia, 2007.

How well did you do?

85% and above, congratulations! This score shows application of test-taking principles and adequate content knowledge.

75%–85%, keep working! Review test-taking principles and try again.

65%–75%, hang in there! Spend some time reviewing concepts and test-taking principles and try the test again.

Chapter 18: *Hematological and Immune Problems*

Lynne M. Dunphy
Jill E. Winland-Brown

Questions

18-1 Which ethnic group has the highest overall cancer incidence rate?

A. Native Americans

B. Asian and Pacific Islanders

C. Hispanics

D. African Americans

18-2 *Physiological changes in the immune system of older adults include*

A. an increase in immunoglobulin A and G antibodies.

B. a high rate of T-lymphocyte proliferation.

C. an increase in the number of cytotoxic T cells.

D. an increase in CD8, which affects regulation of the immune system.

18-3 *The first choice of therapy for a client who is positive for HIV and has oral candidiasis is*

A. fluconazole (Diflucan) 100 mg PO daily.

B. ketoconazole (Nizoral) 200 mg PO daily.

C. clotrimazole troches (10 mg) five times daily or nystatin (Mycostatin) suspension 500,000–1,000,000 units three to five times daily.

D. griseofulvin (Grisactin) 500 mg bid.

18-4 *Which of the following is a benign neoplasm?*

A. Leiomyoma

B. Osteosarcoma

C. Glioma

D. Seminoma

18-5 *You suspect that your new client Doug has hepatitis C, although he is currently* asymptomatic. *Your suspicion is based on his medical history, which includes which of the following factors that has been identified as a red flag for this disease?*

A. Lactose intolerance

B. Frequent sore throats and upper respiratory infections

C. A history of mononucleosis at age 17

D. Unsafe sexual behaviors

18-6 *Tobacco has been linked to which of the following types of cancer?*

A. Colon cancer

B. Bladder cancer

C. Prostate cancer

D. Cervical cancer

18-7 *Prostate cancer is associated with which of the following viruses?*

A. Herpes simplex virus types 1 and 2

B. Human herpesvirus 6

C. Human cytomegalovirus

D. Human T-lymphotropic viruses

18-8 *What does shift to the left or left shift mean?*

A. A rise in basophils

B. A rise in monocytes

C. A rise in neutrophils

D. A rise in lymphocytes

18-9 *What is the earliest visual sign of oral and pharyngeal squamous cell carcinomas?*

A. Leukoplakia

B. Mucosal erythroplasia

C. Loss of sensation in the tongue

D. Difficulty chewing or swallowing

459

18-10 *Select a statement that is true about the erythrocyte sedimentation rate (ESR).*

A. It is a very specific indicator of inflammation.

B. A rise in the ESR is a normal part of aging.

C. It is useful in detecting pancreatic cancer.

D. It is diagnostic for rheumatoid arthritis.

18-11 *Samantha is being given platelets because of acute leukemia. One "pack" of platelets should raise her count by how much?*

A. 2,000–4,000 mm³

B. 5,000–8,000 mm³

C. 9,000–12,000 mm³

D. About 15,000 mm³

18-12 *Pernicious anemia is a result of*

A. not enough folic acid.

B. not enough intrinsic factor.

C. not enough vitamin D.

D. not enough iron.

18-13 *The gold standard for definitive diagnosis of sickle cell anemia is*

A. a reticulocyte count.

B. the sickle cell test.

C. a hemoglobin electrophoresis.

D. a peripheral blood smear.

18-14 *A client with HIV infection has a CD4 count of 305 and an HIV RNA level of 13,549. The client is asymptomatic. What is your course of action?*

A. Negotiate with your client a time to start therapy.

B. Recheck the laboratory results in 1 month. If the counts remain like this, start treatment.

C. Start therapy now because the client's CD4 count is less than 500 and the HIV RNA level is greater than 10,000.

D. Wait to start therapy until the client becomes asymptomatic.

18-15 *Which of the following indicates that Jim, a 32-year-old client with AIDS, has oropharyngeal candidiasis?*

A. Small vesicles

B. Fissured, white, thickened patches

C. Removable white plaques

D. Flat-topped papules with thin, bluish-white spiderweb lines

18-16 *Systemic lupus erythematosus is diagnosed on the basis of*

A. positive antinuclear antibody (ANA), malar rash, and photosensitivity.

B. positive ANA, weight loss, and night sweats.

C. negative ANA, photosensitivity, and renal disease.

D. leukopenia, negative ANA, and photosensitivity.

18-17 *Which of the following situations might precipitate a sickle cell crisis in an infant?*

A. Taking the infant to visit a relative

B. Hepatitis B immunization

C. Taking the infant to an outdoor event

D. Having the infant sleep on its back

18-18 *Despite successful primary prophylaxis, which infection remains a common AIDS-defining diagnosis?*

A. *Pneumocystis jiroveci* pneumonia (PCP)

B. Cryptococcosis

C. Cryptosporidiosis

D. Candidiasis

18-19 *Jimmy is a 6-month-old with newly diagnosed sickle cell disease. His mother brings him to the clinic for a well-baby visit. Which of the following should you do on this visit?*

A. Tell the parents that Jimmy will not be immunized because of his diagnosis.

B. Tell the parents that Jimmy should not go to day care.

C. Immunize Jimmy with diphtheria, tetanus, and pertussis; *Haemophilus influenzae* type b (HIB); hepatitis B (HBV); and poliomyelitis vaccines.

D. Immunize Jimmy with measles, mumps, and rubella; HIB; and HBV vaccines only.

18-20 *The Centers for Disease Control and Prevention's definition of AIDS includes the presence of which of the following disorders, with or without laboratory evidence of HIV infection?*

A. Pneumonia in clients younger than age 60

B. Dementia in clients younger than age 60

C. Kaposi's sarcoma in clients younger than age 60

D. Primary brain lymphoma in clients older than age 60

18-21   A loss of DNA control over differentiation that occurs in response to adverse conditions is referred to as

A. hyperplasia.

B. metaplasia.

C. anaplasia.

D. dysplasia.

18-22   Clients with AIDS typically experience the neurological symptomatic triad consisting of

A. cognitive, motor, and behavioral changes.

B. seizures, paresthesias, and dysesthesias.

C. Kaposi's sarcoma, cryptococcal meningitis, and depression.

D. seizures, depression, and paresthesias.

18-23   When a neonate is initially protected against measles, mumps, and rubella because the mother is immune, this is an example of which type of immunity?

A. Natural active

B. Artificial active

C. Natural passive

D. Artificial passive

18-24   Your client, Ms. Jones, has an elevated platelet count. You suspect

A. systemic lupus erythematosus.

B. infectious mononucleosis.

C. disseminated intravascular coagulation (DIC).

D. splenectomy.

18-25   Sally has HIV infection and asks which method of birth control, other than abstinence, would be best for her. You suggest

A. latex condoms.

B. the spermicide nonoxynol-9.

C. an intrauterine device (IUD).

D. an oral contraceptive.

18-26   Stu, age 49, has slightly reduced hemoglobin and hematocrit readings. What is your next action after you ask him about his diet?

A. Repeat the laboratory tests.

B. Perform a fecal occult blood test.

C. Start him on an iron preparation.

D. Start him on folic acid.

18-27   Which of the following is an X-linked recessive disorder commonly seen in African American men?

A. Sickle cell anemia

B. Glucose-6-phosphate dehydrogenase deficiency

C. Pyruvate kinase deficiency

D. Bernard-Soulier syndrome

18-28   Jan is having biological therapy for her pancreatic cancer. What kind of treatment is this?

A. Surgery

B. Radiation therapy

C. Immunotherapy

D. Chemotherapy

18-29   One major approach to cancer prevention is

A. colonoscopy.

B. new drug trials.

C. Pap smears for women of all ages.

D. host modification.

18-30   Tina, age 2, had a complete blood count (CBC) drawn at her last visit. It indicates that she has a microcytic hypochromic anemia. What should you do now at this visit?

A. Obtain a lead level.

B. Instruct Tina's parents to increase the amount of milk in her diet.

C. Start Tina on ferrous sulfate (Feosol) and check the CBC in 6 weeks.

D. Recheck the CBC on this visit.

18-31   Which is the most abundant immunoglobulin (Ig) found in the blood, lymph, and intestines?

A. IgG

B. IgA

C. IgM

D. IgD

18-32 Your client, Mr. Jones, has Sjögren's syndrome. Which treatment do you suggest?

A. Artificial tears and chewing sugarless gum

B. Frequent rinsing out of the mouth with mouthwash

C. Drinking at least one glass of milk per day

D. Removing wax from the ears at regular intervals

18-33 Your client, George, age 60, presents with pruritus and complains of lymphadenopathy in his neck. He also complains of night sweats and has noticed a low-grade fever. He has not lost any weight and otherwise feels well. He is widowed and has been dating a new women recently. On physical exam, you find enlarged supraclavicular nodes. You suspect

A. lung cancer.

B. hodgkin's lymphoma.

C. a lingering viral infection from a bout of flu he had 6 weeks ago.

D. non-Hodgkin's lymphoma.

18-34 Your client, Jeannie, age 64, comes to you complaining of tinnitus and lightheadedness without loss of consciousness. On physical exam, you note splenomegaly. To sort out your differential diagnosis, you order an alkaline phosphatase and vitamin B_{12} level because you are ruling out a diagnosis of

A. liver cancer.

B. pancreatic cancer.

C. mononucleosis.

D. polycythemia vera.

18-35 You are examining Joseph, age 9 months, and note a palpable right supraclavicular node. You know that this finding is suspicious for

A. candidiasis.

B. cryptococcosis.

C. lymphoma of the mediastinum.

D. abdominal malignancy.

18-36 When Judy tells you that she has hemophilia, you know that

A. both of her parents also have the disease.

B. her maternal grandfather probably had the disease and it skipped a generation.

C. her father had the disease and her mother was a carrier.

D. her mother had the disease.

18-37 Julie's brother has chronic lymphatic leukemia. She overheard that he was in stage IV and asks what this means. According to the Rai classification system, stage IV is a stage

A. at which the lymphocytes are greater than 10,000 mm^3.

B. with an absolute lymphocytosis, in which the client may live 7–10 years or more.

C. of thrombocytopenia, in which the life expectancy may be only 2 years.

D. of anemia.

18-38 Your client, Jackson, has decreased lymphocytes. You suspect

A. bacterial infection.

B. viral infection.

C. immunodeficiency.

D. parasitic infections.

18-39 Your 18-year-old client, Mandy, has infectious mononucleosis. What might you expect her blood work to reflect?

A. Thrombocytopenia and elevated transaminase

B. Elevated white blood cells (WBCs)

C. Decreased WBCs

D. Decreased serum globulins

18-40 Marsha states that a relative is having a carcinoembryonic antigen (CEA) test done to detect some type of cancer. She wants to know what kind. You tell her a CEA is performed to detect

A. adenocarcinoma of the prostate.

B. medullary cancer of the thyroid.

C. adenocarcinomas of the colon, lung, breast, ovary, stomach, and pancreas.

D. multiple myeloma.

18-41   *Prophylaxis for the first episode of*
Pneumocystis jiroveci *pneumonia in an adult or*
adolescent client infected with HIV is

A. isoniazid (Nydrazid) 300 mg PO and pyridoxine
    (vitamin B$_6$ [Beesix]) 50 mg PO daily for 12 days.

B. clarithromycin (Biaxin) 500 mg PO twice daily
    for 2 weeks.

C. rifampin (Rimactane) 600 mg PO daily for
    12 months.

D. trimethoprim-sulfamethoxazole (TMP-SMZ)
    (Bactrim) DS 1 tablet PO daily for 10 days.

18-42   *Which of the following is a genotoxic*
carcinogen?

A. Vinyl chloride polymers

B. Chemotherapy drugs

C. Asbestos

D. Wood and leather dust

18-43   *Which tumor marker may detect a tumor*
of the ovary or testis?

A. Alpha fetoprotein

B. Carcinoembryonic antigen

C. Human chorionic gonadotropin

D. Cancer antigen 125

18-44   *Caroline, an older adult, is homeless and has*
iron-deficiency anemia. She smokes and drinks when
she can and has an ulcer. Which of the following is
not one of the risk factors of iron-deficiency anemia?

A. Smoking

B. Poverty

C. Ulcer disease

D. Age older than 60

18-45   *Pernicious anemia is a result of*

A. not enough folic acid.

B. not enough intrinsic factor.

C. not enough vitamin D.

D. not enough iron.

18-46   *Thalassemia is caused by*

A. blood loss.

B. impaired production of all blood-forming
    elements.

C. increased destruction of red blood cells.

D. autoimmune antibodies.

18-47   *Which type of leukemia produces symptoms*
with an insidious onset including weakness, fatigue,
massive lymphadenopathy, pruritic vesicular skin
lesions, anemia, and thrombocytopenia?

A. Acute lymphocytic leukemia

B. Acute myelogenous leukemia

C. Chronic lymphocytic leukemia

D. Chronic myelogenous leukemia

18-48   *Bladder cancer can be detected early by*

A. an annual urine culture.

B. a bladder tumor marker blood test.

C. an annual cystoscopy.

D. none of the above; there is no early detection.

18-49   *Multiple myeloma is a plasma cell*
malignancy in which the bone marrow is
replaced, and there is bone destruction and
paraprotein formation. Myeloma is a disease
of older adults overall (median age at
presentation, 65 years). Common presenting
symptoms include

A. nausea and vomiting and chronic cough.

B. fatigue and splenomegaly.

C. lower back pain and hypercalcemia.

D. nausea and vomiting and fatigue.

18-50   *When should you order a complete blood*
count for your client?

A. Routinely

B. Before dental work

C. In the case of infection

D. If she is pregnant

18-51   *Which is the best serum test to perform*
to spot an iron-deficiency anemia early before it
progresses to full-blown anemia?

A. Hemoglobin

B. Hematocrit

C. Ferritin

D. Reticulocytes

18-52   *Julia asks how smoking increases the risk for folic acid deficiency. You respond that smoking*

A. causes small-vessel disease and constricts all vessels that transport essential nutrients.

B. decreases vitamin C absorption.

C. affects the liver's ability to store folic acid.

D. causes nausea, thereby inhibiting the appetite and ingestion of foods rich in folic acid.

18-53   *Joan had a modified mastectomy with radiation therapy 10 years ago. She asks when she can have her blood pressure or needle sticks taken in the affected arm. How do you respond?*

A. "If it's been 10 years and you've had no problems, you can discontinue those precautions."

B. "Because you didn't have a radical mastectomy, you can do those things now."

C. "You must observe these precautions forever."

D. "As long as you do limb exercises and have established collateral drainage, you can discontinue these precautions."

18-54   *Samuel, age 5, is receiving radiation therapy for his acute lymphocytic leukemia. He is at increased risk of developing which type of cancer as a secondary malignancy when he becomes an adult?*

A. Chronic lymphocytic leukemia

B. Brain tumor

C. Liver cancer

D. Esophageal cancer

18-55   *Pregnant women may be prone to thrombophilias, which may be inherited or acquired. Which of the following is an example of a factor that predisposes pregnant women to acquired thrombophilic states in pregnancy?*

A. Factor V Leiden

B. Homocystine

C. Immobilization and malignancy

D. Protein S and protein C

18-56   *Which of the following laboratory studies is used to determine if a client has had hepatitis?*

A. Serum protein

B. Protein electrophoresis

C. Antibody testing

D. Globulin levels

18-57   *Kathy, age 64, is a sun worshipper. She tells you that because she did not get skin cancer in her youth, she certainly will not get it now. How do you respond?*

A. "You're probably right; if you haven't had it by now, you're probably safe."

B. "As you age, you have decreased pigment in your skin, which puts you at more risk."

C. "Your skin elasticity is decreased, so you have more of a chance of contracting skin cancer as you age."

D. "Skin cancer is not dependent on age; anyone can get it."

18-58   *Nancy recently had a mastectomy and refuses to look at the site. Her husband does all the dressing changes. When she comes into the office for a postoperative checkup, what would you say to her?*

A. "You'll look at it when you're ready."

B. "You must look at it today."

C. "Everything's going to be OK. It looks fine."

D. "You have to accept this eventually; just glance at it today."

18-59   *Hemolytic anemia may be an inherited condition. Which of the following is not an inherited condition related to hemolytic anemia?*

A. Hereditary spherocytosis

B. Pernicious anemia

C. Glucose-6-phosphate dehydrogenase deficiency

D. Sickle cell anemia

18-60   *Sickle cell anemia is an autosomal recessive disorder caused by the hemoglobin S gene. An abnormal hemoglobin leads to chronic hemolytic anemia with numerous clinical manifestations and becomes a chronic multisystem disease, with death from organ failure, usually between ages 40 and 50. The hemoglobin S gene is carried by*

A. approximately 4% of the U.S. population.

B. approximately 8% of American blacks.

C. approximately 4% of Latinos.

D. approximately 12% of Native Americans.

18-61   *A client with HIV infection has a fever of unknown origin (FUO). Which of the following is a possible cause of an FUO in a client with HIV?*

A. Drug fever

B. Upper respiratory infection

C. Nothing specific; this is a systemic disease manifestation

D. Urinary tract infection

18-62   *The primary reason for newborn screening for sickle cell disease is to*

A. present the parents with the option for genetic screening in the future.

B. test siblings if it is proved that the newborn has sickle cell disease.

C. allow for the prevention of septicemia with prophylactic medication.

D. prevent a sickle cell crisis.

18-63   *Allie, age 5, is being treated with radiation for cancer. Her mother asks about the effect radiation will have on Allie's future growth. Although she knows that a specialist will be handling Allie's care, her mother asks for your opinion. How do you respond?*

A. "Let's worry about the cancer first, then see how her growth is affected."

B. "Chemotherapy may affect her future growth, but radiation will not."

C. "She will probably have growth hormone problems, in which case she can then begin growth hormone therapy."

D. "That's the least of your worries now; everything will turn out OK."

18-64   *Barbie, age 27, had her spleen removed after an automobile accident. You are seeing her in the office for the first time since her discharge from the hospital. She asks you how her surgery will affect her in the future. How do you respond?*

A. "Your red blood cell production will be slowed."

B. "Your lymphatic system may have difficulty transporting lymph fluid to the blood vessels."

C. "You'll have difficulty storing the nutritional agents needed to make red blood cells."

D. "You may have difficulty salvaging iron from old red blood cells for reuse."

18-65   *Which of the following increases the risk of pancreatic cancer?*

A. A high-carbohydrate diet

B. Cigarette smoking, diabetes, and a high-fat diet

C. Diabetes and lack of activity

D. Yo-yo dieting

18-66   *Sam is being worked up for pancreatic cancer. He states that the doctor wants to put a "scope" in and inject dye into his ducts. He wants to know more about this. What procedure is he referring to?*

A. Percutaneous transhepatic cholangiography

B. An endoscopic retrograde cholangiopancreatography

C. An angiography

D. An upper gastrointestinal (GI) series

18-67   *Screening infants for anemia should occur at what age?*

A. 6 months

B. No screening is recommended.

C. 9 months

D. 12 months

18-68   *A platelet count less than 150,000/mm³ may indicate*

A. possible hemorrhage.

B. hypersplenism.

C. polycythemia vera.

D. malignancy.

18-69   *Your client Mrs. Young, age 64, is here to see you because she has pain in her left breast. She reports no pain in right breast and no noted lesions or masses on breast self-exam, which she performs monthly. You know that*

A. at her age, you do not need to worry about breast cancer.

B. initial presentation of breast pain is usually not suspicious for a malignancy.

C. she must be sent for a mammogram as soon as possible.

D. she has no personal or family history of breast cancer; therefore, you are not concerned.

18-70   *Maurice is an intravenous drug abuser with chronic hepatitis B (HBV). The development of which type of hepatitis poses the greatest risk to a client with HBV?*

A. Hepatitis A

B. Hepatitis C

C. Hepatitis D

D. Hepatitis E

18-71   *Sandra, age 19, is pregnant. She is complaining of breathlessness, tiredness, weakness, and is pale. After diagnosing anemia, you order medication and tell her to take it*

A. only with meals because it can be irritating to the stomach.

B. in the morning if she experiences morning sickness.

C. 1 hour before eating or between meals.

D. at bedtime.

18-72   *Under which of the following circumstances is the reticulocyte count elevated?*

A. Aplastic anemia

B. Iron-deficiency anemias

C. Poisonings

D. Acute blood loss

18-73   *Antibodies (inhibitors) directed against factor VIII can arise spontaneously in a number of situations. These include*

A. clients who have mitral regurgitation.

B. as sequelae to a strep infection.

C. clients on antibiotics.

D. women who are several weeks postpartum after a normal labor and delivery.

18-74   *Which of the following is not an effective strategy to prevent the nausea and vomiting associated with the effects of radiation and chemotherapy?*

A. Decreasing the amount of liquids

B. Eating a soft, bland diet low in fat and sugar

C. Relaxation

D. Distraction

18-75   *Mandy's 16-year-old daughter has hepatitis A. Which of the following statements made by Mandy indicates that she understands the teaching you've just completed?*

A. "I guess she needs to be hospitalized until she's recovered."

B. "We'll keep her at home with strict isolation precautions."

C. "We'll stop at the store and buy plastic eating utensils."

D. "We'll stop at the drugstore and pick up prescription medications immediately."

18-76   *Sara comes today with numerous petechiae on her arms. You know that she is not taking warfarin (Coumadin). What other drugs do you ask her about?*

A. Aspirin or aspirin compounds

B. Antihypertensive agents

C. Oral contraceptives

D. Anticonvulsants

18-77   *Sue has sickle cell anemia. In regulating her and monitoring her hemoglobin and hematocrit levels, you want to maintain them at*

A. slightly below normal.

B. strictly at normal.

C. slightly above normal.

D. around normal with only minor fluctuations.

18-78   *A metastatic tumor from below the diaphragm is suspected when you palpate which of the following nodes in the left supraclavicular space?*

A. Wringer's node

B. Sims' node

C. Wiskott-Aldrich node

D. Virchow's node

18-79   *Health maintenance in adults with sickle cell anemia includes which of the following?*

A. Early sterilization should be performed to prevent transmission of the disease.

B. Administer hepatitis A vaccine.

C. Avoid use of oral contraceptives because of increased risk of clotting.

D. Give folic acid 1 mg PO daily.

18-80   The three most common signs and symptoms of primary HIV infection are

A. weight loss, pharyngitis, and fatigue.

B. fever, fatigue, and pharyngitis.

C. night sweats, rash, and headache.

D. myalgias, fatigue, and fever.

18-81   The T in the TNM staging system refers to

A. tolerance.

B. primary tumor.

C. tumor marker.

D. turgor.

18-82   When the donor and recipient of a transplant are identical twins, this is referred to as a(n)

A. isograft.

B. autograft.

C. allograft.

D. xenograft.

18-83   Shelley has esophageal cancer and asks you if alcohol played a part in its development. How do you respond?

A. "Your cancer was caused by your cigarette smoking, nothing else."

B. "Alcohol is also a carcinogen."

C. "Alcohol directly alters the DNA and causes mutations."

D. "Alcohol modifies the metabolism of carcinogens in the esophagus and increases their effectiveness."

18-84   Jill has just been given a diagnosis of HIV infection and has a normal initial Pap test. When do the Centers for Disease Control and Prevention (CDC) guidelines state that she should have a repeat Pap test?

A. In 3 months

B. In 6 months

C. In 1 year

D. She should have a colposcopy every year rather than a Pap test.

18-85   Which cancer can be cured with chemotherapy alone?

A. Breast cancer

B. Malignant melanoma

C. Bladder cancer

D. Testicular cancer

18-86   Lorie, age 29, appears with the following signs: pale conjunctiva and nailbeds, tachycardia, heart murmur, cheilosis, stomatitis, splenomegaly, koilonychia, and glossitis. What do you suspect?

A. Vitamin B_{12} deficiency

B. Folate deficiency

C. Iron-deficiency anemia

D. Chronic fatigue syndrome

18-87   Mindy, age 6, recently was discharged from the hospital after a sickle cell crisis. You are teaching her parents to be alert to the manifestations of splenic sequestration and tell them to be alert to

A. vomiting and diarrhea.

B. decreased mental acuity.

C. abdominal pain, pallor, and tachycardia.

D. abdominal pain and vomiting.

18-88   You have a new client, Robert, age 67, who presents with a generalized lymphadenopathy. You know that this is indicative of

A. disseminated malignancy, particularly of the hematological system.

B. cancer of the liver.

C. Sjögren's syndrome.

D. pancreatic cancer.

18-89   Maria asks if being overweight predisposes her to cancer. How do you respond?

A. "No, you have the same risk as a normal-weight individual."

B. "You have less of a risk of cancer than normal-weight individuals because you have protein stores to combat mutant cells."

C. "Yes, you have an increased risk for hormone-dependent cancers because of your obesity."

D. "Yes, you have an increased risk because you have many more cells in all the organs of your body."

18-90   *What is the most significant reason alcohol use is discouraged in persons with HIV infection or AIDS?*

A. Alcohol interferes with the pharmacokinetics of most AIDS drugs.

B. Filling up on the empty calories of alcohol replaces the desire for food.

C. Alcohol decreases the ability of persons to adhere to a prescribed medical regimen.

D. If clients become addicted to alcohol, when AIDS advances, they will become addicted to painkillers.

18-91   *An increase of which immunoglobulin (Ig) signifies atopic disorders such as allergic rhinitis, allergic asthma, atopic dermatitis, and parasitic infestation?*

A. IgG

B. IgM

C. IgA

D. IgE

18-92   *Sickle cell anemia affects African Americans. Approximately 1 in 400 African Americans in the United States has sickle cell disease (SCD). Advances in treatment have been made, but life expectancy is still limited. The mean survival time for men with the disease is approximately*

A. 24 years.

B. 34 years.

C. 42 years.

D. 52 years.

18-93   *Some pharmacological adjuncts to analgesics in clients with uncontrolled cancer pain include*

A. anticonvulsants and tricyclic antidepressants.

B. anticonvulsants, tricyclic antidepressants, and corticosteroids.

C. selective serotonin receptor inhibitors.

D. benzodiazepines.

18-94   *Which of the following white blood cell types is elevated in parasitic infections, hypersensitivity reactions, and autoimmune disorders?*

A. Neutrophils

B. Eosinophils

C. Basophils

D. Monocytes

18-95   *Fecal occult blood testing (FOBT) is most effective in identifying*

A. cancers in the right colon.

B. polyps.

C. cancers in the sigmoid colon.

D. cancers in the transverse colon.

18-96   *Mrs. Jameson complains of unilateral blurry vision and partial blindness in the left eye. On physical examination, you find decreased peripheral vision on her left side. Funduscopic examination reveals cotton-wool spots. Your most likely diagnosis is*

A. cryptococcosis.

B. toxoplasmosis.

C. cytomegalovirus infection.

D. herpes simplex virus infection.

18-97   *Before initiating cancer therapy, the first crucial step is to*

A. stage the disease.

B. define the goals of therapy.

C. confirm the diagnosis using tissue biopsy.

D. choose a treatment plan from the many therapeutic options.

18-98   *Frank, a 66-year-old white male who is on diuretic therapy, presents with an elevated hematocrit. He also has splenomegaly on examination, as well as subjective complaints of blurred vision, fatigue, headache, and tinnitus. You suspect*

A. multiple myeloma.

B. Waldenström's macroglobulinemia.

C. dehydration related to use of diuretics.

D. polycythemia vera.

18-99   *Robin has HIV infection and is having a problem with massive diarrhea. You suspect the cause is*

A. cryptococcosis.

B. toxoplasmosis.

C. cryptosporidiosis.

D. cytomegalovirus.

18-100   Which of the following cancers is associated with Epstein-Barr virus?

A. Burkitt's lymphoma

B. Kaposi's sarcoma

C. Lymphoma

D. Adult T-cell leukemia

18-101   Skip, age 4, is brought in to the office by his mother. His symptoms are pallor, fatigue, bleeding, fever, bone pain, adenopathy, arthralgias, and hepatosplenomegaly. You refer him to a specialist. Which of the following tests do you expect the specialist to perform to confirm a diagnosis?

A. An enzyme-linked immunosorbent assay

B. A monospot test

C. A prothrombin time, partial thromboplastin time, bleeding time, complete blood count, and peripheral smear

D. A bone marrow smear

18-102   The test in which a small, radioactive tracer dose of cyanocobalamin is given by mouth and then a 24-hour urine sample is collected and assayed for radioactivity is the

A. Coombs' test.

B. oligonucleotide probe test.

C. spherocytic test.

D. Schilling test.

18-103   Sherri's blood work returns with a decreased mean cell volume (MCV) and a decreased mean cellular hemoglobin concentration (MCHC). What should you do next?

A. Order a serum iron and total iron binding capacity (TIBC).

B. Order a serum ferritin.

C. Order a serum folate level.

D. Order a serum iron, TIBC, and serum ferritin level.

18-104   Which bone tumor arises from cartilage and is usually located in the pelvis, femur, proximal humerus, or ribs?

A. Osteosarcoma

B. Chondrosarcoma

C. Ewing's sarcoma

D. Fibrosarcoma

18-105   Which hypersensitivity reaction results in a skin test that is erythematous with edema within 3–8 hours?

A. Anaphylactic reaction

B. Cytotoxic reaction

C. Immune complex–mediated reaction

D. Delayed hypersensitivity reaction

18-106   Your client, Shirley, has an elevated mean cell volume (MCV). What should you be considering in terms of diagnosis?

A. Iron-deficiency anemia

B. Hemolytic anemias

C. Lead poisoning

D. Liver disease

18-107   Macrocytic normochromic anemias are caused by

A. acute blood loss.

B. an infection or tumor.

C. a nutritional deficiency of iron.

D. a deficiency of folic acid.

18-108   In teaching your client about the American Cancer Society's CAUTION model, which identifies signs of many cancers, you teach her that the N stands for

A. night sweats.

B. nagging cough.

C. nausea and vomiting.

D. noxious odor.

18-109   What is the mechanism of action of steroid hormones in cancer chemotherapy?

A. They interfere with DNA or RNA synthesis.

B. They interfere with DNA replication by attacking DNA synthesis throughout the cell cycle.

C. They inhibit protein synthesis.

D. They alter the host environment for cell growth.

18-110 *The placement of a high dose of radioactive material directly into a malignant tumor and giving a lower dose to the normal tissues is referred to as*

A. radiotherapy.

B. teletherapy.

C. brachytherapy.

D. ionization therapy.

Answers

18-1   Answer D

African Americans have the highest overall cancer incidence rate and the highest overall cancer mortality rate. Native Americans have the lowest overall cancer incidence and mortality rate of all of the populations in the United States. Asian and Pacific Islanders have a high rate of nasopharyngeal cancer. There is a high rate of gallbladder cancer among New Mexico Hispanics of Native American ancestry; liver cancer is more prevalent among Mexican Americans; and cervical cancer is more prevalent among women from Central and South America.

18-2   Answer A

Older adults have a change in their immunoglobulin (Ig) balance and a marked increase in IgA and IgG antibodies. Other physiological changes in the immune systems of older adults include a low rate of T-lymphocyte proliferation in response to a stimulus, a decrease in the number of cytotoxic (killer) T cells, and a decrease in the relative production of CD4 (T4 or helper T cells) and CD8, affecting regulation of the immune system.

18-3   Answer C

The first choice of therapy for a client who is HIV positive and has oral candidiasis would be clotrimazole troches (10 mg) five times daily or nystatin (Mycostatin) suspension 500,000–1,000,000 units three to five times daily. Because of the common recurrence of oral candidiasis and increased rates of drug resistance, systemic fungicides, such as fluconazole, ketoconazole, and griseofulvin, should be reserved for severe cases, such as esophageal candidiasis and clients with dysphagia. Clotrimazole troches and nystatin

suspension are the only nonsystemic medications listed.

18-4   Answer A

A leiomyoma is a benign neoplasm of the smooth muscle. An osteosarcoma is a malignant neoplasm of the bone tissue, a glioma is a malignant neoplasm of the neuroglia cells, and a seminoma is a malignant tumor of the germ cells of the ectoderm and endoderm.

18-5   Answer D

Identified risk factors for hepatitis C virus (HCV) are intravenous drug use and, to some extent, unsafe sexual behaviors. Previously associated with transfusions before 1990 and with dialysis, the proportion of the population with these risk factors is now less common. High-risk sexual behaviors, particularly sex with someone infected with HCV, and the use of illegal drugs such as cocaine or marijuana have also been associated with increased risk. Lactose intolerance, a history of mononucleosis, and a history of sore throats and frequent upper respiratory infections are not documented risk factors for HCV.

18-6   Answer B

Tobacco use has been linked to an increased risk for bladder, pancreatic, laryngeal, esophageal, oropharyngeal, and some types of gastric cancer. Persons who smoke pipes and cigars are especially susceptible to oropharyngeal and laryngeal cancers. Those who chew tobacco are especially susceptible to oral and esophageal cancers. Colon cancer, cervical cancer, and prostate cancer have not been linked to tobacco use.

18-7   Answer C

Prostate cancer is associated with the human cytomegalovirus. Carcinoma of the lip, cervical carcinoma, and Kaposi's sarcoma are all associated with herpes simplex virus types 1 and 2; lymphoma is associated with human herpesvirus 6; and adult T-cell leukemia and lymphoma, T-cell variant of hairy cell leukemia, and Kaposi's sarcoma are associated with human T-lymphotropic viruses.

18-8   Answer C

A *shift to the left* or *left shift* indicates an elevated white blood count (WBC) count and a relative increase in segmented and band neutrophils. Usually seen in acute bacterial infections, it indicates clinically that the body is responding to an acute need before the neutrophils can fully mature in the bone marrow. The term originated from the Shilling hemogram, which charted the maturation of the granulocytes from the least mature (blasts) on the left to most mature (segmented neutrophils) on the right. To represent the border between the bone marrow and the circulating blood, a line was drawn between the band neutrophils and the segmented ones. When the body releases immature cells into the circulating blood, there is an·increase in the cells in the circulating blood from the left of the line (left shift). Early hand devices for counting blood cells in a differential had the keys lined up in such a way that the technicians had to move their hand to the left to hit the keys for the more immature granulocytes.

18-9   Answer B

Mucosal erythroplasia (red inflammatory lesions) is the earliest visual sign of oral and pharyngeal squamous cell carcinomas. Leukoplakia (thickened whitish patches on the tongue or mucous membranes) is the most common premalignant lesion, but only about 30% of people with these lesions are later found to have malignancy. Other symptoms, which typically appear after mucosal erythroplasia, include pain in the face, jaw, or ear; bleeding; stuffy nose; sore throat; loss of sensation in the tongue; difficulty chewing or swallowing; or a feeling of a mass in the mouth or throat.

18-10   Answer B

The erythrocyte sedimentation rate (ESR) is a very nonspecific indicator of inflammation and is often elevated in inflammatory musculoskeletal conditions; it is not, however, diagnostic for rheumatoid arthritis. Additionally, anemia can cause an increased ESR. As people age, their "normal" sedimentation rate increases.

18-11   Answer B

One pack of platelets should raise the count by 5,000–8,000 mm^3. One pack equals about 50 mL. A "6-pack" is a pool of platelets from six units of blood. Platelets may be given for decreased production of or destruction of platelets, such as occurs in aplastic anemia, acute leukemia, or after chemotherapy.

18-12   Answer B

Pernicious anemia is a result of the parietal cells of the stomach lining failing to secrete enough intrinsic factor to ensure intestinal absorption of vitamin B$_{12}$. A deficiency of folic acid in a pregnant woman can contribute to the development of neural tube defects in the fetus. It can also lead to a slowly progressive type of anemia known as megaloblastic anemia in which the red blood cells are larger than normal and deformed and have a diminished rate of production and a diminished life span. A deficiency in vitamin D interferes with use of calcium and phosphorus in bone and tooth formation and can lead to osteomalacia in adults and rickets in children. A deficiency in iron results in iron-deficiency anemia with insufficient hemoglobin; symptoms include pallor of the skin and nailbeds, fatigue, and weakness.

18-13   Answer C

The gold standard for definitive diagnosis of sickle cell anemia is a hemoglobin electrophoresis, a test that determines the presence of hemoglobin S. The client with sickle cell anemia has a decreased hematocrit level, as well as sickled cells on the smear. The baseline reticulocyte count is markedly elevated in sickle cell anemia, but that is not specific to the condition. The sickle cell test is a screening test. A peripheral blood smear is used for red cell morphology. Additional testing is always required to define the hemoglobin phenotype.

18-14   Answer C

Regardless of whether the client is symptomatic, the Centers for Disease Control and Prevention standards call for therapy to be started when a client with HIV infection has a CD4 count less than 500 and a HIV RNA level greater than 10,000.

18-15   Answer C

Oral candidiasis (thrush) appears as white plaques that can be scraped off (removed), revealing an erythematous mucosal surface. Because of this, it is often referred to as a pseudomembranous lesion. Herpes simplex is an acute viral disease that causes small vesicles on the lip borders (cold sores). Leukoplakia is a disease of the mucous membranes of the cheeks, gums, or tongue with white, thickened, fissured patches that may become malignant. Flat-topped papules with thin, bluish-white spiderweb lines are lesions of lichen planus, an inflammatory pruritic benign disease of the skin and mucous membranes.

18-16   Answer A

Systemic lupus erythematosus (SLE) is a multisystem autoimmune disease of unknown etiology. According to the American College of Rheumatology, 4 of 11 criteria must be present at some point through the course of the disease. These include positive antinuclear antibody; malar rash; photosensitivity; renal disease; neurological disorders, especially seizures and psychosis; oral or nasal ulcers; nonerosive arthritis with inflammation; pleuritis or pericarditis; hematological disorder, specifically hemolytic anemia with reticulocytosis, leukopenia (WBC less than 4,000 on two occasions), lymphopenia (less than 1,500 on two occasions), or thrombocytopenia (less than 100,000 on two occasions); and immunological disorder, specifically anti-DNA antibody, anti-Sm antibody, and antiphospholipid antibody, including false-positive syphilis. Weight loss and night sweats are not diagnostic for SLE.

18-17   Answer C

Certain precautions must be taken for infants with sickle cell disease to prevent vaso-occlusive crisis. Any activity or situation that would cause dehydration should be avoided. An example is sitting in a stroller in the heat for any length of time. Children with the disease should always have access to fluids. Exposure to cold temperatures slows the circulation and can cause sickling, as can any activity that can lead to hypoxia. Immunization for hepatitis B should be done. The infant can be taken to visit relatives, although some care should be taken to avoid exposure to children and adults with upper respiratory infections (URIs).

18-18   Answer A

Before the appearance of AIDS, *Pneumocystis jiroveci* pneumonia (PCP) was a rare disease that immunosuppressed persons and clients with leukemia sometimes developed. Today, PCP is usually the defining characteristic in clients with AIDS in both the United States and Europe. Cryptococcosis is a life-threatening systemic fungal infection that usually targets the central nervous system and the lungs, although it may attack anywhere. Cryptosporidiosis is a protozoal infection responsible for diarrhea in clients with AIDS. Candidiasis is the most common fungal infection, affecting 90% of all clients with AIDS, although it is common in the general population as well.

18-19   Answer C

At 6 months of age, Jimmy should be immunized with diphtheria, tetanus, and pertussis (DTP); *Haemophilus influenzae* type b (HIB); hepatitis B (HBV); and poliomyelitis vaccines. Children with sickle cell disease should receive all the standard well-baby care, but in addition to the standard immunizations, they should receive the pneumococcal vaccine at age 2 years. There is no cure for this disease. Children should be treated like other children, and their activities should not be limited unless they are experiencing a painful sickle cell crisis.

18-20   Answer C

Kaposi's sarcoma in a client younger than age 60 is considered conclusive evidence of AIDS under the Centers for Disease Control and Prevention's definition. Other disorders, with or without laboratory evidence of HIV infections that also define AIDS, include *Pneumocystis jiroveci* pneumonia; candidiasis of the esophagus, trachea, bronchi, or lungs; extrapulmonary cryptococcosis; cryptosporidiosis with persistent diarrhea; cytomegalovirus infection; herpes simplex virus infection with persistent skin lesions; *Mycobacterium avium* infection; progressive multifocal leukoencephalopathy; toxoplasmosis of the brain; and primary lymphoma of the brain in a client younger than age 60.

18-21   Answer D

A loss of DNA control over differentiation occurring in response to adverse conditions is referred to as dysplasia. Dysplastic cells show an abnormal degree of variation in size, shape, and appearance and a disturbance in the usual arrangement. An example of dysplasia is a change in the cervix in response to the human papillomavirus. Hyperplasia is an increase in the number or density of normal cells. Hyperplasia occurs in response to stress, increased metabolic demands, or elevated levels of hormones. An example of hyperplasia is the change in uterine cells in response to rising levels of estrogen during pregnancy. Metaplasia is a change in the normal pattern of differentiation such that dividing cells differentiate into cell types not normally found in that location in the body. An example of metaplasia is the replacement of normal columnar ciliated cells in the bronchial epithelium by stratified squamous cells in response to inhaled pollutants, primarily cigarette smoke. Anaplasia is the regression of a cell to an immature or undifferentiated cell type. Anaplastic cell division is no longer under DNA control. It usually occurs when a damaging or transforming event takes place inside the dividing, but still undifferentiated, cell. An example of anaplasia may be a response to an overwhelmingly destructive condition inside the cell or in the surrounding tissue.

18-22   Answer A

Certainly all of the possible answer options listed may occur in clients with AIDS. However, the key word in the stem of the question is *neurological*. The neurological symptomatic triad that clients with AIDS typically experience consists of cognitive, motor, and behavioral changes. These changes are present to a greater or lesser degree in all clients with AIDS. Kaposi's sarcoma is not neurological; it is a multifocal neoplasm with vascular tumors in the skin and other organs.

18-23   Answer C

When a neonate is initially protected against measles, mumps, and rubella (MMR) because the mother is immune, this is an example of natural passive immunity. This type of immunity is acquired by the transfer of maternal antibodies to the fetus or neonate via the placenta or breast milk. Chickenpox and hepatitis A are examples of natural active immunity, which is acquired by infection with an antigen, resulting in the production of antibodies. MMR, polio, diphtheria, pertussis, tetanus, and hepatitis B vaccines are examples of artificial active immunity, which is acquired by immunization with an antigen, such as attenuated live virus vaccine. A gamma globulin injection following hepatitis A exposure is an example of artificial passive immunity, which is acquired by administration of antibodies or antitoxins in the immune globulin.

18-24   Answer D

Increased platelet count is seen in myeloproliferative leukemias, polycythemia vera, and status postsplenectomy. Platelets are decreased in coagulation disorders such as disseminated intravascular coagulation (DIC), septicemia, and eclampsia; increased destruction of platelets is seen in idiopathic thrombocytopenic purpura, systemic lupus erythematosus (SLE), and infectious mononucleosis; and decreased production of platelets is seen in aplastic anemia, most leukemias, and secondary to radiation and chemotherapy.

18-25   Answer A

The latex condom, when used consistently and correctly, is the preferred contraceptive method for the client infected with HIV because it provides the most effective barrier between partners. The spermicide nonoxynol-9 has not been shown to prevent viral transmission in humans, especially when used alone. Because intrauterine devices increase menstrual blood flow, they expose a woman's partner to a greater viral load. Although the effect of oral contraceptive pills on HIV transmission is not known, the estrogen and progestin can promote HIV disease progression through opportunistic infections, as well as cervical neoplasia by their immunomodulating effects.

18-26   Answer B

Tests for fecal occult blood in the stools should be done on all clients suspected of having iron-deficiency anemia. In the early stages of iron-deficiency anemia, both the hemoglobin and hematocrit measures are normal to slightly reduced. It is necessary to determine whether the iron deficiency is related solely to inadequate dietary intake, decreased absorption, or chronic blood loss.

18-27   Answer B

Glucose-6-phosphate dehydrogenase (G6PD) deficiency is an X-linked recessive disorder commonly seen in African American men. It is an enzyme defect that causes episodic hemolytic anemia because of the decreased ability of red blood cells to deal with oxidative stresses. The other disorders listed are not X-linked. Sickle cell anemia is an autosomal recessive disorder in which an abnormal hemoglobin leads to chronic hemolytic anemia with a variety of severe clinical consequences. Pyruvate kinase deficiency is a rare autosomal recessive disorder that causes chronic hemolytic anemia, usually with the onset in childhood. Bernard-Soulier syndrome is a rare autosomal recessive intrinsic platelet disorder causing bleeding.

18-28   Answer C

Immunotherapy is also called biological therapy. It is a form of treatment that uses the body's natural ability (immune system) to fight disease or to protect the body from adverse effects of treatment. Radiation therapy uses high-energy rays to damage cancer cells and prevent them from growing and dividing. Chemotherapy uses drugs to kill cancer cells.

18-29   Answer D

Although drug trials and research and development with new drug products are important ways to work toward eradicating a disease, they do nothing for prevention. The three major approaches to cancer prevention are education, regulation, and host modification. Education reduces the cancer-causing behaviors of individuals, such as smoking. Regulations and guidelines help by prohibiting introduction of carcinogens and include methods such as encouraging nonsmoking areas, not selling cigarettes to minors, and workplace environmental guidelines. Host modification refers to increasing knowledge about cancer genetics. Health-care providers are instrumental in educating the public and sharing decisions that may be made concerning the appropriate use of genetic testing. Colonoscopy is a screening measure aimed at detecting disease, not preventing it. The same is true of a Pap smear.

18-30   Answer A

The provider should always check a lead level before starting iron supplementation in children because an elevated lead level will cause anemia despite a normal iron level. Supplementation can cause iron overload. Regular milk (cow's milk) is often the cause of anemia in children; thus, a thorough diet history must be obtained. Children younger than age 1 year are usually on iron-fortified infant formulas, and when they switch to cow's milk, they do not receive sufficient iron.

18-31   Answer A

Also known as gamma globulin, immunoglobulin (Ig) G (IgG) is the most abundant Ig (75%) found in the blood, lymph, and intestines. IgG is active against bacteria, bacterial toxins, and viruses. IgA (10%–15%) is found in the blood, lymph, saliva, tears, as well as bronchial, gastrointestinal (GI), prostatic, and vaginal secretions. IgA provides local protection on exposed mucous membrane surfaces

and potent antiviral activity by preventing binding of the virus to cells of the respiratory and GI tracts. IgM (5%–10%) is found in the blood and lymph and has high concentrations early in infection, decreasing within about a week. IgD (less than 1%) is found in the blood, lymph, and surfaces of B cells.

18-32   Answer A

Sjögren's syndrome is a multisystem autoimmune disease characterized by dysfunction of the exocrine glands, specifically notable for dry eyes and dry mouth. Treatment is aimed at increasing comfort and lubrication. Artificial tears can be self-administered as needed; preservative-free products are usually better tolerated. For dry mouth, increasing hydration and chewing sugarless gum may be helpful. Rinsing frequently with mouthwash, which contains alcohol, can prove more drying. Oral pilocarpine (Salagen), 5 mg four times a day, and cevimeline (Evoxac), 30 mg three times a day, have been shown to increase saliva production. Drinking milk is not recommended. Frequent removal of earwax is irrelevant to this problem.

18-33   Answer B

This presentation is classic for Hodgkin's lymphoma. Although often seen in younger adults, this disease has a bimodal incidence that peaks at ages 15–35 and over age 50. Pruritus is not uncommon, and up to 40% of clients have low-grade fever with recurrent night sweats. These constitutional symptoms are not as commonly seen in cases of non-Hodgkin's lymphoma. Although supraclavicular nodes may be present in lung cancer, one does not typically see these other symptoms.

18-34   Answer D

Polycythemia vera causes a hyperviscosity of the blood, which leads to decreased cerebral blood flow resulting in the symptoms of tinnitus, lightheadedness, and occasionally stroke and thrombosis. Alkaline phosphatase and serum vitamin B_{12} levels are elevated; leukocytosis and thrombocytosis are also present. Red blood cell mass is elevated, and arterial oxygen saturation is more than 92% (i.e., the erythrocytosis is not secondary to hypoxia).

18-35   Answer C

Palpable supraclavicular lymph nodes are not normal in infants, children, or adults. A right-sided palpable node is more commonly associated with lymphoma of the mediastinum, whereas a palpable left-sided node is more commonly associated with an abdominal malignancy. Different lymph nodes will be palpable in the presence of infectious processes such as candidiasis and cryptococcosis.

18-36 Answer C

Hemophilia is a classic example of an X-linked recessive disease, and as a rule, only males are affected. In rare instances, female carriers are clinically affected if their normal X chromosomes are disproportionately inactivated. Women such as Judy may also become affected if they are the offspring of a father with hemophilia and a mother who is a carrier.

18-37 Answer C

Stage IV in the Rai classification system for chronic lymphatic leukemia (CLL) is the stage of thrombocytopenia where the life expectancy may be only 2 years. CLL is the only leukemia in which a staging system is commonly used because CLL has prognostic implications. A client with only an absolute lymphocytosis (Rai stage 0) may live 7–10 years or more. In the Rai classification system, stage 0 indicates a lymphocyte count greater than 10,000 mm^3, stage I indicates enlarged lymph nodes, stage II indicates an enlarged liver and/or spleen, stage III indicates anemia, and stage IV indicates thrombocytopenia.

18-38 Answer C

A decrease in lymphocytes would be most consistent with immunodeficiency disorders, long-term corticosteroid therapy, or debilitating diseases such as Hodgkin's lymphoma or lupus erythematosus. Lymphocytes are increased primarily in viral infections (hepatitis, infectious mononucleosis, CMV, herpes zoster) and only occasionally in bacterial infections (pertussis, brucellosis). Eosinophils are elevated in parasitic infections such as malaria, trichinosis, and ascariasis.

18-39 Answer A

Infectious mononucleosis is a lymphocytic leukocytosis that may be confused with leukemia and other disorders. The presence of heterophile antibodies (monospot test) in the context of appropriate clinical and hematological findings is diagnostic; false-positive reactions are rare. Atypical lymphocytes usually account for more than 10% of the leukocytes in the peripheral blood smear. Detection of viral capsid antigen antibody IgM (elevated) is the most accurate test confirming acute infection. White blood count may be high, normal, or low; a relative and absolute neutropenia is present in many clients. Thrombocytopenia is common, and an elevated transaminase in most clients is related to hepatic involvement.

18-40 Answer C

Carcinoembryonic antigen is a tumor marker for adenocarcinomas of the colon, lung, breast, ovary, stomach, and pancreas. Prostate-specific antigen (PSA) is the tumor marker for adenocarcinoma of the prostate; calcitonin is the tumor marker for a medullary cancer of the thyroid; and an immunoglobulin test will detect a multiple myeloma.

18-41 Answer D

Prophylaxis for the first episode of *Pneumocystis jiroveci* pneumonia in an adult or adolescent client infected with HIV is trimethoprim-sulfamethoxazole (TMP-SMZ) (Bactrim) DS 1 tablet PO daily for 10 days. Clarithromycin (Biaxin) is the first choice for *Mycobacterium avium* complex infection; rifampin (Rimactane) is the first choice for combating isoniazid-resistant organisms; and isoniazid (Nydrazid) and pyridoxine (Beesix) are the first choices for combating *Mycobacterium tuberculosis* organisms.

18-42 Answer B

Chemotherapy drugs are genotoxic carcinogens. Carcinogens can be classified in two groups: genotoxic and promotional carcinogens. Genotoxic carcinogens directly alter DNA and cause mutations. Other examples of genotoxic carcinogens include polycyclic hydrocarbons (smoke, soot, tobacco), arsenic, and methylaminobenzene. Promotional carcinogens cause other adverse biological effects, such as hormonal imbalances, altered immunity, or chronic tissue damage. Examples include vinyl chloride polymers, asbestos, and wood and leather dust.

18-43 Answer A

Alpha-fetoprotein levels may be elevated with embryonal cell tumors of the ovary or testis, hepatocellular carcinoma, and choriocarcinoma.

Carcinoembryonic antigen detects colon, rectal, pancreatic, stomach, lung, breast, and ovarian tumors. Human chorionic gonadotropin detects choriocarcinoma, germ cell carcinoma, testicular teratoma, and hydatidiform moles. Cancer antigen 125 (CA 125) is the tumor marker for epithelial ovarian neoplasms and breast and colorectal malignancies.

18-44   Answer A

Smoking is not one of the risk factors for iron-deficiency anemia. The risk for iron-deficiency anemia increases in persons older than age 60; those who live in poverty; and those with a recent illness, such as an ulcer, diverticulitis, colitis, hemorrhoids, or gastrointestinal tumors. Iron supplements should be taken.

18-45   Answer B

Pernicious anemia is a macrocytic anemia marked by achlorhydria. The parietal cells of the stomach fail to secrete enough intrinsic factor to ensure intestinal absorption of vitamin B_{12}, the extrinsic factor. This leads to a deficiency of B_{12}. Folic acid deficiency also causes a macrocytic anemia, but the B_{12} levels are normal, and there are not the associated neurological symptoms seen in pernicious anemia. Vitamin D is not essential for the absorption of vitamin B_{12}. A deficiency of iron results in iron-deficiency anemia, a microcytic hypochromic anemia.

18-46   Answer C

Thalassemia is caused by a decreased synthesis of hemoglobin and malformation of red blood cells (RBCs) that increases their hemolysis (increased destruction of RBCs). It is an inherited disorder that occurs primarily in Asians or persons of Mediterranean ancestry. Aplastic anemia is a depression or cessation of all blood-forming elements. An acquired hemolytic disorder is most often drug induced or autoimmune; in such cases antibodies that cause premature destruction of RBCs are produced.

18-47   Answer C

Chronic lymphocytic leukemia (CLL) has an insidious onset with weakness, fatigue, massive lymphadenopathy, pruritic vesicular skin lesions, anemia, and thrombocytopenia. Acute lymphocytic leukemia (ALL) produces fever, respiratory infections, anemia, bleeding mucous membranes, lymphadenopathy, fatigue and weakness, and a tendency to infection. Acute myelogenous leukemia has the same symptoms as ALL but less lymphadenopathy. Chronic myelogenous leukemia produces weakness, fatigue, anorexia, weight loss, splenomegaly, anemia, thrombocytopenia, and fever and can have a fulminant stage.

18-48   Answer D

There are no generally accepted guidelines for the prevention or early detection of bladder cancer. The first problem is usually gross hematuria, followed by dysuria, frequency or urgency, and symptoms of urethral obstruction. Bladder cancer comprises approximately 4%–5% of all cancers in the United States. It is three times more common in men than women and two times more common in whites than blacks. Smoking should be discouraged and exposure to certain chemicals used in the textile and rubber industries eliminated. There is no bladder tumor marker, and annual cystoscopies are not recommended.

18-49   Answer C

Bone pain is a common presenting symptom, most frequently manifested as low back pain or pain in the rib, and may present as a pathological fracture, especially in the femoral neck. Hypercalcemia is often present related to the leakage of calcium occurring from bone destruction. These clients are also prone to infections and fatigue. Examination may reveal pallor, bone tenderness, and soft tissue masses. Splenomegaly is absent unless amyloidosis is present. There is seldom a chronic cough. Nausea may be present related to hyperviscosity syndrome but typically not vomiting.

18-50   Answer C

Routine ordering of a complete blood count (CBC) is not indicated in asymptomatic adults; it should be ordered only when a specific condition is suspected, such as an infection or a hematological disorder. Hemoglobin or hematocrit determination is recommended in pregnant women and high-risk infants, but not necessarily a CBC. There are no current recommendations for healthy adults to have a CBC as part of a routine preadmission or preoperative physical examination if little or no blood loss is anticipated, as is the case in most dental procedures.

18-51   Answer C

A serum measurement of ferritin, the body's iron-storing protein, can tell exactly how much iron is on hand in the body. It is the best way to spot an iron deficiency early before it progresses to full-blown anemia. If the ferritin level is borderline, a dietary and supplemental regimen of iron will rebuild the iron stores. Hemoglobin is the iron-containing pigment of the red blood cells that carries oxygen from the lungs to the tissues. Hematocrit is the volume of erythrocytes packed in a given volume of blood. The hemoglobin and hematocrit values give the values only at a given time, without regard for the body's stores. Reticulocytes are the last immature stage of red blood cells.

18-52   Answer B

Smoking decreases vitamin C absorption, which is necessary for folic acid absorption. Smoking increases vitamin requirements. Clients with a folic acid deficiency should be encouraged to eat foods that are high in folic acid (asparagus spears, beef liver, broccoli, mushrooms, oatmeal, peanut butter, and red beans) daily because the liver can store folic acid for a limited time only.

18-53   Answer C

Lymphedema may occur many years after a mastectomy (whether radical or modified) or radiation therapy on the affected side. Procedures such as venipuncture and blood pressure measurements should never be done on the affected arm because there is a greater risk for infection and compromised wound healing in that limb. About 15%–20% of women develop lymphedema after treatment for breast cancer by surgery or radiation, some not until many years later. Several interventions have been tried with lymphadenopathy, ranging from nothing to aggressive surgical procedures, and have met with limited success. Most interventions include elevation, exercises, and pneumatic compression devices.

18-54   Answer B

Children receiving radiation therapy for acute lymphocytic leukemia are at an increased risk for developing a brain tumor as a secondary malignancy. This has been seen more often in children who were treated with radiation at age 5 or younger. In general, about 3%–12% of children treated for cancer will develop a new cancer within 20 years of being treated for the primary cancer.

18-55   Answer C

Risk factors for the development of acquired thrombophilias in pregnancy include immobilization, an underlying malignancy, trauma, high estrogen levels, nephrotic syndrome, CHF and atrial fibrillation, postoperative states, and pregnancy and postpartum periods. Factor V Leiden, homocystine, protein C, and protein S are all examples of inherited thrombophilias.

18-56   Answer C

Antibody testing may be ordered to determine whether a client has developed antibodies in response to an infection, such as hepatitis, or immunization. Antibody titers evaluate antibody-mediated responses. Serum protein is a measurement of the total protein in the blood. Albumin is a protein primarily responsible for the osmotic pressure of the blood. Globulins account for the majority of remaining serum protein. Globulins include all of the immunoglobulins and the antibodies they contain. Decreased globulin levels are noted with immunological deficiencies. Protein electrophoresis further breaks down globulin into its specific components. Analysis of specific levels of each provides cues about the immune status of the client.

18-57   Answer B

Although anyone can get skin cancer, older adults have an increased risk because of decreased pigment in their skin. People of northern European ancestry with very fair skin, blue or green eyes, and light-colored hair seem to be the most vulnerable to skin cancer, but it is a problem for all people.

18-58   Answer D

With the loss of a body part, there is an initial stage of shock and denial. It is a protective mechanism and should be neither challenged nor promoted. The best response to Nancy, who refuses to look at her mastectomy scar, would be to say: "You have to accept this eventually; just glance at it today." Then every day she could spend a little more time looking at it until she is able to care for the wound herself. Saying, "You'll look at it when you're ready" may mean that she'll never be ready. She should not be forced, but you should take a matter-of-fact approach with an empathetic attitude that will assist in her eventual acceptance of the change in body image. Practitioners should always avoid saying "Everything's going to be OK" because sometimes it is not.

18-59   Answer B

Pernicious anemia is caused by an inadequate absorption of vitamin B$_{12}$. The symptoms of pernicious anemia develop slowly and subtly and may not be recognized right away. In contrast, hemolytic anemias caused by the premature destruction of red blood cells (hemolysis) occur when the bone marrow cannot produce red blood cells fast enough to compensate for those being destroyed. These anemias can be acquired or congenital. Inherited conditions include hereditary spherocytosis, glucose-6-phosphate dehydrogenase deficiency, sickle cell anemia, and thalassemia.

18-60   Answer B

The hemoglobin S gene is carried by approximately 8% of American blacks, and 1 birth in 400 in American blacks will produce a child with sickle cell. Prenatal diagnosis is now available for couples at risk of producing a child with sickle cell. DNA from fetal cells can be examined, and the presence of the sickle cell mutation can be accurately and definitively diagnosed. Genetic counseling should be made available to such couples.

18-61   Answer A

A fever of unknown origin (FUO) in clients with HIV is defined as temperature greater than 101°F on multiple occasions over 4 weeks in an outpatient and over 3 weeks in an inpatient, with an uncertain diagnosis after three appropriate investigations of cultures and the like. Common causes of FUO of clients with HIV include drug fever, tuberculosis, sinusitis, cryptococcosis, lymphoma, histoplasmosis, *Pneumocystis jiroveci* pneumonia (PCP), disseminated cytomegalovirus, esophageal candidiasis, and disseminated *Mycobacterium avium*–intracellular complex. Upper respiratory infection will either resolve and/or become something more severe; likewise, a urinary tract infection has more specific, identifiable, and treatable symptoms. Although the cause of FUO may in some cases never be identified, it is not merely a systemic manifestation of disease but more likely has a specific cause.

18-62   Answer C

The primary reason for newborn screening for sickle cell disease is to allow the prevention of septicemia with prophylactic medication (penicillin) and prompt clinical intervention for infection and future crises. Early detection will not prevent future crises. Although providing information to the parents will allow them to make future decisions and have the benefit of possible genetic testing, as well as testing siblings, this is not the primary reason for early screening.

18-63   Answer C

Growth complications depend on the direct damage to the endocrine tissue. Children with acute lymphocytic leukemia, brain tumors, nasopharyngeal cancers, and orbital tumors who have received radiation therapy are at the highest risk. Approximately 50%–90% of these children will have some evidence of growth hormone deficiency. They may benefit from growth hormone therapy. Spinal radiation inhibits the vertebral body growth. Chemotherapy may result in a decrease in linear growth, but usually the child catches up when the chemotherapy is discontinued. Assuring the mother that "everything will be OK" is always a poor choice, as is negating her concern by saying, "Let's worry about the cancer first, then see what happens."

18-64   Answer D

The spleen is not essential for life. When it is removed, the liver and bone marrow assume the spleen's functions. Although the bone marrow will produce and store hematopoietic stem cells, from which all cellular components of the blood are derived, it will not remove iron from old red blood cells for reuse.

18-65   Answer B

Smoking, diabetes, and a high-fat diet are risk factors for pancreatic cancer. Persons who smoke develop pancreatic cancer two to three times more often than nonsmokers. Diabetes is also a risk factor. Twice as many people with diabetes develop pancreatic cancer compared with people without diabetes. The risk of pancreatic cancer is also higher among people whose diet is high in fat and low in fruits and vegetables. Occupational exposure to petroleum and other chemicals also increases the risk of pancreatic cancer. Although a high-carbohydrate diet and lack of activity may predispose one to obesity, which may lead to diabetes, this has not been documented as a risk factor for pancreatic cancer. Yo-yo dieting is not a documented risk factor.

18-66 Answer B

An endoscopic retrograde cholangiopancreatography uses an endoscope, which is inserted via the mouth and passed by the stomach and into the small intestine, where dye is injected into the pancreatic ducts and x-rays are taken to determine if any obstruction is apparent. A percutaneous transhepatic cholangiography is a procedure in which a thin needle is put into the liver through the skin on the right side of the abdomen. Dye is injected into the bile ducts to visualize any blockages. An angiography is a procedure in which x-rays are taken of the blood vessels after dye is injected. An upper gastrointestinal series is a series of x-rays of the upper digestive system taken after barium is ingested. It shows the outline of the digestive organs. All four of these procedures are used to produce pictures of the pancreas and nearby organs to assist in the diagnosis of pancreatic cancer.

18-67 Answer C

All infants should be screened for anemia using either hemoglobin or hematocrit testing at approximately 9 months of age. The cutoff points for a diagnosis of anemia at this age are a hemoglobin below 11 g/dL or a hematocrit below 33%. Cutoff points should be adjusted upward for children who live at high altitudes. You should consider repeat screening at age 3–4 years. Cutoff points for children this age are a hemoglobin of 11.2 g/dL or a hematocrit of 34%.

18-68 Answer B

A platelet count less than 150,000/mm³ may indicate hypersplenism as well as possible bone marrow failure or accelerated consumption of platelets. A count greater than 350,000/mm³ may indicate hemorrhage, polycythemia vera, or malignancy.

18-69 Answer C

Pain in one breast in postmenopausal women is highly suggestive of a malignant process, despite past personal and/or family history. Additionally, you know that age 64 puts this client at a high risk of occurrence of breast cancer. You send her for a mammogram as soon as possible, even if she has had one less than a year before that was negative.

18-70 Answer C

Hepatitis D (delta) virus (HDV) poses the greatest risk to a client with chronic hepatitis B (chronic HBV). Chronic HBV carriers who acquire HDV infection have a much higher incidence of cirrhosis, approaching 70%–80% compared with a 15%–30% chance of liver cirrhosis with chronic HBV alone. Modes of transmission for HDV are similar to those of HBV.

18-71 Answer C

Sandra's symptoms indicate anemia, which is probably caused by a poor diet. She probably has an iron and folic acid deficiency. You should order iron, folic acid, and other supplements and tell her that for better absorption, she should take the iron supplement 1 hour before eating or between meals. You should also suggest that she eat foods high in vitamin C, such as citrus fruits and fresh, raw vegetables, because vitamin C makes iron absorption more efficient. Iron also will turn bowel movements black and often cause constipation, so you may want to discuss this with Sandra.

18-72 Answer D

The reticulocyte count indicates the percentage of newly maturing red blood cells released into the circulating blood from the bone marrow. As the red blood cell (RBC) matures, it loses its endothelial reticulum. The reticulocyte count is elevated in cases of blood loss, as the body tries to replace the loss; it might also be elevated during treatment of anemias (e.g., iron, folic acid, vitamin B_{12}), and bone marrow disorders, when immature RBCs are displaced by other proliferating cells. It is decreased in aplastic anemia because the bone marrow has shut down all production of cells; it is also decreased in poisonings and disorders of red blood cell maturation such as iron-deficiency anemias.

18-73 Answer D

Acquired inhibitors of coagulation are found in women who are several weeks postpartum after a normal labor and delivery, in clients with collagen vascular disease such as systemic lupus erythematosus, in older clients, and in clients with known inherited coagulation disorders, particularly factor VIII deficiency. There is no evidence that this is associated with mitral regurgitation, antibiotic usage, or as a sequela to a streptococcal infection.

18-74   Answer A

It is important to maintain an adequate fluid intake to prevent dehydration, which may result in vomiting; therefore, decreasing the amount of liquids in the client's diet is not an effective strategy to prevent the nausea and vomiting associated with the effects of radiation and chemotherapy. Causes of nausea and vomiting include the effects of radiation and chemotherapy, obstruction of the gastrointestinal tract by tumor growth and metastasis, other metabolic abnormalities, and stress. Nausea and vomiting should be expected and anticipatory antiemetic therapy initiated before treatment and continued around the clock after starting the cancer treatment according to the anticipated length of symptoms. It can then be used on an as-needed basis. A soft, bland diet low in fat and sugar, as well as relaxation, distraction, and guided imagery, help to reduce the adverse effects of nausea and vomiting.

18-75   Answer C

Clients with hepatitis A should have separate eating and drinking utensils or use disposable ones. Most clients can be cared for at home without undue risk; strict isolation is not necessary. There is no specific medicine to treat hepatitis A.

18-76   Answer A

If your client has numerous petechiae, ask about the use of aspirin or aspirin compounds. Aspirin is a very effective antiplatelet agent. The recommended dosage for clients with chronic stable angina and certain other conditions is 325 mg (one tablet) per day. Many clients assume that if one tablet a day is good, two are better. Depending on the individual clotting time, even 325 mg per day may result in bleeding into the tissues. Antihypertensive agents, oral contraceptives, and anticonvulsants by themselves do not affect platelet activity.

18-77   Answer A

Clients with sickle cell anemia should have their hemoglobin and hematocrit levels maintained at a level slightly below normal because this protects from some of the vaso-occlusive infarctive

complications related to the viscosity characteristic of sickle cell anemia. When there is a painful sickle cell crisis, the client should be placed at rest, hydrated, given oral analgesics, and have the blood alkalinized mildly with an intravenous bicarbonate solution. Oxygen should be given to keep the hemoglobin well oxygenated, and the amount of deoxyhemoglobin must be kept low.

18-78   Answer D

A metastatic tumor from below the diaphragm is suspected when you palpate Virchow's node in the left supraclavicular space. Virchow's node is an enlarged left supraclavicular node usually infiltrated with a metastatic tumor from below the diaphragm, especially of gastrointestinal origin. The other nodes listed do not exist. A wringer-type injury is seen in children who put their hands between the rollers of older washing machines still in use. Sims' position is a side-lying position, and Wiskott-Aldrich syndrome is a childhood immunodeficiency disease.

18-79   Answer D

Clients with sickle cell anemia should be given folic acid 1 mg PO daily. Genetic counseling, not early sterilization, is recommended for all clients with sickle cell disease; there is no routine risk in the use of oral contraceptives by women with the disease.

18-80   Answer B

The most common signs and symptoms of primary HIV infection and their frequency are fever (95%), fatigue (90%), and pharyngitis (70%).

18-81   Answer B

One of the most commonly used staging systems to label the extent of a cancer is the TNM staging system. The T is for primary tumor, N is for regional lymph nodes, and M is for distant metastasis. In an example of colorectal cancer, a person classified as T1N1M0 would have a tumor that invaded the submucosa, metastasis in one to three pericolic or perirectal lymph nodes, but no distant metastasis.

18-82   Answer A

An isograft is a transplant in which the donor and recipient are identical twins. An autograft is a transplant of the client's own tissue; it is the most successful type of tissue transplant. An allograft is a graft between members of the same species, but who have different genotypes and, in the case of humans, human leukocyte antigens. A xenograft is a transplant from an animal species to a human, such as pigskin used as a temporary covering after a massive burn.

18-83   Answer D

Alcohol acts as a promoter by modifying the metabolism of carcinogens in the esophagus and liver, thereby increasing the effectiveness of the carcinogens in some tissues. Because Shelley smoked cigarettes and drank alcohol, she has an increased risk for oral, esophageal, and laryngeal cancers.

18-84   Answer B

The Centers for Disease Control and Prevention guidelines state that if a woman infected with HIV has a normal initial Pap test, then a second evaluation should be done in 6 months to reduce the likelihood of a false-negative initial test. If the initial two Pap smears are both negative, annual Pap smears are then adequate. If severe inflammation with reactive squamous cellular change is found, another Pap smear should be done within 3 months.

18-85   Answer D

Cancers with macroscopic disease that can be cured with chemotherapy include testicular and ovarian cancer and Hodgkin's disease. Bladder and breast cancers are cancers with microscopic disease that can be cured with adjuvant chemotherapy. A malignant melanoma has a low response rate or can be unresponsive to chemotherapy.

18-86   Answer C

Lorie has the classic signs of iron-deficiency anemia: pale conjunctiva and nailbeds, tachycardia, heart murmur, cheilosis (reddened lips with fissures at the angles), stomatitis, splenomegaly, koilonychia (thin and concave fingernails with raised edges), glossitis, esophageal webs (Plummer-Vinson syndrome), melena, and menorrhagia. Signs of vitamin B_{12} deficiency include weakness of the extremities, ataxia, pallor, loss of vibratory and position sense, memory loss, changes in mood, and hallucinations. Signs of a folate deficiency include weakness, pallor, and glossitis, with congestive heart failure occurring if the anemia is severe. A person with chronic fatigue syndrome might have a fever, a sore throat, muscle discomfort and myalgia, and generalized headaches.

18-87   Answer C

Abdominal pain, pallor, and tachycardia are all manifestations of splenic sequestration. Early recognition of splenic sequestration can be a lifesaving skill. Parents can be taught to recognize signs of increasing anemia and enlarging spleen. Part of the educational plan for the parent is teaching them how to recognize increasing abdominal girth or abdominal pain, as well as how to palpate the spleen. Vomiting and diarrhea do not necessarily accompany this complication, nor does a decrease in mental acuity.

18-88   Answer A

Generalized lymphadenopathy is usually indicative of disseminated malignancy, usually hematological in nature (such as lymphoma or leukemia), collagen vascular disease, or an infectious process such as mononucleosis, syphilis, cytomegalovirus, tuberculosis, AIDS, toxoplasmosis, to name some examples.

18-89   Answer C

Persons who are obese have an increased risk of hormone-dependent cancers because of their excessive body fat. Because sex hormones are synthesized from fat, these people have excessive amounts of the hormones that feed hormone-dependent malignancies such as cancer of the breast, bowel, ovary, endometrium, and prostate.

18-90   Answer C

The most significant reason alcohol use is discouraged in persons with HIV infections or AIDS is that alcohol decreases the ability of persons to adhere to a prescribed medical regimen. Current treatment regimens involve complex pharmacological schedules with accurate dosing, strict compliance, and regular checkups that are crucial to the success of the treatment and prevention of complications. Alcohol calories are empty and also fill up the person so that he or she may not eat essential food. If the client has liver disease (which may have been caused by alcohol), it may be aggravated by the potentially hepatotoxic effects of various drugs that are commonly used.

18-91   Answer D

An increase in immunoglobulin (Ig) E signifies atopic disorders such as allergic rhinitis, allergic asthma, atopic dermatitis, and parasitic infestation. An increase of IgG may signify bacterial infections, hepatitis A, glomerulonephritis, rheumatoid arthritis, systemic lupus erythematosus (SLE), and AIDS. An increase in IgM would occur with hepatitis A and B infections, chronic infections, SLE, rheumatoid arthritis, Sjögren's syndrome, and AIDS. An increase in IgA would occur with SLE, rheumatoid arthritis, glomerulonephritis, and chronic liver disease.

18-92   Answer C

The mean survival time for people with sickle cell disease in the United States is 42 years for men and 48 for women.

18-93   Answer B

Pain that is poorly controlled with opioids and NSAIDs is often neuropathic in nature, meaning that it is a result of direct nerve injury, such as nerve compression. This pain may be controlled with anticonvulsants, tricyclic antidepressants, and corticosteroids. Corticosteroids may also be effective for severe bone pain. SSRIs have not had the proven results with neuropathic pain that tricyclics have, although they may prove effective in clients with cancer in general. Benzodiazepines are not usually recommended because of their sedativelike effects. The goal with cancer clients who experience chronic pain is to provide adequate pain control while keeping the client awake and able to interact with those around them and maintain as normal a life as possible.

18-94   Answer B

Eosinophils are elevated in parasitic infections, hypersensitivity reactions, and autoimmune disorders. Neutrophils are increased in acute infections, the stress response, myelocytic leukemia, and inflammatory or metabolic disorders. Basophils are increased in hypersensitivity responses, chronic myelogenous leukemia, chickenpox or smallpox, after a splenectomy, and in hypothyroidism. Monocytes are increased in chronic inflammatory disorders, tuberculosis, viral infections, leukemia, Hodgkin's disease, and multiple myeloma.

18-95   Answer C

Fecal occult blood testing (FOBT) is accurate in identifying 25%–40% of colorectal cancers, specifically those in the sigmoid colon. It is less effective for identifying cancers of the right colon or transverse colon. It is not effective for identifying polyps. Persons older than age 40 should have an annual stool examination performed because this can help decrease colorectal cancer mortality rates by 33%–57%. FOBT has a false-negative and a false-positive possibility. Certain medications such as aspirin and other NSAIDs, eating red meat or raw vegetables, or bleeding hemorrhoids may cause a false-positive reading. These medications and foods should be avoided for 3 days before the administration of the test. False-negative results may occur because of polyps or the fact that some cancers do not bleed or may bleed only occasionally.

18-96   Answer C

The classic signs and symptoms of cytomegalovirus infection include cotton-wool spots ("cottage cheese and ketchup" appearance), hemorrhage, and exudates on funduscopic examination. Decreased peripheral vision, blurriness, and partial blindness are other clinical manifestations. Referral to an ophthalmologist is imperative. Cryptococcosis is a systemic fungus infection that may involve any organ of the body, including the lungs or skin, but it has a marked predilection for the brain and its meninges. In the cerebral type, headache, dizziness, vertigo, and stiffness of the neck muscles are present. Toxoplasmosis produces symptoms that may be so mild as to be barely noticeable or may be more severe and include lymphadenopathy, malaise, muscle pain, or little, if any, fever. It may result in brain deterioration. Herpes simplex is characterized by thin-walled vesicles that tend to recur in the same area, usually at a site where the mucous membrane joins the skin; however, they may be limited to the gingiva, oropharynx, or conjunctiva.

18-97   Answer C

Before initiating cancer therapy, the first crucial step is to confirm the diagnosis using tissue biopsy. This sounds simplistic, but some practitioners "diagnose" unconfirmed cancer that cannot then be effectively treated. The next step is to stage the disease using appropriate diagnostic means. The stage or the extent of the disease determines the prognosis and treatment. The third step is to define the goals of therapy— whether it is curative, adjuvant, or palliative—because that will influence the extent and aggressiveness of treatment. The last step before initiating therapy is to choose a treatment plan from the many therapeutic options, depending on many different client characteristics such as age, goals, wishes of the client and family, and extent of the cancer.

18-98   Answer D

An elevated hematocrit due to contracted plasma volume, rather than increased red blood cell mass, may be due to diuretic use or may occur without obvious cause. However, the associated signs and symptoms of splenomegaly, blurred vision, fatigue, headache, and tinnitus lead you to suspect polycythemia vera. An elevated hematocrit due to contracted plasma volume is often called *spurious polycythemia*, and a number of conditions such as hypoxia and high altitude exposure can cause a secondary polycythemia, but splenomegaly is absent in these cases. Primary polycythemia vera is an acquired myeloproliferative disorder that causes an overproduction of all three hemapoietic cell lines. In multiple myeloma, there is a malignancy of the plasma cells, not typically characterized with an elevated hematocrit. Waldenström's macroglobulinemia is a malignant disorder of B cells that appear to be a hybrid of lymphocytes and plasma cells; these cells characteristically secrete an IgM paraprotein, and the disorder does not manifest itself with an elevated hematocrit.

18-99   Answer C

When clients with HIV infection have massive diarrhea, a protozoa of the *Cryptosporidium* genus is the most likely cause. The organism affects primarily the small intestine and produces massive diarrhea accompanied by nausea and fatigue. The diarrhea may exceed 4 L/day and can easily lead to dehydration and electrolyte imbalance if not treated promptly. Cryptococcosis is a fungal infection that usually appears as meningitis. Toxoplasmosis is a protozoal infection that causes encephalitis in persons with AIDS. Cytomegalovirus is a significant opportunistic infection of the herpesvirus family that can be acquired during the perinatal period, in the preschool years, or during the sexually active years.

18-100   Answer A

Burkitt's lymphoma is associated with Epstein-Barr virus. Kaposi's sarcoma is associated with human cytomegalovirus, a lymphoma is associated with the human herpesvirus 6, and adult T-cell leukemia is associated with human T-lymphotropic viruses.

18-101   Answer D

Skip has the characteristic symptoms of acute lymphoblastic leukemia. Diagnosis is made by the characteristic appearance found on a bone marrow smear. The enzyme-linked immunosorbent assay is the best test for rotavirus infection because it detects viral antigens. The monospot test is a latex agglutination test that measures production of heterophile antibodies during acute and recent episodes of Epstein-Barr virus infection. Its use is limited because of false-negative readings of 10%–20%. A prothrombin time, partial thromboplastin time, bleeding time, complete blood count, and peripheral smear are included in an initial work-up of bleeding disorders.

18-102   Answer D

The Schilling test is performed by giving a small, radioactive tracer dose of cyanocobalamin (about 0.5–2 mg) by mouth and then collecting and assaying a 24-hour urine sample for radioactivity. This is diagnostic of cobalamin deficiency (vitamin B_{12} deficiency). Coombs' tests ascertain the presence or absence of immunoglobulin and complement in the coating of red blood cells. The tests (direct and indirect) can differentiate between various types of hemolytic anemias; determine minor blood types, including the Rh factor; and test for erythroblastosis fetalis. The oligonucleotide probe test is a method used to diagnose antenatal thalassemia. Spherocytes are round, rather than discoid, cells.

18-103   Answer D

A decreased MCV and MCHC is indicative of a microcytic, hypochromic anemia. To make a more final diagnosis, you need to order both a serum iron and total iron binding capacity (TIBC) level and a serum ferritin level. You would order a folate level if you had an elevated MCV and a normal MCHC, indicative of macrocytic anemia.

18-104   Answer B

A chondrosarcoma arises from cartilage and is usually located in the pelvis, femur, proximal humerus, or ribs. It is the second-most common bone malignancy, seen most frequently in men between ages 30 and 60. An osteosarcoma is the most common primary bone-forming tumor, usually affecting children and young adults. It arises from osteoblast cells that multiply rapidly during periods of skeletal growth. More common in men, osteosarcomas are usually located around the knee joint, with the proximal humerus also being a common site. Ewing's sarcoma is a marrow-originating tumor consisting of small round cells. It is seen primarily in male children and adolescents. It arises most commonly in the diaphysis of long bones and in flat bones. A fibrosarcoma is a rare type of bone tumor that consists of interlacing bundles of collagen cells. It is more common in men ages 20–60 and is commonly found in the femur and tibia.

18-105   Answer C

An immune complex–mediated hypersensitivity reaction results in a skin test that produces erythema and edema within 3–8 hours. It may result from serum sickness, systemic lupus erythematosus, or rheumatoid arthritis. An anaphylactic reaction may occur with allergic rhinitis or asthma. The mediator of injury is histamine and the skin test appears as a wheal and flare. A cytotoxic reaction, such as a transfusion reaction, does not produce any reaction from a skin test. A delayed hypersensitivity (cell-mediated) reaction, such as contact dermatitis or after a tuberculosis test, produces erythema and edema within 24–48 hours.

18-106   Answer D

MCV indicates the average size of individual RBCs. Normal range, also referred to as normocytic, is 76–96 femtoliters. The MCV is increased (macrocytic) in megaloblastic anemias (vitamin B_{12} deficiency, folate deficiency), liver disease (alcohol abuse), and some drugs (e.g., zidovudine). The MCV is decreased (microcytic) in iron-deficiency anemia, defects in porphyrin synthesis (lead poisoning), and hemolytic anemias.

18-107   Answer D

A folic acid and/or vitamin B_{12} deficiency causes macrocytic normochromic anemias in which the cell size is large and irregular. Acute blood loss and most hemolytic processes cause normocytic normochromic anemias in which the cell size is normal. Infections or tumor may cause an anemia of chronic disease that produces a normocytic red blood cell. Iron-deficiency anemias are hypochromic microcytic and may result from dietary insufficiencies as well as acute blood loss.

18-108   Answer B

In the American Cancer Society's CAUTION model to help individuals be alert to many cancers, the C is for change in bowel or bladder habits, the A is for a sore that does not heal, the U is for unusual bleeding or discharge, the T is for thickening or lump in the breast or elsewhere, the I is for indigestion or difficulty in swallowing, the O is for obvious change in wart or mole, and the N is for nagging cough or hoarseness.

18-109   Answer D

Steroid hormones (androgens, such as fluoxymesterone [Halotestin]; estrogens, such as ethinyl estradiol [Estinyl]; and progestins, such as megestrol acetate [Megace]) are useful in cancer chemotherapy because they alter the host environment for cell growth. Antibiotics, such as doxorubicin (Adriamycin) and bleomycin (Blenoxane), interfere with DNA or RNA synthesis depending on the drug. Alkylating agents, such as chlorambucil (Leukeran) and melphalan (Alkeran), interfere with DNA replication by attacking DNA synthesis throughout the cell cycle. Other agents, such as asparaginase (Elspar) and cisplatin (Platinol), inhibit protein synthesis.

18-110   Answer C

Radiation therapy consists of delivering ionizing radiations of gamma and x-rays in one of two ways. In brachytherapy, radioactive material is placed directly into a tumor site and delivers a high dose to the tumor and a lower dose to the normal surrounding tissues. It is also called internal, interstitial, or intracavitary radiation. Teletherapy is external radiation that involves placing the source of radiation at a distance from the client and delivering a relatively uniform dosage. Radiotherapy is another name for radiation therapy. Ionization involves the passage of radioactive particles.

Bibliography

AIDS Education and Training Centers (AETC): Opportunistic infection prophylaxis: Guide for HIV/AIDS clinical care. HRSA HIV/AIDS Bureau, January 2011. www.aidsetc.org/aidsetc?page=cg-306_oi_prophylaxis.

Dambro, MR: *Griffith's 5-Minute Consult.* Lippincott, Williams & Wilkins, Philadelphia, 2011.

Dunphy, LM, et al: *Primary Care: The Art and Science of Advanced Practice Nursing,* ed 3. FA Davis, Philadelphia, 2011.

Gates, RA, and Fink, RM: *Oncology Nursing Secrets*, ed 3. Hanley & Belfus, Philadelphia, 2007.

Goolsby, MJ: *Nurse Practitioner Secrets*. Hanley & Belfus, Philadelphia, 2002.

Goolsby MJ, and Grubbs, L: *Advanced Assessment: Interpreting Findings and Formulating Differential Diagnoses*. FA Davis, Philadelphia, 2006.

Hay, WW, et al: *Current Pediatric Diagnosis and Treatment*. Appleton & Lange, Stamford, CT, 2008.

Lin, TL, and Rypkema, SW: *The Washington Manual of Ambulatory Therapeutics*. Lippincott, Williams & Wilkins, Philadelphia, 2008.

Mangione, S: *Physical Diagnosis Secrets* ed 2. Hanley & Belfus, Philadelphia, 2007.

Piccini, JP, and Nilsson, K: *The Osler Medical Handbook*, ed 2. Mosby, Philadelphia, 2006.

Speicher, CE: *The Right Test: A Physician's Guide to Laboratory Medicine*, ed 4. WB Saunders, Philadelphia, 2007.

Swartz, MH: *Textbook of Physical Diagnoses: History and Examination*, ed 6. Saunders/Elsevier, Philadelphia, 2011

Tallia, AF, et al: *Swanson's Family Practice Review*, ed 4. Mosby, St. Louis, 2001.

Taylor, RB: *Manual of Family Practice*, ed 2. Little, Brown, Boston, 2002.

Tierney, LM, McPhee, SJ, and Papadakis, MA (eds): *2011 eCurrent Medical Diagnosis and Treatment (CMDT)*, ed 47. Lange Medical Books/McGraw Hill, New York, 2011.

Varricchio, C (ed): *A Cancer Source Book for Nurses*. American Cancer Society/Jones and Bartlett, Sudbury, MA, 2003.

Weber, J, and Kelley, J: *Health Assessment in Nursing*, ed 3. Lippincott, Williams & Wilkins, Philadelphia, 2007.

How well did you do?

85% and above, congratulations! This score shows application of test-taking principles and adequate content knowledge.

75%–85%, keep working! Review test-taking principles and try again.

65%–75%, hang in there! Spend some time reviewing concepts and test-taking principles and try the test again.

ISSUES IN PRIMARY CARE

Chapter 19: *Issues in Primary Care*

Lynne M. Dunphy
Jill E. Winland-Brown
Karen Rugg

Questions

19-1 *What factors primarily determine the ability of an Advanced Practice Registered Nurse (APRN) to obtain clinical privileges in an institution?*

A. The desires of the collaborating physician

B. Education, certification, and continuing education credits

C. Institutional policy, medical staff bylaws, state law, and Joint Commission on Accreditation of Healthcare Organizations accreditation standards

D. Reimbursement and prescriptive privileges

19-2 *In the outpatient office setting, the most common reason for a malpractice suit is failure to*

A. properly refer.

B. diagnose correctly in a timely fashion.

C. obtain informed consent.

D. manage fractures and trauma correctly.

19-3 *The primary nursing responsibility during a crisis situation is to*

A. provide for psychotherapeutic intervention.

B. refer.

C. establish a therapeutic relationship.

D. encourage hospitalization.

19-4 *What is the best way to monitor compliance?*

A. Obtain drug levels.

B. Use clinical judgment.

C. Ask the client.

D. Monitor the responses to treatment.

19-5 *To reinforce client teaching, a useful strategy is to*

A. model or demonstrate the desired behavior.

B. have repeated discussions of the need for behavioral change.

C. provide additional written materials.

D. quiz the client periodically while monitoring the client's progress.

19-6 *Concrete strategies used to keep your client's attention as you institute client education include*

A. providing the education session immediately after lunch.

B. going over the materials more than once.

C. translating theoretical information into practical terms.

D. using repetition.

19-7 *Legal authority for advanced-practice nursing rests with*

A. the Health Care Financing Administration.

B. federal statutes.

C. state laws and regulations.

D. certifying bodies.

19-8 *Which of the following statements is true regarding the consultative aspects of the APRN role?*

A. The APRN provides an ongoing supportive and educational relationship to a more junior clinician.

B. The problem is identified by the clinician who then may decide to call in a consultant, a recognized expert, and a nonhierarchical relationship ensues or is established.

C. The APRN consultant assumes responsibility for the client once he or she is called into a clinical situation.

D. The person who has contracted with the consultant must take the recommendations of the APRN consultant.

19-9 *When caring for a client who speaks a language different than yours, the ideal strategy is to*

A. use gestures to convey the meaning of words and use a foreign-language dictionary of medical terms.

B. rely on family members to interpret.

C. review the case first with an interpreter before beginning the clinical visit.

D. use a pad and pencil to pass information back and forth with an interpreter.

19-10   Some sources suggest that you create a marketing portfolio with documents that support what you have to offer as an APRN. These documents include

A. your personal mission statement.

B. your scores on the certification examination or your college transcript.

C. the state nurse practice act and regulations, prescriptive authority legislation, third-party reimbursement rules and regulations, and practice protocols.

D. letters of reference.

19-11   According to the Joint Commission on Accreditation of Healthcare Organizations, decisions regarding policy and client care should be made based on

A. experience.

B. clinical expertise.

C. consultation and collaboration.

D. research findings.

19-12   Which of the following statements related to statistical techniques and their usage in research is true?

A. Statistical significance and clinical significance are the same.

B. If a journal article you are writing is required to be limited in length, you should delete the descriptive statistics and keep the inferential statistics.

C. Correlational coefficients infer causality.

D. To determine the appropriate statistical test to use, consider sample size, level of measurement, and data type.

19-13   According to the health belief model, motivation, or readiness to act, is determined by which of the following components?

A. Perceived threat, efficacy, benefits of action, and perceived barriers to action

B. Education and positive reinforcement

C. Predisposing factors, reinforcing factors, and enabling factors

D. Self-efficacy theory and perceived ability to act

19-14   The Agency for Healthcare Research and Quality (AHRQ) was established to

A. mandate treatment protocols.

B. dictate health-care policy based on voluminous research.

C. promote evidence-based practice.

D. develop cost-effective interventions.

19-15   The primary purpose of an institutional review board is to

A. protect human subjects.

B. evaluate the scientific merit of proposed research.

C. oversee and coordinate the research efforts of an institution.

D. oversee and coordinate the research efforts of an individual.

19-16   The primary purpose of professional licensure is to

A. protect the public by ensuring a minimum standard for competency.

B. ensure high nursing care standards.

C. standardize nursing programs.

D. grant prescriptive privileges.

19-17   There are advantages to owning your own practice. However, there are also barriers to the ability to do this. These barriers include which of the following?

A. Getting and keeping a collaborative physician if required by law, getting on managed care panels, and getting privileges at hospitals

B. Getting privileges in hospitals, getting referrals from hospital emergency departments, and lack of knowledge

C. Inability to find a collaborating physician, inability to find clients, and lack of empathy

D. Lack of legal authority to admit clients to nursing homes, to order home care, and to direct hospice services; lack of ability to manage client care without clear medical oversight and supervision

19-18   The best way in which you, as an individual APRN, can make a difference or true impact is by

A. reading about issues in the newspaper.

B. writing letters to the editor supporting APRNs.

C. thinking positively about the work you do.

D. supporting a Democratic candidate.

19-19   Schedule IV drugs include which of the following?

A. Morphine, codeine, fentanyl, and hydromorphone

B. Depressants such as alprazolam, clonazepam, diazepam, and flurazepam

C. Amphetamines and pentobarbital

D. Methaqualone

19-20   "Advanced-practice nurse" refers to

A. nurse practitioners, physician assistants, and nurse anesthetists, on the basis of CMS (Centers for Medicare and Medicaid) reimbursement practices.

B. nurse practitioners, nurse anesthetists, clinical nurse specialists, and nurse midwives.

C. only nurse practitioners.

D. clinical nurse specialists, nurse midwives, and nurse anesthetists.

19-21   According to standards of care and legal prescribing, which of the following questions must you ask each client before prescribing any medication?

A. Are you breastfeeding? Are you allergic to any medications? Are you pregnant? Have you taken this medication before? Do you have kidney or liver problems? What other medications are you taking? What medical problems do you have?

B. Are you allergic to any medications?

C. What other medications are you on?

D. Have you taken this medication before?

19-22   Ethical responsibilities of the nurse practitioner as employee include

A. protecting the employer's "trade secrets," such as client mailing lists, and remaining unimpaired by drugs or alcohol.

B. advertising the practice using one's own funds.

C. never indulging in any criticism of the practice regardless of the circumstances.

D. attempting to promote the role of the nurse practitioner above all else.

19-23   An emancipated minor is a client who is younger than age 18 but who is considered a competent adult with the authority to accept or refuse medical treatment. How do you determine if the 16-year-old you are seeing is an "emancipated minor"?

A. No one age 16 would be defined as an emancipated minor.

B. Although definitions vary among states, the term usually implies that the minor has entered into a valid marriage, is a member of the military, or has been granted this status by a court.

C. The client claims that he is free from all parental control.

D. The client is accompanied by an older friend who states that he or she will accept legal responsibility and is the client's "guardian."

19-24   Indemnity insurer *refers to an insurer*

A. in a health maintenance organization.

B. in a preferred provider organization.

C. that pays for the medical care of the insured but does not provide that care.

D. that pays using a fee-for-service plan.

19-25   "Do not resuscitate" orders are decided by the

A. physician.

B. health-care facility.

C. physician in consultation with the client, family, or surrogate decision maker.

D. interdisciplinary health-care team.

19-26   The stages of grief include

A. shock, reality, and recovery.

B. awareness and resolution.

C. numbness, loss, and reawakening.

D. pain and loss.

19-27 *Motivational interviewing is a technique that can be useful in implementing behavior change because it*

A. gets clients to do what you want them to do.

B. assists clients to acknowledge and verbalize the change(s) they need to make.

C. helps the practitioner determine what motivates them to help others.

D. dictates a list of tasks or steps a client must take to create change.

19-28 *The purpose of a block grant is to*

A. provide more comprehensive services for Medicaid recipients.

B. encourage individuals to obtain their own health insurance so that they will not need government assistance.

C. allow states to have greater flexibility in providing services to the poor.

D. decrease the proportion of state taxes that are allocated to paying for Medicare.

19-29 *You are seeing your client for the first time, and he says, "I like that you are a physician assistant." You tell him that you are a nurse practitioner, and he asks you how they are different. Your best answer is*

A. the nurse practitioner has much more training than the physician assistant.

B. nurse practitioners can't practice independently.

C. physician assistants do not have the breadth of knowledge that nurse practitioners have.

D. Physician assistants are health-care professionals who are authorized by the state to practice medicine under the license of a physician, whereas the nurse practitioner has an independent base of knowledge—advanced nursing knowledge—and independent licensure to practice.

19-30 *The type of health-care delivery system that allows the client the greatest freedom of choice is a*

A. health maintenance organization.

B. preferred provider organization.

C. managed care plan.

D. fee-for-service plan.

19-31 *The majority of Medicaid enrollees are*

A. young women and children.

B. unemployed, homeless clients.

C. older adults.

D. clients with a disability.

19-32 *The research function of the APRN may be operationalized as both a consumer of research findings and a researcher. Being a consumer of research findings involves a number of activities, including*

A. reading the literature, analyzing its clinical applicability, and using new interventions.

B. organizing and conducting a research study.

C. collecting data.

D. ensuring protection of human subjects.

19-33 *The marketing process is guided by a number of factors. These include*

A. the prospective pool of clients.

B. your advertising budget and what you have to offer.

C. cost, benefit, and barriers.

D. product, price, place, and promotion.

19-34 *Goals and objectives for* Healthy People 2020 *include*

A. improving access to health care for all Americans, increasing the life span for all Americans, and mandatory emergency care.

B. instituting a nationalized health insurance plan.

C. reducing disparities in health care, increasing healthy life span, and increasing access to health care for all Americans.

D. preserving choice of provider and health-care plans for all Americans.

19-35 *What is a strategy that can help to foster client compliance?*

A. In-depth client education

B. Frequency of medication dosing

C. Providing positive feedback and reinforcement

D. Performing serum drug levels to assess therapeutic range

19-36 *It is important to prepare for your interview as an APRN. You should be prepared to answer which of the following?*

A. How old you are and how many children you have because your child-care responsibilities might affect how you are able to do your job

B. Whether you are prepared to advertise the practice from your own funds as well as other things that you can bring to the practice

C. What you can bring to the practice and whether you will be able to see clients in a 10–15 minute block of time to make yourself revenue producing

D. Why you should be hired, how many clients per day you will see, what you can bring to the practice, your willingness to work evenings and/or weekends and to take calls, and how independent you are in your practice

19-37 *Sally, an APRN, sees Mr. Bell, who is suffering from congestive heart failure. She increases his diuretic but makes no note of his potassium and orders no replacement potassium. Mr. Bell returns a week later for routine laboratory testing. His potassium level is found to be low; however, Mr. Bell has no complaints. Sally orders a potassium supplement to begin immediately and a follow-up potassium level measurement. Is Sally guilty of malpractice?*

A. Yes, because she breached the standard of care

B. No, because no harm came to the client

C. No, because she took remedial action

D. Yes, because she was negligent

19-38 *As an APRN, you begin a new job in a small practice with two other physicians. You have been hired to be a partner in the practice, but the eldest partner is reluctant to allow you to take on new clients. This is an example of*

A. role stress.

B. role strain.

C. role insufficiency.

D. role conflict.

19-39 *You are attempting to elicit a history from Mr. Barnes during his first visit to your office. He is becoming increasingly angry and belligerent. He says, "Can't you hurry up? Dr. Smith never takes this long! Why are all these questions necessary?" You respond,*

A. "I'm sorry, Mr. Barnes, but I need these questions answered."

B. "I want to provide the best possible care for you, Mr. Barnes."

C. "Perhaps your wife can assist with some of these questions."

D. "You seem very upset, Mr. Barnes. Could you share with me what is bothering you?"

19-40 *Credentialing means that*

A. an individual is permitted to practice advanced-practice nursing.

B. the practitioner has met certain criteria through licensure, certification, and education.

C. an individual has completed a program of study.

D. an individual has prescriptive authority.

19-41 *Which of the following is the best method for evaluating the efficacy of a new clinical intervention?*

A. A case report

B. A descriptive study

C. A randomized, controlled clinical trial

D. A correlational study

19-42 *According to the Center for Medicare and Medicaid Services (CMS), one of core reasons for the adoption of the electronic health record is to*

A. increase computer literacy among health care professionals.

B. allow all health professionals access to a client record.

C. reduce the incidence of medical error by improving the accuracy and clarity of medical records.

D. speed up client charting.

19-43 *Mrs. Smith, age 85, lost her husband 6 months ago. Since that time, she has been overwhelmed and has had difficulty coping. Today, she is in your office, tearful, weak, and discouraged. Her mobility is also becoming increasingly limited because of her need for a hip replacement. She is indecisive, expresses fear about the surgery, and tells you that she does not want the surgery. Your action is to*

A. treat the client's psychological problems and provide support.

B. respect the client's wishes.

C. consider placing the client in an assisted-living facility.

D. explain to the client that she is depressed and will feel better after the surgery.

19-44 *If conflict arises during a job negotiation, you should consider*

A. separating the issue from the person.

B. always standing your ground.

C. getting a legal opinion.

D. basing your actions on the contract a friend of yours has secured in a local practice.

19-45 *The requirements for reportable communicable disease vary among states. Which of the following lists includes diseases that must be reported in every state?*

A. Syphilis, tuberculosis, and hepatitis

B. HIV infection, *Chlamydia* infection, and syphilis

C. Gonorrhea, syphilis, and *Chlamydia* infection

D. Hepatitis, syphilis, and HIV

19-46 *When applying for a new position, a nurse practitioner is counseled to assess the work environment. What does this include?*

A. Call time; support staff and what they will do; supervising relationships; whether you will be building your own panel of clients and/or seeing those overbooked

B. Administrative support and call time

C. Research opportunities and the nature of the supervising relationship

D. Time off and whether you will be building your own panel of clients and/or attending to the overbooked

19-47 *Collaboration is best defined as*

A. interdisciplinary teamwork.

B. a protocol arrangement with a physician.

C. case management.

D. cooperation with another to achieve mutual goals while not losing sight of one's own interests.

19-48 *Mr. Brill, age 50, is a house painter who has smoked two to three packs of cigarettes per day since he was 20 years old. He comes into the clinic complaining of a chronic cough. When you discuss his smoking behavior, he states, "I know I need to*

stop smoking, but I'm under too much stress right now." Mr. Brill is at which stage of learning?

A. The precontemplative stage

B. The contemplative stage

C. The action stage

D. The maintenance stage

19-49 *Mr. Griffin, age 85, has been given a diagnosis of bowel cancer, and surgery is indicated. He is mentally alert; however, he is refusing to give consent for the procedure. You respond by*

A. ordering a psychiatric consultation.

B. having your collaborating physician talk with the client.

C. respecting his wishes.

D. talking with his family.

19-50 *You are interviewing a client who becomes tearful. An appropriate response is to*

A. ask if the client has a support person with them.

B. sit quietly with the client and offer a tissue.

C. offer a glass of water to help the client compose himself or herself.

D. let the client have privacy, and spend the time reviewing the chart and the background of the client.

19-51 *What must you do as an APRN before billing for visits?*

A. Establish a collaborative agreement with a physician

B. Obtain a provider number and familiarize yourself with the rules and policies of the third-party payer

C. Provide evidence of continuing medical education

D. Have a Drug Enforcement Agency (DEA) number

19-52 *Your Native American client is convinced that her illness has been caused by the ill will of a fellow tribeswoman. Her description of her illness is an example of her*

A. explanatory reasoning.

B. lack of understanding of scientific medicine.

C. delusional ideation.

D. cultural bias.

19-53   Which of the following statements is true about Medicaid?

A. Medicaid is a federal plan to provide care for all indigent persons.

B. Medicaid pays for family planning services, dental care, and eyeglasses.

C. Eligibility requirements for Medicaid are mandated by the Health Care Financing Administration.

D. Medicaid is a program for the indigent financed jointly by the federal and the state governments.

19-54   Reviewing the literature refers to the ability to research existing literature about a specific problem, whether clinical or policy. The most important skill necessary to performing a thorough review of the literature is

A. talking with colleagues about the sources.

B. attending a research conference.

C. critiquing the findings and synthesizing the results.

D. reviewing clinical journals.

19-55   What is the NPI (national provider identifier)?

A. A number assigned to all nurse practitioners at graduation

B. A number required to sit for the national certification exam for the APRN

C. A unique identifying number for health-care providers required by CMS (Centers for Medicare and Medicaid)

D. A number required to get reimbursement from third-party private insurers

19-56   APRNs are affected by laws and rules, although these vary by state. Which of the following is affected by state law and regulation?

A. Delegation of authority by physicians

B. How many clients you must see every hour

C. Universal health-care law

D. Making no more than five referrals for one client

19-57   What is the maximum number of points you should attempt to make in one teaching session?

A. One

B. Two

C. Three to four

D. As many as you need; there is no limit

19-58   Medicare is a federal program administered nationally by the Centers for Medicare and Medicaid Services (CMS) and administered locally by Medicare carrier agencies. The CMS has developed Guidelines for Evaluation and Management Coding, which all Medicare providers, including nurse practitioners, are expected to follow in coding client visits for reimbursement purposes. Which of the following is an important consideration regarding billing practices?

A. It is important to "undercode" so that one does not get charged with Medicare fraud.

B. The practice of "overcoding" is essential in this age of decreasing reimbursements; just provide the appropriate documentation.

C. Failing to bill for billable services will lead to unnecessarily low revenues.

D. Time spent with the client is a very important determinant of billing.

19-59   The gerontological population is designated a vulnerable one when it comes to obtaining informed consent to serving as a research subject because of the potential for exploitation of older adults. Safeguards you should adhere to when conducting research on a geriatric population include which of the following?

A. Assess the competence of the individual before obtaining consent.

B. Obtain permission from the family or staff.

C. Stress how important the research is and why their participation and perspective, as an older adult, are important.

D. Determine if the research is exempt, in which case you do not need to obtain consent to participate.

19-60   What conditions must be met for you to bill "incident to" the physician, receiving 100% reimbursement from Medicare?

A. You must initiate the plan of care for the client.

B. The physician must be on-site and engaged in client care.

C. You must be employed as an independent contractor.

D. You must be the main health-care provider who sees the client.

19-61 *You are working in an emergency department as an APRN. An adolescent boy is brought in, unconscious, with a head injury after being struck by a car. He has no identification, and there is no parent or adult with him. What should you do?*

A. Provide the appropriate medical treatment even if it involves surgery.

B. Do everything except order a blood transfusion, although it is indicated, because you do not know the client's religious preferences.

C. Call the hospital attorney before instituting any care.

D. Contact all local police stations in an attempt to identify the client and find his parents before instituting treatment.

19-62 *The primary purpose of certification is to*

A. document competence and specialization.

B. regulate advanced-practice nursing.

C. enable the practitioner to obtain third-party reimbursement.

D. assure the public that an individual has a special set of skills.

19-63 *An effective method used to assess a client's retention and understanding of educational materials is*

A. asking the client to restate what you have reviewed.

B. providing a pathophysiology book for your client to take home and read.

C. repeating your explanations of disease pathology.

D. objective testing.

19-64 *According to the 2008 APRN Consensus Model, a nurse should refer to himself or herself as an APRN if his or her specialty role is*

A. a professor of nursing, a nurse midwife, or a nurse anesthetist.

B. a nurse practitioner, an RN with CCRN certification, or a nurse midwife.

C. a nurse anesthetist, a psychiatric nurse, or a clinical nurse specialist.

D. a primary care nurse practitioner (CNP), a certified nurse midwife (CNM), or a certified registered nurse anesthetist (CRNA).

19-65 *Prescriptive authority for APRNs*

A. is permitted only under protocol.

B. is mandated by law in more than 40 states.

C. varies by state.

D. includes the ability to prescribe controlled substances.

19-66 *Which of the following statements is true about case management?*

A. Case management oversees the client throughout acute care hospitalization.

B. Case management is organized around a system of interdisciplinary resources and services.

C. Case management depends on physician-driven leadership to oversee the illness episode.

D. Case management is applicable to the rehabilitative portion of the episode of the illness.

19-67 *Strategies for developing cultural competence include which of the following?*

A. Disregarding folk beliefs because they are not scientific.

B. Learning basic words and sentences in the client's language.

C. Explaining the pathophysiology of the disease process to the client so that he or she understands what is happening to him or her.

D. Explaining your cultural beliefs to the client.

19-68 *Medicare is divided into Part A and Part B. What is the difference between these two parts?*

A. Medicare Part A provides coverage for hospital care and skilled nursing facility and home care; Part B pays for outpatient fees at 80% of what Medicare determines to be reasonable.

B. Medicare Part A covers health-care expenses for individuals younger than age 65; Part B pays for individuals older than age 65.

C. Medicare Part A covers disabled individuals younger than age 65, but they are not eligible for Part B.

D. Medicare Part A pays for outpatient fees including home care; Part B provides coverage for hospital care only.

19-69   *Most health maintenance organizations (HMOs) use a reimbursement mechanism called capitation. This means that the*

A. HMO reimburses the provider on a fee-for-service basis.

B. HMO reimburses the provider a predetermined fee per client, per month, based on the client's age and sex.

C. fee paid to the provider fluctuates with the treatment.

D. provider is reimbursed by each individual client or family.

19-70   *Advance directives, such as health-care proxies and durable powers of attorney, are important for all clients to consider. In particular, persons who are unable to marry legally and those who are single by choice or circumstances may preserve their health-care wishes by*

A. executing a durable power of attorney for health care.

B. drafting a letter stating that their next of kin is not the surrogate decision maker.

C. signing an institutional document stating that the health-care provider is allowed to make all health-care decisions for the client.

D. having one partner declared legally incompetent.

19-71   *Mr. Jones, age 44, is admitted to the emergency department complaining of chest pain. Which of the following actions would be the best way to establish a therapeutic relationship with Mr. Jones?*

A. Ask several quick and specific questions in rapid succession to establish the exact nature of this emergent clinical situation.

B. Ask open-ended questions to elicit pertinent clinical data.

C. Reassure the client that he is in good hands in a well-equipped emergency department and that all will be OK.

D. Ask the client about his anxiety level.

19-72   *Health behaviors can be difficult to change. Which of the following is most important in influencing behavioral change?*

A. Motivation

B. Health beliefs

C. Cognitive knowledge

D. Social supports

19-73   *Human research subjects are entitled to all of the following EXCEPT*

A. the right to informed consent.

B. the right to compensation for their participation.

C. the right to withdraw from the research without being penalized.

D. the right to alternative treatments other than the experimental treatment.

19-74   *Which of the following are third-party payers?*

A. Indemnity insurance companies and businesses that contract for certain services

B. Free clinics

C. The Commission on Mental Retardation

D. Social organizations

19-75   *A good way to use an interpreter is to*

A. try to use an interpreter who is of the same sex as and older than the client.

B. have the interpreter translate word for word so that you do not receive any misinformation.

C. use more than one interpreter if necessary.

D. attempt no communication with the client other than through the interpreter.

19-76   *The levels of evaluation and management (E/M) services are based on which types of histories?*

A. Medical-surgical

B. Psychosocial

C. Expanded problem focused

D. Preoperative

19-77   *There are a number of barriers to full implementation of an autonomous role for APRNs in primary care. Major barriers are*

A. the need for medical specialists because of rapidly changing technologies.

B. the increasingly complex health problems of vulnerable populations.

C. prescriptive authority, scope of practice, and reimbursement.

D. managed care organizations' views of APRNs.

19-78   *You have seen a client who has tested positive for syphilis. You have treated the client, tested the client for other potential sexually transmitted diseases including HIV infection, counseled the client about safe sexual practices, and scheduled the client to return at 3 and 6 months for repeat serological testing. The tests at those times demonstrated that no further syphilis was present. Should you have taken any other action?*

A. No, you have treated the client appropriately.

B. Yes, you must report the case to the local health authorities.

C. Yes, you need to notify all sexual contacts.

D. Yes, you must follow up on the client's HIV status.

19-79   *Elder abuse and neglect are increasing concerns, and it is estimated that 4%–10% of older Americans are abused or neglected. What is the legal responsibility of the health-care provider in reporting elder abuse and neglect?*

A. The health-care provider should discuss the suspected abuse or neglect with the client.

B. The health-care provider should discuss the suspected abuse or neglect with the client's family.

C. The health-care provider must report the suspected abuse or neglect to the appropriate state protective agency.

D. The health-care provider must confirm the suspected abuse or neglect before reporting it to the appropriate state protective agency.

19-80   *When negotiating a contract for employment as a nurse practitioner, there are a number of important factors to consider. What are some important questions to ask?*

A. What is the most frequently billed current procedural terminology (CPT) code for this practice, and what amount does the practice bill and receive, on average, for that CPT code?

B. What is the cultural mix of clients seen in this practice?

C. What is the age and sex of my supervising physician?

D. What are the arrangements for child care in this practice?

19-81   *One of the two organizations that offer certification to the FNP (family nurse practitioner) is*

A. the Organization for the Advancement of Nurse Practitioners.

B. the American Academy of Nurse Practitioners.

C. the Nursing Organizations Alliance.

D. the American Board of Nursing Specialties.

19-82   *When teaching your client about medication that you are prescribing, the most important point(s) to discuss initially is (are)*

A. the action of the drug and its adverse effects.

B. whether to take the drug on a full or empty stomach.

C. what it is for, how much to take, and when to take it.

D. what to do if the client experiences any adverse effects.

19-83   Usual and customary *refers to*

A. an insurance term for how a charge compares with charges made to other persons receiving similar services and supplies.

B. how an insurer evaluates the need for an ordered diagnostic test.

C. a comparison of interventions across populations.

D. how much an insurer will charge to provide coverage.

19-84   *Who oversees the APRN's prescribing of controlled substances?*

A. The federal government

B. The pharmaceutical board of the state

C. The practice protocols of the hospital

D. Practice agreements

19-85   *Regulation of the APRN consists of four essential elements. They are*

A. licensure, certification, education and accreditation.

B. clinical performance, prescriptive privilege, preceptorship, and practice setting.

C. examination, continuing education, discipline, and awards.

D. workplace, collaborations, licensure, and prescriptive privilege.

19-86 *A situation in which medical information may be passed on without client consent is when*

A. the client has a gunshot wound.

B. a potential employer asks for it.

C. certifying absence from work.

D. talking to another health-care provider.

19-87 *What are some important negotiating points for the nurse practitioner seeking a job?*

A. Practice philosophy of the physician-owner

B. Salary and benefits

C. Salary

D. Salary, benefits, and work environment

19-88 *Which of the following are ways one may risk breaching client confidentiality?*

A. Leaving a client's record within view

B. Discussing the client with the consulting surgeon

C. Shredding duplicate records

D. Confirming the client's diagnosis over the telephone with a pharmacist

19-89 *Mrs. Hernandez, age 79, is insisting on discharge from the skilled nursing facility where she is receiving rehabilitation after a left hip replacement. She lives alone and has very little support. You do not think she is ready for discharge. Mrs. Hernandez's insistence on discharge is an example of your client exercising her right to*

A. self-determination.

B. beneficence.

C. justice.

D. utilitarianism.

19-90 *A good résumé can be crucial to your success in obtaining a job. It should include*

A. religious activities.

B. community service.

C. demographic data, including marital status and age.

D. number of children.

19-91 *As measured by the Center for Medicare and Medicaid (CMS), national health expenditures are grouped into which two categories?*

A. Medicare A and B

B. Medicare and Medicaid

C. Research and medical facilities construction and payments for health services and supplies

D. Long-term care and medications

19-92 *When caring for clients from a different culture, which of the following is an important piece of assessment data?*

A. Determining the ultimate decision maker

B. Making decisions based on your general knowledge about the cultural background of the client

C. Determining the family's perception of the client's problem

D. Understanding that clients from other cultures expect their health-care provider to be an authority figure

19-93 *Certain characteristics differentiate research from quality improvement. Which of the following is an example of research?*

A. Client satisfaction is evaluated relative to existing practice.

B. An intervention, well supported in the literature, is implemented and evaluated.

C. A standard assessment tool (e.g., risk assessment for falls) is implemented and evaluated.

D. A new intervention is implemented and compared with current practice to determine which is better.

19-94 *Denial-of-provider status is something that seriously impedes a nurse practitioner's ability to practice. If that occurs, some steps one can take include*

A. requesting that your clients lobby on your behalf, going to the newspapers, and reapplying.

B. requesting that your physician colleagues intervene on your behalf and writing critical letters to the organization in question.

C. "bashing" the organization to others, reapplying, and contacting an attorney.

D. writing letters to the organization's president and CEO, activating others to lobby on your behalf, and reapplying after a 6-month period.

19-95 *Negotiating a salary in a practice is important. A factor to consider is*

A. the practice philosophy of the physician-owner.

B. what payment method will be used—straight salary, percentage of net receipts, base salary plus percentage, or hourly rate.

C. the socioeconomic status of the surrounding community.

D. hourly salary only.

19-96 *Relapse is a common phenomenon seen during behavioral change. Useful strategies for the health-care provider to institute to aid the client in a relapse situation include*

A. using fear to reinforce the need to change.

B. telling the client that the relapse is a learning opportunity in preparation for the next action stage.

C. stressing the need to stay on "the straight and narrow."

D. involving the family in stressing the need to stay "straight."

19-97 *A comprehensive history includes which of the following elements?*

A. Chief complaint; review of systems; history of present illness; and past, family, and social history

B. Chief complaint, psychosocial assessment, and risk factor analysis

C. History of present illness, immunizations, and exposure to chemicals

D. Coping mechanisms, social support, and review of systems

19-98 *What is the responsibility of the primary care provider?*

A. The primary care provider is the coordinator of the client's health care.

B. Once the client is referred to another provider for ongoing treatment, the responsibility of the primary health-care provider is relieved.

C. The primary care provider should dictate all aspects of the client's plan of care.

D. The primary care provider turns over care of the client to the specialist.

19-99 *Which of the following nonverbal communication techniques is important to the establishment of rapport with the client?*

A. Taking notes only while the client is talking

B. Making direct eye contact with the client with periodic breaks to check or take notes

C. Having a desk between you and the client

D. Wearing jeans in the clinical setting to ensure your comfort

19-100 *Multiple regression and analysis of variance and covariance are tests of*

A. prediction.

B. statistical significance.

C. association.

D. correlation.

19-101 *Techniques used to enhance a client's adherence to a treatment plan include*

A. stressing the dangers of missing medications.

B. giving clear written instructions and simplifying the drug regimen.

C. allowing plenty of time between follow-up visits so that the client has time to adjust to the regimen.

D. explaining the importance of the regimen to the family.

19-102 *What is important to do before negotiating a contract?*

A. Do your homework.

B. Hire a lawyer.

C. Plan a signing-of-contract dinner.

D. Stand your ground.

19-103 *Zero-base budgeting refers to a budgeting system that*

A. accounts for unexpected budget variances.

B. accounts for expected budget variances only.

C. justifies each budget on its own merits, not on the basis of the previous period's budget.

D. justifies each budget based on the previous period's budget.

19-104 *Which of the following verbal communication techniques is helpful in establishing rapport with the client?*

A. Not calling the client by name because you do not want to appear intrusive

B. Speaking directly to the client, introducing yourself by name, and establishing the purpose of the interaction

C. Communicating slowly and quietly so as not to upset the client

D. Very thoroughly discussing every detail of the client's history with the client

Answers

19-1   Answer C

Although the desires of the collaborating physician; education, certification, and continuing education credits; and reimbursement and prescriptive privileges may influence institutional policy and medical staff bylaws, the factors that primarily determine the ability of an APRN to obtain clinical privileges in an institution are institutional policy, medical staff bylaws, state law, and the Joint Commission on Accreditation of Healthcare Organizations accreditation standards.

19-2   Answer B

In the outpatient office setting, the most common reason for a malpractice suit is failure to diagnose correctly. Approximately one-third of malpractice cases brought against general practitioners involve cases of failure to diagnose in a timely manner. These cases usually involve cancer, particularly cancer of the breast (failure to diagnose promptly accounts for the highest number of liability cases), lung, colon, or testes. Failure to refer and failure to manage fractures and trauma are among the top seven allegations in malpractice cases. Failure to obtain informed consent accounts for approximately 10% of the cases.

19-3   Answer C

The primary nursing responsibility during a crisis situation is to establish a therapeutic relationship. Other nursing responsibilities include providing education regarding the recovery process, stress management and reduction, and integration of the crisis experience. The establishment of support mechanisms and the development of coping mechanisms frequently enable the client to mobilize effectively and move beyond the crisis stage. Occasionally hospitalization may be necessary during an acute crisis, and psychotherapy may be a useful intervention.

19-4   Answer C

Although obtaining drug levels, using clinical judgment, and monitoring the responses to treatment will all assist you in assessing the degree of the client's compliance, the best way to monitor compliance is to ask the client. Most clients will be truthful.

19-5   Answer A

To reinforce client teaching, a useful strategy is to model the healthy behaviors. Role modeling is a very successful reinforcement strategy. Many people learn best by imitating the behavior of others. For example, if you are teaching exercises to your client, demonstrate them and then have the client practice them. Videos or pictures of others performing the exercises can also be helpful. Repeated discussions of the need for behavioral change are not often effective. Although providing some written materials is helpful, providing them without behavioral support may not add to the client's motivation. Likewise, although quizzing the client may provide information about his or her knowledge base, it does not positively reinforce behavior or lead to positive behavioral change.

19-6   Answer C

Concrete strategies used to keep your client's attention as you institute client education include making your point clear from the start; varying your tone of voice (speaking in a monotone may communicate a lack of interest); using various teaching methods (visual aids work best); and translating theoretical information into practical terms. Repetition is usually not an effective strategy for keeping your client's attention. Providing an educational session immediately after eating lunch is also not necessarily conducive to learning.

19-7   Answer C

Legal authority for all nursing practice, including advanced-practice nursing, rests with the individual state boards of nursing that administer the legal statutes that define nursing practice in that state.

The Health Care Financing Administration oversees the administration of federal Medicare and Medicaid funds. Legal authority for professional practice was delegated to the states and territories by the Constitution and is not regulated by federal statutes. Some states require national certification for licensure as an APRN, but not all.

19-8   Answer B

Principles of consultation include the identification of a problem by a professional, such as an APRN, who calls in a consultant with documented expertise in a given area; the consultant making recommendations based on his or her assessment of the situation; and the APRN remaining free to accept or reject these recommendations and retaining responsibility for the outcome of care. Classically, there is a nonhierarchical relationship between the consultant and consultee. The issue of responsibility for the outcome of care is what separates collaboration from consultation. A situation in which a senior clinician provides a supportive and educative relationship with a junior clinician is defined as "clinical supervision" and implies that responsibility for the outcome of care remains in the hands of the senior clinician.

19-9   Answer C

Reviewing the case with an interpreter before seeing the client is the *ideal* strategy to enhance cross-cultural communication if you are in a setting where an interpreter is available. Information about the reason for the visit and the purpose of the health-care encounter can be exchanged beforehand, potentially enhancing communications. It may be necessary to rely on family members to translate, but it is not the best strategy. For example, it is often the school-age child who has the best grasp of English; however, relying on the child to interpret reverses parent-child roles and places unnecessary and sometimes inappropriate burdens on the child. It also lessens the client's sense of authority and privacy. Gesturing and relying on a dictionary may be necessary but distracts from the general flow of communication and slows the speed and comprehension of the communication.

19-10   Answer C

A marketing portfolio that will support what you have to offer as an APRN or nurse practitioner should include the state nurse practice act and regulations, prescriptive authority legislation, third-party reimbursement rules and regulations, and practice protocols. This type of information provides concrete data to potential employers and reimbursers concerning the range of services you can offer. Your personal mission statement should be used to help you personally focus your job search and options. Your scores on the certification examination and the specifics of your transcript are usually not relevant. Letters of reference should be provided only when requested.

19-11   Answer D

According to the Joint Commission on Accreditation of Healthcare Organizations (JCAHO), decisions regarding policy and client care should be based on research findings. The JCAHO mandates that decisions be based on research and rooted in and supported by scientific literature. Experience, clinical expertise, and consultation and collaboration are no longer acceptable as the rationale for policy and client-care decisions. This supports evidence-based practice.

19-12   Answer D

To determine the appropriate statistical test to use, consider sample size, level of measurement, and data type, as well as other factors. Statistical significance and clinical significance are not the same. If a journal article you are writing is limited in length, you should not delete the descriptive statistics and keep the inferential statistics. You must describe your sample and possibly a number of other things before explaining your inferences. Correlational coefficients measure the strength of the relationship between variables; correlation does not infer causality, nor can you make firm predictions based on these data.

19-13   Answer A

An underlying assumption of the health belief model (HBM) is that behavior is determined more by a person's perceived reality than by environmental factors. Components include perceived threat, efficacy, benefits of action, and perceived barriers to action. People take actions to change their lifestyle to prevent a disease only to the extent that the disease exists in their perception. They must also perceive the benefits of action as well as feel the confidence (often referred to as efficacy) to act. These benefits must outweigh the barriers to action. Benefits and barriers are people's beliefs rather than objective facts about the effectiveness of action. Education and positive reinforcement are not concepts associated with the HBM. Predisposing factors, reinforcing factors, and enabling factors are concepts from the precede-proceed model, which is used for comprehensive planning in health education and health promotion with individuals and communities. Self-efficacy theory and the perceived ability to act are one and the same and form only part of the HBM.

19-14 Answer C

The Agency for Healthcare Research and Quality (AHRQ) was established to promote evidence-based practice and develop databases for research and clinical guidelines. The AHRQ routinely publishes reviews of studies on clinical problems with summaries of treatment protocols and effectiveness. It does not mandate these in practice, although the provider may be held to these as a standard of care. It also does not dictate health-care policy or develop cost-effective interventions, although it does do cost-benefit analysis of the interventions.

19-15 Answer A

The purpose of an institutional review board (IRB) is to protect human subjects. The primary purpose of the IRB is ethical; it does not evaluate the scientific merit of proposed research, nor does it oversee and coordinate the research efforts of an institution or an individual. These functions are usually performed by the institution's research committee. It is your obligation as a researcher to obtain some form of IRB approval any time you are conducting research on human subjects. If you are planning a research project in a private practice setting, approval should be obtained from the IRB of some affiliating institution such as a hospital where you are credentialed and permitted to admit clients.

19-16 Answer A

The primary purpose of professional licensure is to protect the public from unsafe practitioners by ensuring a minimum standard for competency. Licensure is a legal status granted by a regulating authority (in the case of nursing, by individual state boards of nursing). In nursing, this is accomplished by mandating passage of the National Council Licensure Exam (NCLEX-RN) by an individual before state licensure. Licensure does not ensure

high nursing standards; passage of the NCLEX is designed to assess minimum competency to practice safely. The curriculum of a nursing program, although providing a foundation of nursing knowledge that will graduate a safe and competent practitioner, is not specifically geared to the NCLEX exam. Nursing programs retain autonomy over their own curricula. Although the licensing statutes may spell out prescriptive privileges for APRNs, they do not necessarily do that, nor is that the primary purpose of professional licensure.

19-17 Answer A

Barriers to independent practice include getting on managed care panels; getting and keeping a collaborating physician if mandated in the state where one is practicing; getting referrals from hospital emergency rooms and getting privileges in hospitals; lacking legal authority in the state of practice to admit to nursing homes, offer home care services, and/or to direct hospice services. Lack of knowledge and lack of empathy should not be barriers to practice. A nurse practitioner should be able to manage client care without direct and specific physician oversight, although collaboration in some situations is essential to nurse practitioner practice just as it is when physicians call for a referral.

19-18 Answer B

As an individual APRN, you can make a difference in advancing the role of all APRNs by writing letters to the editor on health-care issues that outline the positive impact of APRNs. Although reading newspapers keeps you well informed, it is not enough to affect others unless you also speak out in a knowledgeable fashion. Likewise, thinking positive thoughts about your role may help you communicate a positive attitude, but the communication element is essential if you are to affect others. Supporting a Democratic candidate may or may not help advance the cause of advanced-practice nursing. The stances of candidates of both parties need to be researched to ascertain each one's personal stance on this issue. There is no one "party line" on this issue.

19-19 Answer B

Schedule IV drugs are all those listed in answer B, plus some stimulants such as phentermine. Schedule IV drugs include depressants such as alprazolam, clonazepam, diazepam, and flurazepam; stimulants such as phentermine; and other substances such as pentazocine. Schedule I drugs include substances with little or no approved medical usage that have a high abuse potential, such as LSD and marijuana. Schedule II drugs are those with a high abuse potential with severe psychic or physical dependency but with clinical utility, such as meperidine, morphine, and methadone, to name just a few. Stimulants such as amphetamines are also included in schedule II. Schedule III drugs have a potential for abuse, but the potential is lower than for schedule II drugs. These drugs often contain a combination of controlled and noncontrolled substances such as Tylenol with codeine #3.

19-20   Answer B

The term *advanced-practice nurses* refers to nurse practitioners, clinical nurse specialists, nurse anesthetists, and nurse midwives.

19-21   Answer A

Answers to all questions listed in answer A must be ascertained before prescribing medication for a client.

19-22   Answer A

It is the ethical responsibility of the nurse practitioner to add to the goodwill that the employer has developed within the community; protect the employer's "trade secrets," such as client mailing lists; remain unimpaired by drugs and/or alcohol; provide one's best customer services at all times; maintain one's credentials and adherence to the "standard of care"; and maintain client confidentiality. The APRN has an ethical and legal responsibility to follow the standard of care. There is no ethical responsibility to advertise the practice from one's own funds; nor should the nurse practitioner promote that role above all others. The nature of the practice should be collaborative.

19-23   Answer B

To treat this client as an emancipated minor, you need some proof of marriage, active military status, or papers from a court attesting to the minor's status as emancipated. To petition a court for emancipation, a minor must be a certain age (from 14–16, depending on the state law), not live with his or her parents or guardian, be capable of managing financial affairs, and have the ability to provide for his or her well-being. Accepting the word of someone accompanying the client, or the client himself, is not enough data for you to make the appropriate decision.

19-24   Answer C

Indemnity insurer refers to an insurer that pays for the medical care of the insured but does not provide that care. A health maintenance organization provides the medical care as well as the insurance of the insurer. A preferred provider organization is a network of health-care providers linked together through similar reimbursement mechanisms. A fee-for-service plan refers to reimbursement for health-care services under a fee schedule.

19-25   Answer C

Do not resuscitate (DNR) orders are decided by the physician in consultation with the client, family, or surrogate decision maker. Advance directives may help clarify end-of-life decisions, but the lack of a documented DNR order in the chart presumes that the client desires full intervention and holds health-care providers legally responsible to initiate life-sustaining treatment. A DNR order, written by the physician, relieves the health-care providers of that responsibility. The individual decision is never made by the health-care facility, although the facility may draft generic guidelines to assist procedurally in end-of-life situations.

19-26   Answer A

The stages of grief include shock, reality, and recovery. The shock stage is characterized as numbness, the reality stage as deep pain, and the recovery stage as beginning to live again. Numbness, pain, loss, and resolution are all components of the process of grief. A grieving person shares many behavioral similarities with a depressed individual; however, grieving is a natural, not a pathological, process and is usually time limited.

19-27   Answer B

Motivational interviewing (MI) is well suited for the profession of nursing and the role of nurse practitioner as coach because it encompasses the holistic therapeutic communication principles of empathy, active listening and acceptance. It uses techniques such as asking open-ended questions, affirmation, and reflection to gain trust and establish a therapeutic relationship with the client. Using

MI, the client can verbalize how he or she might be able to take the necessary steps needed to make a positive change. MI does not dictate or make mandates to the client, and it is a nonthreatening form of communication.

19-28   Answer C

The purpose of a block grant is to allow states to have greater flexibility in providing services to the poor. Accelerating costs of the Medicaid program have prompted state-based initiatives for reform of the program. The federal government has considered converting Medicaid funds to block grants to allow states greater flexibility in providing Medicaid services.

19-29   Answer D

According to the National Commission on Certification of Physician Assistants Web site, physician assistants are health-care professionals who are authorized by the state to practice medicine as part of a team with, and under the direction of, a physician. As licensed independent practitioners, APRNs practice autonomously and in collaboration with health-care professionals and other individuals to assess, diagnose, treat, and manage the client's health problems and needs. Like APRNs, PAs do participate in an educational program but may have varied clinical experiences. PA program applicants must complete 2 years of college courses in basic and behavioral sciences as prerequisites. Most students have a bachelor's degree and about 3 years of health-care experience before entering a PA program. APRNs are nurses from different clinical backgrounds and are from a bachelor's-prepared accredited nursing school, who must obtain a master's degree to sit for national certification as an APRN.

19-30   Answer D

The type of health-care delivery system that allows the client the greatest freedom of choice is a fee-for-service plan. A health maintenance organization, a preferred provider organization, and a managed care plan all have greater restrictions.

19-31   Answer A

The majority of Medicaid enrollees are young women and children. The majority of Medicaid funds, however, go to long-term care services for older adults and clients with disabilities.

19-32   Answer A

A consumer of research findings engages in a number of activities that include reading the literature, analyzing clinical applicability, and using new interventions. Organizing and conducting a research study, as well as ensuring the protection of human participants, are tasks of the researcher. Collecting data may be done by anyone trained to do it and does not necessarily require advanced knowledge of the research process. Research utilization, on the other hand, involves reading the current literature; critically evaluating the study, including its methods and conclusions, to evaluate applicability to practice; introducing relevant findings into clinical practice; evaluating the results of the new treatments on clients; and disseminating those results in clinical practice.

19-33   Answer D

The marketing process is guided by a number of factors, including product, price, place, and promotion. Referred to as the "4 P's of the marketing process," *product* stands for the service you offer; *price* is identification of the right cost for the service; *place* is where the services are delivered or the demands of the market where the service will be offered; and *promotion* is your ability to increase your market's awareness of what you have to offer. The prospective pool of clients, your advertising budget, and what you have to offer are only portions of a marketing plan. Cost, benefit, and barriers do not describe the marketing process in a meaningful or coherent way.

19-34   Answer C

The goals and objectives contained in *Healthy People 2020* include reducing disparities in health care, increasing healthy life span, and increasing accessibility to health care for all Americans. They do not include mandatory provision of emergency care. *Healthy People 2020* does not advocate instituting a nationalized health insurance plan. Preserving choice of provider for all Americans is not one of the goals and objectives of *Healthy People 2020*.

19-35   Answer C

Strategies that help to prevent client noncompliance include providing positive feedback and reinforcement and performing careful follow-up on canceled and missed appointments.

In-depth client education does not help prevent client noncompliance. Instead, client education that is short, uses multiple ways of learning, and is meaningful to the client's situation is usually more effective. Likewise, a high frequency of medication does not foster compliance but rather leads to a greater likelihood that the client will miss a dose. Monitoring blood levels to assess therapeutic efficacy does not involve the client as a partner in their health care.

19-36   Answer D

You must be prepared to answer what you will bring to the practice, although it does not have to be put in writing. You must be prepared to answer whether you will be on call on the weekends or evenings. You may not be willing to do this, but you must have an answer for this question. You must be able to share how many clients you may be able to see in one day as well as how independently you are willing to practice. You do not have to share your age or the number of dependents you have and/or any arrangements in caring for them, and you are not expected to advertise the practice out of your own revenues. You must, however, be willing to positively promote the practice in the community.

19-37   Answer B

Sally is not guilty of malpractice because no harm came to Mr. Bell as a result of her actions. For malpractice to occur, the provider must have a duty to the client (which Sally had), a standard of care must have been breached (which Sally did when she did not check his potassium level when she increased the dosage of diuretic), and harm or damage must occur as a result of the duty and the breach of the standard of care (which did not occur). Because all of the components were not met, malpractice has not been established.

19-38   Answer D

Interprofessional role conflict can result from perceived differences in the expected role of nurse practitioner (NP) joining a practice. The NP can often be perceived as a threat of competition, and some may view the NP as an extender of medical care and not as an independent practitioner.

19-39   Answer D

The most important aspect of communicating with clients is acknowledging their feelings. By responding, "You seem very upset, Mr. Barnes. Could you share with me what is bothering you?" you're acknowledging Mr. Barnes's discomfort by reflecting back his feelings, and you offer to assist him. If you respond by saying, "I'm sorry, Mr. Barnes, but I need these questions answered" or "I want to provide the best possible care for you, Mr. Barnes," you have not acknowledged Mr. Barnes's feelings. If you respond by saying, "Perhaps your wife can assist with some of these questions," you violate Mr. Barnes's autonomy and right to self-determination.

19-40   Answer B

Credentialing means that the practitioner has met certain criteria through licensure, education, and certification. The criteria for credentialing vary depending on the credentialing body. Hospitals, for example, may use credentialing to grant hospital privileges. An individual is permitted to practice basic or advanced-practice nursing by licensure. An academic degree is awarded when one has completed a program of study. Prescriptive authority is mandated by state statutes.

19-41   Answer C

The best method for evaluating the efficacy of a new clinical intervention is a randomized, controlled clinical trial. Case reports, descriptive studies, and correlational studies are methodological approaches that are less reliable in establishing causal relationships, and thus the attribution of an effect to the new clinical intervention would be less clear. The effect might be attributable to other confounding variables.

19-42   Answer C

According to CMS (Centers for Medicare and Medicaid Services), the purpose of the electronic health record (EHR) is to have an electronic version of a client's medical history that is maintained by the provider over time and may include all of the key administrative clinical data relevant to that person's care under a particular provider, including demographics, progress notes, problems, medications, vital signs, past medical history, immunizations, laboratory data, and radiology reports. The EHR automates access to information and has the potential to streamline the clinician's workflow. The EHR can improve client care by reducing the incidence of medical error by improving the accuracy and clarity of medical records, making the health information available, reducing duplication of tests, reducing delays in treatment, keeping clients well informed to make better decisions, and reducing medical error by improving the accuracy and clarity of medical records. Not all clinicians are embracing the EHR or feel that it is speeding up their charting or recording responsibilities.

19-43   Answer A

Your action is to treat the client's psychological problems and provide support. With Mrs. Smith, there are enough symptoms to warrant evaluation and possible intervention for psychological problems, most likely depression. Then it would be appropriate to support the client's decision. There are not enough data to evaluate the need for placement in an assisted-living facility at this point. To try to convince the client that she is in need of surgery would be coercive and would violate the client's autonomy.

19-44   Answer A

Seeking a legal opinion might be prudent but is usually not necessary and can set up additional roadblocks in some situations. You should not base your actions or decisions on a similar situation that someone you know may have experienced. Although the experiences of others may be useful sources of comparisons, your decisions should be based on your analysis of your own situation. Standing your ground is important but not if it means being unreasonable. During the process of negotiation, an honest difference of opinion can arise. Resolving the issue is wise and prudent behavior. Always separate the issue from the person. It is about achieving a mutually satisfying outcome—a win-win situation. Clarifying misconceptions and focusing on what has been achieved thus far can be an effective strategy. You want to leave the process with positive feelings even if a work agreement is not achieved.

19-45   Answer A

Of the lists presented, the communicable diseases that must be reported in every state include syphilis, tuberculosis, and hepatitis. The diseases that are notifiable by law vary by state and over time. Criteria for determining notifiable diseases have generally been based on the potential for control or prevention of additional cases of the disease. Practitioners should be familiar with which diseases need to be reported in their state; for example, invasive *Haemophilus influenzae* infection, meningitis, encephalitis, giardiasis, measles, and Reye's syndrome are reportable in more than 40 states.

19-46   Answer A

Although research opportunities and administrative support may be important components of the work environment for an individual nurse practitioner, the most general and inclusive answer is A. The number and role of support staff, on-call time, nature of supervision, reporting relationships, and clarification regarding which clients will be seen during the course of a day are all important parameters of the work environment.

19-47   Answer D

Collaboration is best defined as cooperation with another to achieve mutual goals while not losing sight of one's own interests. True collaboration combines the activities of cooperation or concern for another's interests with assertiveness. The interest considered most important in nurse-physician collaboration is the professionals' concern for the care of the client rather than the provider's personal agenda. Collaboration is essential in interdisciplinary teamwork but is not the definition of collaboration. Collaboration may include a protocol arrangement with a physician, but it is not solely defined that way. Case management is defined as managing an entire episode of illness from the standpoint of coordination of resources and services. This will involve collaboration but is a different concept.

19-48   Answer A

To assess Mr. Brill's readiness to learn, ask, "What do you think you should do about your smoking?" If Mr. Brill answers, "I have no problem," he is in the precontemplative stage of learning. You would focus your teaching on increasing his awareness of his condition. Mr. Brill's response indicates that he is in the contemplative stage of learning. He is considering change but has not taken any action. You would focus your teaching on reinforcing his understanding of the need to change, teaching him the skills needed to make the change, pointing out the positive aspects of making the change, and stressing his ability to do so. If the client had already begun to change his behavior, he would be in the action stage. You would focus your teaching on reinforcing his behavior with modeling and reward. This is a crucial stage because you do not want the client to stop the behavioral change. You must support his actions in every way possible. A client in the maintenance stage is practicing the behavior regularly. Your intervention is to continue to reinforce the new behavior and the need to maintain the change.

19-49   Answer C

Respecting the client's wishes is the most correct response to this situation. You may want to consider a psychological overlay, such as depression, and be sure this is not a driving component of the client's behavior. If the client appears to be of sound mind, his wishes should be respected. Ordering a psychiatric consult or having your collaborating physician talk with the client is not necessary. Talking to his family interferes with the client's autonomy, a primary value of care.

19-50   Answer B

The most important thing the practitioner can do for a crying client is to accept his or her feelings. If the client is on the verge of tears during the interview, pausing, gently probing, or responding with empathy gives him or her permission to cry. Asking if a support person has accompanied the client deflects from the expression of his or her feelings, and such expression is itself therapeutic. Leaving the client to get a glass of water, or to review the record, or to allow the client time to compose himself or herself also shuts down the expression of feelings. Offering a tissue and waiting for the client to recover is appropriate and your best initial response.

19-51   Answer B

To bill your clients for services, you must obtain a provider or panel membership as needed and familiarize yourself with the rules and policies of each payer. Some, but not all, states require a collaborative agreement with a physician for you to practice; some states require national certification to practice, but not all do. In some states you are able to provide controlled substances, which requires that you have a DEA number; other states do not allow you to prescribe controlled substances. Currently, there is not a requirement that you have

a specific number of continuing medical education credits to bill for services provided.

19-52   Answer A

Explanatory reasoning—reasoning that explains, in the client's view, the cause of the client's illness—has been attributed to anthropologist Arthur Kleinam as the *explanatory model*. The client may have a cognitive understanding of scientific medicine but reject it. The client's view, in this situation, is not necessarily delusional or a cultural bias.

19-53   Answer D

Financed jointly by the federal and state governments, Medicaid is a program to pay for health-care services for the indigent. Each state defines income eligibility and the benefit structure. Minimally, Medicaid must provide inpatient, skilled nursing facility, and home care; physician services; outpatient care; family planning services; and periodic screening, detection, and treatment care of children under age 12. As for services such as dental care, eyeglasses, and prescription drugs, each state makes its own decisions concerning payment.

19-54   Answer C

Although talking with colleagues, attending a research conference, and reviewing your own clinical journals may all help identify relevant databases, the most important skill necessary to performing a thorough review of the literature is critiquing the findings and synthesizing the results.

19-55   Answer C

The national provider identifier (NPI), instituted in 1994, is a unique identifying number for health-care providers required by CMS (Centers for Medicare and Medicaid Services). The purpose of the NPI is to uniquely identify a health-care provider in standard transactions, such as health-care claims. NPIs may also be used to identify health-care providers on prescriptions, in coordination of benefits between health plans, in client medical record systems, in program integrity files, and in other ways. This number must be applied for by the practitioner.

19-56   Answer A

APRNs must abide by laws and rules, such as those related to scope of practice, reimbursement for health-care services, delegation of authority by physicians, quality of care, and requirements for collaboration. However, the number of clients seen per hour, universal health-care law, and number of referrals are not regulated by law.

19-57   Answer C

The maximum number of points you should attempt to make in one teaching session is three to four. The average adult can remember only five to seven points at a time. Therefore, to enhance your client's recall, limit your instructions to three to four major points in any one teaching session. Teaching more points may overwhelm even the most advanced learner. Additionally, health-care situations are often charged with anxiety, which can further interfere with learning. Be specific about what you want the client to know, and use simple, everyday language.

19-58   Answer C

It is important to bill for the appropriate services and support that with appropriate documentation. Time spent with the client is not always the determining factor because it may have been time spent inappropriately. Billing is based on history taking, examination, and medical decision making. Each of these activities has specific measures and parameters to be documented. When selecting the appropriate code for ambulatory care, only face-to-face time is considered.

19-59   Answer A

Safeguards to follow when conducting research on a geriatric population include assessing the competence of the individual before obtaining consent, making sure the consent form is in understandable language, and obtaining verbal consent (in some situations, verbal consent is all that is required). Permission must be obtained from the client. Obtaining permission from the family or staff is usually not acceptable because it may interfere with client autonomy. Additionally, stressing the importance of the research to encourage participation is coercive. Even research deemed exempt requires consent from participants.

19-60   Answer B

The term *incident to* implies that your services as an APRN are performed in connection with a physician. The reimbursement rate for Medicare

billing "incident to" a physician is 100%. The physician must be on-site when the care is provided and must be providing medical services rather than performing administrative work. The physician must have previously seen the client and initiated the plan of care, and the physician must see the client frequently enough to provide ongoing input into the care of the client.

19-61   Answer A

The emergency treatment exception allows you to treat minors in emergency or life-threatening situations when a parent or guardian cannot be reached to give consent for treatment. This includes transfusions when necessary. The legal definition of an emergency medical condition is any condition that threatens the loss, impairment, or serious dysfunction of life or limb or causes severe pain.

19-62   Answer A

The primary purpose of certification is to document competence and specialization. Certification is a voluntary process by which a nongovernmental agency or association certifies that an individual has met certain predetermined standards for competency and specialization in a particular area. Although some states mandate that an APRN pass a national certification examination before granting licensure to practice at an advanced level, this is not the case in all states. National certification may be necessary to obtain third-party reimbursement; however, that is not the primary purpose of certification, either. Although certification at the national level does provide the public with information about the skills of the practitioner, that is the realm of licensure, not the primary purpose of certification.

19-63   Answer A

Methods used to assess your client's retention and understanding of educational materials include asking your client to restate or do a return demonstration of what you have reviewed, having your client keep a diary or record of his or her behaviors, and reviewing written materials with your client. Providing a pathophysiology book to your client does not help assess your client's retention and understanding of educational material. Repeated explanations of pathophysiology of disease will most likely not increase your client's retention, nor will objective testing.

19-64   Answer D

According to the 2008 APRN Consensus Model, the focus of the defining factor for all APRNs is that a significant component of the education and practice focuses on direct care of individuals. According to the model, there are four major titles or roles associated with the APRN title. They are the CRNA (certified registered nurse anesthetist), the CNM (certified nurse midwife), CNS (clinical nurse specialist), and the CNP (certified nurse practitioner). Competencies, education, and accreditation process arespecified for each individual role.

19-65   Answer C

Prescriptive authority for APRN varies by state. Some states mandate the filing of a protocol that documents physician oversight, but other states do not. It is not mandated by law in more than 40 states. The ability to prescribe controlled substances varies among states.

19-66   Answer B

Case management is organized around a system of interdisciplinary resources and services; the clinical and financial aspects of care are overseen by a case manager who has a financial incentive to manage risk and maximize the quality of care. It is not physician driven. Case management is applicable to the entire episode of the illness, not just the client's acute care, hospitalization, or rehabilitative care.

19-67   Answer B

Strategies for developing cultural competence include learning basic words and sentences in the client's language, attending special cultural events and celebrations, and relating a client's belief to your own even if it is different. It is important to recognize that clients who have English as a second language may regress to their first language under the stress of an illness. Learning a few key phrases in the client's native language and knowing how to address the client properly can go a long way in establishing rapport and trust. Disregarding folk beliefs because they are not scientific is not a strategy to develop cultural competence. Folk beliefs must be taken into consideration because they can profoundly affect the course of the client's illness. If the client believes his or her illness is the result of a "curse," you may need to strategize ways to "undo" the curse. Explaining the pathophysiology

of a disease process is not necessarily effective in countering the client's deeply held cultural beliefs.

19-68   Answer A

Medicare Part A provides coverage for inpatient care, including hospital care, skilled nursing facility care, and home health care; Part B pays for outpatient fees at 80% of what Medicare determines to be reasonable. Disabled individuals younger than age 65 are eligible for Medicare A and B.

19-69   Answer B

The reimbursement mechanism called *capitation* that some health maintenance organizations (HMOs) use is one in which the HMO reimburses the provider a set fee per client, per month, based on the client's age and sex. HMOs are prepaid, comprehensive systems of health benefits that combine both financing and delivery of services to subscribers. They may pay providers on a capitated or fee-for-service basis. Capitation is a set fee that does not fluctuate. The provider is reimbursed by the HMO and not the client. Most plans require clients to make a copayment at the time of the visit. Capitated fees for primary care range from $5 to $35 per month depending on the client's age and sex and, thus, relative risk. Fee for service refers to reimbursement for health-care services under a fee schedule that is based on a complex variety of factors. These include the number and type of services provided, the current procedural terminology, International Classification of Disease (ICD-9) codes, the geographic area (the "usual and customary" fee), and certain office and training expenses of the provider.

19-70   Answer A

A durable power of attorney for health care (DPAHC) authorizes another person or agent to make medical decisions on behalf of an individual if and when that client becomes unable or unwilling to make those decisions. It is a version of the power of attorney used in commercial transactions. In the absence of such a document, in most cases, the client's next of kin (typically a spouse, parent, or child, depending on individual circumstances) is legally mandated to assume that role. Unlike the "living will," which is used for end-of-life decisions, a DPAHC is used to make decisions when the client is incapacitated.

19-71   Answer B

Asking open-ended questions is essential to establishing a therapeutic relationship, even in an emergency situation, and it is a good interviewing technique. Asking several questions in rapid succession may help establish the nature of the clinical situation, but it will not facilitate a therapeutic relationship or communication. To reassure the client may be unrealistic. False reassurance is considered a block to therapeutic communication. Asking the client about his anxiety level will probably only increase the client's anxiety. It is also an irrelevant question because the client would most certainly be anxious.

19-72   Answer A

Motivation is the most important factor influencing behavioral change. Health beliefs and self-efficacy may underlie motivation for change, but it is motivation that is most strongly correlated with actual behavioral change. Cognitive knowledge and social supports have some relationships to the concept of self-efficacy, but not directly to motivation.

19-73   Answer B

Human research subjects are entitled to the right to informed consent, the right to withdraw from the research without being penalized, and the right to treatments other than the experimental treatment. Subjects are not guaranteed any compensation for participation, although some research studies do provide compensation.

19-74   Answer A

Medicare, Medicaid, indemnity insurance companies, managed care organizations, and businesses that contract for certain services (e.g., colleges that provide health-care services) are the major categories of third-party payers. Clients who pay their own bills are not, strictly speaking, third-party payers but still are a source of reimbursement.

19-75   Answer A

The role of an interpreter in a health-care setting is often one of cultural broker, to act as a translator not just of words but also of cultural concepts and beliefs. Cultural values may make it more difficult for the client to discuss certain issues in the presence of an interpreter. It is helpful for the practitioner to

face the interpreter and client together, maintaining eye contact with both if possible. It also facilitates observation of nonverbal cues. Using a trained same-sex interpreter, preferably one older than the client, has been found to work best. The client also needs to be reassured about the confidentiality of the information shared. For this reason, it is best to use only one interpreter and for the provider to establish rapport with the client in any way possible.

19-76   Answer C

The levels of evaluation and management (E/M) services are based on four types of histories: (1) problem focused, (2) expanded problem focused, (3) detailed, and (4) comprehensive.

19-77   Answer C

The limitation on prescriptive authority and the scope of practice and reimbursement issues are major barriers to full implementation for an autonomous role for APRNs in primary care. The complex health problems of vulnerable populations are frequently rooted in lifestyle issues such as poverty, violence, and poor housing. These social problems are often more amenable to traditional nursing-based approaches. Managed care organizations' views are currently shifting and variable. Managed care organizations' support for advanced nursing practice continues to be variable. In some settings it is one barrier; in other settings it is something else.

19-78   Answer B

The practitioner is also responsible for reporting the case of syphilis to the local health authorities. All sexual partners of the client should be contacted; however, it is the health department that has trained staff who will perform the investigation of contacts and follow-up. Syphilis is easily treated and controllable if its presence is reported. It is not necessary to retest the client's HIV status unless there is a new clinical reason on subsequent visits.

19-79   Answer C

If a health-care provider suspects elder or dependent-adult abuse or neglect, the provider, in most states, must report it to the appropriate state protective agency. The goals of intervention are to protect the client and prevent further injury. Although data regarding the abuse may have come from the client, depending on the situation, it is not always advisable to confront the client or the family directly. Most state laws mandate reporting of suspected abuse or neglect, not just confirmed abuse or neglect. Trained investigators can then be called in to make a more detailed assessment. Health-care providers should be involved in educating the public about the problems of elder abuse and neglect and should be aware of community resources and supports that might help clients and their families.

19-80   Answer A

There are many important questions that a nurse practitioner seeking employment in a practice needs to ask; however, the cultural background of clients, the age and sex of the supervising physician, and specific arrangements for child care are not always appropriate questions. Things to consider are many, such as how many clients do I see per hour, day, month, and year and how much physician consultation time is necessary, and will provide evidence about the speed needed in this practice setting; also important is basic information about how the practice gets its revenues. This is why the information on frequently billed CPT codes is important and relevant. Another important question is what percentage of practice income goes to support practice expenses, as well as the collection rate for the practice (90% is considered good). Additionally, self-assessment as to what terms of employment are essential and which can be given up helps position the nurse practitioner to be in the best negotiating position. Vacation time, sick time, health insurance, consideration of malpractice insurance, support for continuing professional education, and on-call time, as well as hospital privileges and responsibilities, are also important considerations.

19-81   Answer B

There are two governing boards that issue certification for the FNP: the American Academy of Nurse Practitioners and the American Nurses Association.

19-82   Answer C

It can be difficult to find time to do client teaching; therefore, apply the rule of three S's: short, specific, and simple. The most important points you need to teach your client initially about a new drug are what the medication is for, how much to take, and when to take it. The specifics of taking the medication and what to do if there are adverse effects are also important but should be explained after the other information. Discussing the action and adverse

effects of the drug might distract the client from what he or she really needs to know initially.

19-83   Answer A

The term *usual and customary* refers to comparing charges with other like charges for services and supplies received in the immediate vicinity, as well as in a broader geographic area. It does not refer to the "usual and customary" charge to obtain insurance but rather to how much the insurer will reimburse for a service. Whether to order a diagnostic test is up to the provider's discretion, although the payer may hold the provider to the standard of care. *Usual and customary* is not a term used to compare interventions across populations.

19-84   Answer A

The federal government, specifically the Drug Enforcement Agency (DEA), oversees the APRN's prescribing of controlled substances. State laws vary, as do physician oversight and scope of practice from state to state. Federal registration is based on the applicant's complying with state and local laws. If a state requires a separate controlled-substance license, the APRN must obtain that license and submit a copy with an application for a DEA number. If state law does not authorize the APRN to prescribe controlled substances, the DEA will not issue a DEA number.

19-85   Answer A

The acronym given to the four essential areas of focus for the APRN Consensus Model are LACE, which stands for licensure, accreditation, certification, and education. Each of these core elements plays an essential part in the implementation of the model.

19-86   Answer A

One situation in which medical information may be passed on without client consent is when the client has a gunshot wound. Other situations include when the client has a sexually transmitted or communicable disease. All other situations require the client's consent for release of medical records and information.

19-87   Answer D

The physician may not be the owner of the practice, and although the philosophy of the "owner" is important, there are other important, concrete considerations—salary, benefits, working hours, and work environment. The neglect of one of these areas over the others may lead to discontent.

19-88   Answer A

Leaving a client's record within view, talking about a client within earshot of others, discarding unshredded duplicate records, discussing a client's condition with family members, releasing a client's medical information without written permission, and leaving a telephone message on a client's answering machine are all ways one may risk breaching client confidentiality.

19-89   Answer A

Mrs. Hernandez's insistence on discharge is an example of her exercising her right to self-determination or autonomy. The principle of beneficence implies doing the greatest good for the client and preventing harm; justice implies treating individuals fairly; and utilitarianism implies doing the greatest good for the greatest number of individuals.

19-90   Answer B

A good résumé should include name, address, telephone and fax numbers, e-mail address, educational background and degrees, professional employment, community service, research interests, grants written, publications, speaking engagements, consulting activities, honors and awards, professional memberships, and military history. Religious and demographic data, including number of children, should not be included to prevent candidates from being ruled out by any of these noncontributing factors.

19-91   Answer C

As measured by the Center for Medicare and Medicaid Services (CMS), national health expenditures are grouped into two categories: research and medical facilities construction and payments for health services and supplies. Medicare and Medicaid account for more than 76% of personal health-care services. Long-term care and medications are subsumed under the other categories. Public spending for research and facilities construction totals approximately $17 billion, only a small fraction of the approximately $900 billion spent on all health care in recent years. Of that,

more than 75% was dedicated to research paid for at the federal level.

19-92   Answer A

When caring for clients from a different culture, important pieces of assessment data include determining the ultimate decision maker (it may be someone other than the client; e.g., it may be the male patriarch of the family); determining the client's perception of the cause of his or her problem (e.g., some clients may view it as fate or a curse); and ascertaining the client's, not the family's, expectations of the provider. It is not appropriate to make decisions based on your general knowledge about the cultural background of the client. Assuming that the client expects an authoritarian health-care provider is cultural stereotyping. The practitioner should not fall into this common trap. Each clinical visit needs to be evaluated in light of the general cultural background of the client as well as the specific reasons for the visit.

19-93   Answer D

One characteristic that differentiates research from quality improvement is that research compares a new intervention with current practice to determine which is better. Research asks new questions that generate new knowledge when answered with a degree of generalizability. Additionally, there may be a risk implied to a human subject. Clients receiving the new and untested interventions may be at risk. Quality improvement evaluates things such as client satisfaction, for example, or the implementation and evaluation of new interventions already well-supported in the literature. It is not new knowledge but evaluation of existing knowledge. Similarly, with the implementation and evaluation of a standardized assessment tool, new knowledge is not gained.

19-94   Answer D

There are many steps a nurse practitioner can take if denied provider status by a third-party reimburser. Going to an attorney or contacting the newspapers may be strategies to resort to over time, but there are many more immediate and constructive strategies to try first. "Bashing" an organization is never smart; first one should ascertain the reasons for this stance and determine whether it is the same across the board regarding nurse practitioners. If it is a consistent policy, attempt to find out why and begin marshalling evidence to overturn this stance in a constructive way. This may include having both clients and physician colleagues "lobby" on your behalf. Find out who the decision maker in the organization is and attempt to communicate directly with that person. Ascertain if there is a law in the state mandating this policy. Be prepared to testify at hearings and speak out at community meetings about this issue. Request language changes that specify "ask your doctor" and lobby to have these changes adopted. Reapplication in 6 months is reasonable. Repeated applications without attempt to change policy will not be effective.

19-95   Answer B

The practice philosophy of the owner-physician is important, but it is essential that the nurse practitioner ascertain the payment methods, as listed in answer B.

19-96   Answer B

Useful strategies for the health-care provider to institute to aid the client in a relapse situation include telling the client that the relapse is a learning opportunity in preparation for the next action stage (positive reframing). Involving the family is not usually appropriate, and stressing the need to stay "straight" may be punitive and not helpful. Using fear to reinforce the need to change usually does not work for behavioral issues.

19-97   Answer A

A comprehensive history includes a chief complaint (CC); history of present illness (HPI); review of systems (ROS); and past, family, and/or social history. Although aspects of other data mentioned in the other answer options may be present, they do not include *all* the elements necessary for a comprehensive history.

19-98   Answer A

The primary care provider is the coordinator of all care that the client receives. The primary care provider does not necessarily dictate all aspects of the client's care—for example, the cardiologist may decide on the antihypertensive regimen, and the primary care provider may continue to monitor the client's response. But neither does the primary care provider turn over all aspects of the care to the specialist.

19-99   Answer B

Nonverbal communication techniques important to the establishment of rapport with the client include making direct eye contact with the client, with periodic breaks to check or take notes; avoiding having a desk between you and the client; and having personal grooming appropriate to the setting. Taking notes only while the client is talking does not help establish rapport with the client because making direct eye contact with the client aids in establishing trust. A break in eye contact, however, is important because some cultures view staring as disrespectful. Other nonverbal communication techniques that help establish rapport include sitting while interviewing the client rather than standing; standing or sitting near the client but not invading the client's personal comfort zone; and maintaining a friendly, helpful expression.

19-100   Answer A

Multiple regression and analysis of variance and covariance are tests of prediction. They are statistical techniques of inferences and imply causality, not just correlation. Statistical significance is a level set by the researcher to establish when results are sufficient to make inferences. A test of association does not exist.

19-101   Answer B

Techniques used to enhance a client's adherence to the treatment plan include giving clear written instructions, simplifying the drug regimen (such as once-a-day dosing), and having the client be an active participant (the factor most highly correlated to adherence). Negative statements that generate fear, such as stressing the dangers of missing medications, have not been found to be conducive to adherence. Positive reinforcement is best. Frequent and convenient appointments have also been correlated with higher levels of adherence. You must deal directly with the client to increase adherence, not the family.

19-102   Answer A

You need to do your homework. This means being prepared to present the facts clearly and succinctly. Talk with your colleagues by networking with other nurse practitioners in your area. Write down an optimal salary and benefits, as well as your required bottom-line salary and benefits to help establish a reasonable range. You do not necessarily need to hire a lawyer; you can handle most or all of this process yourself with proper preparation. It is premature and is not your best use of time to plan a signing dinner. Standing your ground is important but not if it means being unreasonable. Negotiate for agreement, not for winning or losing.

19-103　Answer C

Zero-based budgeting refers to a budgeting system that justifies each budget on its own merits, not on the basis of the previous period's budget. It is a process in which the budgets for succeeding budget periods are unrelated to those of earlier budget periods but rather are justified on their own merits, as if no previous budgets had ever been prepared.

19-104　Answer B

Verbal communication techniques helpful in establishing rapport with the client include verifying the name of the client and using it throughout the conversation; speaking directly to the client, introducing yourself by name, and establishing the purpose of the interaction; and communicating in a tone of voice, speed, and choice of words that are similar to the client's. Very thoroughly discussing every detail of the client's history with the client, unless absolutely necessary, can be disturbing to the client. It is important to take cues from the client. Some areas of the history will be much more important than others. You must be astute and attuned to the client without missing important information.

Bibliography

American Academy of Physician Assistants: The PA profession. www.aapa.org/the_pa_profession.aspx, accessed February 15, 2012. http://www.nursecredentialing.org/.accessed March 2012.

American Association of Colleges of Nursing: *The Essentials of Master's Education for Advance Practice Nursing.* American Association of Colleges of Nursing, Washington, DC, 2011.

American Nurses Association: *Nursing Social Policy Statement,* ed 3. American Nurses Association, Washington, DC, 2010.

American Nurses Credentialing Center: Home page. www.nursecredentialing.org/, accessed March 3, 2012.

APRN Consensus Work Group and the National Council of State Boards of Nursing APRN Advisory Committee: Consensus model for APRN regulation: Licensure, accreditation, certification & education, July 7, 2008. http://nonpf.com/associations/10789/files/APRNConsensusModelFinal09.pdf.

Buppert, CK: Justifying nurse practitioner existence: Hard facts to hard figures. *Nurse Practitioner* 20(8):43–48, 1995.

Buppert, CE: *Nurse Practitioner's Business Practice and Legal Guide,* ed 3. Aspen, Gaithersburg, MD, 2008.

Burke, CE, and Bair, JP: Marketing the role. In Sheehy, CM, and McCarthy, M, *Advanced Practice Nursing: Emphasizing Common Roles.* FA Davis, Philadelphia, 1998.

Centers for Medicare and Medicaid Services: Electronic health records. www.cms.gov/EHealth Records/, accessed March 3, 2012.

Centers for Medicare and Medicaid Services: Frequently asked questions. https://questions.cms.gov, accessed February 12, 2012.

Cronenweit, L: Molding the future of advance practice nursing. *Nursing Outlook* 43(3):112–118, 1995.

Dart, MA: *Motivational Interviewing in Nursing Practice-Empowering the Patient.* Jones and Bartlett, Boston, 2011.

Dunphy, LM, et al: *Primary Care: The Art and Science of Advanced Practice Nursing,* ed 3. FA Davis, Philadelphia, 2011.

Goolsby, MJ: *Nurse Practitioner Secrets.* Hanley & Belfus, Philadelphia, 2002.

Hamric, AB, Spross, JA, and Hanson, CM: *Advanced Practice Nursing. An Integrative Approach,* ed 4. Saunders/Elsevier, St. Louis, MO, 2009.

Hickey, JV, Ouimette, RM, and Venegoni, SL (eds): *Advance Practice Nursing,* ed 3. Lippincott-Raven, Philadelphia, 2007.

www.healthypeople.gov/2020/topicsobjectives2020/overview.aspx?topicid=39

Kovner, AR, and Jonas, S (eds): *Jonas and Kovner's Health Care Delivery in the United States,* ed 6. Springer, New York, 2007.

Mahoney, DF: Employer resistance to state authorized prescriptive authority for nurse practitioners. *Nurse Practitioner* 20(1):58–61, 1995.

Medicare Benefit Policy Manual. CMS Services, Washington, DC, 2010.

National Organization of Nurse Practitioner Faculties: *Curriculum Guidelines and Program Standards for Nurse Practitioner Education*. National Organization of Nurse Practitioner Faculties, Washington, DC, 2000.

Pearson, LJ: Annual update of how each state stands on legislative issues affecting advance nursing practice. *Nurse Practitioner* 37(1), 2012.

Pew Health Professions Commission: *Interdisciplinary Collaborative Teams in Primary Care: A Model Curriculum and Resource Guide*. University of California, San Francisco Center for the Health Professions, San Francisco, 1995.

Pew Health Professions Commission: Nurse practitioners: Doubling graduates by the year 2000. In *Commission Policy Papers*. Pew Health Professions Commission, San Francisco, 1994.

Schaffner, JW, Ludwig-Beymer, P, and Wiggins, J: Utilization of advance practice nurses in health care systems and multispecialty group practice. *Journal of Nursing Administration* 25(12):37–43, 1995.

Snyder, M, and Mirr, MP: *Advanced Practice Nursing: A Guide to Professional Development*. Springer, New York, 2000.

US Department of Health and Human Services: Social determinants of health: Overview. www.healthy-people.gov/2020/topicsobjectives2020/overview.aspx?topicid=39, accessed August 2012.

How well did you do?

85% and above, congratulations! This score shows application of test-taking principles and adequate content knowledge.

75%–85%, keep working! Review test-taking principles and try again.

65%–75%, hang in there! Spend some time reviewing concepts and test-taking principles and try the test again.

PRACTICE EXAMINATIONS

Examination 1

Jill E. Winland-Brown
Lynne M. Dunphy

Questions

1-1 *What is the most common presentation of a client with a sprained ankle?*

A. Point tenderness over a ligament, ecchymoses, edema, and pain

B. General achiness, reddened skin, and no edema

C. Bony deformity, no edema, and cool skin

D. Crepitus, ecchymoses, severe pain, and no point tenderness

1-2 *Anticipatory guidance for the parents of a child with molluscum contagiosum should include that the condition will*

A. result in small circular scars.

B. develop hypopigmented areas.

C. remain contagious until all of the lesions are gone.

D. respond easily to treatment.

1-3 *Which of the following is a urological emergency?*

A. Testicular torsion

B. Epididymitis

C. Varicocele

D. Hydrocele

1-4 *Which of the following topical preparations should not be used in intertriginous areas or in the perineum because they increase maceration?*

A. Gel solutions

B. Ointments

C. Emollient creams

D. Powders

1-5 *Your client Mrs. Jones, age 78, is brought to your primary care office by her son, James. He is describing recent changes in Mrs. Jones's behavior and affect. You are trying to differentiate between depression and dementia. You know that*

A. the person with dementia usually tries to conceal memory problems.

B. the person with depression has wide mood swings.

C. dementia has a sudden onset.

D. agitation always accompanies depression.

1-6 *Auscultation of the chest of a client with congestive heart failure typically reveals*

A. an S_3 gallop.

B. a pericardial rub.

C. bronchial vesicular breath sounds.

D. S_4 sounds.

1-7 *Ethel, age 72, lives by herself quite capably. Her daughter feels that she is sometimes forgetful and needs to move in with her. She calls Ethel's physician to try to convince him that he should persuade Ethel to move in with her. This is*

A. a violation of Ethel's personal autonomy.

B. evidence of a thoughtful daughter.

C. evidence of a daughter who feels ethically obliged to take care of her mother.

D. not the daughter's decision; the physician should decide Ethel's competency.

1-8 *The most common pathogen for bronchiolitis in children younger than age 2 is*

A. parainfluenza.

B. influenza.

C. respiratory syncytial virus.

D. adenovirus.

1-9 *The most common clinical manifestation of heart failure is*

A. tachycardia.

B. syncope.

C. dyspnea.

D. peripheral edema.

1-10 *The process of enabling people to increase control over and to improve their health is referred to as*

A. primary care.

B. health promotion.

C. primary prevention.

D. collaborative care.

1-11 *A bruit in which of the following areas may indicate renal artery stenosis?*

A. Epigastric

B. Aortic

C. Iliac

D. Femoral

1-12 *Which test differentiates iron-deficiency anemia from the anemia of chronic disease in clients with normal or low mean corpuscular volume values?*

A. Ferritin

B. Total iron-binding capacity

C. Folate

D. Erythrocyte sedimentation rate

1-13 *Clinical symptoms of congestive heart failure noted on physical examination may include*

A. collapsed neck veins.

B. splenomegaly.

C. hepatomegaly.

D. hyperactive bowel sounds and diarrhea.

1-14 *When is a magnetic resonance imaging (MRI) scan indicated to rule out a herniated nucleus pulposus (HNP)?*

A. When the client experiences a loss of bowel and bladder function

B. When the client has acute low back pain

C. When there is no improvement after 2 weeks

D. When the client is complaining of spasms in both calves at night

1-15 *Jill's son, Nathan, has asthma, and she cannot decide whether he should play Little League*

baseball or not. She asks for your advice. What do you tell her?

A. "Exercise should be encouraged rather than restricted."

B. "Sports are recommended unless exercise-induced bronchospasm occurs."

C. "He should find some other type of recreational activity."

D. "If he has a nebulization treatment before playing, he should do fine."

1-16 *June, age 24, who started on oral contraceptives several months ago, presents today with pruritic, tender plaques on her hands and elbows. She doesn't take any other medications except for the birth control pill. What do you suspect?*

A. Urticaria

B. Psoriasis

C. Contact dermatitis

D. Erythema multiforme

1-17 *Which type of hepatitis is transmitted by the fecal-oral route; is rare in the United States but endemic in Southeast Asia, India, North Africa, and Mexico; and does not progress to chronic liver disease?*

A. Hepatitis D (HDV)

B. Hepatitis E (HEV)

C. Hepatitis C (HCV)

D. Hepatitis A (HAV)

1-18 *Erythropoietin replacement therapy is indicated in*

A. chronic renal failure.

B. thalassemia minor.

C. sickle cell disorders.

D. aplastic anemia.

1-19 *Which type of communication tends to be misunderstood the most?*

A. Verbal

B. Nonverbal

C. Written

D. Telephone

1-20 Which of the following features at an initial prenatal assessment suggests that a woman is at higher risk for the development of gestational diabetes?

A. Previous cesarean section

B. Decreased urine osmolality

C. Macrosomia

D. Yeast infection

1-21 Separation anxiety and stranger anxiety occur around age

A. 5–6 months.

B. 7–8 months.

C. 8–9 months.

D. 10–11 months.

1-22 When performing a respiratory assessment on a client with pneumococcal pneumonia, you would expect to find

A. increased vocal fremitus.

B. fine crackles.

C. hyperresonance.

D. asymmetric chest expansion.

1-23 Joe has had several kidney stones over the past year. They have been analyzed and determined to be calcium stones. What question might you ask him to help determine prevention recommendations?

A. "Do you use vitamin D supplements?"

B. "Are you on any antidepressants?"

C. "Do you take excessive amounts of vitamin C?"

D. "Do you have a history of frequent urinary tract infections?"

1-24 Matthew, age 3, is rushed into the office with an upper airway obstruction as a result of foreign body aspiration. A partial obstruction is present. What is your next step?

A. Place him facedown over your arm and give him five measured back blows.

B. Use the Heimlich maneuver.

C. Allow him to use his own cough reflex to extrude the foreign body.

D. Blindly probe his airway to dislodge the foreign body.

1-25 "Pustular" is a morphological classification of which skin lesion?

A. Herpes simplex

B. A wart

C. Acne rosacea

D. Impetigo

1-26 Damages covered by the "personal injury" clause in a practitioner's liability insurance might include

A. the practitioner's dog biting the physician.

B. false arrest, detention, or imprisonment.

C. a visitor tripping over the practitioner's child's toy.

D. clients not being able to get an appointment within 24 hours.

1-27 In which Tanner developmental stage is Josh, whose pubic hair is becoming darker and coarser, slightly curled, and spreads over his symphysis; whose penis is starting to lengthen; and whose scrotum shows a little increase in size?

A. Tanner stage 1

B. Tanner stage 2

C. Tanner stage 3

D. Tanner stage 4

1-28 Marnie comes to the clinic with multiple bruises and complaining of low back pain. She answers all questions with monosyllabic answers and averts her gaze. What should be your first response?

A. "Don't worry. We'll take care of everything."

B. "Is someone hurting you at home?"

C. "Are your children bruised also?"

D. "What happened to you?"

1-29 Jenny is a primigravida. You talk to her about "quickening" and tell her to expect it at about

A. 12–14 weeks' gestation.

B. 14–16 weeks' gestation.

C. 18–20 weeks' gestation.

D. 22–24 weeks' gestation.

1-30   *When assessing abdominal pain, determine the severity of the pain by asking the client*

A.   "Is it the worst pain you've ever experienced?"

B.   "Do you feel at the 'end of your rope'?"

C.   "How would you rate it on a scale of 1–10?"

D.   "Please describe it for me."

1-31   *A pharmacological approach for the client with chronic systolic dysfunction includes the use of*

A.   angiotensin-converting enzyme (ACE) inhibitors.

B.   diuretics as monotherapy.

C.   vasoconstrictive agents.

D.   digoxin as monotherapy.

1-32   *Which of the following can trigger a lesion in the client with psoriasis?*

A.   A headache

B.   Salt water

C.   Aspirin

D.   Alcohol

1-33   *The most significant factor in a client developing recurrent urinary tract infections is the*

A.   type of bacteria present.

B.   presence of a urinary obstruction.

C.   type of antibiotic taken.

D.   lack of hydration.

1-34   *Martin is coming in for his examination directly after a dental appointment at which he was told he had gingival overgrowth. What medication do you think he must be taking?*

A.   Phenytoin (Dilantin)

B.   Methyldopa (Aldomet)

C.   Prednisone (Deltasone)

D.   Sertraline (Zoloft)

1-35   *A classic symptom of carpal tunnel syndrome is acroparesthesia, which is*

A.   the relief of tingling and numbness of the fingers by shaking or rubbing the hands.

B.   awaking at night with numbness and burning pain in the fingers.

C.   wrist pain with repetitive motions.

D.   pain on percussion of the median nerve.

1-36   *Jack, age 42, has diabetes and now has a diagnosis of hypertension. He is not tolerating the ACE inhibitor you tried as initial therapy. What would you try next?*

A.   A calcium channel blocker

B.   A beta blocker

C.   An angiotensin receptor blocker

D.   A diuretic

1-37   *Ben, age 72, is complaining of insomnia and asks your advice. You recommend that he*

A.   take alprazolam (Xanax) at bedtime.

B.   go for a walk before bedtime.

C.   eat a large meal before bedtime for relaxation.

D.   refrain from napping during the day.

1-38   *An ultrasound is often the most reliable way of ascertaining the estimated date of confinement (EDC) because a woman's memory regarding the date of her last menstrual period is often unreliable. When performed during the first trimester, ultrasound is able to predict the EDC to within 7–10 days using which measurement?*

A.   Biparietal diameter

B.   Femur length

C.   Skull width

D.   Crown-rump length

1-39   *An expectant mother shares that she is a pescatarian. Which of the following is correct regarding the pescatarian diet?*

A.   It includes fruits, vegetables, beans, grains, seeds, and nuts. All animal sources of protein—including meat, poultry, fish, eggs, milk and cheese, are excluded.

B.   It includes dairy products in addition to fruits, vegetables, beans, grains, seeds, and nuts. Meat, poultry, fish and eggs are excluded.

C.   It includes dairy products and eggs in addition to fruits, vegetables, beans, grains, seeds, and nuts. Meat, poultry, and fish are excluded.

D.   It includes daily products and eggs in addition to fruits, vegetables, beans, grains, seeds, and nuts. Meat and poultry are excluded from the diet, but fish is permitted.

1-40   Which laboratory finding would be indicative of celiac disease?

A. Excessive fecal fat

B. Hyperproteinemia

C. Many villi apparent in the jejunal mucosa on intestinal biopsy

D. A normal carbohydrate metabolism

1-41   Educating the public and industry to use healthy rehabilitated persons to the fullest extent possible is an example of

A. primary prevention.

B. secondary prevention.

C. tertiary prevention.

D. general prevention.

1-42   Jennifer, age 36, has systemic lupus erythematosus. She exhibits erythematous raised patches with adherent keratotic scaling and follicular plugging. This is characteristic of

A. a malar rash.

B. a discoid rash.

C. photosensitivity.

D. an oral ulcer.

1-43   Sandra, a nurse practitioner, tells you that she has a collaborative practice as described in the American Nurses Association's Social Policy Statement. You know that she misunderstands the term when she tells you that it is

A. the exchange of ideas and knowledge.

B. the recognition of expertise of others within and outside of one's expertise.

C. shared functions and a common focus on the same mission.

D. the NPs and PAs in the practice group working together under the physician's direction.

1-44   For borderline dyslipidemia, a sensible nutritional approach is the best recommendation. Which of the following would be one of the recommendations?

A. Reducing total fat to 10%

B. Limiting dietary cholesterol to less than 100 mg/day

C. Having a daily intake of fewer than 1,000 calories

D. Reducing saturated fat to less than 7% of calories

1-45   In trying to determine which type of urinary incontinence Mona, age 56, has, you order a postvoid residual urine. The results come back with a low reading. Which type of incontinence would this indicate?

A. Hypoactive bladder (neurogenic bladder)

B. Outlet incompetence (stress incontinence)

C. Outlet obstruction (overflow incontinence)

D. All types of incontinence result in a high level (amount) of postvoid residual urine.

1-46   John, age 46, has AIDS. He comes to the office with white lesions in his oropharynx. What do you suspect?

A. Kaposi's sarcoma

B. Herpes simplex virus

C. Thrush or oral hairy leukoplakia

D. Gingivitis

1-47   How often should a CD4 count be evaluated in a client with AIDS if the client's previous levels have been greater than 500?

A. Every month

B. At every visit

C. Every 6 months

D. Annually

1-48   The O'Leary family is taking a trip to Florida. They ask you which sunscreen you recommend for their 4-month-old daughter. What is the best advice to give this couple?

A. Apply products with Zinc oxide every 2 hours.

B. Keep the baby out of the sun, use protective clothing, and apply a minimal amount of SPF 15 sunscreen to small areas, such as the face and the back of the hands.

C. Apply products with titanium dioxide and stay in the shade from 10 a.m. until 2 p.m.

D. Apply products with octinoxate 7% every 2–3 hours.

1-49   You are examining a pregnant woman. Measuring from the symphysis pubis, you find that the fundal height is palpable at the umbilicus. As a rule of thumb, you would estimate this woman to be at

A. 12 weeks' gestation.

B. 16 weeks' gestation.

C. 20 weeks' gestation.

D. 24 weeks' gestation.

1-50 *Which of the following foods has the highest amount of calcium and should be recommended to your client with osteoporosis?*

A. Swiss cheese

B. Cottage cheese

C. Eggs

D. Yogurt

1-51 *Lorie has been given a diagnosis of Cushing's disease. You tell her that 80% of all cases are cured by*

A. subtotal transsphenoidal hypophysectomy.

B. irradiation.

C. adrenal enzyme inhibitors.

D. adrenalectomy.

1-52 *A class III Pap test result indicates*

A. a normal Pap test.

B. carcinoma in situ.

C. adenocarcinoma.

D. mild dysplasia.

1-53 *Certain drugs have enhanced effects when combined with oral contraceptives. This is true for which of the following drugs?*

A. Beta blockers

B. Phenytoin (Dilantin)

C. Antacids

D. Oral anticoagulants

1-54 *Clinical manifestations of headache, drowsiness, agitation, slowed thinking, and confusion all characterize the most common type of intracranial hematoma. This is a (an)*

A. meningeal.

B. subdural.

C. intracerebral.

D. epidural.

1-55 *Your 68-year-old client has just been diagnosed with type 2 diabetes. There are many aspects of the client's health that need careful inspection. Which of the following could you hold off on until a later visit?*

A. Has my client received a foot exam and instruction in routine foot care?

B. Are liver function tests normal or not?

C. What is the client's cardiovascular risk?

D. What is the degree of obesity?

1-56 *Martha is experiencing an acute clinical syndrome characterized by fever, night sweats, lethargy and malaise, myalgias, arthralgias, general lymphadenopathy, pharyngitis, maculopapular rash, and a headache. You suspect this to be an acute primary infection that usually follows exposure to HIV. How many weeks ago do you think she was exposed to HIV?*

A. 1 week

B. 2–4 weeks

C. 1–2 months

D. 2–4 months

1-57 *You are auscultating Mr. Harris' (age 78) heart. You hear a short, high-frequency click (opening snap) after S_2 during the beginning of diastole. You know that this indicates*

A. nothing unusual for a client of this age.

B. aortic regurgitation.

C. mitral regurgitation.

D. mitral stenosis.

1-58 *What is the most common cause of progressive dementia in persons older than 55?*

A. Alzheimer's disease

B. Vascular disease

C. Huntington's disease

D. Parkinson's disease

1-59 *Lacresha is a 6-year-old who recently returned from a trip to Jamaica. A rash developed shortly after her time playing on the beach. The rash is on the dorsa of the feet and the interdigital spaces of the toes and her thumbs. It is extremely pruritic, linear, and serpiginous. The clinician knows that the following condition should be considered until proven otherwise?*

A. Tinea pedis

B. Larva migrans

C. Sea lice

D. Hand-foot-mouth disease

1-60 Sally, age 8, has frequent episodes of epistaxis. What prevention strategy do you suggest to her mother?

A. Vigorously blow her nose before going to bed to ensure a patent airway.

B. Start low-dose daily aspirin therapy.

C. Humidify the bedroom.

D. Tilt her head back and pinch her nose.

1-61 To what specialty would the NP refer clients for nutrition therapy, medication management, and to gain increased skill in self-management of their diabetes?

A. Fitness trainer

B. Board-certified endocrinologist

C. Certified diabetic educator

D. Medical doctor

1-62 Which type of seizure is initiated from both cerebral hemispheres?

A. Generalized seizures

B. Partial complex seizures

C. Partial simple seizures

D. Temporal lobe seizures

1-63 Mason has chronic nonbacterial prostatitis. He is predisposed to develop

A. infertility.

B. decreased fertility.

C. benign prostatic hypertrophy.

D. prostate cancer.

1-64 In examining a child with possible rheumatic fever, you may note

A. a murmur consistent with valvular sufficiency.

B. subcutaneous nodules on the extensor surfaces of the lower extremities.

C. an erythematous rash over the trunk and proximal part of the limbs.

D. confusion caused by low fevers.

1-65 Lymphedema may be differentiated from venous edema by

A. being a soft pitting edema with skin of normal texture.

B. affecting the foot but not the toes.

C. being a firm edema that pits poorly, with thickened skin.

D. showing an increase in the superficial venous pattern.

1-66 Johnny, age 2, is brought in by his mother with painless rectal bleeding with dark red and black stools. You suspect

A. Hirschsprung's disease.

B. chylous ascites.

C. duplications of the gastrointestinal tract.

D. Meckel's diverticulum.

1-67 Your client Sally has had significant diarrhea for several days. What laboratory values would you expect to be increased?

A. Serum chloride

B. Serum potassium

C. Serum sodium

D. Serum bicarbonate

1-68 At what age should medication be considered for children with LDL cholesterol levels of 190 or higher if changes in diet and exercise haven't been successful?

A. 5 years

B. 6 years

C. 8 years

D. 10 years

1-69 Gestational diabetes occurs in what percentage of all pregnancies?

A. 0.5%

B. 1%–2%

C. 5%

D. 7%

1-70 Jacob, age 56, is started on finasteride (Proscar) to improve his benign prostatic hyperplasia symptoms by reducing the size of his prostate. Which of the following statements is true regarding finasteride?

A. Liver function tests should be done every 3–6 months to assess for potential liver damage.

B. The dose should be started low initially, then titrated upward.

C. For a complete therapeutic trial, the medication should be continued for a full 12 months.

D. If not effective by 6 months, the drug should be discontinued.

1-71 *Signs of elder mistreatment may include*

A. minimal visits from family members at a nursing home.

B. polypharmacy.

C. clean dry skin.

D. decubitus ulcer.

1-72 *Marie has a 9-month-old daughter whose first tooth has not erupted yet. She asks you when she should take her daughter to the dentist. You tell her*

A. "She should go to the dentist now."

B. "Wait until her first tooth erupts."

C. "She should go at 1 year of age even if her first tooth has not come in or as soon as it does."

D. "When she's 1½ years old and ready to brush her teeth, she should go to the dentist."

1-73 *Jeff, a nurse practitioner, is pressing down on the client's prostate with his index finger, moving from the base to the distal end of the gland. He is sweeping the gland's entire surface in a series of longitudinal strokes. What is he doing?*

A. A digital rectal examination

B. Checking for induration of the prostate

C. Assessing for benign prostatic hypertrophy

D. Prostatic massage

1-74 *In the screening portion of a routine physical, you ask a child to copy a cross after observing you do so; to stand on one leg for at least 10 seconds; to hand you two sticks from a pile of four tongue depressors; and to draw a man (expecting a head, two appendages, and possibly two eyes but probably not a torso). What age would you expect the child to be?*

A. 2–3 years

B. 3–4 years

C. 4–5 years

D. 5–6 years

1-75 *How does phenytoin (Dilantin) cause megaloblastic anemia?*

A. It interferes with vitamin B_{12} metabolism.

B. It interferes with vitamin C metabolism.

C. It interferes with vitamin D_3 metabolism.

D. It interferes with vitamin B_1 metabolism.

1-76 *In which age group does the highest incidence of rape and other sexual assaults occur?*

A. Age younger than 10 years

B. Ages 14–19

C. Young and middle-aged adults

D. Older adults

1-77 *Latoya is a 38-year-old investment banker, pregnant with her second child. She is a single mother and lives in the city with her son and cat. Her diet is vegan. The clinician knows that Latoya is at risk for toxoplasmosis due to her*

A. employment setting.

B. vegan diet.

C. living with a cat.

D. advanced maternal age.

1-78 *Joyce is hypothyroid and has been taking levothyroxine (Synthroid) 112 mcg. She is now pregnant. What should you change her dose to?*

A. 75 mcg

B. 88 mcg

C. 125 mcg

D. 137 mcg

1-79 *Susan is 36 weeks pregnant, and during a routine examination you test her urine and note a 3+ proteinuria. Her blood pressure is normal. Your next step is to*

A. refer her to an obstetrician.

B. monitor her blood pressure and urine 2 days later.

C. obtain a clean-catch midstream urine specimen for culture and sensitivity.

D. have her drink several glasses of water and test a second urine specimen.

1-80 Which of the following is a component of metabolic syndrome?

A. An HDL-C less than 40 mg/dL in women

B. A BP greater than 140/90

C. A waist circumference greater than 35 in. in women

D. A fasting glucose greater than 120 mg/dL

1-81 At which disk levels of the lumbar spine do most herniations occur?

A. L1–L3

B. L2–L4

C. L3–L5

D. L4–S1

1-82 Samantha, age 35, states that she wants to be tested for "thyroid disease" because it runs in her family. Her thyroid-stimulating hormone level comes back mildly high, and she has normal T_3 and T_4 levels. What is the diagnosis?

A. Primary hypothyroidism

B. Subclinical hypothyroidism

C. Primary hyperthyroidism

D. Subclinical hyperthyroidism

1-83 A positive Phalen's sign indicates

A. splenomegaly.

B. carpal tunnel syndrome.

C. a fractured hip.

D. rheumatoid arthritis.

1-84 What is the term for pain or discomfort during or after intercourse?

A. Metrorrhagia

B. Dyspareunia

C. Dysmenorrhea

D. Dysphagia

1-85 Your client of many years calls you for advice because she states that her obstetrician just told her that her newborn has breast milk jaundice. She wants to know if she has to stop breastfeeding. What do you tell her?

A. "Yes, you should start the infant on a bottle."

B. "You should stop breastfeeding for a week, pump your breasts, then resume feedings when the jaundice clears up."

C. "The jaundice clears before 3 months in almost all infants, even when breastfeeding is continued."

D. "You need to stop breastfeeding for at least 1 month but may resume after that."

1-86 Ms. Peterson shares concerns about having a child with a disability because her sister's child has recently been diagnosed with Rett's syndrome. The clinician knows that Rett's syndrome usually occurs in

A. boys.

B. girls.

C. a equal number of boys and girls.

D. Ashkenazi Jews.

1-87 Which of the following exercises would you recommend as being the best for your client with osteoporosis?

A. Swimming

B. Walking

C. Chair aerobics

D. The client should avoid any exercise that might cause an injury.

1-88 The expected change in weight in the neonate (physiological weight loss) is the result of a loss of

A. intracellular fluid.

B. extracellular fluid and meconium.

C. blood through the umbilical cord.

D. blood, fluid, and meconium.

1-89 Mr. Albert has chronic leukemia and currently is experiencing a low platelet count. This is usually manifested as

A. multiple macular lesions in sun-exposed area.

B. red, flat, nonblanchable petechiae.

C. numerous brown, nonscaly macules that become more prominent after exposure to the sun.

D. an irregular border and a black lesion.

1-90 When examining the newborn, what is the minimum number of café-au-lait spots that should be of concern?

A. Any number

B. 1–3

C. 4–5

D. More than 5

1-91   *Which document "drives" the health-care agenda for the nation?*

A. The Pew Health Professions Commission Report

B. The World Health Organization report

C. *Healthy People 2020*

D. The ANA Social Policy Statement

1-92   *Which positive sign on physical examination is indicative that the client may have appendicitis?*

A. McBurney's

B. Phalen's

C. Tinel's

D. Chvostek's

1-93   *Which of the following statements is true regarding eye disease and persons with diabetes?*

A. Cataracts occur at the same rate in people with diabetes and those without diabetes.

B. Closed-angle glaucoma is more common in people with diabetes.

C. Cataracts occur at a younger age and progress more rapidly in people with diabetes.

D. Eye surgery must be approached with caution in people with diabetes because of poor healing.

1-94   *Which type of cancer has the highest mortality rate of all cancers and yet is one of the most preventable?*

A. Cervical cancer

B. Bladder cancer

C. Breast cancer

D. Lung cancer

1-95   *Barbara has type 2 diabetes and now has dyslipidemia. Which drug should be added to her regimen to lower the triglycerides into an acceptable range?*

A. Gemfibrozil (Lopid)

B. Nicotinic acid (Niacin)

C. Cholestyramine (Questran)

D. Bile acid sequestrant (Colestid)

1-96   *What is the most common complication experienced by the largest percentage of clients with type 2 diabetes?*

A. Neuropathies

B. Blindness

C. Kidney failure

D. Urinary tract infections

1-97   *Which person or group stated that health reflects a philosophic ideal, encompassing optimal mental, physical, and emotional well-being, and not merely the absence of disease?*

A. Nola Pender

B. The World Health Organization

C. Betty Newman

D. The American Nurses Association

1-98   *Allison is scheduled for her annual school physical. The client looks older than what is indicated on her chart. The clinician knows that puberty is considered precocious if it occurs*

A. in boys or girls 8 years of age or less.

B. before 6 years of age in African American girls.

C. before 9 years of age in Caucasian girls.

D. before 10 years of age in boys.

1-99   *Allergic rhinitis results from which immunoglobulin-mediated type I hypersensitivity?*

A. IgA

B. IgD

C. IgG

D. IgE

1-100   *Which of the following is an indication for a lumbar diskectomy?*

A. Pain controlled by large doses of NSAIDs

B. Cauda equina syndrome

C. A rapid onset of a neurological deficit

D. Sciatica

1-101   *The most common ocular manifestation with rosacea is*

A. blepharitis.

B. conjunctivitis.

C. hordeolum.

D. tearing.

1-102 *National guidelines recommend that which one of the following screening tests does not need to be performed every year on a type 1 diabetic client?*

A. A hearing test

B. A dilated eye exam

C. A foot exam

D. Microalbuminuria spot testing

1-103 *Which of the following statements is true about cluster headaches?*

A. They predominantly affect middle-aged women.

B. There is always a family history of headache or migraine.

C. Alcohol may trigger an attack.

D. The episodes usually awaken the client at night and then last for about 4 hours.

1-104 *Which type of skin cancer is most common in adults?*

A. Basal cell

B. Squamous cell

C. Melanoma

D. Actinic keratosis

1-105 *Marta, age 52, is scheduled for sclerotherapy. She asks you what to expect during her recovery. You tell her that she will*

A. be able to walk out of the office wearing shorts and looking great.

B. have to go home and put her feet up (either in bed or in a lounge chair) for several days.

C. be in the hospital for several days.

D. have her legs wrapped afterward with graduated compression stockings.

1-106 *Your client brings her daughter to the clinic with her. She says three words over and over again. About what age do you think she is?*

A. 10 months

B. 13 months

C. 15 months

D. 18 months

1-107 *The most common cause of erectile dysfunction is*

A. prostate surgery.

B. generalized atherosclerosis.

C. drug use (antihypertensives, antidepressants).

D. diabetes.

1-108 *While doing an assessment of a baby in the newborn nursery, the clinician knows that up to 20% of newborns present with*

A. cysts and nodular lesions.

B. neonatal acne.

C. truncal acne.

D. *Malassezia* species colonization.

1-109 *Your client with a colostomy seems to have excessive flatus. In teaching him some strategies to help decrease the flatus, you know he misunderstands your teaching when he tells you which of the following?*

A. "I'll stop smoking and chewing gum."

B. "I'll eliminate beer from my diet."

C. "I'll avoid broccoli, brussels sprouts, cabbage, cauliflower, cucumbers, mushrooms, and peas."

D. "I'll poke multiple holes in the bottom of the bag to let the air out."

1-110 *Secondary amenorrhea is*

A. the failure to menstruate by age 14 in girls with no secondary sex characteristics (breast development).

B. the failure to menstruate by age 16 in girls who may or may not have developed secondary sexual characteristics.

C. the absence of menstruation for 3 or more consecutive months in a woman who has achieved menarche.

D. the absence of menstruation during a second pregnancy.

1-111 *Susan, age 46, states that she has a slowly developing, painless, hard mass on her right eye. Physical examination with eversion of the eyelid reveals a red, elevated mass that is quite large on the meibomian gland pressing against the eye, causing nystagmus. What is your diagnosis?*

A. Hordeolum

B. Blepharitis

C. Sebaceous cell carcinoma

D. Chalazion

1-112   *Maura, age 36, has just been given a diagnosis of Bell's palsy and asks you about her chances for a complete recovery. How do you respond?*

A. "Don't worry; I'm sure you'll have a complete recovery."

B. "You have about a 50-50 chance of complete recovery; otherwise, you may have some minor problems."

C. "About 80% of clients have a complete recovery within 2 months."

D. "Although you won't recover completely, the residual effects are minor."

1-113   *Lynne asks you about the site selection for a blood specimen on her newborn. You tell her that the best site is*

A. the most lateral surface of the plantar aspect of the infant's heel.

B. the central area of the newborn's foot.

C. the newborn's finger.

D. a previous puncture site.

1-114   *Sam, age 72, has dry eye with a triad presentation of burning, itching, and a foreign body sensation in the eye. You know this as keratoconjunctivitis sicca (KCS). This symptom is frequently associated with the diagnosis of*

A. Reuter's syndrome.

B. Sjögren's syndrome.

C. temporal arteritis.

D. glaucoma.

1-115   *Which bacterial infection in children appears as a firm, dry crust, surrounded by erythema that exudes purulent material?*

A. Ecthyma

B. Impetigo

C. Bullous impetigo

D. Cellulitis

1-116   *Which nerve root is responsible for the Achilles reflex?*

A. L4

B. L5

C. S1

D. S2

1-117   *A client has a diagnosis of bronchiectasis. When he asks what caused this, the nurse practitioner tells him that the structural changes in the bronchi are usually associated with*

A. chronic bronchitis.

B. lung tumors.

C. bacterial infections.

D. congenital defects.

1-118   *Which of the following is the best statement regarding diastolic blood pressure in pregnancy?*

A. The diastolic blood pressure is lower during the second trimester and increases to prepregnancy levels by about week 36.

B. The diastolic blood pressure tends to be somewhat higher during the second and third trimester.

C. The diastolic blood pressure tends to be somewhat lower during the second and third trimesters.

D. The diastolic blood pressure is higher during the second trimester because of weight gain and lower during the third.

1-119   *A rule of thumb for the growth guideline of children is that their birth weight triples by age*

A. 6 months.

B. 9 months.

C. 12 months.

D. 15 months.

1-120   *A woman shares concerns that the baby she is carrying may have osteogenesis imperfecta (OI) because a distant family member has OI. The majority of cases of OI occur due to which of the following?*

A. A small section of a chromosome is missing.

B. A chromosomal rearrangement called a balanced translocation

C. A dominant mutation to type 1 collagen (COL1A1 or COL1A2) genes

D. Two, or occasionally more, X chromosomes along with a Y chromosome

1-121 *Chronic urinary retention may result in*

A. total incontinence.

B. stress incontinence.

C. urge incontinence.

D. overflow incontinence.

1-122 *Sandy, age 9, has seizures with brief, jerking contractions of her arms, legs, and trunk. Which seizure type is this?*

A. Myoclonic

B. Clonic

C. Tonic

D. Tonic-clonic

1-123 *Liability insurance that covers claims made against the practitioner only while the policy is in force is referred to as*

A. an occurrence policy.

B. an annual aggregate policy.

C. a claims made policy.

D. a functional policy.

1-124 *Ginger says she was taught that because she has diabetes, she should carry sweets with her in case she has a hypoglycemic episode. However, she is unsure of how much to take. How much rapidly absorbable carbohydrate do you tell her to take to abort a hypoglycemia episode?*

A. 5–10 g

B. 10–15 g

C. 15–20 g

D. 20–25 g

1-125 *Which of the following symptoms is typical in fibromyalgia?*

A. Widespread pain at multiple sites

B. Sleeping deeply for greater than 8 hours

C. Afternoon fatigue

D. Difficulty with fine motor tasks

1-126 *Which of the following signs might lead you to suspect something other than metabolic syndrome?*

A. Elevated HDL

B. Central abdominal obesity

C. Hypertension

D. Exercise intolerance

1-127 *The type of insulin most commonly used in an insulin pump is*

A. rapid-acting insulin.

B. long-acting insulin such as Lantus.

C. short-acting insulin.

D. NPH.

1-128 *Mrs. Robertson reports that her son Jamal is a "handful." She states that he refuses to do anything she asks him to do, and he blames others for his mistakes. What do you suspect?*

A. Conduct disorder

B. Oppositional defiant disorder

C. Social aggression

D. Attention deficit disorder

1-129 *The TNM staging system for cancer assists in guiding therapeutic choices. The T in TNM stands for*

A. the type of tumor.

B. the extent of the primary tumor.

C. the length of time the tumor has been in existence.

D. how solid the tumor feels to touch.

1-130 *The study of proxemics has identified that personal space is appropriate for close relationships in which touching may be involved and good visualization is desired. Personal space is defined as a distance of*

A. up to 18 inches.

B. 18 inches to 4 feet.

C. 4–9 feet.

D. 9 feet and over.

1-131 *The purpose of administering a vasodilating drug to a client in heart failure is to*

A. reduce contractility.

B. increase preload.

C. increase afterload.

D. reduce afterload.

1-132   Which skin disorder in newborns occurs when the infant is placed on one side and the dependent half develops an erythematous flush while the upper half of the body becomes pale?

A.   Sebaceous gland hyperplasia

B.   Erythema toxicum

C.   Erythema toxicum neonatorum

D.   Harlequin color change

1-133   Which statement by your client with diabetes leads you to believe that he could use some more education on his diabetes?

A.   "I am eating smaller portions of the food I once ate and am now going to the gym."

B.   "I have learned to count my carbohydrates and am beginning to exercise and lose weight."

C.   "I have lost weight, am exercising as instructed, and have made my yearly appointments with my eye doctor, podiatrist, and lab work."

D.   "Management of my diabetes is really a matter of cutting out sweets in my diet."

1-134   Classic psoriasis lesions exhibit

A.   diffuse macules over the torso.

B.   sharply marginated plaques and papules with marked silvery-white scales.

C.   ulcerations on flexor surfaces of the extremities.

D.   transient thin-roofed vesicles with honey-colored crusts.

1-135   What does Trousseau's sign assess for?

A.   Hypocalcemia

B.   Hypercalcemia

C.   Hyponatremia

D.   Hypomagnesia

1-136   Mary is at risk for endometrial cancer because she

A.   is between 40 and 50 years of age.

B.   is underweight.

C.   has a history of hypertension, diabetes, and endometrial hyperplasia.

D.   has a family history of ovarian and breast cancer.

1-137   The majority of ovarian malignancies are caused by

A.   granulosa stromal cell tumors.

B.   germ cell tumors.

C.   undifferentiated tumors.

D.   epithelial tumors.

1-138   Junior can say approximately 900 words and speaks intelligible four-word phrases. How old do you think he is?

A.   2 years old

B.   3 years old

C.   4 years old

D.   5 years old

1-139   According to the American Nurses Association's Social Policy Statement, the authority for the practice of nursing is based on

A.   a social contract that acknowledges professional rights and responsibilities, as well as being a mechanism for public accountability.

B.   the values and assumptions of nursing theorists, with the society as a sounding board.

C.   state regulatory laws and legislation.

D.   legislation set by the state boards of medicine.

1-140   You suspect that Marcia has an eating disorder because she is 5 ft 6 in. tall, weighs 110 lbs, and seems disgusted with herself when you weigh her. During your examination, you suspect bulimia rather than anorexia because of her

A.   sensitivity to cold.

B.   hair loss.

C.   swollen salivary glands.

D.   statement regarding irregular menstruation.

1-141   Mindy is taking levothyroxine (Synthroid) for her hypothyroidism, along with several other medications. She asks if she needs to stop taking any of her medications when she comes in for blood work because she has heard that many drugs affect thyroid function test results. Which drug do you tell her that she can continue taking because it will not affect the results?

A.   Corticosteroids

B.   Cough medications

C. Estrogens

D. Antibiotics

1-142 *A child with slanted eyes with inner epicanthal folds; a short, flat nose; and a thick, protruding tongue probably has*

A. Down syndrome.

B. hypertelorism.

C. craniosynostosis.

D. Marfan's syndrome.

1-143 *Mrs. Lopez brings her 3-year-old daughter, Maria, in for a well-child visit. Maria is drinking liquid from a bottle. The clinician knows that prolonged bottle feeding is associated with*

A. iron deficiency.

B. failure to thrive.

C. decreased intake of solid foods.

D. lower BMI.

1-144 *After performing the cover-uncover test for ocular alignment, you note that a child's right eye turns inward toward the nose. The child does not have a broad flat nasal bridge (epicanthal folds or epicanthus). How would you document your findings?*

A. Pseudostrabismus

B. Right esotropia

C. Right exotropia

D. Congenital ptosis

1-145 *Which of these women who are currently pregnant is at high risk, warranting a referral?*

A. Marcie, age 35, whose first son was delivered by cesarean section

B. Sandra, age 29, who is expecting twins

C. Georgia, age 24, who has a history of osteoporosis

D. Maxine, age 38, whose daughter was born at 39 weeks' gestation

1-146 *A man who is inadequately treated for gonorrhea may develop*

A. a reinfection.

B. an immunity to the microorganism.

C. ureteritis, pyelonephritis, and nephritis.

D. prostatitis, epididymitis, and orchitis.

1-147 *A benign heart murmur, previously undocumented and discovered after an episode of pharyngitis, may be a clue to the diagnosis of*

A. scarlet fever.

B. Reye's syndrome.

C. rheumatic fever.

D. diphtheria.

1-148 *The use of silence when communicating*

A. is never appropriate.

B. implies that the interviewer is unsure.

C. reduces pressure on the interviewee.

D. forces the interviewee to speak.

1-149 *Your type 1 diabetes client voices concern about traveling by air with insulin. Your best response would be,*

A. "Don't worry because airport security is used to seeing diabetic supplies."

B. "I will fill out a form with an explanation of the supplies you will need to have with you."

C. "Check your supplies in your suitcase so that they will not be an issue."

D. "The security people are not allowed to let you take vials and needles on the plane."

1-150 *Mrs. Jay has just been placed on warfarin (Coumadin) therapy. To maintain adequate anticoagulation to reduce the risk of recurrent thrombosis, as well as the potential for hemorrhage, the goal is a(n)*

A. partial thromboplastin time (PT) of 55–80 seconds.

B. prothrombin time ratio of 2.0–2.5 times the control.

C. PT of 17–19.

D. international normalized ratio of 2.0–3.0.

1-151 *Which of the following is an important step to be taken before assisting with a lumbar puncture?*

A. Obtain a complete blood count.

B. Assess the fundi for papilledema.

C. Obtain other diagnostic tests that might preclude the need for a lumbar puncture.

D. Have a cerebrospinal fluid pressure-reading device readily available.

1-152   *Mavis, age 76, comes to the office with a unilateral throbbing headache in the periorbital region. She states that the pain has been gradually increasing over the past several hours and when she went out into the cold weather, the pain was extremely bad. What do you suspect?*

A. Trigeminal neuralgia

B. A migraine

C. Giant-cell arteritis

D. A transient ischemic attack

1-153   *Which of the following conditions includes weakness, muscle atrophy, muscle fasciculations, mixed hyper- and hyporeflexia, and spares the ocular muscles?*

A. Parkinson's

B. Alzheimer's

C. Multiple sclerosis

D. Amyotrophic lateral sclerosis

1-154   *The presence of which type of cast in the urine is not indicative of renal disease?*

A. Red cell casts

B. Hyaline casts

C. Renal tubular cell casts

D. White cell casts

1-155   *Home health services are provided under which part of Medicare?*

A. Part A

B. Part B

C. Parts A and B

D. Home health services are not covered under Medicare.

1-156   *You suspect that a pregnant client with a diagnosis of anemia practices pica. What makes you suspect this?*

A. She smokes when no one is looking.

B. She keeps boxes of starch under her bed.

C. Her breath smells like alcohol.

D. There are many empty vitamin bottles in the trash.

1-157   *Which objective is new to Healthy People 2020?*

A. Increase quality and years of healthy life.

B. Provide health care to all Americans.

C. Decrease some of the health disparities.

D. Increase the proportion of practicing primary care providers.

1-158   *Which of the following indicates an impending complication of influenza?*

A. Myalgia and headache

B. Diffuse crackles in the lungs

C. Sore throat and productive cough

D. Fever of 100.4°F with chills

1-159   *Sue, age 53, comes to your office for a routine examination. In passing, she mentions that she has Sjögren's syndrome. What do you think is her major complaint related to this syndrome?*

A. Fatigue

B. Diarrhea

C. Constipation

D. A dry, gritty sensation in her eyes

1-160   *Your 17-year-old client Hillary has infectious mononucleosis. Which of the following do you expect her blood work to reflect?*

A. Decreased serum globulins

B. Thrombocytopenia and elevated transaminase

C. High potassium and blood urea nitrogen (BUN)

D. Elevated serum protein

1-161   *Alexandra, age 48, has a bad complexion and has been treated for acne unsuccessfully. You suspect rosacea rather than acne because rosacea*

A. appears as blackheads and whiteheads.

B. causes the skin to become oily.

C. appears primarily around the nose and cheeks.

D. appears red and waxy.

1-162   *Monique has type 1 diabetes and states that she always has a blood sugar level of 230 mg/dL before breakfast. Your action is to*

A. increase her neutral protamine Hagedorn (NPH) insulin dosage at bedtime.

B. start her on metformin (Glucophage) 500 mg bid.

C. have her test her blood sugar at 3 a.m.

D. ask when she last changed the batteries in her home glucose monitoring kit.

1-163   You suspect a bladder neck or prostatic urethral problem with Bob because he is complaining of

A. initial hematuria.

B. terminal hematuria.

C. total hematuria.

D. "spotty" hematuria.

1-164   An allergic reaction in the kidney is often characterized by which of the following urinary sediments?

A. Leukocytes

B. Eosinophils

C. Crystals

D. Erythrocytes

1-165   Mrs. Miller is pregnant during the flu season. She asks if she should get the flu shot. How do you respond?

A. "The flu vaccine is not indicated for women who are pregnant."

B. "Yes, you should receive this today."

C. "No, it could harm the baby."

D. "Yes, it will protect you but will not protect the baby."

1-166   When should all pregnant women first be screened for gestational diabetes?

A. Between 16 and 20 weeks' gestation

B. Between 20 and 24 weeks' gestation

C. Between 24 and 28 weeks' gestation

D. Between 30 and 32 weeks' gestation

1-167   The American Urological Association (AUA) Symptom Index is a good tool to follow the course of someone with benign prostatic hyperplasia. Which of the following questions is one of the items on the index?

A. Over the past month, how many times on average do you urinate during the day?

B. Over the past month, how often have you had a sensation of not emptying your bladder completely after you finished urinating?

C. Over the past month, how many times have you not made it to the bathroom to urinate?

D. Over the past month, how many times did you get to the bathroom and were unable to urinate?

1-168   Saul comes today with a history of a sudden headache that started yesterday with a severity never experienced previously. It was followed by nausea and vomiting and a transient loss of consciousness. When he awakened, he was slightly confused and irritable. He exhibits nuchal rigidity. What do you suspect?

A. Subarachnoid hemorrhage

B. Intracranial aneurysm

C. Intracerebral hemorrhage

D. Cerebral infarction

1-169   What assessment finding indicates sarcoidosis?

A. Use of accessory muscles

B. Increased resistance to airflow into the lungs

C. Decreased lung compliance

D. Increased vital capacity and total lung capacity

1-170   The system that is affected in about 75% of all clients with systemic lupus erythematosus and has one of the most serious systemic sequelae, leading to significant morbidity and mortality, is the

A. renal system.

B. cardiovascular system.

C. neuromuscular system.

D. integumentary system.

1-171   You are using a penlight to attempt to transilluminate Tommy's left testicle, which on physical examination revealed a scrotal mass, as well as the testicle being swollen and reddened. Which finding will be translucent?

A. A testicular tumor

B. A hematocele

C. A hydrocele

D. A varicocele

1-172   Permanent teeth begin erupting around age

A. 3 years.

B. 4–5 years.

C. 6–7 years.

D. 7–8 years.

1-173   Which of the following is a risk factor for the development of cervical cancer?

A. A postmenopausal state

B. Nulliparity

C. A history of endometrial, breast, or colon cancer

D. A history of exposure to diethylstilbestrol and smoking

1-174   Which of the following is a "trigger" that may aggravate rosacea?

A. Nonalcoholic beer

B. Salt

C. Mild exercise

D. Caffeine

1-175   Marian has newly diagnosed diabetes, and diet modification has failed. You decide to try sulfonylurea therapy and tell her that it

A. acts as an insulin sensitizer.

B. acts as an antihyperglycemic agent.

C. augments pancreatic insulin secretion.

D. interferes with digestion and absorption of dietary carbohydrates.

1-176   Which type of pharyngitis do you suspect when a client has a sore throat with dysphagia and thin, white nonvesicular diffuse exudative ulcers on the mucosa?

A. Allergic pharyngitis

B. Streptococcal pharyngitis

C. Mononucleosis

D. Candida infection

1-177   Jason, age 14 months, is carried into the examination room screaming and drawing up his knees. His abdomen is tender and distended. You palpate a sausage-shaped mass in the upper midabdomen. Your next step is to order

A. stools for guaiac times three.

B. an ultrasound.

C. a barium enema.

D. a computed tomography scan.

1-178   Which of the following statements about adults in the United States is true?

A. Five percent of all physician visits require hospital admissions.

B. The average client visits a physician about twice a year.

C. Older adults visit their physicians about four times as often as other clients.

D. More than 75% of clients visit a physician's office at least once per year.

1-179   Which legislation is the basis for the federal Medicare program?

A. Title XVIII of the amendments to the Social Security Act

B. The original Social Security Act

C. The Health Insurance Association of America Act

D. Title XIX of the amendments to the Social Security Act

1-180   George, age 62, just had a carotid Doppler scan done to determine what type of cerebrovascular accident (CVA) he suffered. If the results show an occlusion of the carotid artery, which type of CVA is suspected?

A. Transient ischemic attack

B. Ischemic CVA

C. Embolic CVA

D. Hemorrhagic CVA

1-181   What are the components of Cushing's triad?

A. Hypertension, bradycardia, irregular respirations

B. Hypotension, tachycardia, regular respirations

C. Normotension, bradycardia, regular respirations

D. Hypertension, tachycardia, irregular respirations

1-182   Joan, age 24, has chronic fatigue syndrome. She is so frustrated with her family and friends thinking that it is all in her head that she tells you that she has actually thought about suicide. Knowing which of the following would be most helpful in assessing Joan's suicidal risk?

A. If there is a history of suicide in the family

B. If Joan lives alone

C. If Joan uses any alcohol or recreational drugs

D. If Joan has developed a plan for the suicide

1-183 *Which nerve root is responsible for the patellar reflex?*

A. L2

B. L3

C. L4

D. L5

1-184 *Constipation in older adults is commonly caused by which of the following?*

A. A high-fiber diet

B. An excessive fluid intake

C. Caffeine intake

D. Chronic laxative use

1-185 *Judy has been on hemodialysis for several years and wants to try continuous ambulatory peritoneal dialysis (CAPD). In teaching her about this, you tell her that the major complication is*

A. dehydration.

B. hemorrhage.

C. peritonitis.

D. electrolyte imbalance.

Answers

1-1   Answer A
Content area: Musculoskeletal Problems (chap. 16)

1-2   Answer C
Content area: Health Counseling (chap. 6)

1-3   Answer A
Content area: Male Genitourinary Problems (chap. 14)

1-4   Answer B
Content area: Integumentary Problems (chap. 8)

1-5   Answer A
Content area: Neurological Problems (chap. 7)

1-6   Answer A
Content area: Cardiovascular Problems (chap. 11)

1-7   Answer A
Content area: Issues in Primary Care (chap. 19)

1-8   Answer C
Content area: Respiratory Problems (chap. 10)

1-9   Answer C
Content area: Cardiovascular Problems (chap. 11)

1-10   Answer B
Content area: Health Promotion (chap. 3)

1-11   Answer A
Content area: Renal Problems (chap. 13)

1-12   Answer A
Content area: Hematological and Immune Problems (chap. 18)

1-13   Answer C
Content area: Cardiovascular Problems (chap. 11)

1-14   Answer A
Content area: Musculoskeletal Problems (chap. 16)

1-15   Answer A
Content area: Respiratory Problems (chap. 10)

1-16   Answer D
Content area: Integumentary Problems (chap. 8)

1-17   Answer B
Content area: Abdominal Problems (chap. 12)

1-18   Answer A
Content area: Hematological and Immune Problems (chap. 18)

1-19   Answer B
Content area: Health Counseling (chap. 6)

1-20   Answer C
Content area: Care of the Emerging Family (chap. 4)

1-21   Answer C
Content area: Growth and Development (chap. 5)

1-22   Answer A
Content area: Respiratory Problems (chap. 10)

1-23   Answer A

Content area: Renal Problems (chap. 13)

1-24   Answer C

Content area: Respiratory Problems (chap. 10)

1-25   Answer C

Content area: Integumentary Problems (chap. 8)

1-26   Answer B

Content area: Issues in Primary Care (chap. 19)

1-27   Answer C

Content area: Growth and Development (chap. 5)

1-28   Answer B

Content area: Health Counseling (chap. 6)

1-29   Answer C

Content area: Care of the Emerging Family (chap. 4)

1-30   Answer C

Content area: Abdominal Problems (chap. 12)

1-31   Answer A

Content area: Cardiovascular Problems (chap. 11)

1-32   Answer D

Content area: Integumentary Problems (chap. 8)

1-33   Answer B

Content area: Renal Problems (chap. 13)

1-34   Answer A

Content area: Head and Neck Problems (chap. 9)

1-35   Answer B

Content area: Musculoskeletal Problems (chap. 16)

1-36   Answer C

Content area: Endocrine and Metabolic Problems (chap. 17)

1-37   Answer D

Content area: Health Counseling (chap. 6)

1-38   Answer D

Content area: Care of the Emerging Family (chap. 4)

1-39   Answer D

Content area: Female Genitourinary Problems (chap. 15)

1-40   Answer A

Content area: Abdominal Problems (chap. 12)

1-41   Answer C

Content area: Health Promotion (chap. 3)

1-42   Answer B

Content area: Hematological and Immune Problems (chap. 18)

1-43   Answer D

Content area: Issues in Primary Care (chap. 19)

1-44   Answer D

Content area: Cardiovascular Problems (chap. 11)

1-45   Answer B

Content area: Renal Problems (chap. 13)

1-46   Answer C

Content area: Hematological and Immune Problems (chap. 18)

1-47   Answer C

Content area: Hematological and Immune Problems (chap. 18)

1-48   Answer B

Content area: Health Counseling (chap. 6)

1-49   Answer C

Content area: Care of the Emerging Family (chap. 4)

1-50   Answer D

Content area: Health Promotion (chap. 3)

1-51   Answer A

Content area: Endocrine and Metabolic Problems (chap. 17)

1-52   Answer D

Content area: Female Genitourinary Problems (chap. 15)

1-53   Answer A

Content area: Female Genitourinary Problems (chap. 15)

1-54   Answer B

Content area: Neurological Problems (chap. 7)

1-55   Answer D

Content area: Endocrine and Metabolic Problems (chap. 17)

1-56   Answer B

Content area: Hematological and Immune Problems (chap. 18)

1-57   Answer D

Content area: Cardiovascular Problems (chap. 11)

1-58   Answer A

Content area: Neurological Problems (chap. 7)

1-59   Answer B

Content area: Integumentary Problems (chap. 8)

1-60   Answer C

Content area: Head and Neck Problems (chap. 9)

1-61   Answer C

Content area: Health Counseling (chap. 6)

1-62   Answer A

Content area: Neurological Problems (chap. 7)

1-63   Answer B

Content area: Male Genitourinary Problems (chap. 14)

1-64   Answer C

Content area: Cardiovascular Problems (chap. 11)

1-65   Answer C

Content area: Hematological and Immune Problems (chap. 18)

1-66   Answer D

Content area: Abdominal Problems (chap. 12)

1-67   Answer A

Content area: Abdominal Problems (chap. 12)

1-68   Answer C

Content area: Cardiovascular Problems (chap. 11)

1-69   Answer B

Content area: Care of the Emerging Family (chap. 4)

1-70   Answer C

Content area: Renal Problems (chap. 13)

1-71   Answer D

Content area: Health Promotion (chap. 3)

1-72   Answer C

Content area: Health Counseling (chap. 6)

1-73   Answer D

Content area: Male Genitourinary Problems (chap. 14)

1-74   Answer C

Content area: Growth and Development (chap. 5)

1-75   Answer A

Content area: Hematological and Immune Problems (chap. 18)

1-76   Answer B

Content area: Female Genitourinary Problems (chap. 15)

1-77   Answer C

Content area: Care of the Emerging Family (chap. 4)

1-78   Answer C

Content area: Endocrine and Metabolic Problems (chap. 17)

1-79   Answer C

Content area: Care of the Emerging Family (chap. 4)

1-80   Answer C

Content area: Cardiovascular Problems (chap. 11)

1-81   Answer D

Content area: Musculoskeletal Problems (chap. 16)

1-82   Answer B

Content area: Endocrine and Metabolic Problems (chap. 17)

1-83   Answer B

Content area: Musculoskeletal Problems (chap. 16)

1-84   Answer B

Content area: Female Genitourinary Problems (chap. 15)

1-85   Answer C

Content area: Abdominal Problems (chap. 12)

1-86   Answer B

Content area: Care of the Emerging Family (chap. 4)

1-87   Answer B

Content area: Health Promotion (chap. 3)

1-88   Answer B

Content area: Growth and Development (chap. 5)

1-89   Answer B

Content area: Integumentary Problems (chap. 8)

1-90   Answer D

Content area: Integumentary Problems (chap. 8)

1-91   Answer C

Content area: Issues in Primary Care (chap. 19)

1-92   Answer A

Content area: Abdominal Problems (chap. 12)

1-93   Answer C

Content area: Endocrine and Metabolic Problems (chap. 17)

1-94   Answer D

Content area: Health Promotion (chap. 3)

1-95   Answer A

Content area: Endocrine and Metabolic Problems (chap. 17)

1-96   Answer A

Content area: Endocrine and Metabolic Problems (chap. 17)

1-97   Answer B

Content area: Health Promotion (chap. 3)

1-98   Answer B

Content area: Health Counseling (chap. 6)

1-99   Answer D

Content area: Head and Neck Problems (chap. 9)

1-100   Answer B

Content area: Musculoskeletal Problems (chap. 16)

1-101   Answer A

Content area: Integumentary Problems (chap. 8)

1-102   Answer A

Content area: Endocrine and Metabolic Problems (chap. 17)

1-103   Answer C

Content area: Neurological Problems (chap. 7)

1-104   Answer A

Content area: Integumentary Problems (chap. 8)

1-105   Answer D

Content area: Health Counseling (chap. 6)

1-106   Answer B

Content area: Growth and Development (chap. 5)

1-107   Answer B

Content area: Male Genitourinary Problems (chap. 14)

1-108   Answer B

Content area: Care of the Emerging Family (chap. 4)

1-109   Answer D

Content area: Abdominal Problems (chap. 12)

1-110   Answer C

Content area: Health Promotion (chap. 3)

1-111   Answer D

Content area: Head and Neck Problems (chap. 9)

1-112   Answer C

Content area: Neurological Problems (chap. 7)

1-113   Answer A

Content area: Health Counseling (chap. 6)

1-114   Answer B

Content area: Head and Neck Problems (chap. 9)

1-115   Answer A

Content area: Integumentary Problems (chap. 8)

1-116   Answer C

Content area: Musculoskeletal Problems (chap. 16)

1-117   Answer C

Content area: Respiratory Problems (chap. 10)

1-118   Answer A

Content area: Care of the Emerging Family (chap. 4)

1-119   Answer C

Content area: Growth and Development (chap. 5)

1-120   Answer C

Content area: Care of the Emerging Family (chap. 4)

1-121   Answer D

Content area: Renal Problems (chap. 13)

1-122   Answer A

Content area: Neurological Problems (chap. 7)

1-123   Answer C

Content area: Issues in Primary Care (chap. 19)

1-124   Answer B

Content area: Endocrine and Metabolic Problems (chap. 17)

1-125   Answer A

Content area: Female Genitourinary Problems (chap. 15)

1-126   Answer D

Content area: Cardiovascular Problems (chap. 11)

1-127   Answer A

Content area: Endocrine and Metabolic Problems (chap. 17)

1-128   Answer B

Content area: Growth and Development (chap. 5)

1-129   Answer B

Content area: Hematological and Immune Problems (chap. 18)

1-130   Answer B

Content area: Health Counseling (chap. 6)

1-131   Answer D

Content area: Cardiovascular Problems (chap. 11)

1-132   Answer D

Content area: Integumentary Problems (chap. 8)

1-133   Answer D

Content area: Health Counseling (chap. 6)

1-134   Answer B

Content area: Integumentary Problems (chap. 8)

1-135   Answer A

Content area: Endocrine and Metabolic Problems (chap. 17)

1-136   Answer C

Content area: Female Genitourinary Problems (chap. 15)

1-137   Answer D

Content area: Female Genitourinary Problems (chap. 15)

1-138   Answer B

Content area: Growth and Development (chap. 5)

1-139   Answer A

Content area: Issues in Primary Care (chap. 19)

1-140   Answer C

Content area: Neurological Problems (chap. 7)

1-141   Answer D

Content area: Endocrine and Metabolic Problems (chap. 17)

1-142   Answer A

Content area: Growth and Development (chap. 5)

1-143   Answer A

Content area: Growth and Development (chap. 5)

1-144   Answer B

Content area: Head and Neck Problems (chap. 9)

1-145   Answer B

Content area: Care of the Emerging Family (chap. 4)

1-146   Answer D

Content area: Male Genitourinary Problems (chap. 14)

1-147   Answer C

Content area: Head and Neck Problems (chap. 9)

1-148   Answer C

Content area: Health Counseling (chap. 6)

1-149   Answer B

Content area: Health Counseling (chap. 6)

1-150   Answer D

Content area: Cardiovascular Problems (chap. 11)

1-151   Answer B

Content area: Neurological Problems (chap. 7)

1-152   Answer C

Content area: Neurological Problems (chap. 7)

1-153   Answer D

Content area: Neurological Problems (chap. 7)

1-154   Answer B

Content area: Renal Problems (chap. 13)

1-155   Answer C

Content area: Issues in Primary Care (chap. 19)

1-156   Answer B

Content area: Health Counseling (chap. 6)

1-157   Answer D

Content area: Health Promotion (chap. 3)

1-158   Answer B

Content area: Respiratory Problems (chap. 10)

1-159   Answer D

Content area: Head and Neck Problems (chap. 9)

1-160   Answer B

Content area: Hematological and Immune Problems (chap. 18)

1-161   Answer C

Content area: Integumentary Problems (chap. 8)

1-162   Answer C

Content area: Endocrine and Metabolic Problems (chap. 17)

1-163   Answer B

Content area: Renal Problems (chap. 13)

1-164   Answer B

Content area: Renal Problems (chap. 13)

1-165   Answer B

Content area: Respiratory Problems (chap. 10)

1-166   Answer C

Content area: Care of the Emerging Family (chap. 4)

1-167   Answer B

Content area: Male Genitourinary Problems (chap. 14)

1-168   Answer A

Content area: Neurological Problems (chap. 7)

1-169   Answer C

Content area: Respiratory Problems (chap. 10)

1-170   Answer A

Content area: Hematological and Immune Problems (chap. 18)

1-171   Answer C

Content area: Male Genitourinary Problems (chap. 14)

1-172   Answer C

Content area: Growth and Development (chap. 5)

1-173   Answer D

Content area: Female Genitourinary Problems (chap. 15)

1-174   Answer D

Content area: Integumentary Problems (chap. 8)

1-175   Answer C

Content area: Endocrine and Metabolic Problems (chap. 17)

1-176   Answer D

Content area: Head and Neck Problems (chap. 9)

1-177   Answer C

Content area: Abdominal Problems (chap. 12)

1-178   Answer D

Content area: Health Promotion (chap. 3)

1-179   Answer A

Content area: Issues in Primary Care (chap. 19)

1-180   Answer B

Content area: Neurological Problems (chap. 7)

1-181   Answer A

Content area: Endocrine and Metabolic Problems (chap. 17)

1-182   Answer D

Content area: Neurological Problems (chap. 7)

1-183   Answer C

Content area: Musculoskeletal Problems (chap. 16)

1-184   Answer D

Content area: Abdominal Problems (chap. 12)

1-185   Answer C

Content area: Renal Problems (chap. 13)

Good Luck on Your Certification Examination!

Examination 2

Jill E. Winland-Brown
Lynne M. Dunphy

Questions

2-1 Anne has a history of hyperlipidemia, and today you note a soft, yellowish, raised, waxy lesion beneath her right eyelid. You diagnose this as a

A. xanthelasma.

B. hordeolum.

C. chalazion.

D. lagophthalmos.

2-2 Marjorie has a Bartholin's cyst. What is the most common offending pathogen?

A. Gonococcus

B. Staphylococcus aureus

C. Streptococcus faecalis

D. Escherichia coli

2-3 You have just seen Mrs. Hill with her 4-month-old infant boy for a well-baby visit. You would schedule the next appointment in

A. 1 month.

B. 2 months.

C. 3 months.

D. 4 months.

2-4 Mrs. Hill's 4-month-old infant son is formula fed. An infant that age should have approximately how much formula per day?

A. 8–9 oz given in four feedings per day

B. 6–7 oz given in four to five feedings per day

C. 5–6 oz given in six feedings per day

D. 5 oz given in seven feedings per day

2-5 Judy has come to have an influenza immunization today. Which of the following would be a contraindication for her to receive the injection?

A. She is pregnant.

B. She has a temperature of 102°F (38.8°C).

C. She has a history of neurological reaction.

D. She had a previous anaphylactic reaction to neomycin and streptomycin.

2-6 Marsha, age 36, comes for a physical. Her chart mentions a swan-neck deformity. You will be sure to assess her

A. hands.

B. neck.

C. shoulders.

D. ankles.

2-7 Betsy, age 23, is 38 weeks pregnant and has a urinary tract infection. Which drug is the best choice for treatment?

A. Cefprozil (Cefzil)

B. Tetracycline (Achromycin)

C. Nitrofurantoin (Furadantin)

D. Amoxicillin (Amoxil)

2-8 Thyroxine (T_4) level may be influenced by a number of factors, thus giving an inaccurate result. These factors include

A. pregnancy, malnutrition, and alcohol use.

B. pregnancy, birth control pills, and malnutrition.

C. birth control pills, alcohol use, and use of opiates.

D. physical activity level, malnutrition, and alteration in liver function.

2-9 The most common cause of disability in clients younger than age 45 is

A. stress-related psychological disturbances.

B. low back pain.

C. severe migraine headaches.

D. alcohol and drug-related problems.

2-10 *Karen, age 43, was recently in a car accident but is now up and about. She comes into the office with vague complaints of being tired. You assess Cullen's sign and Grey Turner's sign. You assume therefore that she has*

A. anemia.

B. retroperitoneal bleeding.

C. portal hypertension.

D. liver dysfunction.

2-11 *Spoon-shaped, thin nails are often seen in clients with*

A. psoriasis.

B. a fungal infection.

C. anemia.

D. eczema.

2-12 *You are assessing the direction of Jim's abdominal venous blood flow and note a centrifugal venous return radiating outward from his umbilicus. This may be a sign of*

A. inferior vena cava obstruction.

B. normal blood flow.

C. portal hypertension.

D. an abdominal aortic aneurysm.

2-13 *The majority of clients affected with inflammatory bowel disease are*

A. older adults, with men and women equally affected.

B. young adults, with men and women equally affected.

C. older adults, with women affected twice as frequently as men.

D. young adults, with women affected twice as frequently as men.

2-14 *You suspect that Bill, age 44, is abusing alcohol. There are several effective ways of eliciting sensitive information from such a client. Which of the following is the most effective way of eliciting meaningful information?*

A. Ask Bill directly, "How much do you drink?"

B. Ask Bill if he has had a drink in the past 24 hours.

C. Ask Bill if he has ever tried to cut down on his drinking.

D. Ask Bill if he has ever had health, legal, or personal problems as a result of alcohol, and if the response is yes, ask him "When was the last time you had a drink?"

2-15 *All of the following are common discomforts of pregnancy except*

A. leg cramps.

B. edema of the face and fingers.

C. varicosities.

D. urinary frequency.

2-16 *Jane, age 74, is incontinent of urine about 50% of the time. Which of the following is the absolute last resort in management of incontinence?*

A. Incontinence pads

B. Intermittent catheterization

C. A bladder training program (because of her age)

D. Indwelling catheterization

2-17 *Cranial nerve XI is tested by*

A. touching the pharynx with a cotton applicator.

B. asking the client to say "ah."

C. having the client shrug his or her shoulders while you resist movement.

D. having the client stick out his or her tongue and move it from side to side.

2-18 *Julie says that her doctor told her to participate in 20–30 minutes of vigorous activity at least three times per week and asks you to qualify "vigorous." How do you respond?*

A. "Exercise that makes you sweat is vigorous, as long as you sweat for the entire 20–30 minutes."

B. "It's vigorous if the heart rate is elevated to at least 60% of maximum for your age with the maximum heart rate calculated as 220 minus your age."

C. "If your heart rate is increased to 1.5 times your walking rate, the exercise is vigorous."

D. "If your heart rate is increased to twice your resting rate and is no more than 160, the exercise is vigorous."

2-19 In a 4-year-old child, the ideal glucose level after 2 or more hours of fasting should be

A. 80–180 mg/dL.
B. 100–200 mg/dL.
C. 70–150 mg/dL.
D. 120–220 mg/dL.

2-20 The initial diagnostic procedure for the evaluation of a deep venous thrombosis is

A. a contrast venography.
B. a duplex ultrasound.
C. an arteriogram.
D. an MRI of the affected limb.

2-21 The most important activity that the care provider performs is

A. taking the history.
B. the ordering of appropriate tests.
C. disease follow-through.
D. the ordering of appropriate medications.

2-22 Mrs. Graves, age 38, has been on birth control pills for approximately 15 years. She is a smoker, has a blood pressure of 110/70 mm Hg, and has lipid levels within normal limits. You advise that she should

A. discontinue the birth control pills because of her smoking.
B. remain on the pill because her blood pressure and lipids are within normal limits.
C. remain on the pill until her follicle-stimulating hormone level is greater than 30.
D. discontinue the pill because of her age.

2-23 Angie, age 17, is complaining of nasal congestion, sneezing, and itchiness of the eyes that worsens when she does yard work. She has been self-medicating with an over-the-counter nasal decongestant spray. Although this has been temporarily helpful, she reports that her symptoms are now worsening. You should

A. counsel her to avoid yard work.
B. advise her of the rebound effect of the nasal spray.

C. order a nonsedating antihistamine and a corticosteroid nasal spray.
D. advise a combination nonsedating antihistamine and decongestant tablet.

2-24 Timmy, age 5, comes for a preschool physical. You note that his urethral meatus opens on the ventral surface of the penis and document this as

A. epispadias.
B. paraphimosis.
C. phimosis.
D. hypospadias.

2-25 David, age 19, has end-stage renal disease and needs to continue on dialysis, which he started 2 years ago. He is on a waiting list for a kidney transplant, but his chance to receive one is slim because of his rare blood type. He has made the choice to stop dialysis. How do you respond?

A. "You're crazy. Any life is better than no life at all."
B. "You don't have the right to make that decision. I'm your health-care provider."
C. "Let me talk to your parents about this."
D. "Let's discuss the risks and consequences."

2-26 About what percentage of children have congenital anomalies of the genitourinary tract, with severity ranging from abnormalities that remain asymptomatic through adulthood to malformations incompatible with life?

A. Less than 3%
B. 5%
C. 10%
D. More than 10%

2-27 Sigrid, age 78, is given a diagnosis of bacterial meningitis. What is the most probable offending pathogen?

A. Neisseria meningitides
B. Staphylococci
C. Streptococcus pneumoniae
D. Gram-negative bacilli

2-28   *When percussing the chest, hyperresonance often is heard with*

A. lung cancer.

B. pneumonia.

C. pleural effusion.

D. emphysema.

2-29   *A variety of drugs have been implicated in erectile dysfunction. These include but are not limited to*

A. diuretics, beta blockers, and ACE inhibitors.

B. vasodilators, anticholinergic agents, and antihistamines.

C. cimetidine (Tagamet), beta blockers, and diuretics.

D. ACE inhibitors, calcium channel blockers, estrogens, and digoxin.

2-30   *What is the major cause of chronic renal failure?*

A. Hypertension

B. Glomerulonephritis

C. Diabetes mellitus

D. Obstructive uropathy

2-31   *Janice is 28 weeks pregnant and makes an emergency visit complaining of painful vaginal bleeding. You palpate a tender, boardlike uterus. What is this most indicative of?*

A. Placenta previa

B. Abruptio placentae

C. Gestational trophoblastic disease

D. Emboli

2-32   *The most common cause of a chronic cough that is more severe early in the morning and produces a yellowish-brown mucus is*

A. cigarette smoking.

B. asthma.

C. bronchogenic carcinoma.

D. angiotensin-converting enzyme (ACE) inhibitor use.

2-33   *Delirium in the older adult typically presents with which of the following behaviors?*

A. Agitation and wandering behavior

B. Acute change in mental status and apathy, lack of response to stimuli

C. Agitation and restlessness

D. Absence of purpose and apathy

2-34   *The term pica refers to*

A. an insatiable craving for such substances as laundry starch, clay, and ice and is thought to suggest iron deficiency.

B. poverty and violence.

C. mental retardation in children.

D. a folic acid deficiency.

2-35   *Ms. Clancy, age 28, is complaining of a "cold that won't go away." She "thinks" that she has had a fever (she is afebrile in your office) and reports a nasal discharge that has become greenish in color. She also reports a cough. You decide that she has an acute, uncomplicated sinusitis and order*

A. amoxicillin (Amoxil) 500 mg PO tid for 14–21 days.

B. sulfamethoxazole and trimethoprim (Bactrim) 1 DS tab PO bid for 7–10 days.

C. amoxicillin (Amoxil) 500 mg PO bid for 3–4 weeks.

D. ciprofloxacin (Cipro) 500 mg bid for 14 days.

2-36   *A good technique for assessment of the supraclavicular nodes is*

A. to have the client sit up and perform Valsalva's maneuver.

B. to use the diaphragm of the stethoscope.

C. to palpate the axilla.

D. to use the bell of the stethoscope.

2-37   *Sandy says that her baby can now roll from side to side and from back to front. How old do you suspect her baby to be?*

A. 3 months

B. 4 months

C. 5 months

D. 6 months

2-38   *At what age can children use scissors, draw stick figures, and fasten and unfasten simple buttons?*

A. 3 years

B. 4 years

C. 5 years

D. 6 years

2-39   An 18-month-old child is able to demonstrate which of the following competencies and characteristics?

A. Walks up steps, puts two words together, and performs simple tasks

B. Walks down steps, puts two words together, and has stranger anxiety

C. Throws overhand, zips and unzips, and points to and vocalizes wants

D. Kicks ball, puts four to six words together, and turns doorknob

2-40   It can be difficult to assess nausea in a young child. A good question to ask to determine if the child has nausea is

A. "Are you hungry?"

B. "Are you sick to your tummy?"

C. "Are you nauseous?"

D. "Are you eating the way you normally eat?"

2-41   Jeremy, age 18, comes in for a visit. His left arm is in a cast, and he tells you that he has a comminuted fracture of his humerus. This means that

A. the bone is crushed.

B. bony fragments are in many places.

C. bone breaks cleanly but does not penetrate the skin.

D. broken ends of the bone protrude through the soft tissues and skin.

2-42   Prophylaxis for the first episode of Pneumocystis jiroveci pneumonia, an opportunistic disease in HIV-infected adults and adolescents, is

A. rifampin (Rimactane) 600 mg PO daily.

B. isoniazid (Nydrazid) 300 mg PO plus pyridoxine (Beesix) 50 mg PO daily.

C. trimethoprim-sulfamethoxazole (TMP-SMZ) (Bactrim) 1 PO daily.

D. clarithromycin (Biaxin) 500 mg PO bid.

2-43   You are trying to make a diagnosis of a lung problem described by your client Mr. Fry, age 65. In making the distinction between emphysema and chronic bronchitis, you know that chronic bronchitis

A. usually presents with a mild cough.

B. has an insidious progressive dyspnea and usually occurs after age 50.

C. demonstrates a markedly increased residual volume.

D. presents with wheezing and rhonchi.

2-44   Mark has a diagnosis of bullous myringitis. What might you expect to see during an otoscopic examination?

A. Bulging of the tympanic membrane (TM)

B. Serous amber fluid and air behind the TM

C. Vesicles on the TM

D. Perforation of the TM

2-45   Mary is here to see you to discuss many concerns she has about toilet training her daughter. Which of the following is important information for you to convey?

A. Boys are usually toilet trained 2.5 months earlier than girls.

B. The majority of children are bowel trained prior to bladder training.

C. About 85% of children are completely trained after age 3.

D. Girls are usually toilet trained an average of 2.5 months earlier than boys.

2-46   In infants and children, the cardinal sign of right-sided congestive heart failure is

A. cyanosis.

B. edema of the lower extremities.

C. tachypnea.

D. hepatomegaly.

2-47   Beulah, age 86, has stasis dermatitis of her left lower leg. Her ankle is edematous and there is a rusty, brownish discoloration of the skin. What is your diagnosis?

A. Arterial valvular insufficiency

B. Venous valvular insufficiency

C. Cellulitis

D. Diabetic nephropathy

2-48   Mrs. Garvey brings her 10-year-old son, Steve, to your primary care office. He has a 3-in. laceration on his leg that occurred over 24 hours before this visit. He did not tell his mother about this injury when it happened, and the bleeding has stopped. No special efforts had been taken to cleanse the wound until the evening, when his mother discovered it. The wound edges are in close approximation. You should

A. cleanse, suture, and dress the wound and then have Steve return in 5 days for suture removal.

B. cleanse the wound and apply Steri-Strips.

C. cleanse and dress the wound, then have the client return in 3–5 days.

D. irrigate and cleanse the wound with antiseptic agents.

2-49   Immunizations in adults age 65 and older should include

A. diphtheria, tetanus, and pertussis every 5 years and pneumococcal vaccine every 6 years starting at age 65.

B. pneumococcal vaccine at age 65 and tetanus and diphtheria every 10 years.

C. diphtheria, tetanus, and acellular pertussis every 10 years and pneumococcal vaccine at age 65.

D. influenza immunization every fall, tetanus, diphtheria, and acellular pertussis every 10 years, and pneumococcal vaccine at age 65.

2-50   Mrs. Greene scheduled an appointment for her 50-year-old husband for a routine check of his blood pressure. He is currently taking enalapril (Vasotec) 5 mg PO daily. She tells the receptionist that she would really like the nurse practitioner to talk with her husband about his alcohol use and smoking. When you press Mr. Greene for details about his alcohol and tobacco use during his visit, he becomes irritated and defensive. What stage of change is Mr. Greene exhibiting regarding the possibility of behavioral change?

A. Contemplation

B. Precontemplation

C. Lack of awareness

D. Prepreparation

2-51   Most persons who are advised to perform monthly self-examinations do not do so. Which of the following statements is true regarding self-examination?

A. Women perform a monthly breast self-examination 50%–60% of the time.

B. Adults perform a routine self-examination 20% of the time.

C. Men perform a testicular self-examination 10%–15% of the time.

D. Adults check their skin on a routine basis.

2-52   You have asked Tim, age 16, to walk a straight line, placing heel to toe. You are assessing

A. the proprioceptive system.

B. cranial nerve function.

C. sensory function.

D. cerebellar function.

2-53   Social support is important for every age group. For adults, research has shown that which of the following is the most significant source of social support?

A. Close friends

B. Parents (if living)

C. Spouse or significant other (if applicable)

D. Children

2-54   Tonsils that touch the uvula are graded in which way?

A. Grade 1+

B. Grade 2+

C. Grade 3+

D. Grade 4+

2-55   Urinary incontinence in older adults is widely underreported. It affects which of the following?

A. 15%–30% of those living in the community and as high as 50% of those in institutional settings

B. 10%–15% of all those living in the community and 35% of those in institutional settings

C. 40% of those living in the community and 60% of those in institutional settings

D. 7%–10% of those living in the community and 40% of those in institutional settings

2-56   You suspect that Marvin has digitalis toxicity. What is the most dangerous manifestation that you will be on the alert for?

A. Seizures

B. Diarrhea

C. Delirium

D. Arrhythmias

2-57   The treatment of choice for an adult with a diagnosis of group A beta-hemolytic streptococcal pharyngitis is

A. ofloxacin (Floxin) 500 mg PO bid for 5 days.

B. sulfamethoxazole and trimethoprim (Bactrim) DS 1 tab PO bid for 10 days.

C. penicillin V (Pen-Vee K) 500 mg PO bid for 10 days.

D. cefaclor (Ceclor) 500 mg PO for 7 days.

2-58   Your client Annie had a normal vaginal delivery approximately 24 hours ago. The charge nurse calls you stat to say that Annie cannot breathe and is extremely agitated. You suspect

A. a panic attack.

B. sudden onset pneumonia.

C. a stroke.

D. pulmonary embolism.

2-59   The most common risk factors for thromboembolism include

A. fractures and prolonged immobilization.

B. myocardial infarction and atrial fibrillation.

C. cardiomyopathy and pregnancy.

D. abnormal fibrinolysis and congestive heart failure.

2-60   Betty states that she is infertile because of polycystic ovary syndrome. She asks you what causes the symptoms of amenorrhea, hirsutism, acne, and obesity. You tell her they are related to

A. androgen excess.

B. estrogen deficiency.

C. inadequate gonadotropin stimulation.

D. excessive adrenocorticotropic hormone.

2-61   The aging process results in a variety of physiological changes. One change is

A. a decreased absorption of fat-soluble vitamins.

B. an increase in pupil size.

C. an increase of enzymatic activity.

D. an increase in liver size.

2-62   Countries that have socialized medicine have more cost-effective health-care systems than the United States, partly because

A. they have fewer nurses.

B. they have more primary care physicians than specialists.

C. they have a lower cost of living.

D. they have no health maintenance organizations.

2-63   Shane, age 15, arrives in your office with a chief complaint of a sore throat. Upon examination you observe tonsillar exudates, a fever of 102°F, an absence of a cough, and anterior cervical adenopathy. Which causative agent is a high probability?

A. Rhinovirus

B. Epstein-Barr virus

C. Group A beta-hemolytic streptococcus

D. *Haemophilus influenzae*

2-64   Irritable bowel disease is commonly seen in the primary care setting. It affects what percentage of all clients?

A. 10%

B. 15%

C. 20%

D. 30%

2-65   The proper technique for measuring the fundal height in a pregnant client is to have the client

A. empty her bladder and then lie supine with legs flexed.

B. empty her bladder and then lie supine with legs extended.

C. empty her bladder and then assume a semi-Fowler's position with legs flexed.

D. lie in a completely flat position with legs extended.

2-66 Your client Anna, who is of an average height and weight, is 5 months pregnant. She wants to know how many extra calories she should be adding to her diet each day now that she is pregnant. You tell her she should be adding

A. 700 calories.
B. 500 calories.
C. 300 calories.
D. 200 calories.

2-67 Which of the following is a risk factor for dorsal kyphosis?

A. Older age
B. Adolescence
C. Obesity
D. Pregnancy

2-68 Of the abnormalities that might show up on an ultrasound during pregnancy, all of the following warrant a referral except

A. hydramnios.
B. placenta previa (after 28 weeks).
C. breech position at 28 weeks.
D. oligohydramnios.

2-69 Scott, age 22, has cryptorchidism and was never treated. To what is he more susceptible than men who do not have this?

A. Malignant neoplasm of the testes
B. Epididymitis
C. Prostate cancer
D. Diverticular disease

2-70 An area of deep abrasion, including a "road burn," on the left forearm is best treated by doing which of the following?

A. Icing the wound after irrigation
B. Cleansing it several times a day and leaving it open to air
C. Prescribing prophylactic antibiotic therapy
D. Removing ground-in dirt using forceps

2-71 Jean wonders whether her 2-year-old son is developing normally. She is concerned because he seems to have a lot of temper tantrums. About what percentage of all children between the ages of 2 and 3 have a daily temper tantrum?

A. 10%
B. 20%
C. 50%
D. 70%

2-72 Jill is perimenopausal and asks you about the relationship between exercise and preventing osteoporosis. You tell her that

A. exercise has no effect; she should take calcium supplements.
B. weight-bearing exercise prevents bone mass loss.
C. all types of exercise assist in preventing osteoporosis.
D. after one has exercised regularly for 5 years, even after stopping, bone mass decreases slowly.

2-73 What is the age when an infant listens to talking, can respond to simple commands, and can begin to differentiate among words?

A. 3–5 months
B. 6–8 months
C. 9–12 months
D. 11–14 months

2-74 Your client has no signs or symptoms other than a fever and coarse crackles. What must you assess for further?

A. Congestive heart failure
B. Pneumonia
C. Bronchitis
D. Pulmonary fibrosis

2-75 The Miller Assessment for Preschoolers screens all the following domains except

A. sensory.
B. motor.
C. language.
D. cognitive.

2-76   John, age 18, has a seizure disorder. He has been taking a combination of phenytoin (Dilantin) and phenobarbital (Luminal) to treat his seizures. He reports a new rash. You know that

A.   the phenobarbital should be discontinued.

B.   the phenytoin should be discontinued.

C.   either of these drugs could cause a rash.

D.   you must begin John on an entirely new drug regimen.

2-77   When doing a pelvic examination on Tara, age 19, you note painful, raised, reddened lesions filled with fluid around the labia. You diagnose these as

A.   lesions associated with syphilis.

B.   a vaginal infection.

C.   condyloma.

D.   herpetic vesicles.

2-78   Your client, Mr. Lane, who suffers from chronic obstructive pulmonary disease (COPD), calls to say that, while visiting his daughter, he was exposed to influenza. He had received a flu shot in your office less than a week ago. He is calling because he is concerned that it is not working as yet. You tell him that

A.   the flu shot will be sufficient to protect him.

B.   because the flu shot will not be fully effective for several weeks, he should wash his hands frequently and get adequate rest.

C.   he should start oseltamivir (Tamiflu) because it has been less than 48 hours since exposure to the infected person.

D.   he should start oseltamivir (Tamiflu) immediately because the time since exposure has been over 72 hours.

2-79   The primary screening test for thyroid abnormalities is

A.   thyroid-stimulating hormone level.

B.   thyroxine (T_4)

C.   free thyroxine index.

D.   thyrotropin-releasing factor.

2-80   Ginny, age 62, comes to the office with a sudden onset of severe, throbbing eye pain and unilateral vision loss. Even before you examine her, you suspect

A.   a unilateral cataract.

B.   iritis.

C.   a detached retina.

D.   acute angle-closure glaucoma.

2-81   Clients with refractive asthma should be evaluated along a number of parameters. These include

A.   continued exposure to known causes, evaluation of compliance with treatment, examination of behavioral aspects, and evaluation of possible other causes of airway obstruction.

B.   underlying, unresolved infectious processes; behavioral aspects of the disease; and compliance with treatment.

C.   environmental aspects, family support systems, and socioeconomic status.

D.   compliance with treatment, an evaluation of underlying nutritional status, family structure, and behavioral aspects of the disease.

2-82   Which type of tremor is goal directed, more prominent with willful action, and may be located in proximal as well as distal extremities?

A.   Cerebellar

B.   Physiological

C.   Parkinsonian

D.   Essential

2-83   Marissa is going to have a splenectomy for her idiopathic thrombocytopenic purpura (ITP). Which of the following statements about this is true?

A.   Splenectomy produces permanent remission in 70%–90% of children with ITP.

B.   Splenectomy is a first-line therapy.

C.   Vitamin B_{12} supplementation is essential.

D.   Anticoagulant therapy is indicated postoperatively when the platelet count rises.

2-84 Rose, age 66, comes in with an intractable headache accompanied by weakness, difficulty chewing, and visual changes. You note some swelling and tenderness on her left forehead. What do you suspect?

A. A migraine headache

B. Temporal arteritis

C. A cluster headache

D. A cerebral aneurysm

2-85 The single most reliable indicator of readiness to return to work after an episode of back pain is

A. cessation of pain.

B. full mobility.

C. work satisfaction.

D. personal motivation.

2-86 Ms. Stanley is in your primary care office today complaining of burning on urination that has persisted for 3 days. She has no fever and no flank pain. This is the second urinary tract infection that she has reported this year, and she thinks that the infections are related to increased sexual activity. She does not use a diaphragm for contraception and has tried drinking cranberry juice to offset this problem, something she read about in a women's magazine. You order

A. sulfamethoxazole and trimethoprim (TMP-SMZ) (Septra or Bactrim) 1 DS tab PO bid for 3 days.

B. TMP/SMZ 1 DS tab PO bid for 7–14 days.

C. TMP/SMZ 1 DS tab PO bid for 3 weeks.

D. a single dose of TMP/SMZ 1 DS tab PO.

2-87 Diabetic clients who are most at risk for hypoglycemic episodes include which of the following?

A. Older adults, alcohol abusers, and those with hepatic and/or renal dysfunction

B. Clients with insulin pumps

C. Clients who are taking certain antifungal agents concurrently with oral hypoglycemic drugs and eating a diet of complex carbohydrates

D. Clients who exercise regularly or take birth control pills

2-88 When examining a client's chest wall, you note crepitus. What condition might you suspect?

A. Emphysema

B. Pleuritis

C. Pulmonary edema

D. Pneumonia

2-89 The most common trigger of rosacea is

A. cold weather.

B. skin care products.

C. sun exposure.

D. dust.

2-90 Early descriptions of this disease were centered on the cutaneous manifestations. In fact, the word means "wolf" and was used to describe the destructive eating away of the skin that was a result of the rash. Which disease is this?

A. Systemic lupus erythematosus

B. Herpes zoster (shingles)

C. Malaria

D. Rubeola

2-91 Which type of stroke has a gradual onset and results in a pure motor or pure sensory stroke?

A. Thrombotic

B. Embolic

C. Hemorrhagic

D. Lacunar

2-92 Andrea, age 16, is seen in your office for an injury to her eye. You remove a small foreign body from her cornea. There is no rust ring. In preparation for discharge, you would

A. patch her eye.

B. prescribe anesthetic eye drops.

C. prescribe steroid eye drops.

D. tell her that she may return to normal activity and take an NSAID for pain if needed.

2-93 Many Americans have their urine tested for illegal drugs for different purposes. What is the estimated percentage of false-positives?

A. Less than 10%

B. 10%–30%

C. 30%–60%

D. More than 60%

2-94 *Previous full-term pregnancies, even if uncomplicated, may cause a woman to lose approximately how much iron?*

A. 1,500–1,700 mg

B. 500–1,000 mg

C. 250–500 mg

D. 1,200–1,500 mg

2-95 *In a woman who is premenopausal, the biggest risk factor for heart attack is*

A. family history.

B. sedentary lifestyle.

C. obesity.

D. cigarette smoking.

2-96 *What is the name of a bone tumor that arises from the cartilage and often affects the pelvis, ribs, femur, or proximal humerus?*

A. Fibrosarcoma

B. Malignant melanoma

C. Chondrosarcoma

D. Ewing's sarcoma

2-97 *Sara, age 57, comes in with a complaint of pain and swelling in her right lower leg. The pain is worse if she tries to walk or stand on the leg. She smokes a half pack of cigarettes a day and takes a hormone replacement pill every night. She states that she returned from Tokyo 3 days ago and still feels jet-lagged. Her vital signs are normal. Her physical examination reveals a warm and slightly reddened right lower leg with marked edema extending from the knee to the foot; intact popliteal, dorsalis pedis, and posterior tibial pulses; and an unremarkable Homans' sign. You suspect*

A. edema from increased salt intake from the foods she had been eating while in Tokyo.

B. acute arterial occlusion.

C. deep venous thrombosis.

D. dependent edema from sitting for long periods of time during her flight home.

2-98 *Food sources rich in iron include*

A. potatoes; bananas; and green, leafy vegetables.

B. enriched grain cereals, cabbage, and sweet potatoes.

C. liver, red meats, prunes, apples, and raisins.

D. enriched grain cereals, strawberries, watermelon, and honeydew melons.

2-99 *Max, age 28, has a normal cholesterol level of 186 mg/dL. How often should he be screened for hypercholesterolemia?*

A. Whenever blood work is done

B. Every year

C. Every 2 years

D. Every 5 years

2-100 *Mr. Hughes is a 46-year-old African American man who is in your primary care office for a physical examination. You recommend which of the following as screening for prostate cancer?*

A. A digital rectal examination (DRE)

B. None; there is no conclusive evidence for screening until age 75 and older

C. A DRE and prostate-specific antigen (PSA) level test

D. A PSA test

2-101 *Mr. Brown is 50 years old. His prostate-specific antigen (PSA) level the year before was 2.8 ng/mL. His PSA this year is 4.3 ng/mL. Your first course of action would be to*

A. refer him for possible biopsy.

B. wait for 2 weeks, then repeat the test.

C. prescribe sulfamethoxazole and trimethoprim (Bactrim) PO bid or doxycycline (Vibramycin) 100 mg PO bid for 4 weeks and repeat the PSA 1 week after completion of the medication.

D. refer him for transrectal ultrasound.

2-102 *George has ischemic changes and gangrene of the hands and fingers. This may be a result of*

A. Raynaud's disease.

B. Buerger's disease.

C. Allen's disease.

D. Hodgkin's disease.

2-103   *You are concerned that Ms. Jones is not taking her antihypertensive medication. The best way to assess this situation is*

A.   to perform serum blood levels to monitor therapeutic effectiveness.

B.   to ask her to come in every day for blood pressure checks.

C.   to ask the client.

D.   to do a mini-mental examination and administer a depression index.

2-104   *When auscultating bowel sounds, you note high-pitched tinkling sounds. What might this indicate?*

A.   Peritonitis

B.   Progressive bowel obstruction

C.   Paralytic ileus

D.   Gastric outflow obstruction

2-105   *The term* sensitivity *is most accurately defined as*

A.   the percentage of clients with a positive test result who actually have the disease.

B.   the percentage of clients with the disease in whom the test is positive.

C.   the percentage of clients with a negative test result who really do not have the disease.

D.   a true positive result.

2-106   *Jack had a routine screening and was found to have proteinuria. Your next action would be to*

A.   schedule a renal ultrasound.

B.   refer him to a urologist.

C.   ask the physician to schedule a renal biopsy.

D.   collect a 24-hour urine sample for quantification.

2-107   *Specific conditions demonstrate fluid in the scrotum on transillumination. These include*

A.   testicular cancer.

B.   a varicocele.

C.   a hydrocele.

D.   testicular torsion.

2-108   *Mrs. Hill wonders when she should start her 4-month-old infant on solid foods. You advise her that*

A.   solid foods may be added to liquid formula in formula-fed infants whenever they are unable to be satisfied with formula alone.

B.   formula-fed infants should not begin on solid foods until they are older than 6 months of age.

C.   solid foods may be begun safely in formula-fed infants between 4 and 6 months of age.

D.   solid foods may be begun safely in formula-fed infants between 6 and 8 months of age.

2-109   *You tell your client Mr. Fish, who is 55 years of age, that he should have a routine colonoscopy. This is an example of*

A.   health promotion.

B.   screening.

C.   disease prevention.

D.   tertiary prevention.

2-110   *Menstruating women lose approximately how much iron per day?*

A.   5 mg

B.   10 mg

C.   0.1–1.6 mg

D.   2 mg

2-111   *Mrs. Moore brings her 3-year-old son to your primary care office for evaluation. She is very upset and reports that, after eating dinner last evening, her son seemed to lose consciousness for a brief period. She states that he was sitting up but that his head drooped and he did not respond to calls from her. She could not recall exactly how long this episode lasted but reports that he returned to normal as the evening progressed and is also acting normally today. You suspect that the child had a(n)*

A.   absence seizure.

B.   tonic-clonic seizure.

C.   myoclonic seizure.

D.   atonic seizure.

2-112 *Which valve is most affected in rheumatic heart disease?*

A. Aortic

B. Tricuspid

C. Mitral

D. Pulmonary

2-113 *Goals for management of the client with diabetes mellitus include which of the following?*

A. Maintaining blood glucose near normal (100–150 mg/dL); achieving normal weight; and eating a low-carbohydrate, high-protein diet

B. Exercising 20–30 minutes three times a week; maintaining a glycosylated hemoglobin ($HgbA_{1c}$) greater than 12%

C. Maintaining an $HgbA_{1c}$ between 8% and 10%; minimizing complications; avoiding hypoglycemia; and maintaining normal lifestyle

D. Achieving a weight of 10% less than normal; exercising vigorously 60 minutes a day, five times a week; and minimizing complications

2-114 *In teaching your client about birth control, you tell her that the highest failure rate is with which birth control method?*

A. Spermicide

B. Withdrawal

C. Cervical cap

D. Condoms

2-115 *Routine screening for hypothyroidism is performed*

A. when a client has a family history of thyroid problems.

B. on all clients every 2 years.

C. Screening is not routinely recommended.

D. when a client reaches age 65.

2-116 *Constipation is a frequent and common problem in older adults. Principles of treatment include*

A. beginning supplemental bulk agents and encouraging exercise.

B. suggesting a combination of applesauce, bran, and prunes to be eaten every morning.

C. establishing a routine for early morning defecation and teaching clients not to ignore the urge to defecate.

D. encouraging adequate hydration and exercise and providing client education regarding a high-fiber diet and stopping laxatives.

2-117 *Mackenzie, age 8, is complaining of something being stuck inside her ear. You consider a number of actions. The action you should NOT do is which of the following?*

A. Instill several drops of mineral oil.

B. Use a small ear syringe to suction out the item.

C. Inspect the inside of the ear with your otoscope even though Mackenzie is crying in pain.

D. Reassure her that this will pass.

2-118 *Mr. Smith, age 68, comes to the primary care office complaining of inability to sleep, fatigue, and lack of concentration. As you talk with him, you discover that his wife died less than a year ago. You note that he has lost over 15 lb since his last visit 6 months ago. Although he is taking enalapril (Vasotec) 5 mg PO daily, you measure his blood pressure to be 154/94 mm Hg. An immediate priority would be to*

A. adjust his antihypertensive medication regimen.

B. assess him for suicidal ideation.

C. discuss beginning antidepressant therapy.

D. refer him to a counselor and suggest a grief support group.

2-119 *Abnormal bony growths on the distal and proximal interphalangeal joints are associated with*

A. rheumatoid arthritis.

B. osteoarthritis.

C. scleroderma.

D. Lyme disease.

2-120 *Often clients do not freely admit their difficulties in adhering to a treatment plan. Signs that the client may not be following the treatment plan include*

A. active involvement, asking many questions, inconsistent response to treatment.

B. obedient and passive attitude, inconsistent response to treatment.

C. dissatisfaction with recommendations, attempts at negotiation.

D. consistent and measurable response to treatment.

2-121   *When performing an ophthalmoscopic examination, you note retinal hemorrhages and narrowing, obliteration, dilation, and tortuousness of the retinal vessels. You diagnose this as*

A. macular degeneration.

B. hypertensive retinopathy.

C. diabetic retinopathy.

D. a cataract.

2-122   *James is a high school senior and cannot understand why you will not prescribe testosterone for him. He states that all of his bodybuilding friends take anabolic androgenic steroids to increase their muscle mass. You tell him that you have seen it ordered*

A. for weight loss.

B. for decreased immune function.

C. for fibrocystic breast disease.

D. to increase energy and appetite in older adults.

2-123   *Margaret thinks that her husband has toxoplasmosis and asks you about the symptoms. You tell her that the most common symptom is*

A. confusion.

B. a fever.

C. a headache.

D. lethargy.

2-124   *You should be suspicious of the accuracy of the results of a positive protein dipstick test that you have done in the office under which of the following circumstances?*

A. The urine concentration is very diluted.

B. The urine is very concentrated.

C. The urine has a very high sugar content.

D. The urine has blood in it.

2-125   *Max, age 16, comes into your office after having been in a fight and sustaining a human bite on his fist. Your first course of action is to*

A. give a tetanus injection.

B. thoroughly débride and irrigate the wound.

C. initiate broad-spectrum antibiotics.

D. leave the wound open for drainage.

2-126   *Which organization is a delivery method in the private sector that gives the sponsoring organization discounts from their usual charges?*

A. Health maintenance organization

B. Preferred provider organization

C. Gatekeeper organization

D. Fee-for-service organization

2-127   *Good diabetes management calls for a urine microalbumin level to be done*

A. annually after the condition is first diagnosed.

B. every 2 years.

C. annually after the client has had diabetes for 5 years.

D. every 6 months.

2-128   *When auscultating Marie's heart sounds in the left semilateral position, you hear an atrial gallop. When documenting this sound, you refer to it as*

A. S_1.

B. S_2.

C. S_3.

D. S_4.

2-129   *When palpating lymph nodes, it is essential to also palpate the supraclavicular nodes located*

A. along the chest wall, high in the axilla.

B. superficially on the medial side of the elbow.

C. hidden behind the sternocleidomastoid muscle's clavicular head.

D. directly in the axillary region.

2-130   *Which would be the best question or statement to use to facilitate open communication between yourself and a morbidly obese woman?*

A. "Don't you want to live to dance at your daughter's wedding?"

B. "It took you a long time to get like this; it will take a while to get the weight off."

C. "What steps have you taken to change your patterns of eating and exercising?"

D. "I'm going to come up with some goals that I think you can live with."

2-131   The major risk of a red blood cell transfusion is

A. cytomegalovirus infection.

B. hepatitis B infection.

C. HIV infection.

D. a hemolytic transfusion reaction.

2-132   Sol, age 46, is overweight and comes in with dyspnea. He also has peripheral edema, ascites, and neck vein distention. What do you further evaluate him for?

A. Anemia

B. Pulmonary hypertension

C. Pleural effusion

D. Central nervous system lesion

2-133   When your teenage client Shane asks you about what to do for his knee, which is sprained from playing ice hockey, you tell him to use

A. heat for 30 minutes every hour for the first 48 hours.

B. ice for 20 minutes and then remove for 30–45 minutes for the first 48 hours.

C. alternately heat for 15 minutes followed by ice for 20 minutes for the first 72 hours.

D. ice for 40 minutes followed by heat for 20 minutes for the first 24 hours.

2-134   Tommy, age 5, wants to go to his grandfather's funeral, but his parents have conflicting opinions. They ask you for advice. What do you say?

A. "Children younger than age 7 should not be exposed to funerals."

B. "He should go, but have him sit in the back and do not allow him to view the corpse."

C. "Let him attend, participate as much as he seems to want, and have someone willing to leave with him when he's ready."

D. "All children at this age should be encouraged to view the corpse to say their final good-byes."

2-135   When diagnosing seizures in a child, despite an appropriate work-up, the etiology remains undetermined 50% of the time. Differential diagnoses for seizure disorders in a child include which of the following?

A. Autism

B. Benign paroxysmal vertigo

C. Drug reaction

D. Labyrinthitis

2-136   A low-residue diet is ordered for your client Kristy, who is newly diagnosed with ulcerative colitis. Which foods should Kristy avoid?

A. Potato chips and brown rice

B. Pasta and white rice

C. Veal, pork, and lamb

D. Vegetable juices and canned vegetables

2-137   The leading cause of death in all age groups younger than age 44 is

A. accidents.

B. heart disease.

C. malignant neoplasms.

D. HIV infection.

2-138   Retinopathy is the leading cause of new blindness in the United States. Given this fact, what should you recommend concerning ophthalmological examinations to your clients with diabetes?

A. Clients with insulin-dependent diabetes mellitus (type 1) should have their first ophthalmological examination within the first 5 years of diagnosis and then yearly thereafter; clients with non–insulin-dependent diabetes mellitus (type 2) should have their first ophthalmological examination immediately on diagnosis and yearly thereafter.

B. Clients with type 2 diabetes should be referred to an ophthalmologist within 5 years of diagnosis and have yearly examinations thereafter; clients with type 1 diabetes should be referred immediately on diagnosis and then have an examination every 3 years.

C. Clients with either type 1 or type 2 diabetes should be referred immediately on diagnosis and then have yearly examinations.

D. Clients with either type 1 or type 2 diabetes should be referred on diagnosis and then followed up every other year depending on age.

2-139   *Melissa has multiple sclerosis and has reached the point at which she needs to use a wheelchair. She anticipates that soon she will not be able to do anything for herself and has decided that, when that time comes, she is going to take an overdose of sleeping pills. If her husband supports her decision, which ethical principle is he using?*

A. Beneficence

B. Veracity

C. Autonomy

D. Justice

2-140   *Mrs. Jones, age 58, comes to your primary care office complaining of dull, left-sided chest pain that increases somewhat on inspiration. This has been going on since the previous day and has no relation to movement or exercise. The pain intensifies when she lies down, and she obtains some relief sitting up and leaning slightly forward. On auscultation, you hear a pericardial friction rub. Her electrocardiogram shows ST-segment elevation, a T-wave inversion, and PR-segment depression. The ST elevations are diffuse and across leads. You suspect*

A. an evolving myocardial infarction.

B. angina.

C. pericarditis.

D. costochondritis.

2-141   *Certain drugs have enhanced effects when combined with oral contraceptives. This is true for which of the following drugs?*

A. Beta blockers

B. Phenytoin (Dilantin)

C. Antacids

D. Oral anticoagulants

2-142   *Your client Mr. Lane, who has COPD, reports a worsening of his respiratory symptoms. You review his entire medication list, noting that he is taking a beta blocker for his hypertension and nitrates for his angina in addition to the theophylline that he takes daily for his COPD. You decide to*

A. switch him to a different bronchodilator.

B. discontinue the beta blocker.

C. switch his beta blocker to a calcium channel blocker.

D. discontinue his nitrates.

2-143   *Sam just left your office with a diagnosis of prostate cancer after an extensive work-up. His wife is on the phone demanding to know what his problem turned out to be. How do you respond?*

A. "Don't worry. Everything will be OK after we send Sam to a specialist."

B. "You'll have to ask Sam; I can't tell you."

C. "He has prostate cancer, but you'll have to talk to Sam about what his choices are."

D. You refuse to take the call.

2-144   *Delirium is often acute and reversible. Reversible causes of delirium include*

A. depression, deafness, and use of nitrates.

B. psychosis, vitamin B_{12} deficiency, and migraine headache.

C. sepsis, syphilis, and use of warfarin (Coumadin).

D. subdural hematoma, depression, and use of anticholinergics.

2-145   *Which glomerular disease occurs 10–14 days after an acute illness (commonly streptococcal in children) and is characterized by tea-colored urine, mild to severe renal insufficiency, and edema?*

A. Henoch-Schönlein purpura glomerulonephritis

B. Glomerulonephritis of systemic lupus erythematosus

C. Postinfection glomerulonephritis

D. Immunoglobulin A nephropathy

2-146   *A "liver flap," associated with hepatic encephalopathy, uremia, and respiratory acidosis, refers to*

A. nonrhythmic flapping of the wrists and hands.

B. a palpable liver that "flaps" against the palpating hand.

C. a jaundiced color of the skin.

D. urine that is the color of liver.

2-147   *Marcus, age 60, has just been given a diagnosis of renal cancer. He asks what the risk factors are. You tell him that they include age older than 40, as well as*

A. tobacco and alcohol use.

B. tobacco use and analgesic abuse.

C. exposure to aniline dyes and a low-fiber diet.

D. a diet high in fat and nitrates.

2-148 Pregnancy-induced hypertension occurs in what percentage of pregnant clients?

A. Less than 3%

B. 3%–5%

C. 5%–7%

D. 7%–10%

2-149 Marge comes for a pelvic examination complaining of vaginal burning and itching and painful intercourse. You note strawberry spots on her cervix, along with a greenish-yellow, frothy, foul-smelling vaginal discharge. What is your diagnosis?

A. *Candida albicans* infection

B. *Gardnerella vaginalis* infection

C. *Trichomonas vaginalis* infection

D. Atrophic vaginitis

2-150 Abnormal bony growths on the proximal interphalangeal joints are referred to as

A. Heberden's nodes.

B. Bouchard's nodes.

C. subcutaneous nodules.

D. tophi.

2-151 Which of the following is the most important factor in influencing behavioral change?

A. Social supports

B. Motivation

C. Cognitive knowledge

D. Health beliefs

2-152 A condition with the symptoms of prostatitis but without infection is

A. prostatodynia.

B. acute nonbacterial prostatitis.

C. epididymitis.

D. chemical prostatitis.

2-153 The older adult is at greater risk for developing an eye infection than a younger person. This is because of the age-related

A. change in vitreous humor.

B. decrease in tear production.

C. loss of subcutaneous tissue.

D. greater emotionality.

2-154 Maurice, who is 13, has gynecomastia. His evaluation should include

A. measuring testosterone level.

B. an evaluation of the adequacy of his liver function.

C. ordering a bilateral mammogram stat.

D. reassuring him that this is nothing and will pass.

2-155 The intended purpose of national certification is to

A. ensure quality and competency at an advanced level of practice.

B. assist the nurse in obtaining a higher salary.

C. make APRNs comparable to MDs.

D. assist the nurse in job promotion.

2-156 According to Erikson's 8 Stages of Man schemata for life span development, the chief psychosocial task for children ages 6–12 is

A. initiative vs. guilt.

B. productivity vs. stagnation.

C. generativity vs. boredom.

D. identity vs. confusion.

2-157 Marty, age 7, was brought to your primary care office with dog bites on his right hand and arm. You would send him home on

A. amoxicillin and clavulanate (Augmentin).

B. penicillin (Pentids).

C. amoxicillin (Amoxil).

D. clarithromycin (Biaxin).

Answers

2-1 Answer A
Content area: Head and Neck Problems (chap. 9)

2-2 Answer A
Content area: Female Genitourinary Problems (chap. 15)

2-3 Answer B
Content area: Care of the Emerging Family (chap. 4)

2-4 Answer B
Content area: Care of the Emerging Family (chap. 4)

2-5 Answer B
Content area: Health Promotion (chap. 3)

2-6 Answer A
Content area: Musculoskeletal Problems (chap. 16)

2-7 Answer D
Content area: Care of the Emerging Family (chap. 4)

2-8 Answer B
Content area: Endocrine and Metabolic Problems (chap. 17)

2-9 Answer B
Content area: Musculoskeletal Problems (chap. 16)

2-10 Answer B
Content area: Abdominal Problems (chap. 12)

2-11 Answer C
Content area: Integumentary Problems (chap. 8)

2-12 Answer C
Content area: Abdominal Problems (chap. 12)

2-13 Answer D
Content area: Abdominal Problems (chap. 12)

2-14 Answer D
Content area: Health Promotion (chap. 3)

2-15 Answer B
Content area: Care of the Emerging Family (chap. 4)

2-16 Answer D
Content area: Renal Problems (chap. 13)

2-17 Answer C
Content area: Neurological Problems (chap. 7)

2-18 Answer B
Content area: Health Counseling (chap. 6)

2-19 Answer B
Content area: Endocrine and Metabolic Problems (chap. 17)

2-20 Answer B
Content area: Cardiovascular Problems (chap. 11)

2-21 Answer A
Content area: Issues in Primary Care (chap. 19)

2-22 Answer A
Content area: Female Genitourinary Problems (chap. 15)

2-23 Answer D
Content area: Head and Neck Problems (chap. 9)

2-24 Answer D
Content area: Male Genitourinary Problems (chap. 14)

2-25 Answer D
Content area: Issues in Primary Care (chap. 19)

2-26 Answer C
Content area: Renal Problems (chap. 13)

2-27 Answer C
Content area: Neurological Problems (chap. 7)

2-28 Answer D
Content area: Respiratory Problems (chap. 10)

2-29 Answer C
Content area: Male Genitourinary Problems (chap. 14)

2-30   Answer C

Content area: Renal Problems (chap. 13)

2-31   Answer B

Content area: Care of the Emerging Family (chap. 4)

2-32   Answer A

Content area: Respiratory Problems (chap. 10)

2-33   Answer C

Content area: Neurological Problems (chap. 7)

2-34   Answer A

Content area: Hematological and Immune Problems (chap. 18)

2-35   Answer A

Content area: Head and Neck Problems (chap. 9)

2-36   Answer B

Content area: Hematological and Immune Problems (chap. 18)

2-37   Answer C

Content area: Growth and Development (chap. 5)

2-38   Answer B

Content area: Growth and Development (chap. 5)

2-39   Answer A

Content area: Growth and Development (chap. 5)

2-40   Answer A

Content area: Abdominal Problems (chap. 12)

2-41   Answer B

Content area: Musculoskeletal Problems (chap. 16)

2-42   Answer C

Content area: Hematological and Immune Problems (chap. 18)

2-43   Answer D

Content area: Respiratory Problems (chap. 10)

2-44   Answer C

Content area: Head and Neck Problems (chap. 9)

2-45   Answer D

Content area: Care of the Emerging Family (chap. 4)

2-46   Answer D

Content area: Cardiovascular Problems (chap. 11)

2-47   Answer B

Content area: Integumentary Problems (chap. 8)

2-48   Answer C

Content area: Integumentary Problems (chap. 8)

2-49   Answer D

Content area: Health Promotion (chap. 3)

2-50   Answer B

Content area: Health Counseling (chap. 6)

2-51   Answer B

Content area: Health Promotion (chap. 3)

2-52   Answer A

Content area: Neurological Problems (chap. 7)

2-53   Answer C

Content area: Health Promotion (chap. 3)

2-54   Answer C

Content area: Head and Neck Problems (chap. 9)

2-55   Answer A

Content area: Renal Problems (chap. 13)

2-56   Answer D

Content area: Cardiovascular Problems (chap. 11)

2-57   Answer C

Content area: Head and Neck Problems (chap. 9)

2-58   Answer D

Content area: Care of the Emerging Family (chap. 4)

2-59   Answer A

Content area: Cardiovascular Problems (chap. 11)

2-60   Answer A

Content area: Endocrine and Metabolic Problems (chap. 17)

2-61   Answer A

Content area: Endocrine and Metabolic Problems (chap. 17)

2-62   Answer B

Content area: Issues in Primary Care (chap. 19)

2-63   Answer C

Content area: Head and Neck Problems (chap. 9)

2-64   Answer B

Content area: Abdominal Problems (chap. 12)

2-65   Answer B

Content area: Growth and Development (chap. 5)

2-66   Answer C

Content area: Care of the Emerging Family (chap. 4)

2-67   Answer A

Content area: Musculoskeletal Problems (chap. 16)

2-68   Answer C

Content area: Care of the Emerging Family (chap. 4)

2-69   Answer A

Content area: Male Genitourinary Problems (chap. 14)

2-70   Answer C

Content area: Integumentary Problems (chap. 8)

2-71   Answer B

Content area: Growth and Development (chap. 5)

2-72   Answer B

Content area: Health Promotion (chap. 3)

2-73   Answer C

Content area: Care of the Emerging Family (chap. 4)

2-74   Answer C

Content area: Respiratory Problems (chap. 10)

2-75   Answer C

Content area: Growth and Development (chap. 5)

2-76   Answer C

Content area: Neurological Problems (chap. 7)

2-77   Answer D

Content area: Respiratory Problems (chap. 10)

2-78   Answer C

Content area: Respiratory Problems (chap. 10)

2-79   Answer A

Content area: Endocrine and Metabolic Problems (chap. 17)

2-80   Answer D

Content area: Head and Neck Problems (chap. 9)

2-81   Answer A

Content area: Respiratory Problems (chap. 10)

2-82   Answer A

Content area: Neurological Problems (chap. 7)

2-83   Answer D

Content area: Hematological and Immune Problems (chap. 18)

2-84   Answer B

Content area: Neurological Problems (chap. 7)

2-85   Answer C

Content area: Musculoskeletal Problems (chap. 16)

2-86   Answer A

Content area: Female Genitourinary Problems (chap. 15)

2-87   Answer A

Content area: Endocrine and Metabolic Problems (chap. 17)

2-88   Answer A

Content area: Cardiovascular Problems (chap. 11)

2-89   Answer C

Content area: Integumentary Problems (chap. 8)

2-90   Answer A

Content area: Integumentary Problems (chap. 8)

2-91   Answer D

Content area: Neurological Problems (chap. 7)

2-92   Answer D

Content area: Head and Neck Problems (chap. 9)

2-93   Answer C

Content area: Health Promotion (chap. 3)

2-94   Answer B

Content area: Hematological and Immune Problems (chap. 18)

2-95   Answer D

Content area: Female Genitourinary Problems (chap. 15)

2-96   Answer C

Content area: Hematological and Immune Problems (chap. 18)

2-97   Answer C

Content area: Cardiovascular Problems (chap. 11)

2-98   Answer C

Content area: Hematological and Immune Problems (chap. 18)

2-99   Answer D

Content area: Health Promotion (chap. 3)

2-100   Answer B

Content area: Male Genitourinary Problems (chap. 14)

2-101   Answer C

Content area: Male Genitourinary Problems (chap. 14)

2-102   Answer B

Content area: Musculoskeletal Problems (chap. 16)

2-103   Answer C

Content area: Issues in Primary Care (chap. 19)

2-104   Answer B

Content area: Abdominal Problems (chap. 12)

2-105   Answer B

Content area: Health Promotion (chap. 3)

2-106   Answer D

Content area: Renal Problems (chap. 13)

2-107   Answer C

Content area: Male Genitourinary Problems (chap. 14)

2-108   Answer C

Content area: Care of the Emerging Family (chap. 4)

2-109   Answer B

Content area: Health Counseling (chap. 6)

2-110   Answer D

Content area: Hematological and Immune Problems (chap. 18)

2-111   Answer A

Content area: Neurological Problems (chap. 7)

2-112   Answer C

Content area: Cardiovascular Problems (chap. 11)

2-113   Answer C

Content area: Endocrine and Metabolic Problems (chap. 17)

2-114   Answer C

Content area: Health Counseling (chap. 6)

2-115   Answer C

Content area: Endocrine and Metabolic Problems (chap. 17)

2-116   Answer D

Content area: Abdominal Problems (chap. 12)

2-117   Answer B

Content area: Head and Neck Problems (chap. 9)

2-118   Answer B

Content area: Neurological Problems (chap. 7)

2-119   Answer B

Content area: Musculoskeletal Problems (chap. 16)

2-120   Answer B

Content area: Health Counseling (chap. 6)

2-121   Answer C

Content area: Head and Neck Problems (chap. 9)

2-122   Answer D

Content area: Male Genitourinary Problems (chap. 14)

2-123   Answer C

Content area: Hematological and Immune Problems (chap. 18)

2-124   Answer B

Content area: Renal Problems (chap. 13)

2-125   Answer B

Content area: Musculoskeletal Problems (chap. 16)

2-126   Answer B

Content area: Issues in Primary Care (chap. 19)

2-127   Answer C

Content area: Endocrine and Metabolic Problems (chap. 17)

2-128   Answer D

Content area: Cardiovascular Problems (chap. 11)

2-129   Answer C

Content area: Integumentary Problems (chap. 8)

2-130   Answer C

Content area: Health Promotion (chap. 3)

2-131   Answer A

Content area: Hematological and Immune Problems (chap. 18)

2-132   Answer B

Content area: Respiratory Problems (chap. 10)

2-133   Answer B

Content area: Musculoskeletal Problems (chap. 16)

2-134   Answer C

Content area: Growth and Development (chap. 5)

2-135   Answer D

Content area: Neurological Problems (chap. 7)

2-136   Answer A

Content area: Abdominal Problems (chap. 12)

2-137   Answer A

Content area: Health Promotion (chap. 3)

2-138   Answer A

Content area: Endocrine and Metabolic Problems (chap. 17)

2-139   Answer C

Content area: Issues in Primary Care (chap. 19)

2-140   Answer C

Content area: Cardiovascular Problems (chap. 11)

2-141   Answer A

Content area: Endocrine and Metabolic Problems (chap. 17)

2-142   Answer C

Content area: Respiratory Problems (chap. 10)

2-143   Answer B

Content area: Issues in Primary Care (chap. 19)

2-144   Answer D

Content area: Neurological Problems (chap. 7)

2-145   Answer C

Content area: Renal Problems (chap. 13)

2-146   Answer A

Content area: Abdominal Problems (chap. 12)

2-147   Answer B

Content area: Male Genitourinary Problems (chap. 14)

2-148   Answer C

Content area: Care of the Emerging Family (chap. 4)

2-149   Answer C

Content area: Female Genitourinary Problems (chap. 15)

2-150   Answer B

Content area: Musculoskeletal Problems (chap. 16)

2-151   Answer B

Content area: Issues in Primary Care (chap. 19)

2-152   Answer A

Content area: Male Genitourinary Problems (chap. 14)

2-153   Answer B

Content area: Head and Neck Problems (chap. 9)

2-154   Answer D

Content area: Endocrine and Metabolic Problems (chap. 17)

2-155   Answer A

Content area: Issues in Primary Care (chap. 19)

2-156   Answer A

Content area: Growth and Development (chap. 5)

2-157   Answer A

Content area: Integumentary Problems (chap. 8)

Good Luck on Your Certification Examination!